PROVIDER MANUAL EIGHTH EDITION

TNCC™

TRAUMA NURSING CORE COURSE

An ENA Course

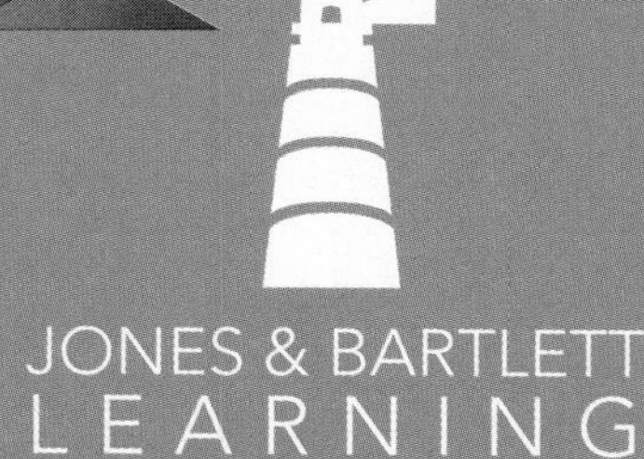

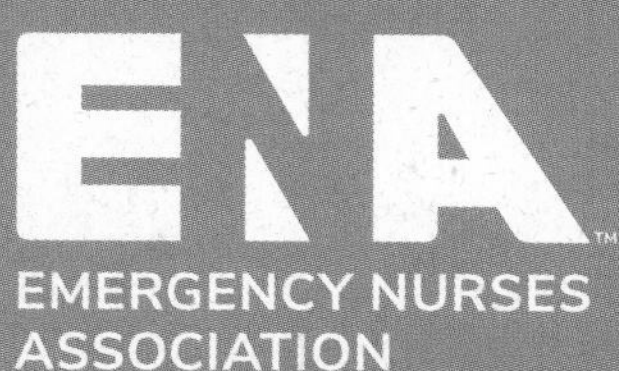

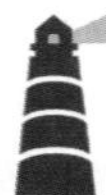

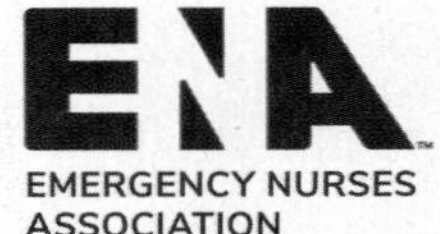

World Headquarters
Jones & Bartlett Learning
5 Wall Street
Burlington, MA 01803
978-443-5000
info@jblearning.com
www.jblearning.com

Emergency Nurses Association
930 E. Woodfield Road
Schaumburg, IL 60173
847-460-4000
education@ena.org
www.ena.org

Jones & Bartlett Learning books and products are available through most bookstores and online booksellers. To contact Jones & Bartlett Learning directly, call 800-832-0034, fax 978-443-8000, or visit our website, www.jblearning.com.

Substantial discounts on bulk quantities of Jones & Bartlett Learning publications are available to corporations, professional associations, and other qualified organizations. For details and specific discount information, contact the special sales department at Jones & Bartlett Learning via the above contact information or send an email to specialsales@jblearning.com.

Production Credits
VP, Product Management: Amanda Martin
Director of Product Management: Matthew Kane
Product Specialist: Christina Freitas
Senior Project Specialist: Vanessa Richards
Product Fulfillment Manager: Wendy Kilborn
Composition: S4Carlisle Publishing Services
Cover Design: Denise Wawrzyniak, Kristin E. Parker
Text Design: Kristin E. Parker
Rights Specialist: John Rusk
Media Development Editor: Troy Liston
Cover Image (Title Page, Part Opener, Chapter Opener): © Antishock/iStock/Getty Images Plus
Printing and Binding: LSC Communications
Cover Printing: LSC Communications

6048

Printed in the United States of America
25 24 23 22 21   10 9 8 7 6 5

Contents

Preface

The eighth edition of the *Trauma Nursing Core Course* (TNCC) continues the long-standing legacy of trauma nursing education that was begun over three decades ago by the Emergency Nurses Association (ENA) and that has become recognized as the international standard for trauma nursing practice. It is both an honor and a humbling responsibility to continue this work. We have built on the solid foundation that others before us have created, and we have listened to the feedback of the members who have taken this course and gone on to teach it.

Just as trauma care has evolved, so have educational methodologies. Indeed, this eighth edition of TNCC is as current as the most recent evidence-based practice published in the literature. Thus, it represents the current state of the art in both trauma care and education. In addition, to be forward looking, we have provided emerging trends sections that offer glimpses into the future of trauma care.

The skills have been updated as well, so that they reflect current practice, and have been consolidated into our unique trauma nursing process format to simulate realistic patient situations. The biggest change related to this edition will be seen in the classroom, where formal didactic presentations have been de-emphasized and facilitated learning is enacted utilizing case studies, group discussions, and other activities to teach the content. We are following the lead set by the Emergency Nursing Pediatric Course (ENPC) team, which has seen early success in this area.

The eighth edition has benefited from the expertise of many dedicated nurses from every aspect of emergency and trauma care. Starting with the work team, chapter authors, and ENA staff, a manual was developed and sent to peer reviewers. Skill stations were revised, and a classroom schedule was created. Item writers were recruited, and an exam template written. The adage, "The whole is greater than the sum of its parts," accurately describes this effort, as a synergy was created that was galvanized at our on-site meeting at ENA headquarters and kept everyone motivated and goal-oriented. The purpose of this course is the same as the goals of those who participate in it—to improve the outcomes of critically ill and injured patients. It is our sincere desire that you find this course helpful in accomplishing this most important mission.

As an old Army guy, I learned that the *infantry* is crucial in a battle. Their role is indispensable in taking ground and holding it. Similarly, *trauma* is the infantry of *emergency care*. We have the opportunity and responsibility to make a difference in the lives of those impacted by injury. This manual is dedicated to all who practice at the "tip of the spear" and work every day to save lives and improve outcomes. Stay sharp!

Joseph S. Blansfield, MS, NP, TCRN
Chair, TNCC Eighth Edition Work Team

Acknowledgments

Lead Editor

Joseph S. Blansfield, MS, NP, TCRN
Trauma and Acute Care Surgery Program Manager
Boston Medical Center
Boston, Massachusetts

ENA Board Liaison

Ron Kraus, MSN, RN, CNS, EMT-B, CEN, ACNS-BC
Clinical Nurse Specialist
Indiana University Health Methodist Hospital
Indianapolis, Indiana

TNCC, Eighth Edition Work Team/Section Editors

Melanie Crowley, MSN, RN, CEN
Trauma Program Manager
Providence Holy Cross Medical Center
Mission Hills, California

Margaret M. McNeill, PhD, RN, APRN-CNS, CCRN-K, CCNS, TCRN, CPAN, NE-BC, NHDP-BC, FAAN
Clinical Nurse Specialist/Nurse Scientist
Department of Professional and Clinical Development
Frederick Regional Health System
Frederick, Maryland

Kellyn M. Pak, MSN, RN, CEN, TCRN, MICN
Senior Nursing Instructor
Disaster Program Manager
Office of Emergency Management
LAC+USC Medical Center
Los Angeles, California

Janis Farnholtz Provinse, MS, BSN, RN, CNS, CEN, TCRN, FAEN
Clinical Nurse Specialist
Highland Hospital—Alameda Health System
Oakland, California

Sheila Silva, DNP, RN, CEN, TCRN
Assistant Professor of Nursing
Emmanuel College School of Nursing
Boston, Massachusetts

Angela M. Westergard, MSN, MBA, RN, CEN
Clinical Nurse Educator
Northwest Medical Center
Tucson, Arizona

Course Administration Faculty Liaison

Paula L. Davis, MSN, ARNP, CEN, CPEN, CFRN, FNP-BC
Emergency Department–Clinical Nurse Educator
NF/SG Veteran's Hospital
Gainesville, Florida

Trauma Committee

Jade Barnes, BSN, RN, CEN, CCRN
Trauma Nurse Clinician
Baylor University Medical Center
Dallas, Texas

Roger M. Casey, MSN, RN, CEN, TCRN, FAEN
Staff Nurse
Freestanding Emergency Department
Kadlec Regional Medical Center
Richland, Washington

Deborah A. Clark, MS, BSN, RN, CEN, CPEN, TCRN
Trauma Program Manager
Geisinger–Community Medical Center
Scranton, Pennsylvania

Chris L. Dellinger, MBA, BSN, RN, FAEN
Director, Trauma Services
Camden Clark Medical Center
Parkersburg, West Virginia

Heidi M. Gilbert, BSN, RN, CEN, SANE
Emergency Department Educator
SANE Program Coordinator
Stillwater Medical Center
Stillwater, Oklahoma

Tim Murphy, MSN, RN, CEN, TCRN, FAEN
PI Coordinator, Trauma and Injury Prevention
Robert Wood Johnson University Hospital
RWJ Barnabas Health
New Brunswick, New Jersey

ENA Staff

Katrina Ceci, MSN, RN-BC, TCRN, CPEN, CEN
Nursing Content Manager
Emergency Nurses Association
Schaumburg, Illinois

Beth Ciarrachi, BA
eLearning Manager
Emergency Nurses Association
Schaumburg, Illinois

Shannon Novotny, MFA
eLearning Coordinator
Emergency Nurses Association
Schaumburg, Illinois

Nicole Williams, MSN, RN-BC
Director, Institute of Emergency Nursing Education
Emergency Nurses Association
Schaumburg, Illinois

Chris Zahn, PhD
Developmental Editor
Emergency Nurses Association
Schaumburg, Illinois

Contributing Authors

Cynthia M. Bratcher, MSN, APRN, FNP-C, CEN
Emergency Medicine Nurse Practitioner
Envision Physician Services
Bowling Green, Kentucky

Shelley A. Calder, DNP, RN, CEN
Clinical Nurse Specialist, Program Director of Ambulatory and Emergency Nursing Education
Beth Israel Deaconess Medical Center
Boston, Massachusetts

Melody R. Campbell, DNP, APRN-CNS, CEN, CCNS, CCRN, TCRN
Trauma Program Manager/Critical Care Clinical Nurse Specialist
Kettering Medical Center
Kettering, Ohio

Roger M. Casey, MSN, RN, CEN, TCRN, FAEN
Staff Nurse
Freestanding Emergency Department
Kadlec Regional Medical Center
Richland, Washington

Angela W. Clarkson, BSN, RN-TCRN
Trauma Outreach and Injury Prevention Coordinator
Novant Health–Presbyterian Medical Center
Charlotte, North Carolina

Kristen M. Cline, BSN, RN, CEN, CPEN, TCRN, CFRN, CTRN, CCRN
Flight Nurse and Base Educator
Sanford AirMed
Instructor and Author
Solheim Enterprises
Sioux Falls, South Dakota

Nancy J. Denke, DNP, RN, ACNP-BC, FNP-BC, CEN, CCRN, FAEN
Nurse Practitioner
Toxicology Consultants of Arizona
Scottsdale, Arizona

Courtney Edwards, DNP, MPH, RN, CCRN, CEN, TCRN
Trauma Outreach Education, Injury Prevention and Research Manager
Parkland Health and Hospital System
Dallas, Texas

Diana Giordano, DNP, RN, FNP-BC
Critical Care/Emergency Department Educator
Franciscan Health
Hammond, Indiana

Richard W. Harley, Jr., BSN, RN
ED Clinical Educator
Porter Regional Hospital
Valparaiso, Indiana

Kyndra P. Holm, MSN, RN, CEN, TCRN
Pediatric Trauma Program Manager
Children's Hospital of Georgia
Augusta University Medical Center
Augusta, Georgia

Steven F. Jacobson, MSN, MS, MBA, RN, CEN, CFRN, NREMT-P
Flight Nurse/Paramedic
Anchorage, Alaska

Cassie A. Lyell, MSN, RN, TCRN
Manager, Trauma and Acute Care Surgery
JPS Health Network
Fort Worth, Texas

Meghan L. McDonald, MSN, RN
Trauma Program Nurse Director
Brigham and Women's Hospital
Boston, Massachusetts

Justin J. Milici, MSN, RN, CEN, CPEN, TCRN, CCRN, FAEN
Clinical Editor
Elsevier, Clinical Solutions
Dallas, Texas

Patricia A. Normandin, DNP, RN, CEN, CPN, CPEN, FAEN
Emergency Department Staff Nurse and Nurse Scientist
Adjunct Faculty Tufts University Medical School
Tufts Medical Center
Adjunct Nursing Faculty
Massachusetts General Hospital Institute of Health Professions
Boston, Massachusetts

Nycole D. Oliver, DNP, APRN, CEN, ACNPC-AG, FNP-C
Advanced Practice Registered Nurse
Baptist Health Fort Smith
Fort Smith, Arkansas

Kristine K. Powell, MSN, RN, CEN, NEA-BC, FAEN
Director of Emergency Services
Baylor Scott & White Health–North Texas
Grandview, Texas

Robin S. Powers-Jarvis, PhD, RNC, CEN, CCRN, TCRN, CPEN
Nurse Educator
West Palm Beach, Florida

Jennifer Radtke, MSN, RN, CEN, TCRN, CIC
Infection Prevention–Manager
University of Tennessee Medical Center
Knoxville, Tennessee

Tiffiny Strever, BSN, RN, CEN, TCRN, FAEN
Trauma Program Manager
Abrazo West Campus
Abrazo Community Health Network
Goodyear, Arizona

Erin Zazzera, MPH, RN, CEN, TCRN
Pediatric Trauma Coordinator
Stony Brook Medicine
Stony Brook, New York

International Authors

Agneta Brandt, MSN, RN, CRNA
Chair
Swedish Association for Trauma Nurses
Saltsjöbaden, Sweden

Joop Breuer, RN, CEN, CCRN, FAEN
Nurse Educator/Charge Nurse
Emergency Department
Leiden University Medical Centre
Leiden, Netherlands

Liz Cloughessy, AM, MHM, RN, FAEN, MACN
Executive Director
Australian College of Emergency Nursing
Sydney, Australia

Darcie Goodman, BSN, MPA
Vice President, Management Consulting
Cope Health Solutions
New York, New York

René C. Grobler, RN, FANSA
National Quality and Systems Manager, Trauma and Emergency Departments
Netcare Hospital Group
President
Emergency Nurses Society of South Africa
Alberton, South Africa

Peggy Wun Man Lee, RN
Nurse Manager
Hospital Authority
Hong Kong

Theo Lighthelm, MPA, B Soc Sc (Hons), RN
Consultant, Disaster Medicine Planning and Training
Gauteng, South Africa

Gabrielle Lomas, BSc (Hons), RN
Matron, Emergency Medicine
Salford Royal Hospital Foundation Trust
Manchester, United Kingdom

Tracey Taulu, BScN, RN, MHS
Director of Operations
University of British Columbia Hospital
Vancouver, British Columbia, Canada

Jill Windle, MSc, BA, RN, FRCN
Lecturer Practitioner in Emergency Nursing
Salford Royal Hospital Foundation Trust
University of Salford
Manchester, United Kingdom

Heather Wong, BSN, MHS, RN
Clinical Nurse Specialist–Emergency and Trauma Services
Interior Health
Kelowna, British Columbia, Canada

Content Reviewers

Melissa Barnes, MSN, RN, FNP-C, CEN
Trauma Nurse Practitioner
Providence Holy Cross Medical Center
Santa Clarita, California

Lucus Christoffersen, MSN-L, RN, CEN, CPEN, CCRN, TCRN
Assistant Professor in Nursing
Idaho State University
Pocatello, Idaho

Audrey S. Cornell, PhD, CNE, RN
Associate Clinical Professor
Western Kentucky University
Bowling Green, Kentucky

Richard Durkee, MSN, RN, CEN, CPEN, TCRN, NREMT
Clinical Nurse Educator
CHA Everett Hospital
Everett, Massachusetts

Nicholas Faoro, MSN, RN
Burn Program Manager
Brigham and Women's Hospital
Boston, Massachusetts

Michelle Galles, MSN, MBA, RN, AGACNP-BC, CEN, TCRN
Trauma Coordinator
Medical Center of Aurora
Aurora, Colorado

Alice Gervasini, PhD, RN, NE-BC
Nurse Director, Trauma and Emergency Surgery Services
Massachusetts General Hospital
Instructor in Surgery
Harvard Medical School
Boston, Massachusetts

Wanda J. Larson, PhD, MEd, RN, CEN, CPEN
Assistant Clinical Professor
University of Arizona
Director of Clinical Nursing Research
Banner University Medical Center
Tucson, Arizona

Sherry Leviner, PhD, RN, CEN, FNP-C
Assistant Professor of Nursing
Fayetteville State University
Hamlet, North Carolina

Jennifer Mattice, MS, BSN, RN
Clinical Nurse Educator
University of California–Davis Medical Center
Sacramento, California

Tracy McDonald, MSN, RN, CCRN-K, NEA-BC
Program Director, Trauma and Acute Care Surgery
Program Director, Gene and Barbara Burnett Burn Center
Program Director, Center for Concussion Management
University of Kansas Health System
Kansas City, Kansas

Laurie M. Nash, MSHS, MA, BSN, RN, NHDP-BC
Clinical Disaster Coordinator
Highland Hospital–Alameda Health System
Oakland, California

Candice Palmisano, MSN, RN, AGCNS-BC, CEN, CPN, MICN
Staff Nurse RN III
Los Angeles County–University of Southern California Emergency Department
Los Angeles, California

Kristopher Pidgeon, DHSc, TCRN, CEN, NREMT-P
Vice President Trauma Services
HCA–South Atlantic Division
Charleston, South Carolina

Deborah J. Schwytzer, DNP, RN, CEN, RN-BC
Associate Professor of Nursing
University of Cincinnati
Cincinnati, Ohio

Dawn M. Specht, PhD, MSN, RN, APN, CPEN, CEN, CCNS, CCRN, AGACNP-BC, FAEN
Associate Professor
American Sentinel University
Aurora, Colorado

Annie D. Stedman, BSN, RN, CEN, TNCC-I
Clinical Consultant
Cheetah Medical, Inc.
Vancouver, Washington

Laura Strickland, MBA, BSN, RN, CEN, TCRN
Pediatric Trauma Program Manager
Grand Strand Medical Center
Myrtle Beach, South Carolina

Juli Verkler, MSN, MFS, RN, CEN, CFN, TCRN
Visiting Assistant Professor
Valparaiso University
Valparaiso, Indiana

Gina Wakelin, MSN, RN, CEN, NREMT-P
Professional Development Director–Emergency Department
Tufts Medical Center
Boston, Massachusetts

CHAPTER 1

Trauma Nursing and Teamwork

Shelley A. Calder, DNP, RN, CEN

OBJECTIVES

Upon completion of this chapter, the learner will be able to:

1. Describe the purpose of the Trauma Nursing Core Course.
2. Describe the philosophy of trauma nursing education.
3. Describe trauma nurse roles and responsibilities.
4. Identify the trauma team structure and roles.
5. Define the qualities of high-performance teams.

Introduction

Excellence in trauma nursing contributes to optimal patient outcomes and the prevention of complications, long-term consequences, and death for patients. The purpose of the Trauma Nursing Core Course (TNCC) is to provide registered nurses with evidence-based core knowledge, assessments, and psychomotor skills involved in the triage and management of injured patients. The trauma nursing process (TNP) reinforces a systematic and standardized approach to trauma nursing care and skills using an integrated approach to trauma teamwork, communication, and collaboration. TNCC is widely recognized as the premier course for hospitals and trauma centers worldwide, empowering nurses with the knowledge, critical thinking skills, and hands-on training to provide expert care for trauma patients.

Trauma Nursing Core Course

TNCC is made up of a number of instructional materials and activities designed to teach essential trauma nursing knowledge and skills. The following sections provide an overview of the course, evaluation process, and learning materials.

Course Description

The program consists of various modes of instruction, including hands-on psychomotor skill stations and interactive online learning. The framework of TNCC is based on the nursing process, which is emphasized throughout the program. Classroom activities highlight critical concepts presented in the chapters and online modules to reinforce learning and the nursing process. The psychomotor skill stations involve applying the TNP to realistic patient scenarios while practicing trauma-specific skills.

Learner Evaluation

Evaluation of learners consists of a written 50-question multiple-choice examination and successful completion of the psychomotor testing station. Only the TNP station is tested in the psychomotor examination, although skills and knowledge from other skill stations are incorporated into the evaluations. These evaluations are designed to assess acquisition of cognitive knowledge, essential psychomotor skills, and critical thinking.

To successfully complete TNCC, the learner must achieve a minimum of 80% on the written examination, actively participate in all psychomotor teaching stations, and demonstrate all of the critical criteria and a minimum of 70% in the psychomotor testing station. Upon successful completion of the course, registered nurses (RNs) are verified as TNCC providers for 4 years. Non-RNs are welcome to attend TNCC but are not eligible for verification. All participants are awarded nursing contact hours after attending the full course.

Course Learners

All nurses involved in the care of trauma patients may benefit from this course. It is expected that the course learner will possess a generic nursing knowledge, have an understanding of emergency care terminology, and be familiar with standard emergency equipment. The curriculum is designed for new trauma nurse learners to acquire essential knowledge and skills. Post-course mentoring and support are essential to further develop and master trauma nursing expertise. Experienced trauma nurses will update their learning to validate and improve established practice.

TNCC Provider Manual

It is ***essential*** that all learners read the TNCC provider manual and complete the online modules prior to attending the TNCC program. This provides learners with a foundational understanding of the concepts that will be applied to scenario-based classroom activities. Chapter content is organized in a consistent format for ease of learning. Each chapter will include the following elements:

- **Objectives**: Within each chapter, the objectives highlight core concepts and critical information that the learner will complete by the end of the chapter.
- **Anatomy and Physiology:** Most chapters provide a brief overview of anatomy and physiology for the convenience of the learner.
- **Pathophysiology as a Basis for Assessment Findings:** Pathophysiologic concepts related to the body's response and associated assessment findings are highlighted.
- **Selected Injuries:** Life-threatening and more frequently occurring injuries associated with the particular system are presented.
- **Nursing Care:** The organization of nursing care is based on the nursing process principles of assessment, diagnosis, planning, implementation, evaluation, and ongoing assessment.
- **Emerging Trends:** This section presents evidence-based information and/or research-related concepts or approaches linked to trauma practice. At the time of publication, these concepts may or may not currently be considered or accepted as the standard of care, they are brought to nurses' attention for discussion.
- **Summary and References:** Each chapter closes with chapter highlights and a complete list of references.

The provider manual also includes an overview of the skills stations and an outline for the TNP psychomotor skills station to assist learners in preparing for these sessions.

Epidemiology

The Centers for Disease Control and Prevention (CDC) estimated that 231,991 people died from injury in 2016, or approximately 1 person every 3 minutes.[1] Trauma is the leading cause of death in individuals ages 1 to 44 years (**Figure 1-1**),[2] and the third leading cause of death across all age groups in the United States. In 2014, approximately 30.6 million people were treated in emergency departments (ED) for injuries associated with trauma.[1] For 2015, the CDC estimated $671 billion was spent on healthcare and lost productivity associated with trauma.[3] Globally, road traffic injuries are projected to become the fourth leading cause of disability-adjusted life years lost by 2030.[4] See **Figure 1-2**.[5]

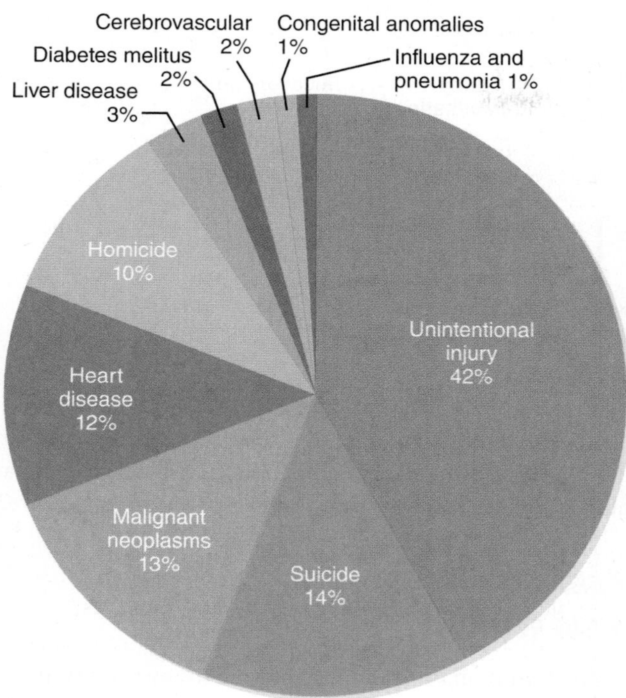

Figure 1-1 *Leading causes of death for individuals younger than age 45, United States.*

Data from Centers for Disease Control and Prevention. (2018). National vital statistics system. Retrieved from https://www.cdc.gov/nchs/nvss/index.htm.

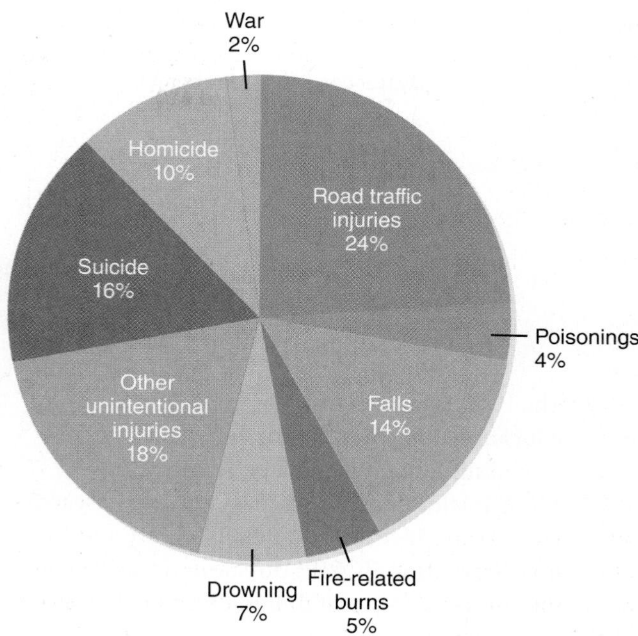

Figure 1-2 *How injuries and violence claim lives: causes of injury deaths, world, 2012.*

Reproduced from World Health Organization. (2014). *Injuries and violence: The facts 2014*. Geneva, Switzerland: Author. Retrieved from http://apps.who.int/iris/bitstream/handle/10665/149798/9789241508018_eng.pdf?sequence=1.

The development of trauma centers, implementation of integrated systems that progress from the point of injury through recovery (**Figure 1-3**),[6] and the systematic and standardized approach to trauma care have been instrumental in saving lives and improving outcomes for those affected by trauma.[7]

Trauma Nursing

Trauma nursing occurs wherever nurses care for injured patients. Nurses play a critical role throughout the continuum of care from the prehospital environment through the resuscitation, surgery, recovery, rehabilitation, and return to the community. Trauma nursing is care-specific and is not dependent on specialized care environments. It includes advocating for patient care (including at the level of the local and national legislatures), providing injury prevention education, and conducting research to further nursing practice.

The practice of the trauma nurse employs a standardized, systematic approach to care, integrating the nursing process as the foundation. Trauma nurses are also skilled in the management of difficult situations; moral agency is applied to advocate for excellence in patient care, even in the face of cultural and administrative obstacles.[8]

The practice of trauma nursing involves core knowledge derived from scientific and evidence-based sources as well as from the nurse's personal/life experiences. As a front-lines provider, it is critical that the trauma nurse gain the appropriate knowledge base and assessment skills to recognize the trauma patient and predict injury patterns and severity.

Emergency Nurses Association's Philosophy of Trauma Nursing Education

The Emergency Nurses Association (ENA) takes the following position regarding trauma nursing education[9]:

1. The optimal care of trauma patients is best accomplished using a standardized and coordinated approach within an organized trauma system.
2. The knowledge and skills presented in the TNCC provide emergency nurses with a standardized approach to assessment and intervention for trauma patients in a trauma team system.
3. TNCC provides essential trauma nursing education and is the educational standard for emergency nurses caring for injured patients.
4. TNCC is a nationally and internationally recognized course of continuing education in trauma care developed by and for nurses.

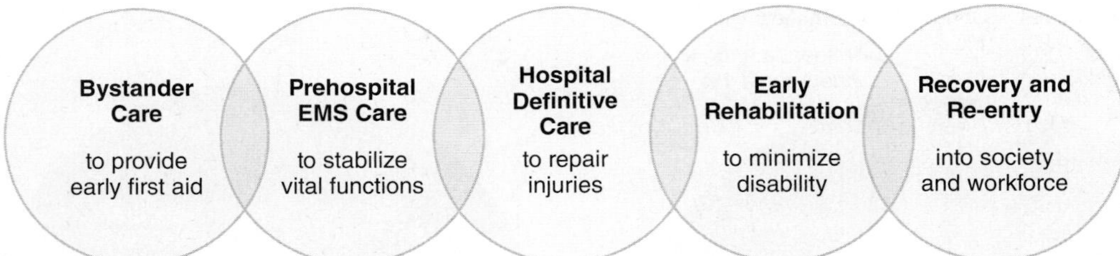

Figure 1-3 *Elements of the trauma system.*

Reproduced from National Academies of Sciences, Engineering, and Medicine. (2016). *A national trauma care system: Integrating military and civilian trauma systems to achieve zero preventable deaths after injury.* Washington, DC: National Academies Press. https://doi.org/10.17226/23511.

5. The ENA facilitates trauma-related continuing education opportunities for emergency nurses providing care for trauma patients.
6. ENA's Institute for Emergency Nursing Research (IENR) and Institute for Quality, Safety and Injury Prevention (IQSIP) pursue and translate injury prevention research into emergency nursing education and practice.

Trauma Nurse Roles and Responsibilities

Trauma nurses are essential members of a multidisciplinary team that is structured to meet the complex needs of the trauma patient. During the trauma resuscitation, the nurse plays a critical role in ensuring team coordination, effective communication, and delivery of systematic, timely care. The trauma nurse also advocates for the patient and family during this incredibly vulnerable time, ensuring that they are treated and cared for with respect and dignity at all times.

Additional trauma nursing responsibilities include ensuring that serial assessments are performed and documented, and reporting all subtle or new findings in the patient's condition. Nurses providing direct care to trauma patients are dynamic and highly skilled professionals who demonstrate the following skills/characteristics:

- Anticipate and determine care priorities
- Maintain order in unpredictable, and at times uncontrolled, situations
- Advocate for patients and families
- Delegate and coordinate trauma team roles and responsibilities
- Formulate efficient and effective decisions based on limited information
- Remain focused in the face of distraction
- Exhibit strong communication and teamwork skills
- Demonstrate resiliency

The trauma nurse is also responsible for ensuring continuity of care throughout the initial phase of care until the patient's admission, discharge, or transfer. The trauma nurse provides continuity and facilitates high-quality care.

Trauma Team Structure and Roles

Trauma resuscitation has been referred to as a team sport—one that requires all team members to perform together for successful results. A team is defined as a set of individuals who are cognizant of one another, interact with each other, and have a shared sense of each other as a group.[10] During the delivery of trauma care, team members respond to and provide specific expertise with a common goal of achieving the best possible outcomes for their patient.

Members of the trauma team may vary based on the clinical setting, time of day, and resources available. Regardless of the situation, a systematic, organized approach is required by all members of the trauma team to provide optimal care for the trauma patient and family. The typical composition of trauma teams includes the following members:

- **Patient:** The trauma nurse's highest priority is to ensure the patient remains the focus of the provision of trauma care. This statement may seem simplistic, but the highly technical nature of trauma care often eclipses the simple human connection with the patient and family. Involving and communicating with the patient and family is a key role of the trauma nurse.
- **Team leader:** The team leader may be a physician, an advanced practice nurse, or a physician assistant. The critical functions of the team leader are maintaining situational awareness, clearly communicating to the team, and encouraging mutual support. The trauma nurse is well suited to lead the core patient-care team and support services, coordinating the care of both the patient and the team in conjunction with the team leader.[11]

Effective leaders in trauma demonstrate the following:
- Organize the team.
- Articulate clear goals.
- Make decisions through collective input of other team members.
- Empower members to speak up and ask questions.
- Allocate resources.
- Provide feedback.
- Model teamwork behaviors.[10]

- **Core team:** This group of care providers works interdependently to manage a trauma patient from assessment to disposition.[12] Roles and responsibilities are often designated for technical skills such as airway management, vascular access, transport, medication administration, and documentation, though they may vary by clinical setting. Institutional guidelines and policies specific to roles, responsibilities, and resources assist in ensuring consistent delivery of high-quality trauma care.
- **Contingency and support services:** These team members provide support to the core team to facilitate optimal trauma care. The contingency team deals with emergencies or specific events. Examples of contingency teams include an airway team (anesthesia, respiratory therapist, paramedic) and a trauma code team, which practices following a standardized response to designated categories of patient injury. Members of the trauma support team may include a pharmacist, radiology, lab, social work, case management, and chaplain.

High-Performance Trauma Teams

Trauma resuscitation requires all team members to be efficient and coordinated, with the common goal of providing high-quality care. Effective trauma teams are dynamic, interdependent, and adaptive, always moving toward a common goal.[13] High-performing teams exhibit the following characteristics[10]:

- Shared mental models
- Optimize resources
- Have strong team leadership
- Engage in a regular discipline of feedback
- Develop a strong sense of collective trust and confidence
- Create mechanisms to cooperate and coordinate their actions
- Optimize performance outcomes

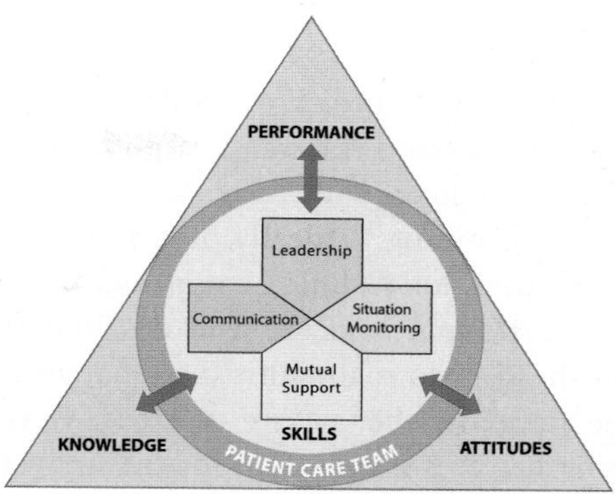

Figure 1-4 *Cornerstones of high-performance teams in trauma care.*

Reproduced from Agency of Healthcare Research and Quality. (2018). TeamSTEPPS 2.0 pocket guide. Retrieved from https://www.ahrq.gov/teamstepps/instructor/essentials/pocketguide.html.

Teamwork and interdisciplinary collaboration directly affect patient care. High-performing trauma teams have been shown to decrease mortality by reducing the time to investigation, total time in the resuscitation room, and the rate of missed injuries.[14] A growing body of supportive evidence also suggests that team training in trauma improves performance and patient outcomes.[15] Nonetheless, skilled communication, cooperation, and coordination are the cornerstones of high-performance teams and high-quality trauma care (**Figure 1-4**).[15,16]

Communication

For decades, the characteristics and behaviors associated with high-performing and low- or poor-performing teams have been observed and dissected. Experts in the fields of aerospace, the military, engineering, and the humanities have found that communication is potentially a team's greatest asset or gravest shortcoming.[17] Despite the general consensus that good communication is critical in healthcare, we continue to fail in the execution of these principles. CRICO Strategies, a division of the risk management foundation of the Harvard Medical Institutions, reported that between 2009 and 2013, communication failures were a factor in 30% of malpractice claims and contributed to 7,149 cases of patient harm.[18]

Team performance is supported by the application of standardized, evidence-based communication tools and practices. The Agency for Healthcare Research and Quality's (AHRQ) Team Strategies and Tools to Enhance Performance and Patient Safety (TeamSTEPPS) curriculum identifies three critical communication points in trauma care: briefs, huddles, and debriefs.[10]

Brief

A brief is a planned teamwork event designed to form the team, designate team roles and responsibilities, establish climate and goals, and engage the team in short- and long-term planning.[10] Ideally, this is done at the beginning of a traditional clinical event such as the start of the shift. Briefs may also occur at designated times throughout the shift to maintain situational awareness. Due to the unpredictable nature of trauma events, a daily briefing helps the team plan for the arrival of an unannounced trauma patient. Many organizations have found the use of a standardized briefing checklist to be helpful. Some hospitals use a whiteboard to facilitate the brief; others have incorporated the brief in an electronic format. Elements of the brief checklist may include the following:

- Introduction
- Staff availability
- Workload and organizational/community situation

Huddle

Another component of teamwork communication is a huddle. Huddles are convened as needed to monitor and modify the plan. The purpose of a huddle is to regain situational awareness, express concerns, and make changes to the plan with reassignment of resources as appropriate. It is important to identify and widely communicate huddle triggers and to ensure that anyone who recognizes a potential critical event has the ability to call a huddle.[20]

Debrief

A debrief can be a quick, informal information exchange or feedback session that occurs after an event and is designed to improve teamwork skills. A debrief checklist can be quite simple:

- What went well?
- What might be done differently next time?
- Does anything need to be fixed right away, and who needs to know?

When the review process is interdisciplinary and encompasses all members of the team, there are increased opportunities for future success. The debriefing can be conducted in a matter of minutes and is standardized to the clinical setting. In one hospital setting, a quick debrief may be held as the patient is being taken to the radiology suite for further studies. In another, it may occur just after the patient is transported to another facility. The timing varies depending on the setting, but the importance of the debrief occurring every time cannot be overstated. If members of the trauma team are not available for the debrief, the team leader assures that the missing team member's feedback and concerns are solicited and included.

Communication before, during, and after a trauma event should be brief, clear, concise, and timely. Many of these tools can be found in the TeamSTEPPS curriculum.[10]

Performance Improvement and Trauma Care

Performance improvement is a system of multidisciplinary reviews with a feedback loop for the purpose of identifying areas for improvement and developing a demonstrated action plan.[19] Effective communication, teamwork, and collaboration with feedback for improvement are the foundations of organized, timely, safe, quality care. These components help the team to provide increasingly excellent care.

Summary

Trauma remains a major threat to the health and socioeconomic well-being of individuals, communities, and countries around the world. Whether a trauma event occurs in a community with a sophisticated multiresource trauma center or a critical access hospital, a coordinated, collaborative, and systematic approach to the initial assessment and management of trauma is essential to ensure optimal outcomes and minimize morbidity and mortality. A high-performance trauma team consistently delivers coordinated and collaborative care by clearly defining roles and responsibilities in addition to ensuring efficiency, safety, and high-quality care delivery.

The trauma nurse is the coordinating member of the team who ensures continuity, consistency and organization among team members. Nurses are essential members of the team and integral to trauma care and resuscitation in the ED. Their contributions through quality clinical care, in addition to effective communication, leadership, and teamwork, ultimately enable optimal patient outcomes.

The ENA believes that the knowledge and skills presented in the TNCC will assist professional nurses in systematically assessing the trauma patient, rapidly intervening and/or assisting with interventions, and functioning within the context of a trauma team. The ENA supports an ongoing commitment and efforts to improve injury surveillance, research, trauma system development, and governmental support for trauma care and injury prevention as a top priority.

References

1. Centers for Disease Control and Prevention, National Center for Injury Prevention and Control. (2018). Web-Based Injury Statistics Query and Reporting System (WISQARS): Fatal injury data. Retrieved from https://www.cdc.gov/injury/wisqars/fatal.html
2. Centers for Disease Control and Prevention. (2018). National vital statistics system. Retrieved from https://www.cdc.gov/nchs/nvss/index.htm
3. Centers for Disease Control and Prevention, National Center for Injury Prevention and Control. (2017). Accidents or unintentional injuries. Retrieved from https://www.cdc.gov/nchs/fastats/accidental-injury.htm
4. Alam, K., & Mahal, A. (2016). The economic burden of road traffic injuries on households in South Asia. *PLoS One, 11*(10), e0164362. http://doi.org/10.1371/journal.pone.0164362
5. World Health Organization. (2014). *Injuries and violence: The facts 2014.* Geneva, Switzerland: Author. Retrieved from http://apps.who.int/iris/bitstream/handle/10665/149798/9789241508018_eng.pdf?sequence=1
6. National Academies of Sciences, Engineering, and Medicine. (2016). *A national trauma care system: Integrating military and civilian trauma systems to achieve zero preventable deaths after injury.* Washington, DC: National Academies Press. https://doi.org/10.17226/23511
7. Ciesla, D. J., Tepas, J. J., Pracht, E. E., Langland-Orban, B., Cha, J. Y., & Flint, L. M. (2013). Fifteen-year trauma system performance analysis demonstrates optimal coverage for most severely injured patients and identifies a vulnerable population. *Journal of the American College of Surgeons, 216*(4), 687–695. https://doi.org/10.1016/j.jamcollsurg.2012.12.033
8. Wolf, L. (2012). An integrated, ethically driven environmental model of clinical decision making in emergency settings. *International Journal of Nursing Knowledge, 24*(1), 49–53. https://doi.org/10.1111/j.2047-3095.2012.01229.x
9. Emergency Nurses Association. (2015). *Trauma nursing education (Position statement).* Des Plaines, IL: Author. Retrieved from https://www.ena.org/docs/default-source/resource-library/practice-resources/position-statements/traumanursing education.pdf?sfvrsn=d7ccdd0a_6
10. Agency for Healthcare Research and Quality. (2014). TeamSTEPPS fundamentals course: Module 2. Team structure. Rockville, MD: Author. Retrieved from http://www.ahrq.gov/teamstepps/instructor/fundamentals/module2/igteamstruct.html
11. Clements, A., Curtis, K., Horvat, L., & Shaban, R. Z. (2015). The effect of a nurse team leader on communication and leadership in major trauma resuscitations. *International Emergency Nursing, 23*(1), 3–7. https://doi.org/10.1016/j.ienj.2014.04.004
12. Geyer, R. (2016). Core team members' impact on outcomes and process improvement in the initial resuscitation of trauma patients. *Journal of Trauma Nursing, 23*(2), 83–88. https://doi.org/10.1097/JTN.0000000000000191
13. Gillman, L., Brindley, P. G., Blaivas, M., Widder, S., & Karakitsos, D. (2016). Trauma team dynamics. *Journal of Critical Care, 32*, 218–221. https://doi.org/10.1016/j.jcrc.2015.12.009
14. Georgiou, A., & Lockey, D. J. (2010). The performance and assessment of hospital trauma teams. *Scandinavian Journal of Trauma, Resuscitation and Emergency Medicine, 18*(66). https://doi.org/10.1186/1757-7241-18-66
15. Peters, V. K., Harvey, E. M., Wright, A., Bath, J., Freeman, D., & Collier, B. (2018). Impact of a TeamSTEPPS Trauma Nurse Academy at a Level 1 trauma center. *Journal of Emergency Nursing, 44*(1), 19–25. https://doi.org/10.1016/j.jen.2017.05.007
16. Agency of Healthcare Research and Quality. (2018). TeamSTEPPS 2.0 pocket guide. Retrieved from https://www.ahrq.gov/teamstepps/instructor/essentials/pocketguide.html
17. Karakitso, D. (2016). Trauma team dynamics (Editorial). *Journal of Critical Care, 32*, 218–221. https://doi.org/10.1016/j.jcrc.2015.12.009
18. CRICO Strategies. (2015). *Malpractice risks in communication failures: 2015 annual benchmarking report.* Boston, MA: Author. Retrieved from https://www.rmf.harvard.edu/Malpractice-Data/Annual-Benchmark-Reports/Risks-in-Communication-Failures
19. American College of Surgeons Committee on Trauma. (2014). Resources for the optimal care of the injured patient 2014: Resources repository. Retrieved from https://www.facs.org/~/media/files/quality%20programs/trauma/vrc%20resources/resources%20for%20optimal%20care.ashx
20. Agency for Healthcare Research and Quality. (2019, March). TeamSTEPPS fundamentals course: Module 4. Leading teams. Retrieved from https://www.ahrq.gov/teamstepps/instructor/fundamentals/module4/igleadership.html

CHAPTER

2

Biomechanics, Kinematics, and Mechanisms of Injury

Richard W. Harley, Jr., BSN, RN, and Diana Giordano, DNP, RN, FNP-BC

OBJECTIVES

Upon completion of this chapter, the learner will be able to:

1. Apply concepts of biomechanics, kinematics, and mechanisms of injury to the traumatic bodily injuries.
2. Describe forms of energy transfer related to trauma.
3. Compare the effects of environmental energy transfer on human tissues.
4. Predict potential injuries from specific mechanisms and patterns of injury.

Introduction

Trauma is the Greek word for "wound"; it is defined as "an injury (such as a wound) to living tissue caused by an extrinsic agent."[1] The potential for traumatic injury is present whenever energy comes into contact with the human body. The laws of physics govern the energy transferred during such events. When the intensity of the applied energy exceeds the capacity of tissue resistance, trauma occurs. Therefore, understanding the laws of physics and applying biomechanics, kinematics, and mechanism of injury (MOI) principles, along with knowledge of anatomy and physiology, can greatly assist the trauma care provider in anticipating the intervention and management needs of the trauma patient (**Table 2-1**).[2-4]

Kinematics: The Physics of Energy Transfer

Energy "at rest" is considered *potential*. However, once an object or mass starts to move, the potential energy becomes *kinetic*, meaning "in motion." Kinematics and the physics of energy transfer can be applied to all mechanical traumas and is considered an essential element when determining traumatic injury.[5] The severity of injury depends on the amount of force that the body absorbs. In relation to Isaac Newton's laws of motion, applying the basic laws of physics to the anatomic and physiologic properties of the human body can illuminate injury patterns experienced by a trauma victim.

TABLE 2-1 Terminology

Term	Definition
Biomechanics	The general study of forces and their effects on a living body
Kinematics	The study of pure motion
Mechanism of injury	How external energy forces in the environment are transferred to the body

Data from the Dictionary.com (n.d.). Biomechanics. Retrieved from https://www.dictionary.com; Dictionary.com (n.d.). Kinematics. Retrieved from https://www.dictionary.com; National Association of Emergency Medical Technicians, & American College of Surgeons, Committee on Trauma. (2016). Kinematics of trauma. In *Prehospital trauma life support* (8th ed., pp. 70–111). Burlington, MA: Jones & Bartlett Learning.

Newton's laws of motion include the following[6]:

- *Newton's First Law of Motion* explains that a body at rest will remain at rest (potential energy) and a body in motion (kinetic energy) will remain in motion unless acted upon by an object.[6] When energy is transferred, alteration can occur to one or both objects.
  - *Example*: When a vehicle is parked, the force of gravity holds the car in a fixed position (potential energy). The vehicle will remain stationary until a force (e.g., collision with another vehicle) sets it in motion. The vehicle will remain in motion until acted upon by another object (e.g., tree).
- *Newton's Second Law of Motion* builds upon the first law and explains that acceleration is dependent upon two variables. An object's acceleration (a) depends directly on the net force (F) and indirectly on the mass (m) of an object. The net force equals the product of the mass multiplied by acceleration: F_{net} = mass × acceleration.[6] This law describes how momentum can either speed up or slow down depending on its acting force. As the force on an object is increased, the acceleration of the object is also increased. However, if the mass of an object is increased, the acceleration of the object is decreased.
  - *Example*: Two vehicles (a sport-utility vehicle and a compact car) have broken down on the road. The drivers are attempting to move their vehicles to the nearest exit ramp. The driver pushing the sport-utility vehicle (larger mass) will have to apply more effort as compared to the driver moving the compact car (smaller mass). Therefore, the driver of the sport-utility vehicle may need greater force (more individuals to help push) to accelerate the vehicle and cause it to move.

CLINICAL PEARL 

Newton's Second Law of Motion

Force is increased = acceleration is increased
Mass is increased = acceleration is decreased

An understanding of this relationship enables the trauma care provider to make an educated prediction regarding the extent of injury and the subsequent care required for a trauma patient.

- *Newton's Third Law of Motion* specifies that for every action (energy impact), there is an equal and opposite reaction resulting from the transfer of energy.[6] When two objects interact, they exert equal force upon each other. For every interaction, two forces are appreciated: (1) The size of the force of the first object equals the force of the second object and (2) the direction of the force of the first object is opposite that of the second object.[5]
  - *Example*: A vehicle is driving down the road and collides with a bird, which strikes the windshield. The bird and the windshield interact with each other (equal and opposite reaction).

Question	Answer	Explanation
According to Newton's third law, which of these two forces is greater: size or force?	Neither. For each force, there is an *equal* and opposite reaction.	The potential demise of the bird results from the difference in the bird's *mass* and its inability to withstand larger acceleration.

- Newton's laws of motion help form the *Law of Conservation of Energy*. Energy cannot be created or destroyed, only changed from one form to another or transferred from one object to another.[6] The total amount of energy must remain constant; that is, it is conserved over time. Therefore, if an object is isolated, the energy it has does not disappear but

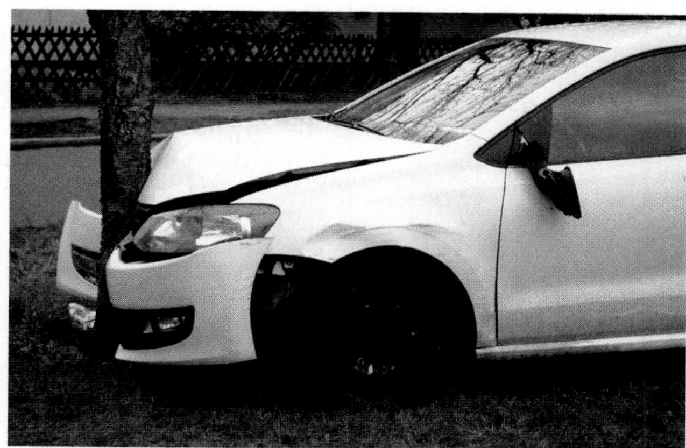

Figure 2-1 *Car versus tree.*

gets conserved, waiting to be acted upon. Trauma care providers must function as energy detectives, identifying where the stored energy put into motion has been transferred to anticipate a patient's physiological condition and needs. The amount of energy inflicted upon a body and the ability to tolerate it will determine injury and severity.[7]

- *Example:* Consider a car-versus-tree scenario (**Figure 2-1**). According to Newton's Law of Conservation of Energy, a car traveling at 60 mph (kinetic energy) collides (transferring its energy) with a tree (conserved energy), thereby creating an equal and opposite reaction that causes the vehicle to come to a sudden stop. However, the person or persons inside the vehicle will continue to travel at that same speed (60 mph), remaining in motion until acted upon by another force, transferring the energy of the person to that object (e.g., steering wheel, windshield, seat belt, air bag). Although the impact may have stopped the forward momentum of the body, the organs within the body remain in motion until they collide with another stationary force, such as the spinal column, abdominal wall, or chest wall.

Biomechanics: Energy Forces and Their Effect

It is useful to consider the energy forces that can affect the human body and their effect so as to better understand what happens during trauma.

Energy Forms

Energy can impact a person in the form of heat, motion, electricity, or some other form (**Table 2-2**). The body composition, preexisting conditions, and concomitant exposure of an individual all affect the intensity of energy transfer absorption. For example, the extent of a thermal burn will vary with the temperature and duration of contact.

TABLE 2-2 Forms of Energy

Energy Form	Source
Chemical	Heat energy transfer from active chemical substances such as chlorine, drain cleaner, acids, or plants
Electrical	Energy transfer from light socket, power lines, or lightning
Mechanical	Energy transfer from one object to another in the form of motion (e.g., a car hitting a tree)
Radiant	Energy transfer from blast sound waves, radioactivity such as a nuclear facility, or rays of the sun
Thermal	Energy transfer of heat in the environment to the host

Kinetic Energy

The energy of a body in motion is identified as kinetic energy (KE). The amount of KE that an object has depends on the relationship between two variables: mass and velocity (speed). KE is equal to one-half the mass (m) multiplied by the square of its velocity (v^2). While mass and velocity contribute to the energy present in a moving object, they do not possess a constant ratio. When mass is doubled, so is the net energy. However, when velocity is doubled, energy is quadrupled. The KE equation is[8]:

$$\text{KE} = \frac{1}{2} mv^2$$

Although this equation may not be used to formally calculate the amount of KE involved in the trauma event when caring for a trauma patient, the comprehension of KE concepts is vital to the healthcare provider. Initial assessments in the aftermath of trauma may not identify a significant injury, but 5% to 15% of those patients may later exhibit significant injuries.[9] Therefore, it is prudent for the trauma care provider to perform serial examinations and reassessments with the understanding that the transfer of energy involved in a collision, whether it was a low- or high-energy event, has the potential to cause harm.

CLINICAL PEARL

KE

Speed increases energy by the square of the velocity and can influence the extent of injury.[10] However, the action of stopping must also be considered. Speed increases the risk of injury, but energy transfer occurs during the "stop," when energy is exerted and applied to the tissues upon impact.

Types of Energy Forces

The degree to which tissues resist destruction under circumstances of energy transfer depends on their proximity to the impact and their structural characteristics. The basic types of forces are identified in **Figure 2-2** and further explained in **Table 2-3**.

In addition to the laws of physics, the distance and total surface area over which the energy is transferred are influential in determining injury patterns.[11] The tissue

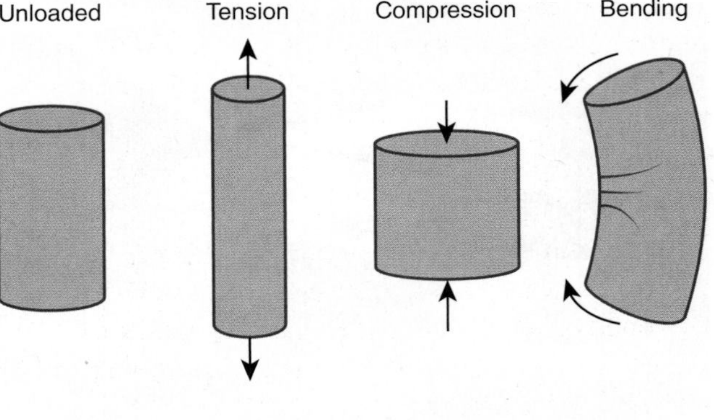

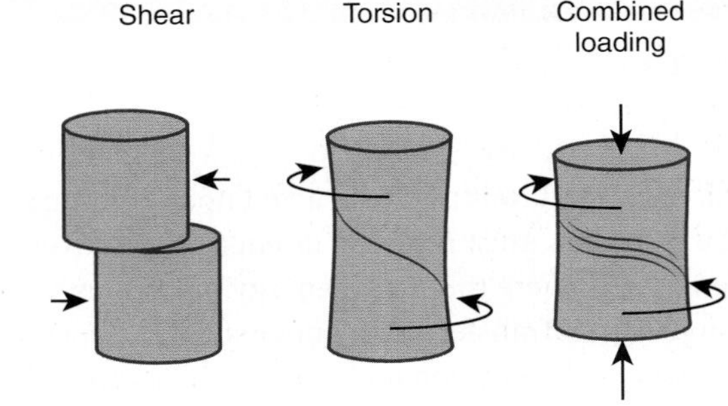

Figure 2-2 *Types of energy forces.*

TABLE 2-3 Energy Forces

Energy Force	Description	Example
Tension	Tension forces stretch by pulling at opposite ends.	Tensile strength describes the tissue's ability to resist pulling apart when stretched. Tendons, ligaments, and muscles can tear when they are overstretched (e.g., Achilles tendon).
Compression	Compression forces crush by squeezing together.	Compression injuries to organs occur when the organs are crushed from surrounding internal organs or structures such as a seat belt worn up across the abdomen, causing compression of the small bowel or a fracture to the lumbar spine.
Bending	Loading about an axis. Bending causes compression on the side the person is bending toward and tension to the opposite side.	A force moves from a straight form to a curved form, such as bending forward from a standing position.
Shearing	Shearing forces damage by tearing or bending by exerting force at different parts in opposite directions at the same time.	Shear strength describes the tissue's ability to resist a force applied parallel to the tissue. An aortic aneurysm is an example: As the aorta is stretched beyond its capacity, the vessel is torn away from the attachment.
Torsion	Torsion forces twist ends in opposite directions.	Twisting motion depends on the body's ability to resist applied torque (e.g., a golfer's spine twisting when swinging a golf club).
Combined loading	Any combination of tension, compression, torsion, bending, and/or shear.	The combination of forces may increase the magnitude of the stress.

most proximal to the point of impact is affected by the amount of energy. As energy traverses across the tissue, it is absorbed by cells. Therefore, the net energy available for transfer is attenuated over distance.[9]

External energy can be exerted by acceleration and deceleration forces.

- *Acceleration force:* Injury from acceleration forces occurs when applied energy causes a sudden and rapid onset of motion. For example, with a forceful blow to the head, the head suddenly accelerates. The stationary brain is struck by the cranium that has been set in motion, causing injury.
- *Deceleration force:* Injury caused by deceleration forces occurs when energy is halted by a sudden stop. The more distance involved, the less likely a severe injury is to occur. Deceleration forces include those applied in falls and collisions where injuries are caused by a sudden stop of the body's motion.

The internal force that resists an applied external force is described as *stress.* When stress is exerted on the body, tissues and organs change their dimensions. The degree to which tissues resist destruction depends on the amount of energy involved (high or low), as well as the structural characteristics and proximity of the organs (or tissue) to the impact. Considerations include:

- *Bone:* Strength and resistance to stress can vary and can be augmented by adjacent muscle systems.
- *Muscle density:* Muscle density surrounding bone absorbs energy. Tensile strength is augmented by the strength of opposing muscles.
- *Organ structures:* Refer to Table 2-3.
  - Solid organs tolerate pressure-wave energy better than air-filled organs.
  - Air-filled organs can resist shear forces better than solid organs.

Types of Injuries

Trauma-related injuries are classified into the following types:

- Blunt trauma
- Penetrating trauma
- Thermal trauma (see Chapter 11, "Surface and Burn Trauma," for more information)
- Blast trauma

Blunt Trauma

Blunt injuries are very common and result from a broad range of energy impacts. Understanding the distance and total surface area over which the energy transfer occurs is important for identifying an injury pattern. The more focused the impact, the greater the damage. However, if an increased distance of energy transfer is experienced, the amount of detrimental injury may diminish. Because blunt trauma may often appear less obvious, with minimal to no outward signs of injury as compared to other mechanisms or types of injuries, its severity may be dismissed initially, resulting in delayed treatment and increased complications. For this reason, early and frequent assessments are crucial for the trauma care provider to identify opportunities for early intervention before the trauma patient becomes unstable. The most common causes of blunt injuries involve both acceleration and deceleration forces such as falls, collisions (motor vehicle, bicycle, and motorcycle), and physical assaults.[12]

CLINICAL PEARL 

Blunt Trauma

Because blunt trauma may often appear less obvious, with minimal to no outward signs of injury as compared to other mechanisms or types of injuries, its severity may be dismissed initially, resulting in delayed treatment and increased complications.

Falls

Falls involve acceleration/deceleration principles as described earlier, as well as Newton's laws of motion. As an example, consider an older adult who becomes dizzy and falls from a standing position. The energy transfer begins as the patient begins to collapse. When the patient collides with the ground, the impact causes energy transfer and injuries related to the following[11]:

- The point of impact on the patient's body determines the major point of energy transfer and underlying injuries or tissues impacted (e.g., head, hip, outstretched arm).
- The type of surface that is hit and the extent to which this surface can absorb the energy affect injuries. Carpet and grass can help to absorb energy better than a hard surface such as tile or concrete.
- The tissue's ability to resist also affects potential injuries. Bone is less flexible than soft tissue. Air-filled organs may rupture; solid organs may fracture.
- The trajectory of force influences the injuries experienced. If a person is pushed or accidentally knocked down, acceleration increases, causing additional transfer of energy, which results in a greater impact on deceleration.

Consider a construction worker who falls from greater than 20 feet: The increased distance increases acceleration, thereby increasing the energy force, transfer of energy, and impact on deceleration. In the pediatric patient, a fall is considered significant if it occurs from three times the child's height.[13]

Motor Vehicle Impact Sequence

Vehicle collisions are reported worldwide as a common cause of blunt abdominal trauma.[14] Several impacts may occur during the progression of a motor vehicle collision (MVC)[9]:

- The first impact occurs when the vehicle collides with another object (e.g., a tree). The occupants experience a relative acceleration as the vehicle comes to an abrupt stop (**Figure 2-3**).
- The second impact occurs after the initial impact. The occupants continue to move in the original direction of travel until they collide with the interior of the vehicle or meet resistance (e.g., steering wheel, windshield, seat belt, or air bag), yet the internal organs continue in motion (**Figure 2-4**). Another factor to consider is air bag deployment, which accelerates toward the occupants at a rate produced by the blast of the deployed device.
- The third impact occurs when internal structures collide within the body cavity. The organs meet resistance from the structures that encapsulate them and/or are torn loose and may continue in motion until they meet the resistance of another structure such as the chest wall or skull (**Figure 2-5**).

The survivability of a collision can be predicted by determining the velocity and stopping distance.[2] When assessing a patient who has been injured in an MVC, the trauma nurse should anticipate potential injuries as a result of the energy transfer. The extent of injuries is influenced by the rate, stopping distance, and deployed safety mechanisms such as seat belts, airbags, and the impact absorbency of the vehicle.

The chemicals used to preserve and deploy air bags may sometimes cause corneal abrasions and minor skin burns as the bag explodes as part of its rapid inflation.[15] Therefore, eye injuries may result and are of particular concern when patients are wearing glasses. Despite the

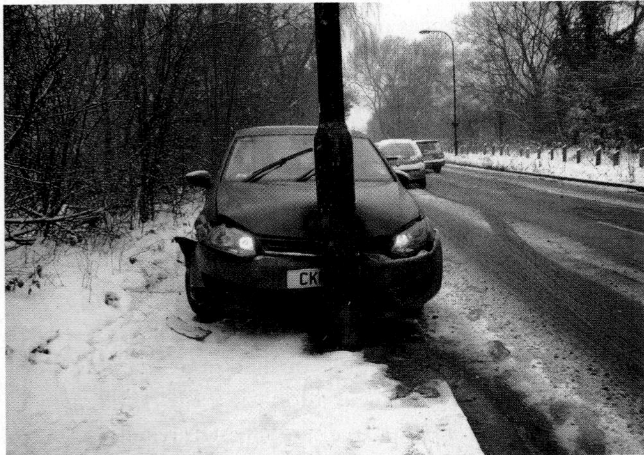

Figure 2-3 *First impact of MVC.*

© DBURKE/Alamy Stock Photo

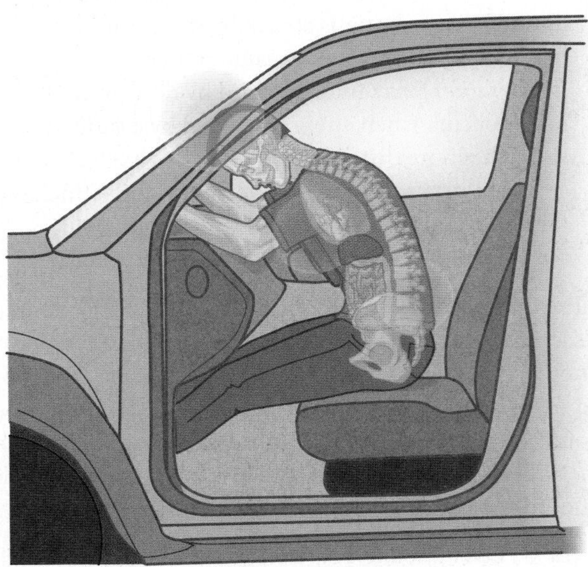

Figure 2-4 *Second impact of MVC: example of an up and over path.*

Note: The body continues in motion until it impacts the inside of the vehicle.

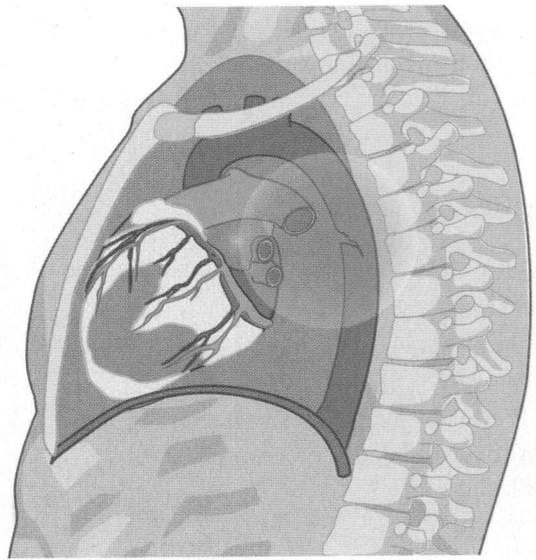

Figure 2-5 *Third impact of MVC.*

Note: Organs continue in motion and are torn away from their attachment. In this example, the aorta is torn at the ligamentum arteriosum until it impacts inside the thoracic cavity.

risks of relatively minor secondary injury patterns, advances in air bag technology have decreased the mortality and morbidity associated with MVCs.[15] While the overall value of the air bag is clear, appropriate-fitting seat belts and proper use of these restraints is required to realize the full benefit of vehicles' safety devices.

The trauma care provider also uses MOI descriptions to anticipate certain injury patterns. See Chapter 3, "Initial Assessment," for more information.

Mechanism of Injury and Potential Injury Patterns in MVCs

Mechanisms of injury and potential injury patterns are associated with the type of motor vehicle involved.

Motor Vehicle (Auto)

Several patterns of pathway injuries are possible with collisions involving automobiles:

- *Up and over* pathway injuries can affect a driver as well as a passenger and occur when the head and chest lead the way over the steering wheel and/or dashboard to the windshield (Figure 2-4). These injuries most commonly involve the head, neck, chest, and/or abdomen.[12]
- *Down and under* pathway injuries occur when the occupants (driver or passenger) move in a downward direction under the steering wheel and/or dashboard (**Figure 2-6**). This type of collision pattern can result from a misplaced seat belt placed above the pelvis, and is associated with lower extremity and pelvis fractures.[9,12]
- *Lateral (T-bone)* impact injury patterns depend on where an individual is located in the vehicle in relation to the impact (**Figure 2-7**). The occupant closest to the point of impact has the potential to incur increased severity of injuries. Lateral impacts may be associated with shear injuries to the aorta and other organs; clavicle, lateral pelvic and abdominal, and lateral head and neck injuries may also be experienced.[16]
- *Rotational* impacts occur when a vehicle is struck on one corner, by either a stationary object or another vehicle going in the opposite direction, causing the rest of the vehicle to move laterally around a pivot point.[12] The impacted corner stops,

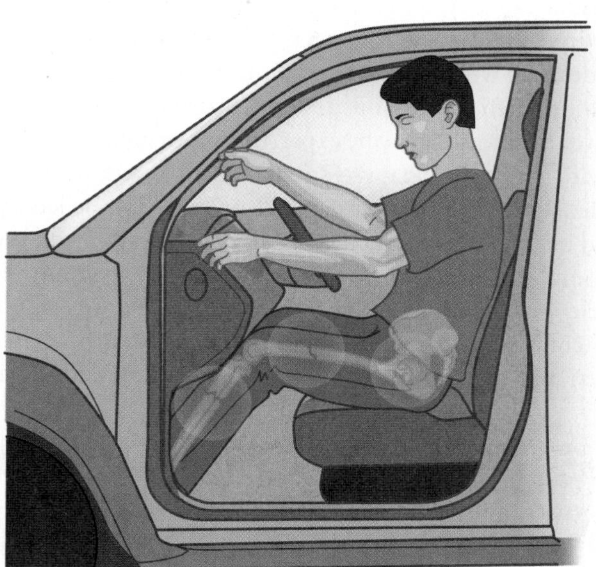

Figure 2-6 *The down and under path.*

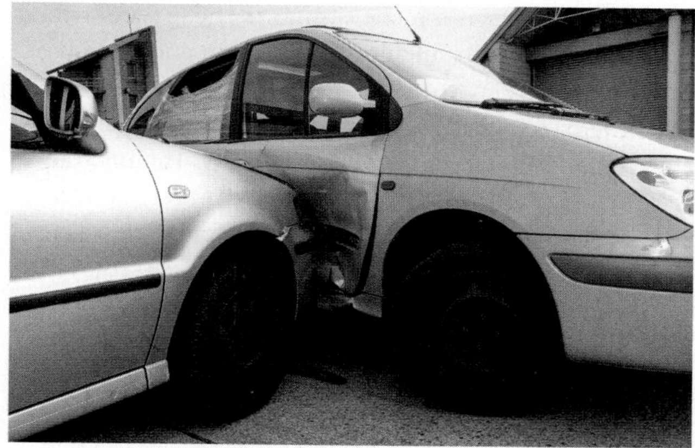

A

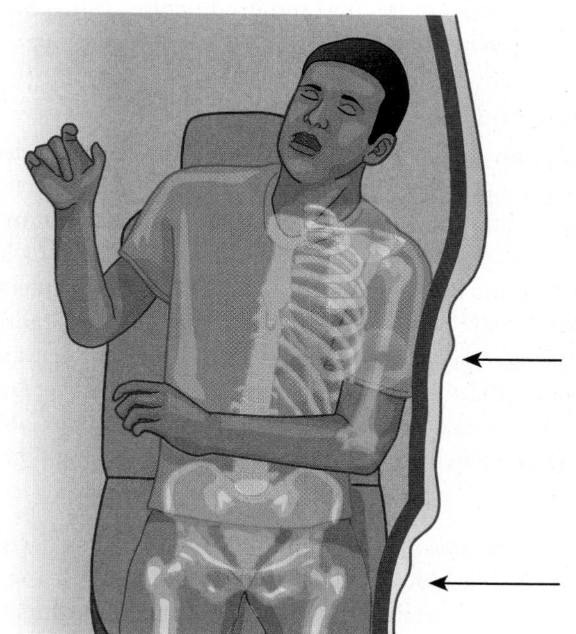

B

Figure 2-7 ***A.*** *Lateral impact.* ***B.*** *Points of contact in a lateral impact motor vehicle collision.*

Note: With a lateral T-bone accident, the greater the amount of intrusion, the greater potential for injury to the vehicle's occupants.

but the rest of the vehicle continues to move until the energy of the vehicle is transferred. The occupant will then travel forward while the lateral side of the car extends inward and collides with the forward-moving body.[9,12] The rotational impact may result in a combination of frontal and lateral impacts.

- *Rear* impacts involve several different forces. As the oncoming vehicle impacts the vehicle in front of it, there is an immediate forward acceleration, resulting in the occupants being forced backward into the seat. The individuals are then propelled forward, colliding with any object located in front of them (e.g., steering wheel, dashboard, windshield). Injury patterns may be similar to those seen with frontal impacts, including extension and flexion of the neck.[9]
- *Rollover* collisions can result in any and/or all of the injury patterns described previously. The Insurance Institute for Highway Safety reports that rollover collisions are rare, accounting for 1% of all crashes; nevertheless, one-third of these crashes result in occupant death.[17]
- *Ejection* from a vehicle can be caused by many factors such as not wearing or inappropriately wearing safety restraints (i.e., seat belts). The centrifugal force of a rollover collision also increases the risk of occupant ejection and head injuries from roof intrusion.[2]

Motorcycles

Collisions involving other types of motorized vehicles—for example, farm tractor, all-terrain vehicles, personal watercraft, and snowmobiles—can also cause traumatic injuries. Concerns with all motorized vehicles include the use and availability of restraint devices and protective gear. Failure to use restraints increases the probability of passenger ejection, especially in those without restraints. It is not the objective of this text to be all inclusive regarding motorized accidents, however. Instead, a few points of interest involving motorcycle collisions are highlighted here[2,12,18]:

- A *low side crash* is commonly referred to as "laying the bike down" and occurs when motorcycle is no longer upright with the tires leading in the direction of travel. Less speed-reducing friction is present when the motorcycle tires are no longer in upright contact with the roadway. A motorcycle sliding on its side may not slow down quickly. Therefore, impact energy experienced before and after the crash can be similar. In a low side crash, abrasions, shoulder and clavicle injuries, lateral head injuries, and lower extremity injuries are common.
- A *high side crash* occurs when a motorcycle begins to fall to the side, but regains traction, placing the motorcycle in an unbalanced position. The force may vault the motorcycle, resulting in the rider being catapulted into the air. Injury patterns include all of those common to low side crashes as well as those associated with the speed and impact of the rider landing onto the surface.
- *Head-on* impacts cause an abrupt deceleration force, ejecting the rider forward with the head and torso leading the way. Depending on the motorcycle design and rider position, the lower extremities can collide with the handlebars, resulting in femur and pelvis fractures and hip dislocations. The remaining injuries depend on the subsequent collisions but are likely to involve the head, neck, chest, and extremities.
- *Lateral or angular* impacts initially result in significant lower extremity injuries, but other patterns can be present as well. The angular impact may initially crush the lower extremities, but will likely cause the motorcycle to rapidly impact the ground, resulting in upper extremity, lateral head, and neck injuries. A T-bone impact to the motorcyclist may result in a lower extremity crush injury followed by side-impact shoulder and head injuries as the rider slams into the hood and windshield of the other vehicle. Then the rider is likely to tumble off of the car and impact the ground.

Vehicle-Versus-Pedestrian Injuries

The height and speed of the vehicle, as well as the height, mental capacity, and distraction of the pedestrian and/or driver, may affect the severity of injuries suffered by a pedestrian who is struck by a vehicle.[12] When the vehicle collides with the adult pedestrian, crushing forces to the lower extremities may be experienced. An adult-sized individual may be catapulted onto the hood and/or windshield of the vehicle, sliding off or being propelled up and over, eventually incurring another collision with the ground (**Figure 2-8**). Adults aware of the oncoming vehicle may respond by turning to escape, resulting in the potential for lateral or posterior injuries. In contrast, children may turn toward the oncoming vehicle, resulting in

CLINICAL PEARL

Rollover Collisions with Ejection

Ejection from the vehicle significantly increases the probability of fatal injury.[9]

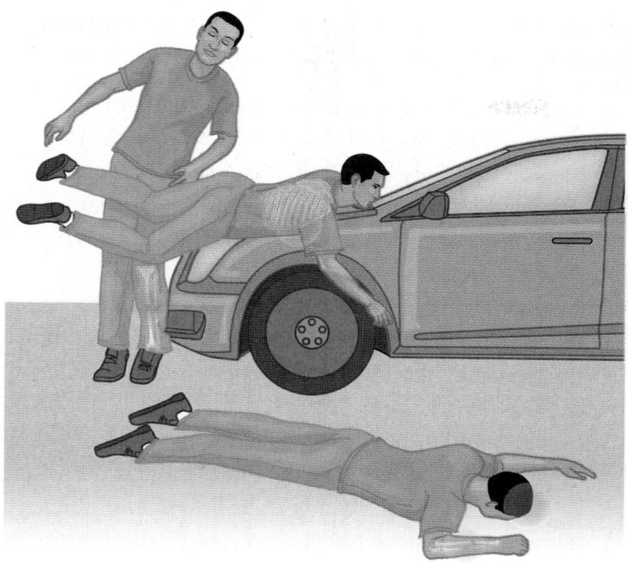

Figure 2-8 *Pedestrian struck by a vehicle.*

anterior impact injuries.[2] The pediatric patient may also be thrown from the vehicle, onto the hood, or slide under the vehicle, incurring a triad of injuries that involve the head, thorax, and lower extremities.[11]

Assault

Interpersonal violence is appreciated across all countries and can result in blunt and/or penetrating injuries. The extent of injuries resulting from assault depends on multiple force factors, including those described in **Table 2-4**.

TABLE 2-4 Assault Force Factors and Results

Force Factor	Result
Amount	The larger the mass, the greater the force.
Distance	Force that travels from a distance is dissipated over that distance.
Object	Which object was used to deliver the force? Was it sharp, dull, large, small, . . . ?
Involved tissue	What is the ability to absorb the force? Consider the difference in the tissue affected, such as the skull versus the abdomen.
Object trajectory	Consider the difference between a boxer who is struck square in the nose versus a boxer who takes a glancing blow as he moves just enough to "roll" with the punch. The direct blow may result in a fractured nose, but the glancing blow may result in only a bruise or contusion.

Penetrating Trauma

Any foreign object that enters through the skin barrier is considered penetrating. This type of injury can involve a victim's internal organs, causing hemodynamic instability (shock) and increased risk for infection.

Penetrating trauma is a notable concern in many countries, with the most common form being assaults from gunshots or stabbings. Risk factors include considerations based on age, race, gender, and geography. The frequency of penetrating trauma from gunshots and stabbings increases significantly with the patient's proximity or access to weapons.[19] For example, blunt abdominal injuries are commonly seen in rural areas, while penetrating injuries are encountered more frequently in urban locations.[14] Approximately 90% of patients with penetrating trauma are male; firearms-related death rates have been reported to be 2 to 7 times greater in the non-Hispanic black male population.[19]

Organs frequently injured during penetrating trauma include the small bowel (50%), large bowel (40%), liver (30%), and intra-abdominal vascular system (25%).[19] The precise damage caused by penetrating mechanisms depends on several variables:

- *Point of impact:* The injury potential of a penetrating object is related to the speed, length of the penetrating object, and point of impact on the body. The density and rigidity of the body, organs, and tissue are significant in terms of determining the amount of energy transfer that occurs with a penetrating injury. The more dense and rigid the receiving area, the more resistance is appreciated, resulting in greater energy transfer and potentially less severe damage.[20]
- *Velocity and speed of impact:* The velocity of the object can be classified by the amount of energy generated. Medium- and high-velocity injuries may result from the use of firearms and explosives. The simplest injury patterns can often be considered the result of low-velocity impacts (e.g., stab wounds). However, this terminology can be misleading. The anatomic area of penetration coupled with the length of the device and angle of bodily entrance of low-velocity mechanisms have the potential to cause significant soft-tissue

injury, as well as damage to vascular structures, nerves, bones, and joints.[20] Although velocity is significant, the speed of the projectile (e.g., bullet) creates high energy transfer.[21] The energy transfer from a projectile is not uniform, as the projectile may ricochet or deform while in transit or upon impact; the point of impact, such as tissue, bone, organs, or protective clothing can also influence the extent of injury.[21]

- *Proximity:* Wounding potential may be influenced by how close an object is to the projectile. Air and objects absorb energy from the projectile while it is in flight, thus slowing its speed. In very close proximity (less than 3 feet), the burning particulate and expanding gases that propel the projectile may also cause injury.[20] While handguns have an effective (lethal) range measured in feet or yards, rifles have an effective range of hundreds to thousands of yards. The longer the barrel of a gun, the more time the expanding gases have to increase bullet acceleration.[20] Therefore, if multiple rounds are ejected, the gun with the shorter barrel (e.g., short-barreled rifle/sawed-off shotgun/handgun) produces a lower-velocity bullet in comparison to a gun with a longer barrel.[20]

CLINICAL PEARL

Velocity and KE Are Positively Correlated with Destruction

KE increases with velocity. Therefore, although velocity is relative, it is the projectile's KE that causes damage by transferring energy to the tissue.

Bullet-Related Considerations

As described earlier in this chapter, in the equation KE $= mv^2/2$, KE is the kinetic energy, m is the projectile mass, and v is the bullet velocity. The velocity is squared, so an increase in velocity has a greater effect on the bullet's energy than an increase in its mass.[22] Bullets travel at their fastest when leaving the muzzle of the firearm, but are then slowed by the effect of drag when they enter the air.[22]

The direction of a bullet is described as its rotational axis, while the deviation is the yaw. The yaw of a bullet is often described as the "wobble" that happens as the bullet is oscillating linearly around the axis of its trajectory.[21-23]

The materials that compose the exterior and interior of the bullet, as well as any modifications made to the bullet, may influence the extent of tissue damage. Characteristics of common bullet types are briefly summarized here[21-23]:

- *Full metal jacket (FMJ)* bullets are made of a dense, heavy metal that covers the bullet from base to tip. They are often seen used in assault rifles, and lose only a small amount of initial velocity as they travel farther from the barrel. The FMJ bullet often penetrates through a target, resulting in minimal tissue deformation on impact. When assessing the patient, the trauma team may notice lead splatter or a snowstorm pattern on radiographic imaging.
- *Soft nose* bullets are non-jacketed. The impact energy of these bullets is designed to expand outward, but at a slower rate than with hollow point bullets. Although soft nose bullets can rapidly disable an individual, they are less likely to penetrate through the body to injure another person.
- *Hollow point* bullets have a hollow cavity in the tip and jacket, and are designed to produce maximal energy transfer upon contact. On impact, the bullet tip is forced backward, flattening and widening, and thereby doubling its surface area. This action is often referred to as an *expanding* round or *mushrooming*. The hollow point bullet design is often seen in law enforcement firearms and in some cases is required in hunting to provide a more humane death for animals.
- *Frangible* bullets are designed to break apart when they impact a surface harder than the bullet. This bullet design disintegrates with rapid energy transfer, dissipating within the target and causing multiple chaotic fragment paths. Scoring a bullet makes it more likely to fragment. These designs can be controversial and were developed for close-quarters defense and law enforcement use.

Cavitation

As indicated by the KE equation, increased velocity of a projectile causes more damage than increased mass; therefore, when a projectile passes through tissue, it transfers its high-pressure KE, creating a cavity (**Figure 2-9**).[24,25] Cavitation may be temporary or permanent.

A temporary cavity is created when a high-pressure object (e.g., bullet) enters the body. As the object decelerates, it transfers its energy to the surrounding tissue. The tissue then accelerates, stretching and displacing outward away from the entering object, creating a vacuum that draws inward air and surface contaminants such as soil, clothing, and skin.[19,24] Although the size of the cavity may diminish, the damage that can occur via cavitation from the crushing, tearing, and shearing forces on the tissue may be significant.

In permanent cavitation, the cavity created by the path of the penetrating object remains, leaving a permanent track and potential loss of tissue.[19,24] Alterations to the body depend on the characteristics of the tissue being affected. For example, the amount of energy transferred may increase with denser tissue.[19,26] Air-filled organs, such as the lungs and stomach, are elastic. Therefore, this type of tissue tolerates high-velocity cavitation relatively well compared to denser tissues. Solid organs, such as the liver, have a greater propensity to shear or tear under the same forces (**Figure 2-10**). If those same energies are instead released inside the cranium, the skull will resist expansion, augmenting soft-tissue crushing until the tensile strength of the bone is exceeded and an explosive release of pressure results.[26]

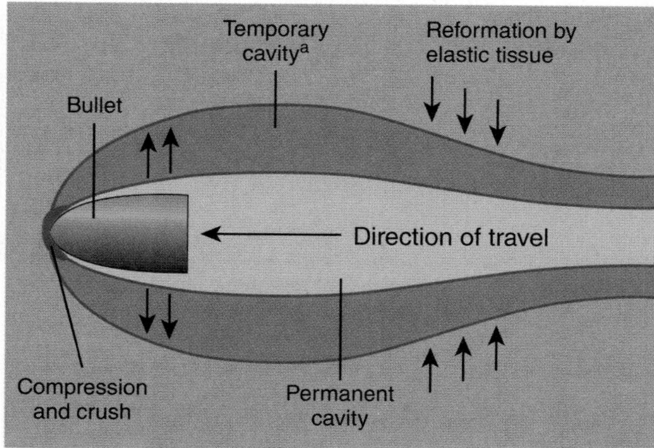

Figure 2-9 *Cavitation caused by a bullet.*

[a] Rigid inelastic organs are more vulnerable to injury.

Reproduced from Imraan Sardiwalla, I., Govender, M., Matsevych, O., & Zacharia Koto, M. (2016). Indirect ballistic injury to the liver: Case report and review of literature. *International Journal of Surgery Open, 5*, 23-26. Retrieved from https://www.sciencedirect.com/science/article/pii/S240585721630050X.

CLINICAL PEARL 

Cavitation can also be seen when an unrestrained driver hits a steering wheel. As the chest pushes inward from the resistance of the steering wheel, a temporary cavity is created.

Thermal Trauma

Chapter 11 discusses the impacts and injuries associated with thermal trauma.

Blast Trauma

Although most commonly associated with the military, blast injuries can strike anywhere. They have occurred in industrial settings, mining industries, shipping industries, and chemical plants. Most recently, blasts have been associated with terrorist attacks. Approximately 53% of the terrorist attacks that occurred in the United States between 2001 and 2011 involved bombs.[27] An explosion

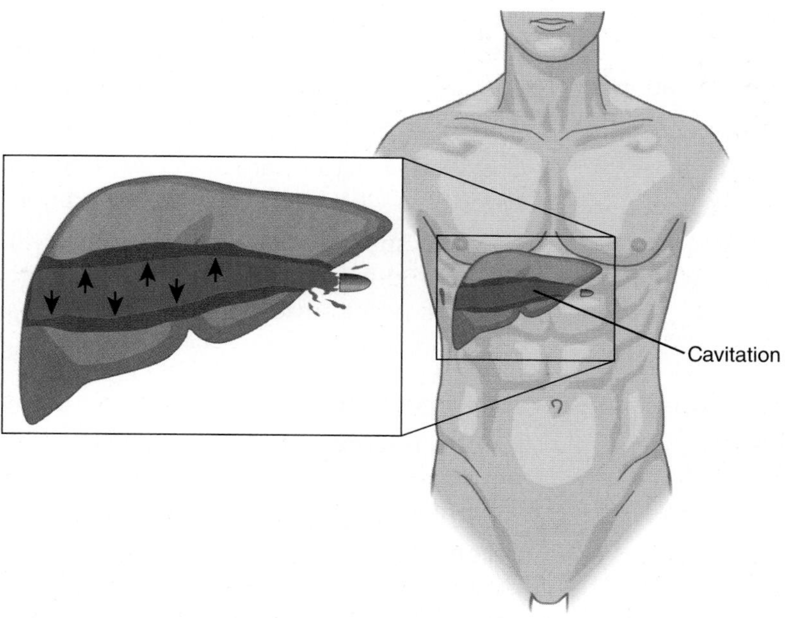

Figure 2-10 *Traumatic cavitation of the liver.*

occurs when energy, in the form of light, heat, and sound, is released rapidly. The blast pressure expands outward in all directions at a rate greater than the speed of sound (**Figure 2-11**).[28,29]

The U.S. Department of Defense classifies blast injuries into five levels.[8] The effects of an explosion on the human body are numerous, as outlined in **Table 2-5**. These injuries can result from a combination of blunt or penetrating trauma and include possible exposure to chemical, thermal, physical, and radioactive agents.

Identifying the space in which an explosion happens can be helpful for the trauma care provider. When a blast occurs within an enclosed space, the release of energy is contained. If an individual is located within the confined

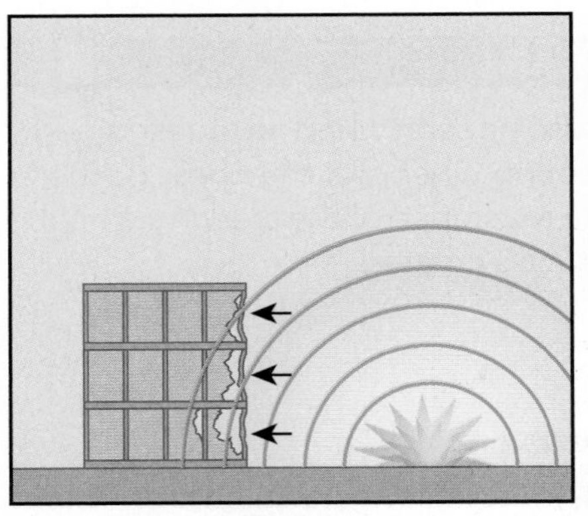

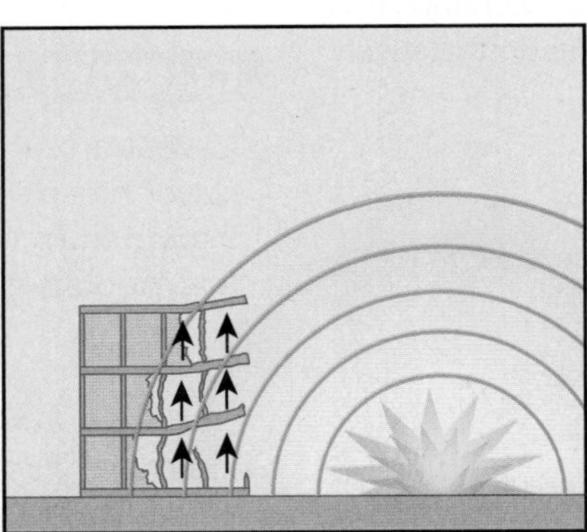

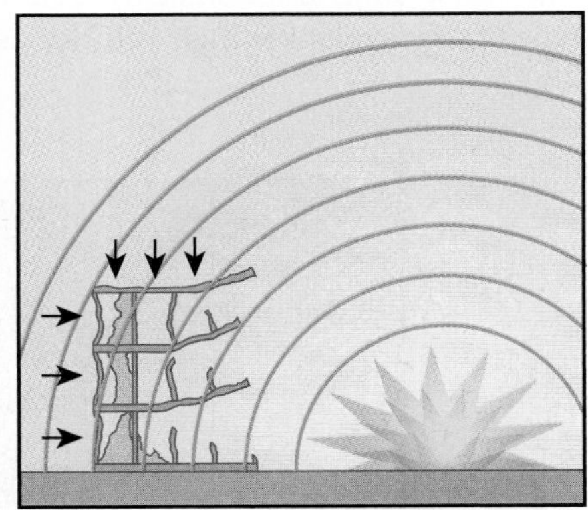

Figure 2-11 *Blast pressure effects on a structure.*

Reproduced from Federal Emergency Management Agency. (2003). Explosive blast. In *Reference manual to mitigate potential terrorist attacks against buildings* (pp. 4-1-4-20). Retrieved from https://www.fema.gov/media-library-data/20130726-1455-20490-6222/fema426.pdf.

TABLE 2-5 Effects of Explosions on the Human Body

Effects	Impact	Mechanism of Injury	Types of Injuries
Primary	Direct blast effects (over- and under-pressurization)	› Direct tissue damage from the blast over-pressure › Interaction of blast effect with body › Gas-filled structures are at high risk › Complex stress and shear waves produce injury or body dismemberment and dissemination	Blast lung (pulmonary barotrauma) Tympanic membrane rupture and middle ear damage Abdominal hemorrhage and perforation Globe (eye) rupture Mild traumatic brain injury (TBI; TBI without physical signs of head injury)
Secondary	Projectiles propelled by explosion	Wounds produced by: › Primary fragments from exploding weapon and shrapnel › Secondary fragments: projectiles from the environment (e.g., debris, vehicular metal)	Penetrating ballistic (fragmentation) or blunt injuries Eye penetration (can be occult) Closed and open brain injury

Effects	Impact	Mechanism of Injury	Types of Injuries
Tertiary	Results from individuals being thrown by the blast wind (propulsion of body onto a hard surface or object)	Displacement of body and structural collapse	Whole or partial body translocation from being thrown against a hard surface: › Blunt/penetrating trauma › Fractures › Traumatic amputations › Closed and open brain injury
Quaternary	All explosion-related injuries, illnesses, or diseases not due to primary, secondary, or tertiary mechanisms (heat and or combustion fumes)	› Burns and toxic injuries from fuel › Metals › Septic syndromes from soil and environmental contamination	All other injuries associated with the blast: › External and internal burns › Crush injuries › Asthma, chronic obstructive pulmonary disease, or other breathing problems from dust, smoke, or toxic fumes › Angina › Hyperglycemia, hypertension
Quinary	Associated with exposure to hazardous materials from radioactive, biologic, or chemical components of a blast (e.g., dirty bomb)	Contamination of tissues from: › Bacteria › Radiation › Chemical agents › Contaminated tissue from bystander or assailant	Variety of health effects depending on the agent

U.S. Department of Defense. (2019, Jun 18). What is blast injury? Blast Injury 101. Retrieved from https://blastinjuryresearch.amedd.army.mil/index.cfm/blast_injury_101; Jorolemon, M. R., & Krywko, D. M. (2019, Jun 22). Blast injuries. StatPearls. Retrieved from https://www.ncbi.nlm.nih.gov/books/NBK430914/

space during an explosion, the resulting injuries may be increased due to the expanded pressure being transferred to the victim.[8,12,28] Suspect the possibility of internal hemorrhage and have a greater concern for fractures when there is evidence of penetrating injuries.[8] It is not uncommon for explosion victims to have a combination of injuries including those involving multiple penetrating and blunt mechanisms; **Table 2-6** provides an overview of injuries commonly associated with explosions.[30]

CLINICAL PEARL 

The explosion that occurs in an enclosed space has an increase in pressure relative to the explosion that occurs in an open environment. The increased pressure compounds the blast effects, and potentially increases internal and external injury severity.

Emerging Trends

In an effort to decrease collision morbidity and mortality, several automotive safety features have been developed. Automotive safety initiatives such as automatic steering, parking, and antilock braking systems have been introduced as well as driving sensors that detect objects located within blind spots and speed limit and lane parameters.[31,32] The inclusion of side-impact air bags as well as decreased air bag deployment time have been implemented in an effort to reduce injuries to vehicle drivers and passengers.[31,32]

However, despite all the automotive advancements, the distracted driver remains an important factor with regard to occupant safety. Technology has improved our electronic devices such as our smartphones and navigational systems. The urge to use them while driving has been reported to be 2 to 3 times greater in individuals younger than the age of 25.[33] The U.S. Department of Transportation's National Highway Traffic Safety Administration (NHTSA) estimates that there are more than

TABLE 2-6 Overview of Explosion-Related Injuries

System	Injury or Condition	System	Injury or Condition
Auditory	Cochlear damage Ossicular disruption Foreign body Tympanic membrane rupture	Circulatory	Blunt cardiac injury Myocardial infarction from air embolism Air embolism–induced injury Shock Vasovagal hypotension Peripheral vascular injury
Eye, orbit, face	Perforated globe Foreign body Fractures Air embolism	Central nervous system	Concussion Spinal cord injury Closed and open brain injury Air embolism–induced injury Stroke
Respiratory	Blast lung Hemothorax Pneumothorax Pulmonary contusion	Renal	Renal contusion Hypotension Laceration Hypovolemia Acute kidney injury due to rhabdomyolysis
Digestive	Bowel perforation Hemorrhage Mesenteric ischemia from air embolism Ruptured liver or spleen	Extremity	Traumatic amputation Lacerations Fractures Crush Acute arterial occlusion Compartment syndrome Air embolism–induced injury Burns

Data from Centers for Disease Control and Prevention. (2009). Blast injuries: Essential facts. Retrieved from https://cdn.ymaws.com/www.amtrauma.org/resource/resmgr/TIIDE/Blast_InjuryEssential_Facts.pdf.

3,000 deaths and approximately 400,000 injuries annually from distracted driving.[33] Other forms of vehicular distraction may include verbal conversation, eating while driving, applying makeup, and being lost in thought. The NHTSA is working toward decreasing the distraction associated with use of electronic devices while driving. Its initiatives include collaboration with the automotive industries to develop hands-free (e.g., Bluetooth) technology in vehicles, as well as laws and restrictions to reduce the use of these technologies while driving.[33]

The motorcycle industry has also experienced advancement in safety devices. One notable change involves improvements in motorcycle helmets. Modern helmets have replaced the older, softer materials such as leather, with improved designs using several layers of foam covered in plastic or fiberglass to protect the head against impact.[34] Despite the lack of global acceptance for requiring helmet use for all riders, helmet laws have been implemented by some U.S. state legislatures.[34]

Recreational equipment has also experienced improvements related to user safety. The multidirectional impact protection system (MIPS) has improved head safety by using a slip plane inside the bicycle helmet. If a collision occurs, this helmet design dissipates energy from the impacting surface away from the head, potentially reducing the severity of a head/brain injury.[35]

Summary

Trauma can be the result of a variety of forces, such as blunt, penetrating, thermal, or blast forces. Energy remains in a potential state until a force acts upon it, turning it into KE. Trauma care providers must function as energy detectives, identifying where the stored energy, now put into motion, has been transferred to anticipate a patient's physiological condition and needs.

The extent of injury can be affected by multiple factors, including the type and amount of force, the object and its distance traveled, and the point of impact and velocity. Cavitation can occur with high-pressure forces; the ensuing changes to the body depend on the characteristics of the tissue being impacted. Depending on the body cavity affected, cavitation may damage hemodynamic stability. The materials that compose the exterior and interior of a projectile determine the extent of tissue damage on impact. Blast injuries can be the result of a direct or indirect exposure to an explosion. Being located in a confined space can also increase the likelihood of injury severity.

Understanding the kinematic concepts associated with the MOI and energy transfer can assist the prepared trauma provider in evaluating and anticipating damage. The ability to predict potential injury and provide early intervention with assessment improves patient survival rates.

As individual awareness and knowledge expand, safety improvements are also anticipated to advance. When an innovation for improved personal safety is developed, there is a human element to consider with its compliance usage: If the technology is present, will the individual actually utilize the safety knowledge and/or device as intended? A trauma care provider has the responsibility to provide required, up-to-date education and guidance on the importance of safety, usage of devices designed to maintain personal and dependent care, and the consequences that may occur if these devices are not utilized.

References

1. *Webster's Dictionary.* (2018). Definition of trauma. Retrieved from https://www.merriam-webster.com/dictionary/trauma
2. National Association of Emergency Medical Technicians, & American College of Surgeons, Committee on Trauma. (2016). Kinematics of trauma. In *Prehospital trauma life support* (8th ed., pp. 70–111). Burlington, MA: Jones & Bartlett Learning.
3. Dictionary.com (n.d.). Biomechanics. Retrieved from https://www.dictionary.com
4. Dictionary.com (n.d.). Kinematics. Retrieved from https://www.dictionary.com
5. Marr, A. B., Stuke, L. E., & Greiffenstein, P. (2017). Kinematics. In E. E. Moore, D. V. Feliciano, & K. L. Mattox (Eds.), *Trauma* (8th ed.). [Kindle version].
6. Newton, I. (1995). *The principia.* Amherst, NY: Prometheus Books.
7. Weigelt, J., Brasel, K. J., & Klein, J. (2009). Mechanism of injury. In K. A. McQuillan, M. Makic, M. B. Flynn, & E. Whalen (Eds.), *Trauma nursing: From resuscitation through rehabilitation* (4th ed., pp. 178–199). St. Louis, MO: Saunders/Elsevier.
8. Federal Emergency Management Agency. (2014). *Medical preparedness for response and bombing incidents: User manual.* College Station, TX: Texas A&M Engineering Extension Service & New Mexico Institute of Mining and Technology.
9. Creel, J. H., Jr. (2016). Scene size up. In J. E. Campbell, R. L. Alson, & American College of Emergency Physicians Alabama Chapter (Eds.), *International trauma life support for emergency care providers* (8th ed., pp. 2–27). Essex, UK: Pearson Education.
10. National Safety Council. (2017). Injury facts. Retrieved from http://viewer.zmags.com/publication/20020222#/20020222/1
11. Wolfe, A. (2014). Biomechanics, kinematics, and mechanisms of injury. In D. Gurney (Ed.), *Trauma nursing core course: Provider manual* (7th ed., pp. 25–37). Des Plains, IL: Emergency Nurses Association.
12. American Academy of Osteopathic Surgeons. (2018). Trauma systems and mechanisms of injury. In A. N. Pollak (Ed.), *Nancy Caroline's emergency care in the street* (8th ed.). Burlington, MA: Jones & Bartlett Learning. [Kindle version].
13. Centers for Disease Control and Prevention. (2012). Guidelines for field triage of injured patients: Recommendations of the National Expert Panel on Field Triage, 2011. *Morbidity and Mortality Weekly Report, 61*(1), 1–21. Retrieved from https://www.cdc.gov/mmwr/pdf/rr/rr6101.pdf
14. Gad, M. A., Saber, A., Farrag, S., Shams, M. E., & Ellabban, G. M. (2012). Incidence, patterns, and factors predicting mortality of abdominal injuries in trauma patients. *North American Journal of Medical Sciences, 4*(3), 129–134. https://doi.org/10.4103%2F1947-2714.93889
15. National Highway Traffic Safety Administration. (2016). NHTSA in action: Air bags. Retrieved from https://www.nhtsa.gov/equipment/air-bags
16. Riley, P. O., Arregui-Dalmases, C., Purtserov, S., Parent, D., Lessley, D. J., Shaw, G., . . . Yasuki, T. (2012). Kinematics of the unrestrained vehicle occupants in side-impact crashes. *Traffic Injury Prevention, 13*(2), 163–171. https://doi.org/10.1080/15389588.2011.637251
17. Insurance Institute for Highway Safety. (2018). Rollover crashes. Retrieved from https://www.iihs.org/iihs/topics/t/rollover-crashes/topicoverview
18. DaCorte, J. (2010). *Motorcycle safety and crashes.* New York, NY: Nova Science Publishers.
19. Bhimji, S. S., & Burns, B. (2017). Penetrating abdominal trauma. Retrieved from https://www.ncbi.nlm.nih.gov/books/NBK459123/
20. Rosen, N., & Dudkiewicz, I. (2011). Wound ballistics and tissue damage. In A. Lerner & M. Soudry (Eds.), *Armed conflict injuries to the extremity: A treatment manual* (pp. 21–33). Heidelberg, Germany: Springer.

21. Nessen, S. C., Lounsbury, D. E., & Hetz, S. (2008). *Forward to resuscitative surgery: An introduction to poly trauma in war surgery in Afghanistan and Iraq: A series of cases, 2003–2007.* Washington, DC: Office of the Surgeon General.
22. Penn-Barwell, J. G., & Helliker, A. E. (2017). Firearms and bullets. In J. Breeze, J. G. Penn-Barwell, D. Keene, D. O'Reilly, J. Jeyanathan, & P. Mahoney (Eds.), *Ballistic trauma: A practical guide* (4th ed., pp. 7–20). Cham, Switzerland: Springer.
23. Stefanopoulos, P. K., Hadjigeorgiou, G. F., Filippakis, K., & Gyftokstas, D. (2014). Gunshot wounds: A review of ballistics related to penetrating trauma. *Journal of Acute Disease, 3*(3), 178–185. https://doi.org/10.1016/S2221-6189(14)60041-X
24. Penn-Barwell, J. G., & Stevenson, T. (2017). The effect of projectiles on tissue. In J. Breeze, J. G. Penn-Barwell, D. Keene, D. O'Reilly, J. Jeyanathan, & P. Mahoney (Eds.), *Ballistic trauma: A practical guide* (4th ed., pp. 35–46). Cham, Switzerland: Springer.
25. Imraan Sardiwalla, I., Govender, M., Matsevych, O., & Zacharia Koto, M. (2016). Indirect ballistic injury to the liver: Case report and review of literature. *International Journal of Surgery Open, 5*, 23–26. Retrieved from https://www.sciencedirect.com/science/article/pii/S240585721630050X
26. Burr, D. B. (2011). Why bones bend but don't break. *Journal of Musculoskeletal & Neuronal Interactions, 11*(4), 270–285. Retrieved from http://www.ismni.org/jmni/pdf/46/01BURR.pdf
27. Rogers, S. (2013). Four decades of US terror attacks listed and detailed. *The Guardian.* Retrieved from https://www.theguardian.com/news/datablog/2013/apr/17/four-decades-us-terror-attacks-listed-since-1970
28. Cartwright, C., Wells, I., Cartwright, J., & Paler, M. C. (2013). Explosions and blast injuries. *Emergency Medical Paramedic.* Retrieved from http://www.emergencymedicalparamedic.com/explosions-and-blast-injuries/
29. Federal Emergency Management Agency. (2003). Explosive blast. In *Reference manual to mitigate potential terrorist attacks against buildings* (pp. 4-1–4-20). Retrieved from https://www.fema.gov/media-library-data/20130726-1455-20490-6222/fema426.pdf
30. Centers for Disease Control and Prevention. (2009). Blast injuries: Essential facts. Retrieved from https://cdn.ymaws.com/www.amtrauma.org/resource/resmgr/TIIDE/Blast_InjuryEssential_Facts.pdf
31. Crash Test. (2018). Vehicle safety and accident prevention. Retrieved from https://www.crashtest.org/
32. Cars Direct. (2012). 10 car safety features. Retrieved from https://www.carsdirect.com/car-safety/5-name-brand-car-safety-features
33. Vegega, M., Jones, B., & Monk, C. (2013). Understanding the effects of distracted driving and developing strategies to reduce resulting deaths and injuries: A report to Congress. Retrieved from https://www.nhtsa.gov/sites/nhtsa.dot.gov/files/understandingeffectsdistractdriving.pdf
34. Robb, T., & Miglietta, M. (2017). Bicycle and motorcycle helmets. Retrieved from https://www.emedicinehealth.com/bicycle_and_motorcycle_helmets/article_em.htm#effectiveness_of_helmets
35. Bell Powersports and Cycling. (2018). Comprehensive protection: Introducing MIPS technology. Retrieved from https://www.bellhelmets.com/mips/

Design credits: Clipboard designed by Vectors Market from Flaticon.

CHAPTER 3

Initial Assessment

Robin S. Powers-Jarvis, PhD, RNC, CEN, CCRN, TCRN, CPEN

OBJECTIVES

Upon completion of this chapter, the learner will be able to:

1. Recognize that the initial assessment process is the foundation of trauma nursing practice.
2. Demonstrate the components of the initial assessment process.
3. Differentiate between the goals of the primary and secondary surveys.
4. Determine actual and potential threats to life and limb using the initial assessment process.
5. Select interventions to manage life-threatening conditions identified during the initial assessment process.

Introduction

The approach to trauma patient care requires a process to identify and treat or stabilize life-threatening injuries in an efficient and timely manner. Time is critical, so an approach that is systematic, yet easy to learn and implement, is most effective. This process is labeled *initial assessment*.

For clarity and ease of flow, initial assessment is divided into the following process points[1]:

- Preparation and triage
- Primary survey (ABCDE) with corresponding interventions as required (FG)
- Reevaluation (consideration of transfer/need for higher level of care)
- Secondary survey (HI) with corresponding interventions as required
- Reevaluation and post-resuscitation care (J)
- Definitive care or transfer to an appropriate trauma center

The A–J mnemonic helps the trauma nurse rapidly assess for and intervene in life-threatening injuries and identify all injuries in a systematic manner; it is the basis for the trauma nursing process (TNP). The steps of the mnemonic are as follows:

- **A:** Across the room assessment for uncontrolled hemorrhage, Airway and Alertness with simultaneous cervical spinal stabilization
- **B:** Breathing and ventilation

- **C:** Circulation and Control of hemorrhage
- **D:** Disability (neurologic status)
- **E:** Exposure and Environmental control
- **F:** Full set of vital signs and Family presence[2]
- **G:** Get monitoring devices and Give comfort (using mnemonic LMNOP):
    - **L:** Laboratory studies (including arterial blood gases [ABGs] and serum lactate) and obtain a specimen for blood type and cross-match
    - **M:** Monitor for continuous cardiac rhythm and rate assessment
    - **N:** Nasogastric or orogastric tube consideration
    - **O:** Oxygenation and ventilation analysis: consider weaning oxygen based on pulse oximetry, end-tidal carbon dioxide ($ETCO_2$) monitoring or capnography for intubated or sedated patients
    - **P:** Pain assessment and management
- **H:** History and Head-to-toe assessment
- **I:** Inspect posterior surfaces
- **J:** Just keep reevaluating—A, B, C, D, E, F, G, H, and I

NOTE

Who Does the Initial Assessment?

We recognize that the initial assessor may be more commonly physicians, advanced practice nurses, or a team of healthcare providers in many settings. However, it is important for all trauma nurses to be competent in performing the initial assessment so that they can anticipate the next steps in care and function more efficiently as members of the trauma team. Additionally, the trauma nurse may not have access to other team members during transfer of patients to other departments within the hospital or transport to another facility. If working in a remote location, it is also important for the trauma nurse to have established the nurse's own baseline assessment to facilitate recognition of changes in patient status, if and when they occur.

Preparation and Triage

Initial assessment starts with preparation and triage.

Preparation

The approach to trauma care typically begins with notification that a trauma patient is or will soon be arriving in the emergency department (ED). Whether notification is from prehospital providers or the triage nurse, it is the trauma nurse's responsibility to prepare to receive that patient.

Safe Practice, Safe Care

When preparing to receive a trauma patient in the ED, keep the following tenet in mind: Safe practice, safe care.

Safe practice means taking into consideration the protection of the team, including the following:

- Observing universal precautions for every patient
- Donning personal protective equipment, such as gown, gloves, mask, and other equipment as necessary, prior to the patient's arrival

Safe practice also includes consideration of any potential patient exposure to hazardous material that may put the trauma team, other patients, and the ED and hospital at risk. Some patients may require decontamination before entering the trauma resuscitation room. See Chapter 18, "Disaster Management," for additional information.

Safe care means assuring the patient gets to the *right* hospital in the *right* amount of time for the *right* care. The trauma triage criteria developed by the American College of Surgeons Committee on Trauma (ACS-COT) serve as the international standard for identifying the trauma patient who would benefit from resuscitation and care at *the right trauma facility* with the appropriate resources. However, it is important to note that the ACS-COT trauma triage criteria are not particularly sensitive to critical injuries, especially in young children and older adults.[3] The trauma nurse calls for trauma team activation as indicated. See Chapter 1, "Trauma Nursing and Teamwork" for additional information.

The *right time* has long been referred to as the "golden hour"; however, patients presenting with some serious injuries will not survive an hour for definitive treatment. Timely, effective, and efficient interventions facilitate improved outcomes for trauma patients.[1] Prehospital providers play a key role in the survival of the trauma patient. Optimal outcomes result when time in the field is minimized and care is focused on airway maintenance, control of hemorrhage, and spinal motion restriction when necessary.[4] Field triage is key to the appropriate use of community resources, with the most severely injured patients being transported directly to the highest level of trauma care available in the community (**Figure 3-1**).[4,5]

The *right resources* to care for the trauma patient are outlined by the ACS-COT and include the right place where essential trauma team members are available during activation, an appropriate skill mix is represented, necessary equipment is on hand in the trauma room, appropriate

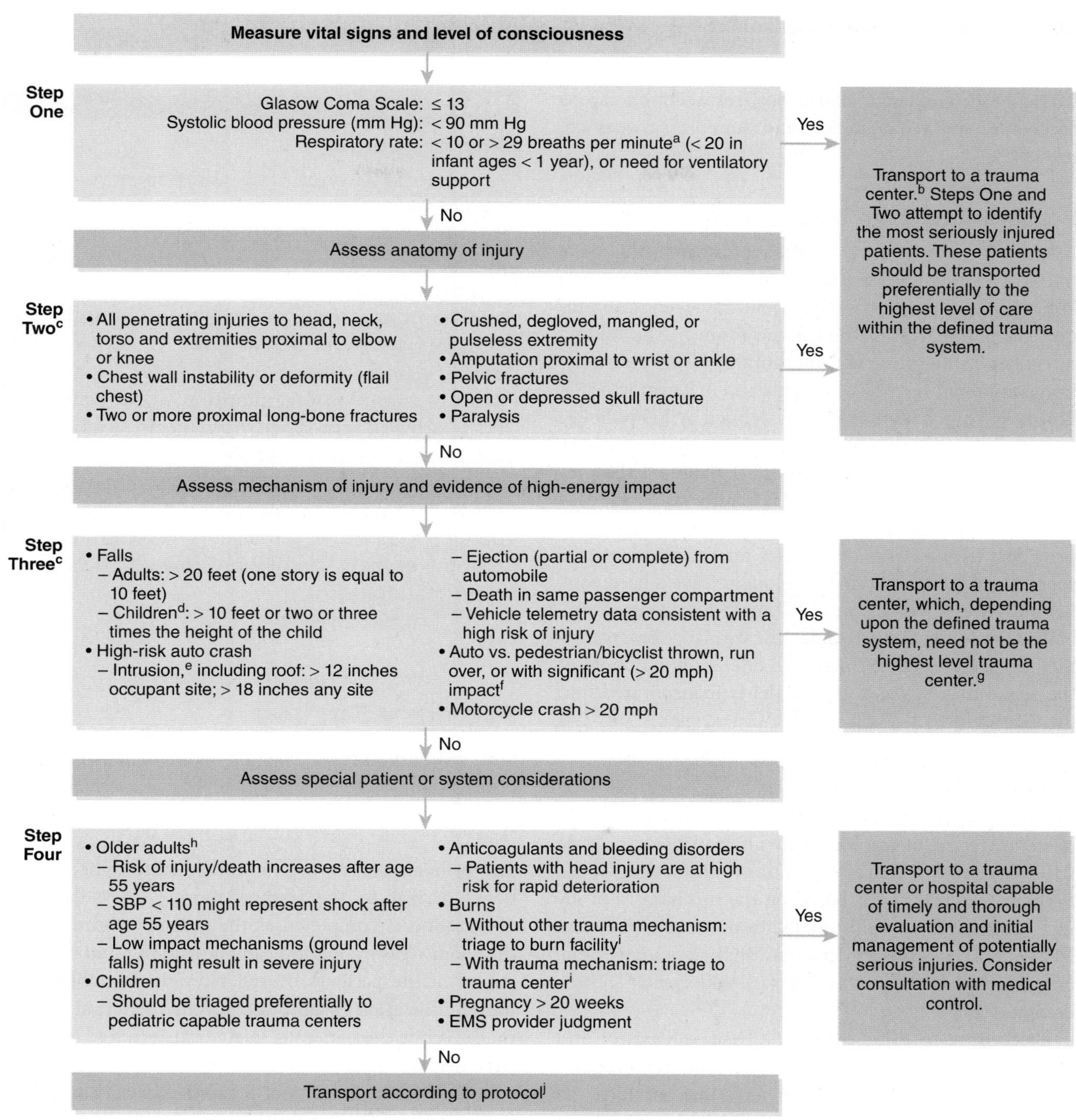

When in doubt, transport to a trauma center

Figure 3-1 *Guidelines for field triage of injured patients.*

Abbreviations: EMS, emergency medical services; SBP, systolic blood pressure.

[a] The upper limit of respiratory rate in infants is more than 29 breaths per minute to maintain a higher level of overtriage for infants.

[b] Trauma centers are designated as Levels I through IV. A Level I center has the greatest amount of resources and personnel for care of the injured patient and provides regional leadership in education, research, and prevention programs. A Level II facility offers similar resources to a Level I facility, possibly differing only in continuous availability of certain subspecialties or sufficient prevention, education, and research activities for Level I designation; Level II facilities are not required to be resident or fellow education centers. A Level III center is capable of assessment, resuscitation, and emergency surgery, with severely injured patients being transferred to a Level I or II facility. A Level IV trauma center is capable of providing 24-hour physician coverage, resuscitation, and stabilization to injured patients before transfer to a facility that provides a higher level of trauma care.

[c] Any injury noted in Step Two or mechanism identified in Step Three triggers a "yes" response.

[d] Age less than 15 years.

[e] Intrusion refers to interior compartment intrusion; deformation refers to exterior damage.

[f] Includes pedestrians or bicyclists thrown or run over by a motor vehicle or those with estimated impact greater than 20 miles per hour with a motor vehicle.

[g] Local or regional protocols should be used to determine the most appropriate level of trauma center within the defined trauma system; it need not be the highest-level trauma center.

[h] Age greater than 55 years.

[i] Patients with both burns and concomitant trauma for whom the burn injury poses the greatest risk for morbidity and mortality should be transferred to a burn center. If the nonburn trauma presents a greater immediate risk, the patient may be stabilized in a trauma center and then transferred to a burn center.

[j] Patients who do not meet any of the triage criteria in Steps One through Four should be transported to the most appropriate medical facility as outlined in local EMS protocols.

Reproduced from Sasser, S. M., Hunt, R. C., Faul, M., Sugerman, D., Pearson, W., Dulski, T., . . . Galli, R. L. (2012). Guidelines for field triage of injured patients: Recommendations of the National Expert Panel on Field Triage, 2011. *MMWR Recommendations and Reports, 61*(RR-1), 1–20. Atlanta, GA: Centers for Disease Control and Prevention. Retrieved from https://www.cdc.gov/mmwr/preview/mmwrhtml/rr6101a1.htm.

surgical care is offered, skilled post-resuscitation care is accessible, and rehabilitation and support services are present.[1]

Preparation in the Trauma Room

Information from the prehospital report can facilitate the initial assessment process and enable the trauma team to anticipate and prepare for interventions likely to be required upon arrival in the trauma room.[1,4] The trauma nurse begins by preparing the room to assure resuscitation equipment is readily available and in working order. This is done on a regular basis as defined by ED policy—minimally at the beginning of the shift and as necessary after each use of the trauma room. Document the prehospital report in a location that is readily visible for easy review by all trauma team members. Many prehospital providers use electronic templates for their patient care reports and, as a result, may no longer leave a hard copy behind. These "perishable data" must be captured verbally by the team to help guide the care given. Emergency medical services (EMS) may also offer a digital photo of the scene that, whenever possible, is incorporated into the record.

Triage

Triage involves the sorting of patients based on their need for treatment and the resources available to provide that treatment.[1] Triage also pertains to the sorting of patients in the field and is based on the mechanism of injury (MOI; head-on collision, fall from more than 20 feet in an adult), physiologic criteria (vital signs), anatomic criteria (flail chest, fractured pelvis), and special considerations (age) (Figure 3-1).[1,5]

According to the Centers for Disease Control and Prevention (CDC) triage criteria, patients who require the highest level of trauma team activation and have the greatest degree of injury will present with physiologic derangements. The next most serious group will be those who present with obvious or suspected anatomic injuries but are relatively hemodynamically stable upon initial assessment. The third group consists of patients who present after sustaining a worrisome MOI where there is suspicion of a high energy transfer that was sustained by the patient. The last group comprises members of special populations who are at increased risk of sustaining injury.[5]

Whether patients present via the EMS system or on their own, the priorities for the identification of life-threatening injuries are guided by the primary survey (ABCDE).

NOTE

Primary Survey

An important tenet of the primary survey portion of the initial assessment is that if any component of the airway, breathing, and circulation is compromised or *absent*, the immediate treatment plan is to *provide* it for the patient—for example, absent airway, insert oropharyngeal airway, endotracheal tube, or some other airway device; absent or ineffective breathing, provide bag-mask ventilations; absent circulation, provide chest compressions; ineffective circulation, identify and treat the cause. Efforts are made to *support and maintain* the primary survey components—for example, airway, assess patency/gag reflex; breathing, provide supplemental oxygen; circulation, provide balanced resuscitation.

Primary Survey

The primary survey begins with across-the-room observation.

Across-the-Room Observation

The primary survey begins immediately upon the patient's arrival to the trauma room. Across-the-room observation is completed as the patient is brought into the room. This evaluation can allow for a rapid determination of the patient's overall physiologic stability and the identification of any uncontrolled external hemorrhage. While the patient is safely transferred to a trauma stretcher, the team is given an update on the patient's condition from prehospital personnel or accompanying family or friends. During the primary survey, the main goal is to immediately identify all life-threatening conditions that can cause death within the first few minutes of presentation. These conditions *must* be treated upon discovery and as such are identified and immediately corrected.[1]

For teaching purposes, the steps in this chapter are presented sequentially in a linear order of importance. In reality, the trauma team will complete the components of assessment and interventions simultaneously as team members function together to accomplish these tasks. The trauma nurse chooses the appropriate examination elements of inspection, auscultation, and palpation for assessment.

NOTE

Uncontrolled Hemorrhage

Uncontrolled hemorrhage is the major cause of preventable death after injury.[1,6,7] If uncontrolled external hemorrhage is noted during the across-the-room observation or as the patient is being transferred to the trauma room stretcher, in some environments, under some circumstances, the priorities may be reordered to <C>ABC. Historically, the standard approach for emergency or trauma care and advanced life support programs has been ABC(D). However, practitioners in the military, through evidence and experience, found that external peripheral hemorrhage is the leading cause of combat casualty death.[5,6] The use of a "bleeding control bundle" can decrease trauma morbidity and mortality.[8] The U.K. military has now replaced ABC with <C>ABC, where <C> signifies catastrophic hemorrhage.[9] Tactical Combat Casualty Care from the U.S. Department of Defense teaches the mnemonic MARCH.[10]

NOTE

The MARCH Mnemonic

The MARCH mnemonic is defined as follows:

- Massive hemorrhage: Control life-threatening bleeding with the use of tourniquet(s); Combat Gauze, Celox Gauze, or Chito Gauze; and replacement of blood loss with whole blood or a 1:1:1 ratio of plasma, red blood cells and platelets to achieve a systolic blood pressure of 80 to 90 mm Hg as soon as possible.
- Airway: Establish and maintain a patent airway.
- Respiration: Decompress suspected tension pneumothorax, seal open chest wounds, and support ventilation and oxygenation as required.
- Circulation: Provide vascular access (intravenous [IV] or intraosseous [IO]) and administer fluids as required to treat shock.
- Head injury/Hypothermia: Prevent or treat hypotension and hypoxia to prevent worsening of traumatic brain injury and prevent or treat hypothermia.

Since civilian trauma care has been guided by military battlefield evidence and practice, present-day civilian trauma care guidelines may, under some circumstances, recommend the <C>ABC approach to trauma care. However, the current civilian approach to trauma resuscitation involves multiple trauma team members, enabling several priorities to be addressed simultaneously, mitigating the need to reprioritize. The first priority remains to *treat the condition posing the greatest threat to life first*.[1,6-11]

NOTE

Assessment: Double-Starred Criteria

The double-starred assessment criteria include the following:

- Alertness
- Airway
- Breathing and ventilation
- Circulation and control of hemorrhage
- Disability (neurologic status)
- Exposure and environmental control

A–E Steps in the Primary Survey

The steps in the primary survey begin with assessing the airway and alertness.

A: Airway and Alertness (with Simultaneous Cervical Spine Protection)

Across-the-room observation also includes assessing the patient's airway and alertness.

Cervical Spinal Stabilization

A cervical spinal injury (CSI) must be suspected in any patient with multisystem trauma, until the patient has a Glasgow Coma Scale (GCS) score of 15 and has been fully evaluated for CSI by an experienced provider or has been cleared of spinal injury via radiography or computed tomography (CT).[12] This is even more critical in the older adult with blunt trauma, as recent studies have indicated that using the National Emergency X-Radiography Utilization Study (NEXUS) criteria may not be sufficient to exclude cervical spine fracture in these patients.[11-13] While in the ED, alignment and protection of the cervical spine can be accomplished by either of the following techniques:

- Manual stabilization: Two hands holding the patient's head and neck in alignment
- Spinal motion restriction: A correctly sized, semi-rigid cervical collar securely fastened

The spine board is primarily a prehospital transportation device; therefore, the patient is removed from the spine board as soon as possible, with the team maintaining cervical spine stabilization during spine board removal and continuing spinal motion restriction with the use of a semi-rigid cervical collar until cervical spine injury has been definitively ruled out. After removing the spine board, consider using a slide board under the patient to facilitate subsequent patient movement from the stretcher.

All spinal motion restriction and transfer devices are removed at the earliest appropriate time. Take extreme care when removing a helmet from patients who have a potentially unstable CSI. Helmet removal requires a coordinated effort by two people, in which one person maintains manual inline stabilization of the patient's head and neck while a second person removes the helmet.[1,11]

During the entire initial assessment and identified required interventions, protection of the cervical spine as described in this section is essential.

Assessment of Alertness

Assessment of alertness is a "double-starred criterion" in the TNP. If an issue with the patient's alertness is identified, it must be appropriately addressed before proceeding to full assessment of the airway. Assessment of alertness will also help in the evaluation of the patient's ability to protect their own airway.

The mnemonic AVPU can help the nurse quickly assess for the patient's level of alertness. Its use at the beginning of the initial assessment can be an important determinant to assist the nurse in selecting the appropriate airway intervention. The components of AVPU are as follows:

- **A:** Alert. If the patient is alert, they will be able to maintain their airway once it is clear. If the patient is alert and interactive, there is no need to proceed beyond this point. If the patient is not alert, go to the V component of the mnemonic.
- **V:** Patient responds to Verbal stimuli. If the patient needs verbal stimulation to respond, an airway adjunct may be needed to keep the tongue from obstructing the airway. If the patient does not respond to voice, proceed to the P component.
- **P:** Patient responds to Pain. Pinching the axillary fold is an effective and minimally obtrusive way to elicit a response to pain. If the patient responds only to pain, they may not be able to maintain their airway, and an airway adjunct may need to be placed while further assessment is made to determine the need for a definitive airway (intubation). If the patient does not respond to pain, proceed to the U component.
- **U:** Patient is Unresponsive. If the patient is unresponsive, announce it loudly to the team and direct someone to *check whether the patient is pulseless* while assessing if the cause of the problem is the airway or something depressing respiratory function in the brain. Consider reprioritizing the assessment priority to <C>ABC.[1,6,14]

> **NOTE**
>
> **AVPU: Assessing Alertness**
>
> **A:** Alert and oriented
> **V:** Responds to verbal stimuli
> **P:** Responds only to painful stimuli
> **U:** Unresponsive

Assessment of Airway: Inspect, Auscultate, and Palpate

Assessment of the airway is a "double-starred criterion" in the TNP. If an issue with the airway is identified, appropriate intervention must be executed, and reassessment of the airway completed before proceeding to the B component of the assessment.

- If the patient is alert or responds to verbal stimuli, ask the patient to open their mouth.
- If the patient is unable to open the mouth, responds only to pain, or is unresponsive, use the jaw-thrust maneuver to open the airway and assess for obstruction (actual or potential). In the patient with suspected CSI, the jaw-thrust procedure is recommended and is performed by two providers: One provides manual stabilization of the cervical spine and the second performs the jaw-thrust procedure.[14]
- Inspect for the following:
  - The tongue obstructing the airway
  - Loose or missing teeth
  - Foreign objects
  - Blood, vomitus, or secretions
  - Edema
  - Burns or evidence of inhalation injury
- Auscultate or listen for the following:
  - Adventitious airway sounds such as snoring, gurgling, or stridor, which may indicate obstruction
- Palpate for the following:
  - Possible occlusive maxillofacial bony deformity
  - Subcutaneous emphysema

If the patient has a definitive airway in place (a tube in the trachea is the definition of a definitive airway), assess for proper placement of the airway device prior to moving to the next step of the primary survey. Assessment for proper placement of a definitive airway includes the following three steps:

1. Attachment of a CO_2 detector device; after 5-6 breaths, assessment for presence of exhaled CO_2.
2. Observation of adequate rise and fall of the chest with assisted ventilation.
3. Auscultation for absence of gurgling over the epigastrium and presence of bilateral breath sounds.

Interventions

The information that follows represents the general approach for all trauma patients. Chapter 4, "Airway and Ventilation," provides additional information regarding specific airway devices and interventions.

If the airway is patent, efforts are aimed at *supporting and maintaining* a patent airway:

- If the patient is awake and has a patent airway, they may be allowed to assume a position that facilitates adequate air exchange. Remember to maintain cervical spine stabilization if CSI is suspected.

If the airway is *not* patent, efforts must be undertaken to *provide* a patent airway. Use of appropriate interventions for airway obstruction and subsequent reevaluation of the airway is a "double-starred criterion" in the TNP.

- Suction the airway.
  - Use care to avoid stimulating the gag reflex.
  - If the airway is obstructed by blood, vomitus, or other secretions, use a rigid suction device to remove these obstructions.
  - If a foreign body is noted, carefully remove it with forceps or by another appropriate method.
- If suctioning does not relieve the airway obstruction, the patient's tongue may be the cause of the obstruction. Insert an airway adjunct, which may be required to alleviate obstruction by the tongue. See Chapter 4 for more information.
  - Use the jaw-thrust maneuver to open the airway while maintaining manual cervical spine stabilization
  - A nasopharyngeal airway (NPA) can be used in patients who are conscious or unconscious. NPAs are used only in patients with *no* evidence of mid-face fractures. Chapter 6, "Head Trauma," provides additional information regarding mid-face fractures.
  - An oropharyngeal airway (OPA) can be used in patients *without* a gag reflex. Proper technique for placement of an OPA is discussed in Chapter 4 and in the airway management skill teaching station.
- Consider use of a definitive airway (endotracheal intubation).
  - A definitive airway is a tube securely placed in the trachea with the cuff inflated.[14]
  - Cuffed tubes are now recommended for use in all patients, including children younger than 8 years of age.[14,15] See Chapter 12, "Special Populations: The Pediatric Trauma Patient," for more information.
  - The following conditions or situations require a definitively secured airway[14-16]:
    - Apnea
    - GCS score of 8 or less
    - Severe maxillofacial fractures
    - Evidence of inhalation injury (facial burns, singed nasal or facial hairs, or a hoarse voice associated with possible pulmonary burn injury and a history of exposure to smoke or products of combustion)
    - Laryngeal or tracheal injury or neck hematoma
    - High risk of aspiration and the patient's inability to protect the airway
    - Compromised or ineffective ventilation
    - Anticipation of deterioration of neurologic status that may result in an inability to maintain or protect the airway

Difficult Airways

Injury or anatomic variations may make it difficult to successfully intubate the patient. In these cases, continue to ventilate the patient with a bag-mask device connected to oxygen at 10–15 L/minute until an alternative airway can be established. See Chapter 4.

B: Breathing and Ventilation

Assessment of breathing and ventilation is a "double-starred criterion" in the TNP.

Assessment

If an issue with the breathing/ventilation is identified, provide the appropriate intervention and reassess breathing/ventilation before proceeding to the C component of the primary survey.

To assess breathing, expose the patient's chest and complete the following steps:

- Inspect for the following:
  - Spontaneous breathing
  - Symmetrical rise and fall of the chest

- Depth, pattern, and rate of respirations
- Signs of respiratory difficulty (increased work of breathing) such as the use of accessory muscles or diaphragmatic breathing
- Skin color (normal, pale, flushed, cyanotic)
- Contusions, abrasions, or deformities that may be a sign of underlying injury
- Open pneumothorax (sucking chest wound)
- Jugular venous distention (JVD) and the position of the trachea (tracheal deviation and JVD are late signs that may indicate a tension pneumothorax)
- Signs of inhalation injury (e.g., singed nasal hairs, carbonaceous sputum)
- Auscultate for the following:
  - Presence, quality, and equality of breath sounds bilaterally at the second intercostal space midclavicular line and the bases at the fifth intercostal space at the anterior axillary line
- Palpate for the following:
  - Integrity or injury to the bony structures and ribs (which may affect ventilation)
  - Subcutaneous emphysema, which may be a sign of a pneumothorax
  - Soft tissue injury
  - Jugular venous pulsations at the suprasternal notch or in the supraclavicular area[15,16]

Intervention

See Chapter 4 for more information.

If breathing is absent, anticipate the need to *provide* it:

- After having opened the airway using the jaw-thrust maneuver (while maintaining manual cervical spinal stabilization) and inserting an oral airway adjunct, if indicated do the following:
  - Assist ventilations with a bag-mask device.
- Prepare for a definitive airway and continued breathing support with mechanical ventilation.

If breathing is present, anticipate the need to *support and maintain* it:

- Administer oxygen at 10–15 L/minute via a nonrebreather mask with reservoir bag.[1,17]
  - Inability to maintain adequate oxygenation causes hypoxemia, resulting in anaerobic metabolism and acidosis.
  - Trauma patients need early supplemental oxygen; however, recent evidence suggests that providers should closely monitor and titrate oxygen delivery for stabilized trauma patients to avoid the detrimental physiologic effects of hyperoxia, especially in patients with significant traumatic brain injury.[18-23] See Chapter 4 for more information.
- Determine whether ventilation is effective.
  - An $ETCO_2$ measurement between 35 and 45 mm Hg shows effective ventilation.[14,16,18,19,24] A level greater than 50 mm Hg signifies depressed ventilation.[24,25]
  - An oxygen saturation (SpO_2) of 94% or higher is associated with effective, adequate oxygenation.[12,14,19]

If ventilation is ineffective, do the following:

- Assist ventilation with a bag-mask device connected to an oxygen source at 10–15 L/minute and administer 10 to 12 breaths per minute (one breath every 5 to 6 seconds).[1,12-14]
- Determine the need for a definitive airway. It is possible that the patient may have an adequate airway, but be unable to effectively ventilate. In this case, the patient will require an airway adjunct to facilitate and assist ventilations.

Life-threatening pulmonary injuries require rapid identification and immediate intervention before proceeding to the next step in the primary survey.[1,16,18,19] See Chapter 7, "Thoracic and Neck Trauma," for more information. Examples of these injuries include the following:

- Open pneumothorax
- Tension pneumothorax
- Flail chest
- Hemothorax

C: Circulation and Control of Hemorrhage

Assessment of circulation and control of hemorrhage is a "double-starred criterion" in the TNP. If an issue with the circulation or hemorrhage is identified, appropriate interventions must be executed, and reassessment of circulation and hemorrhage control completed before proceeding to component D.

Assessment

The major assessment parameters that produce important information regarding the patient's circulatory status within seconds of a patient's arrival are level of consciousness, skin color, and pulse.[1,6] Skin color can be assessed during the across-the-room observation as the patient is brought into the trauma room. The use of AVPU can reveal the patient's level of consciousness and help to determine if the initial assessment may proceed as ABC or be reprioritized as <C>ABC to address hemorrhage control.[6,8-10,26] The assessment of circulation during the primary survey includes early evaluation of the possibility of hemorrhage in the abdomen and pelvis in any patient who has sustained blunt trauma.[1,6] In those cases, an emergent abdominal or pelvic assessment may be performed, including a focused assessment with sonography for trauma (FAST) examination or a radiograph of the pelvis.[1,6,27]

Inspect for the following:

- Uncontrolled external bleeding
- Pale skin color
- Hemorrhage (obvious external hemorrhage)

Auscultate for the following:

- Muffled heart sounds, which may suggest pericardial tamponade[27-29]

Palpate for the following:

- Presence of carotid and/or femoral (central) pulses for rate, rhythm, and strength (bounding or weak)
- Skin temperature and moisture (cool and diaphoretic or warm and dry)

If pulses are absent, be prepared to *provide* interventions to generate pulses:

- Initiate life-supporting measures following the guidelines developed by the American Heart Association (AHA) for basic life support.[14,25]
- If the patient is pulseless, without pausing in the primary survey, another team member may attach the patient to a cardiac monitor to assess for pulseless electrical activity (PEA). Consider and assess for the following as possible causes of PEA:
  - A penetrating wound to the heart
  - Pericardial tamponade
  - Rupture of great vessels
  - Intra-abdominal hemorrhage
- Assess for signs of uncontrolled *internal* bleeding.

Common sites for hemorrhage in the traumatically injured patient are the chest, abdomen, pelvis, long bones, and external bleeding from wounds or amputation. Assessment of the chest, abdomen, and pelvis may be indicated at this time to determine the site of the hemorrhage.[1,27]

If pulses are present, interventions are performed to *support and maintain* circulation. Inspect for the following:

- Any external bleeding
- Skin color
- Palpate for:
  - Central pulses
    - Pulses that are strong, regular, and at a normal rate may indicate normovolemia.
    - A rapid, thready pulse may indicate hypovolemia, and an irregular pulse may warn of potential cardiac dysfunction.[1]
  - Skin temperature and moisture

If pulses are present, but circulation is ineffective, do the following:

- Immediately assess for signs of uncontrolled internal bleeding.
- If the patient has ineffective circulation, consider common sites for hemorrhage such as the chest, abdomen, and pelvis.[1]
  - Administer blood or blood products as ordered.
- Use a rapid infusion device per facility protocol.

Interventions

Control and treat uncontrolled external bleeding by doing the following:

- Apply direct pressure over the site.
- Elevate a bleeding extremity.
- Apply pressure over arterial sites.
- Consider a pelvic binder if an unstable pelvic fracture is suspected. Pelvic binders are used only in instances of high energy traumatic injury with an anterior-posterior force vector.[1,30]
- Consider the use of a tourniquet (see Chapter 5, "Shock," for more information)
- If the patient has signs of bleeding, without pausing in the primary survey, another team member may obtain a blood pressure for baseline and trending.

Cannulate two veins with large-caliber IV catheters[1,6,8,31]:

- If unable to gain venous access quickly, consider IO or central venous access, depending on available resources.[1]
- Obtain a blood sample for type and cross-match. Initiate infusions of warmed isotonic crystalloid solution.[6,7]
- Use blood administration tubing and 0.9% sodium chloride or similar solution to facilitate blood administration, if needed.
- Consider balanced resuscitation needs (Chapter 5 provides more information).
- Administer blood or blood products as ordered.
- Use a rapid infusion device per facility protocol.
- Intervene in life-threatening situations:

    - Prepare and assist with emergency thoracotomy as indicated.
    - Prepare and assist with pericardial needle aspiration to relieve a cardiac tamponade as indicated.
- Be prepared to expedite patient transfer to the operating suite.

Volume Resuscitation

Historically, the traditional approach to treating hypotension in trauma patients has been to replace the volume lost from hemorrhage with isotonic crystalloid solution. More recently, this practice has been recognized as counterproductive. Raising the blood pressure in this manner may dislodge the clots the body has formed and promote further bleeding.[31] In addition, large volumes of IV fluid can lead to dilutional coagulopathy, which worsens metabolic acidosis and may cause hypothermia.[1,6,7,18,32-34]

Component therapy is now suggested as a means of fluid resuscitation to replace patient losses, including administering red blood cells, plasma, and platelets. This balanced approach to resuscitation includes massive transfusion so that oxygen delivery is optimized, acidosis is corrected, coagulopathy is prevented, and damage control surgery may be performed.[1,6-8,32,35,36] See Chapter 5 for more information.

D: Disability (Neurologic Status)

Assessment of disability (neurologic status) using the GCS is a "double-starred criterion" in the TNP. If an issue with the neurologic status is identified, *planning* for appropriate further assessment and intervention must be executed, before proceeding to component E.

Assessment

The GCS offers a standardized method for evaluating level of consciousness. It also serves as an excellent communication tool for members of the trauma team to convey objective information. Scores range from 3 (indicating deep unconsciousness) to 15 (indicating a patient who is alert, converses normally, and is able to obey commands).[37-39]

One limitation of the GCS is that it does not provide for an accurate assessment of patients who are intubated or aphasic and unable to respond to the verbal component.[37-40] Even so, it continues to be the clinical standard against which newer scales are compared and is used widely by emergency and trauma teams, medical and surgical intensive care units (ICUs), and prehospital providers.[37-39] Assess the GCS score upon patient arrival and repeat as necessary and according to policy. Trend analysis of GCS findings is important to detect deteriorating or improving neurologic function. See Chapter 6 for more information.

Assess pupils for equality, shape, roundness, and reactivity (PERRL). Pupil reactivity can be an early indicator of increasing intracranial pressure.[1,19,37,39]

Interventions

Interventions include the following:

- Evaluate for needed CT of the head. Consider any changes in level of consciousness to be the result of CNS injury until proven otherwise.[1,37-40] See Chapter 6 for more information.
- Consider measurement of ABGs. A decreased level of consciousness may be an indicator of decreased cerebral perfusion, hypoxia, hypoventilation, or acid–base imbalance.
- Consider bedside glucose, alcohol level, or toxicology screening. Hypoglycemia, along with other conditions, such as the presence of alcohol, may play a role in the patient's neurologic status and need to be excluded as the primary cause.
- If there is an indication of possible increased intracranial pressure causing decreased level of consciousness, consider elevation of the head or slight reverse Trendelenburg position to facilitate venous return.[41] See Chapter 6 for more information.

E: Exposure and Environmental Control

Performance of patient exposure and environmental control is a "double-starred criterion" in the TNP. If an issue is identified, it must be addressed, and appropriate methods of temperature control must be executed before proceeding to component F.

Assessment

Assess the patient as follows:

- Carefully and completely undress the patient to facilitate a thorough assessment. Cutting the clothing using trauma shears is often the most effective way to remove garments while avoiding manipulation of the patient. Caution is advised to avoid self-injury from something on the patient or in the clothing.
- Inspect for any uncontrolled bleeding and do a quick visual scan of the visible body surfaces for any obvious injuries.

Interventions

Interventions include the following:

- If clothing may be used as evidence, preserve it according to institutional policy. Cut *around* areas of suspected evidence and place clothing in a *paper* bag and label appropriately. Maintain the chain of evidence with law enforcement as indicated. Care of the patient always supersedes evidence collection. See Chapter 16, "Special Populations: The Interpersonal-Violence Trauma Patient," for more information.

- Maintain body temperature as follows:
  - Cover the patient with warm blankets.
  - Keep the ambient temperature warm.
  - Administer warmed IV fluids.
  - Use forced-air warmers.
  - Use radiant warming lights.

Hypothermia, hypotension, and acidosis are a potentially lethal combination in the injured patient.[33,34] The E assessment parameter is intentionally placed in the primary survey to assure that aggressive measures are taken to prevent the loss of body heat and subsequent hypothermia in the trauma patient.

F: Full Set of Vital Signs and Family Presence

Vital signs and the presence of family are both essential components of the assessment of any trauma patient.

Full Set of Vital Signs

To monitor the effectiveness of the resuscitation, obtain and trend vital signs at regular intervals, including blood pressure, pulse, respirations, and temperature.

Family Presence

Facilitate family presence as soon as a member of the trauma team is available to act as liaison to the family. If a social worker, psychiatric nurse, or hospital chaplain is a member of the team, that person may fill this role. Honesty, sensitivity, and a caring approach are important when interacting with the patient's family and friends, as this can be a stressful time. Consider factors such as the patient's age, ethnicity, cultural background, and religion when interacting with the family.

Evidence shows that patients prefer family members present during resuscitation.[42,43] In addition, strong evidence indicates that family members wish to be offered the option to be present during invasive procedures and resuscitation of a family member.[42,43] The Emergency Nurses Association (ENA), along with several other professional organizations, supports the option of family presence during resuscitation.

While some providers may have concerns regarding family presence during resuscitation and invasive procedures, family members are not viewed as a complication, but rather as an extension of the patient.[42,43] Being present at the time of a person's death is viewed in many cultures as a privilege, and trauma teams are encouraged to share this privilege with the patient's family in accordance with the patient's and family's wishes and in accordance with the facility's policies and procedures.[42,43]

G: Get Monitoring Devices and Give Comfort

Consider the mnemonic LMNOP to remember these resuscitation monitoring devices and supports:

- L: Obtain Laboratory studies including ABGs or, in some cases, venous blood gases, and obtain a specimen for blood type and cross-match.
  - Lactic acid is an excellent reflection of tissue perfusion and an endpoint measure of resuscitation.[44]
    - High levels of lactic acid are associated with hypoperfusion.[44]
    - A lactic acid level greater than 2 to 4 mmol/L is associated with poor outcomes.[44]
    - ABGs provide values of oxygen, CO_2, and base excess, which can also be reflective of endpoint measurements of the effectiveness of cellular perfusion, adequacy of ventilation, and the success of the resuscitation.[45] Consider adding a carboxyhemoglobin to the ABGs in patients who have suffered burn trauma.
    - An abnormal base deficit may indicate poor perfusion and tissue hypoxia, which results in the generation of hydrogen ions and metabolic acidosis.
    - A base deficit of less than −6 is associated with poor outcomes.[45]
- M: Monitor cardiac rate and rhythm. Compare the patient's pulse to the monitor rhythm.
  - Dysrhythmias—such as premature ventricular contractions, atrial fibrillation, or S-T segment changes—may indicate blunt cardiac trauma.[1,14,46-48]
  - PEA may point to cardiac tamponade, tension pneumothorax, or profound hypovolemia.[1,14,46,49]
- N: Nasogastric or orogastric tube consideration. The insertion of a gastric tube provides for evacuation of stomach contents and the relief of gastric distention. This intervention may help to optimize inflation of the lungs and prevent vomiting and/or aspiration. If mid-face fractures or head injury are suspected, the oral route is preferred.[16] Maintain cervical spinal stabilization and ensure that suction equipment is readily available. This is considered routine care in the intubated patient to minimize aspiration risk.

- O: Oxygenation and ventilation assessment.
  - Consider weaning oxygen based on pulse oximetry to prevent hyperoxia. Attach patient to capnography if the patient is intubated or sedated.
  - Pulse oximetry detects changes in oxygenation that cannot be readily observed clinically. This noninvasive intervention measures the SpO_2 of arterial blood or percentage of bound hemoglobin. A pulse oximetry reading of 94% or greater is viewed as convincing evidence that peripheral arterial oxygenation is adequate.[1,14,18,20-23,45] However, accurate readings rely on adequate peripheral perfusion. Oximetry offers a measurement of SpO_2; it does not provide evidence of ventilation. Additionally, oximetry readings do not differentiate between O_2 and O_1 (monoxide, which may be present in patients who have been exposed to products of combustion). Monoxide is tightly bound to the hemoglobin molecule and is not available for use by the cells. Patients with high levels of carboxyhemoglobin can have SpO_2 readings of 100%, but still be experiencing cellular hypoxia.[45]
  - $ETCO_2$ monitoring (or capnography) provides instantaneous information about the ventilation, perfusion, and metabolism of carbon dioxide. Normal values are 35 to 45 mm Hg.[24,25,45]
- P: Pain assessment and management.
  - The assessment and management of severe pain is an important part of the treatment of trauma patients, with the goal being to give comfort to the patient while avoiding respiratory depression. Additionally, pain and anxiety cause the release of epinephrine and norepinephrine, which in turn increases myocardial oxygen demand. It is therefore essential to treat or control both pain and anxiety as much as possible to decrease or control this increased demand.[1,40-54]
  - Use of both *pharmacologic* and *nonpharmacologic* pain management techniques is essential in the control of pain in the trauma patient.[52-54] Injuries sustained by the trauma patient may be life-changing for both the patient and family, so it is essential that the trauma team also provide appropriate spiritual and psychosocial support.

Reevaluation

Reevaluation begins with portable radiographs.

Portable Radiograph

A portable anterior–posterior chest radiograph and pelvis radiograph can be obtained at this phase of the resuscitation, if not done previously as part of the primary survey and resuscitation. These studies are performed in the resuscitation area and may help identify or confirm suspected and potentially life-threatening injuries, such as a pneumothorax or pelvic fracture with uncontrolled internal hemorrhage. Radiographs can also be used as part of confirming placement of endotracheal tubes, chest tubes, and gastric tubes. The pelvic radiograph may be withheld if the patient's pelvis is stable on exam and if the patient is moving expeditiously to the radiology department for more definitive abdomen and pelvis imaging (CT scans).

Consider the Need for Patient Transfer

The trauma team leader gathers essential information during the primary survey and resuscitation phase that may indicate the need to transfer the patient to another facility.[1] This consideration requires a deliberate pause and moment of decision. If the patient's injuries are out of the scope or beyond the capabilities of the current facility and require a higher level of care, now is the time to mobilize the transfer resources. This may be accomplished by other team members while the secondary survey is being completed. All life-threatening injuries are identified, addressed, and stabilized to the extent possible by the current facility prior to transferring the patient. The team leader will delegate the initial steps to begin immediate transfer and continue with ongoing evaluation and resuscitation. Follow institutional guidelines for contacting the appropriate facility that has the capability to provide care for the severely injured. See Chapter 19, "Transition of Care for the Trauma Patient," for more information.

If the patient is not being transferred out, this is an opportune time to notify any additional services and support staff (i.e., consult services, resource nurses) who will be needed to assist in managing the patient.

Secondary Survey

The secondary survey (H and I) begins after the completion of the primary survey (ABCDE), after the initiation of resuscitative efforts, once vital functions have been stabilized, and after additional monitoring/interventions have been considered (F and G).

H–J Steps in the Secondary Survey

The secondary survey begins with history taking.

H: History

The patient's condition is greatly influenced by the MOI. Certain injuries can be predicted based on the direction (vector) and amount of energy behind the MOI.[1] See Chapter 2, "Biomechanics, Kinematics, and Mechanisms of Injury," for more information. Additional history includes the following:

- Prehospital report: The mnemonic MIST can be used as a guide:
    - **M:** Mechanism of injury
    - **I:** Injuries sustained
    - **S:** Signs and Symptoms (in the field)
    - **T:** Treatment (in the field)
- Patient history: If the patient's family is present, solicit input regarding the traumatic event and the health history. If the patient is responsive, eliciting answers may assist the trauma nurse in evaluating the patient's level of consciousness and help to identify areas of pain and injury.
- The SAMPLE mnemonic highlights important aspects of patient history:
    - **S:** Symptoms associated with the illness or injury
    - **A:** Allergies
    - **M:** Medications currently used, including anticoagulant therapy
    - **P:** Past medical history (include hospitalizations and/or surgeries)
    - **L:** Last oral intake/Last output (Last menstrual period if female of childbearing age)
    - **E:** Events and Environmental factors related to the illness or injury

Comorbid factors are preexisting conditions that place the patient at greater risk for complications related to the injury. These are important to note and will influence care going forward but do not preempt definitive care. They include the following factors[1,13,15,36]:

- Age: Risk for injury or death increases after age 55, and children require specialized pediatric care.
- Burns: Patients with burns may require early transfer to a burn facility.
- Pregnancy: Pregnant females of any gestational age warrant an early obstetric consult.
- Disabilities: Significant physical and/or mental/emotional disabilities.

H: Head-to-Toe Assessment

During this phase, a complete head-to-toe examination is performed and documented. This information is obtained primarily from inspection, auscultation, and palpation.

In a noisy trauma room, percussion is difficult to perform and has been replaced in some cases by the use of FAST examinations.[27] Systematically move from the patient's head to the lower extremities and posterior surface following the process outlined in this section to identify all injuries.

> **NOTE**
>
> **LACE: Soft-Tissue Injuries**
>
> Inspect for the following:
>
> **L**: Lacerations
> **A**: Abrasions, Avulsions
> **C**: Contusions
> **E**: Edema, Ecchymosis

General Appearance

Note the position and posture of the patient or the presence of any spontaneous guarding. Observe for stiffness, rigidity, or flaccidity of extremities. Document specific odors, such as alcohol, gasoline, or other chemicals. Specific presentations may alert the trauma team to injuries (e.g., shortening and external rotation of a leg might suggest a hip fracture).

Head and Face

Assessment of the head and face includes the following:

- Soft-tissue injuries
    - Inspect for the following:
        - Lacerations, abrasions, avulsions, contusions, edema, or ecchymosis (LACE)
        - Puncture wounds or impaled objects
    - Palpate for the following:
        - Areas of tenderness, step-offs, and crepitus
- Bony deformities
    - Inspect for the following:
        - Asymmetry of facial expression
        - Any exposed tissue or bone that may suggest disruption of the central nervous system (brain matter)
    - Palpate for the following:
        - Depressions, angulations, areas of tenderness

Eyes

Assessment of the eyes includes the following:

- Determine gross visual acuity by holding up fingers and asking the patient to identify how many are being held up. Do this for both eyes independently and both eyes together. Remember, diplopia is a significant finding that can indicate entrapment of cranial nerves III, IV, and VI (oculomotor, trochlear and abducens nerves).[16,18,19]

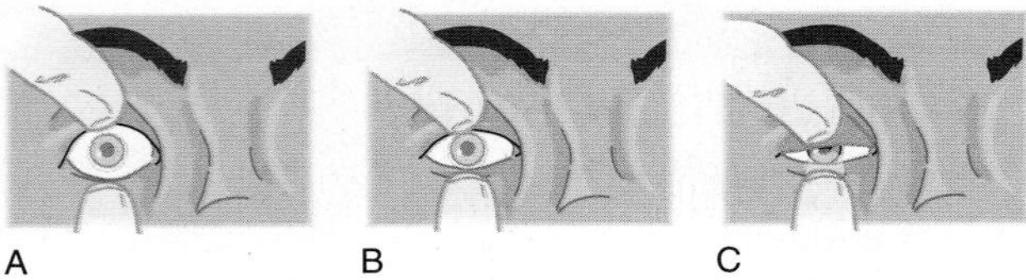

Figure 3-2 *Removal of hard contact lens.*

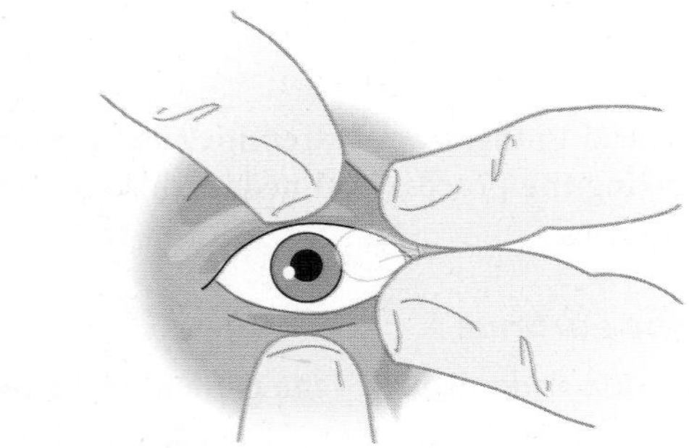

Figure 3-3 *Removal of soft contact lens.*

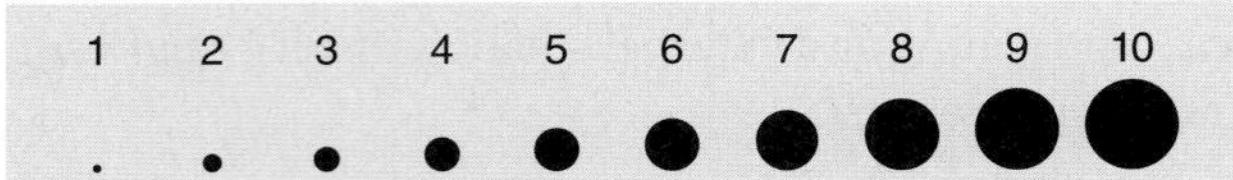

Figure 3-4 *Pupil size.*

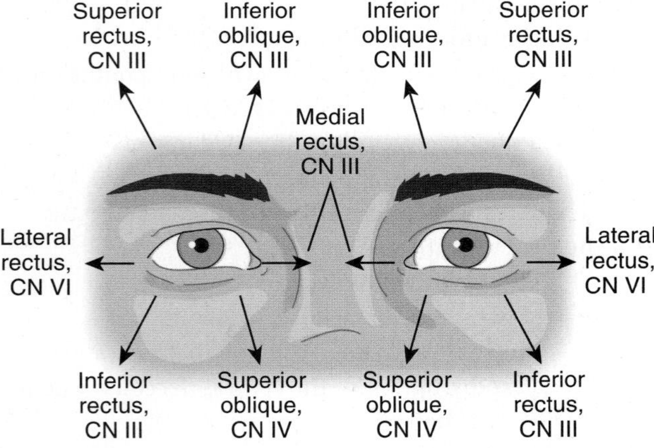

Figure 3-5 *Extraocular eye movements.*

- Assess for prescription eyeglasses or contact lenses. Contact lenses should be removed before edema develops and to decrease the risk of corneal abrasions (**Figure 3-2** and **Figure 3-3**).
- Inspect for the following:
  - Pupils to determine size, equality, shape, and reactivity to light (**Figure 3-4**).
  - Muscle function by asking the patient to follow a moving finger or penlight in the six cardinal positions (**Figure 3-5**). Assessment of eye movement by having the patient follow a finger as it is moved in the shape of an "H" is important to assessing for possible orbital fractures with extraocular muscle entrapment or cranial nerve damage.
  - Presence of foreign bodies as identified by visualization or patient complaint of pain or sensation of something in the eye.

NOTE

Eye Emergency Examples

Specific eye emergencies, while not usually life threatening, can be significantly life altering. Although the initial assessment is not interrupted to immediately address these conditions, they are noted and addressed as soon as the patient is hemodynamically stable. Examples of eye emergencies include the following:

- Lid lacerations (consider repair by an ophthalmologist or oculoplastic surgeon)
- Corneal laceration
- Corneal or intraocular foreign body
- Orbital fracture
- Hyphema
- Retrobulbar hematoma
- Globe rupture
- Ocular burns and ultraviolet keratitis

Ears

Inspect for the following:

- Look for unusual drainage, such as blood or clear fluid from the external ear.
  - Do not pack the ear since a cerebrospinal fluid (CSF) leak may be present and packing could increase the intracranial pressure.
  - Test otorrhea for CSF.
  - If drainage is clear, check it for glucose. Glucose level of CSF is approximately two-thirds of the blood glucose level.[55]
  - β^2-transferrin: This test requires fluid to be sent to the laboratory and is considered the gold standard for identifying CSF otorrhea or rhinorrhea.[56]
- The halo sign (generally considered unreliable) and glucose tests can be done rapidly and provide a general suspicion of CSF leak.[56,57] See Chapter 6 for more information.
- Ecchymosis behind the ear is known as Battle sign; it is usually a later development.
- Ear avulsions or lacerations: Repairs often require the expertise of a plastic surgeon.

Nose

Inspect for the following:

- Look for unusual drainage such as blood or clear fluid.
  - Do not pack the nose to stop clear fluid drainage, as it may be CSF and packing could increase intracranial pressure.
  - Test rhinorrhea for CSF (again, test clear drainage for glucose as described earlier).[55,58]
- If CSF is suspected, notify the physician and do not insert a nasogastric tube.
  - Note the position of the nasal septum.

Neck and Cervical Spine

Assume that patients with maxillofacial or head trauma may also have an unstable CSI (fracture and/or ligament injury). Restrict motion of the cervical spine until adequate studies have been completed and an injury has been excluded. The absence of neurologic deficit does not exclude CSI.[11-14] See Chapter 9, "Spinal Trauma," for more information.

Inspect for the following:

- LACE plus signs of penetrating trauma, including presence of impaled objects or any open wounds
- The position of the trachea and the appearance of the jugular veins

Palpate for the following:

- Cervical tenderness, deformities, or step-offs
- Tracheal deviation, subcutaneous emphysema, and areas of tenderness

Chest

Inspect for the following:

- Presence of spontaneous breathing, respiratory rate, depth, and degree of effort required, use of accessory or abdominal muscles, and any paradoxical chest movement
- Anterior and lateral chest walls—including the axillae—for LACE, puncture wounds, impaled objects, and scars that may indicate previous chest surgery
- Expansion and excursion of the chest during ventilation
- Expressions or reactions that indicate the presence of pain with inspiration and exhalation (facial grimace)

Auscultate for the following:

- *Lung sounds*, noting the presence of any adventitious sounds, such as wheezes or crackles
- *Heart sounds* for the presence of murmurs, friction rubs, or muffled heart tones

Palpate for the following:

- Presence of subcutaneous emphysema
- Bony crepitus or deformities (step-offs or areas of tenderness) to the clavicles, sternum, and *all* ribs

Abdomen/Flanks

Inspect for the following:

- LACE, puncture wounds, impaled objects, and scars that may indicate previous abdominal surgery
- Evisceration
- Distention

Auscultate for the following:

- Presence or absence of bowel sounds

Palpate for the following:

- Note any rigidity, guarding, masses, and areas of tenderness in all four abdominal quadrants.
- Begin light palpation in an area where the patient has not complained of pain or where there is no obvious injury.

Pelvis/Perineum

Inspect for the following:

- LACE, puncture wounds, impaled objects, and scars that may indicate previous surgery
- Bony deformities or exposed bone
- Blood at the urethral meatus (more common in males than females because of the extraperitoneal position of the urethra), vagina, and rectum
- Priapism
- Pain and/or the urge but inability to void (may indicate bladder rupture)
- Scrotal/labial hematoma

Palpate for the following:

- Instability of the pelvis by applying gentle pressure over the iliac wings downward and medially[1]
- Instability of the pelvis by placing gentle pressure on the symphysis pubis

Valid indications for the insertion of a urinary catheter include the following[59,61]:

- Urinary obstruction or retention
- Alteration in blood pressure or volume status
- The need to determine accurate input and output and the patient is unable to use a urinal or bedpan
- Emergency surgery or major trauma
- Urologic procedures or bladder irrigation
- Comfort care for the terminally ill

CLINICAL PEARL

Monitoring Urinary Output

Urinary output reflects end-organ perfusion and is considered a sensitive indicator of the patient's volume status. Continuous or frequent monitoring is best accomplished with an indwelling urinary catheter. However, it is necessary to assess the patient's condition to determine the need for urinary catheter insertion, taking into account indications and contraindications. Urinary tract infection in the healthcare setting is strongly associated with the presence of an indwelling catheter, and alternative methods should be considered before a urinary catheter is placed.[59-61]

Insertion of a urinary catheter is contraindicated if urethral transection is suspected. Signs and symptoms of urethral injury include the following[1]:

- Blood at the urethral meatus
- Perineal ecchymosis
- Scrotal ecchymosis
- High-riding or nonpalpable prostate[62]

Extremities

When performing the extremity assessment, it is important to evaluate the neurovascular status, including circulation, motor function, and sensation (CMS).

Inspect for the following:

- Soft-tissue injuries
  - Bleeding, LACE, puncture wounds, impaled objects, deformity, and any open wounds
- Bony injuries
  - Angulation, deformity, open wounds (with or without evidence of protruding bone fragments), or edema
  - Previously applied splints for correct placement: Leave in place if correctly applied and neurovascular function is intact distal to splint
- Skin color
- Presence of dialysis catheters or dialysis access (fistula or grafts), peripherally inserted central catheters, or other signs of complex medical history

Palpate for the following:

- Circulation
  - Skin temperature and moisture
  - Pulses
    - Always compare one side with the other and note any differences in the quality of the pulses. Assess the femoral, popliteal, dorsalis pedis, and posterior tibialis pulses in the lower extremities; assess the brachial and radial pulses in the upper extremities.
    - Compare pulse quality in the upper extremities to pulse quality in the lower extremities. Weaker pulses in lower extremities could indicate aortic aneurysm.
- Bony injury
  - Crepitus
  - Deformity and areas of tenderness
  - Sensation
    - Determine the patient's ability to sense touch in all four extremities.
- Motor function
  - Elicit the presence or absence of spontaneous movement in the extremities.
  - Determine motor strength and range of motion in all four extremities; compare left to right for strength and quality.

I: Inspect Posterior Surfaces

If pelvic or spinal trauma is suspected, imaging is recommended prior to turning the patient due to the potential for harm from the log roll maneuver. Log rolling can cause secondary injuries, including SCI and hemorrhage from pelvic fractures.[63-65] The head, shoulders, torso, and hips vary in dimensions, and when a body is rolled onto its side, these differences in width make it very difficult to maintain spinal alignment and can cause rotational movement along all axes. The log roll produces significantly greater motion in the unstable cervical spine compared with methods like the lift-and-slide, the straddle lift-and-slide, the 6-plus lift-and-slide, and the scoop stretcher.[63,66] In addition, log rolling a polytrauma patient in the primary survey is potentially life-threatening if the patient has a site of internal hemorrhage because the log roll produces movement that may lead to clot disruption and irretrievable exsanguination.[64] Best practice recommendations are that it is only appropriate to assess the posterior of the patient after a patient has been cleared of spinal injuries, pelvic fracture, or other injuries that may be exacerbated by movement.[65,67-70] If injuries are confirmed, log rolling may be contraindicated.[65,69,70]

If the patient must be turned prior to imaging, do the following while inspecting posterior surfaces:

- Support the extremities, especially those with suspected injuries.

- Log roll the patient with the assistance from members of the trauma team.
  - A designated person, either the team leader or another (at the request of the team leader), is positioned at the patient's head, and is responsible for maintaining cervical spine stabilization and directing the team to turn together.
  - Other team members, positioned at one side of the patient, maintain the torso, hips, and lower extremities.
  - Maintain the vertebral column in alignment during the turning process.
  - When possible, avoid rolling the patient onto the side of an injured extremity. The patient is log rolled away from the examiner, so the back, flanks, buttocks, and thighs can be visually examined.
  - See the section "Emerging Trends" for more information.

Inspect for the following:

- LACE, puncture wounds, impaled objects, and scars along the entire posterior surface
- Presence of blood in or around the rectum

Palpate for the following:

- Deformity and areas of tenderness along the vertebral column, palpating along each spinous process and attempting to determine a vertebral body fracture, including the costovertebral angles
- Deformity and areas of tenderness over the entire posterior surface of the body, including the flanks

A digital rectal examination (DRE) may or may not be indicated. In the awake, cooperative patient, it may not be needed. In the unconscious patient, the presence or absence of rectal tone can indicate spinal cord injury (SCI). A DRE is typically performed by a physician or advanced practice nurse during the secondary survey; however, the sensitivity of this test has been called into question.[71] An alternative is to ask the alert patient to squeeze the buttocks to evaluate spinal cord function. Determine the following assessment parameters:

- Presence or absence of rectal tone
- Presence of a high-riding prostate gland

Promote timely removal of the patient from the spine board if there are no contraindications. Consider placement of a slider board, if not already present, to facilitate patient movement on and off the stretcher.

J: Just Keep Reevaluating

Trauma patients require ongoing monitoring and evaluation. Just because the patient appears stable during the initial assessment, and even if you have successfully identified all life-threatening injuries and appropriately intervened, that does not mean the patient is stable. Once the initial assessment is completed, the nurse must continually reevaluate the patient for response to the injury as well as response to any interventions, treatments, and procedures performed during the initial assessment phase. Reevaluation consists of the following:

- The primary survey (ABCDE)
- The patient's vital signs (F)
- The patient's level of pain (the P in the LMNOP of G)
- The injuries you have identified in H and I

Serial assessments and analyzing trends are essential components of trauma care and the TNP. It is important to continuously reevaluate all your findings when caring for a trauma patient. The major components of the reevaluation can be remembered through use of the mnemonic VIPP:

- **V:** Vital signs
- **I:** Injuries sustained and Interventions performed
- **P:** Primary survey
- **P:** Level of Pain

These are the parameters that you will be continuously reevaluating for your patient.

Additional Tests or Treatments

Upon completion of the secondary survey, the trauma nurse anticipates orders for additional diagnostic tests and interventions to identify or address specific injuries. These include (but are not limited to):

- Additional laboratory studies: ABGs (if not previously done), cardiac enzymes, liver function tests, metabolic profiles, and coagulation studies
- Radiologic imaging
  - Radiographs (of any suspected skeletal injuries)
  - CT scans (of any affected body regions) including the potential for CT angiography
  - Magnetic resonance imaging
- Wound care as required
- Application of splints as indicated
- Application of traction devices as indicated
- Administration of medications:
  - Tetanus prophylaxis
  - Antibiotics

    - Anticoagulation reversal agents
    - Pain medications (part of ongoing assessment)
    - Anxiolytics
    - Neuromuscular blocking agents
- Angiography
- Contrast urography and angiography
- Bronchoscopy or esophagoscopy
- Preparation for the operating room
- Preparation for admission or transfer
- Psychosocial support

These procedures may require transportation of the patient out of the ED; therefore, nurses should ensure the appropriately trained personnel, necessary medications, and resuscitative equipment are available during transport of the patient. Ideally, many of these procedures will not be performed until the patient is hemodynamically stabilized. Injuries identified in the primary and secondary surveys continue to be reassessed along with pain and response to analgesics (the VIPP). Many of these interventions are metrics that are measured as part of a performance improvement program and are time sensitive, such as time of antibiotics and time to operative intervention.

Additional considerations include the following:

- Documentation: Careful and accurate documentation of the assessment, interventions, resuscitation, and the patient's response is an expectation of the trauma nurse. Remember that any trauma patient is a potential legal case (criminal or civil), so accurate and complete documentation is vitally important.
- Family support: The trauma nurse with primary responsibility for the patient can contribute to the ongoing psychosocial support of both the patient and family. Collaboration with the family support person (who is chosen by the family) will assure needs are met and information is shared. Whenever possible, allow the family to stay with the patient and give adequate time for them to have their questions answered.

Post-Resuscitation Care

The post-resuscitation phase of trauma assessment includes the trauma nurse's ongoing reevaluation of the patient's response to the injury and the effectiveness of all the interventions—the "J" of the A–J mnemonic. Achievement of expected outcomes is evaluated, and the treatment plan is adjusted accordingly to enhance patient outcomes.

Post-resuscitation care parameters are the same as the "J" in your initial assessment mnemonic. The nurse will continually reevaluate:

- Components of the primary survey (ABCDE)
- Vital signs (F)
- Pain and response to pain medications and non-pharmacologic interventions (an item in G)
- All identified injuries and the effectiveness of the treatment or interventions (identified in H and I)

See Chapter 20, "Post-Resuscitation Care Considerations," for more information.

Definitive Care or Transport

Definitive care includes the need for specific subspecialty care such as neurosurgery or orthopedics, monitoring and care in an ICU, or the need for evaluation and operative intervention by a trauma surgeon. The decision to transfer a patient to another facility depends on the patient's injuries, facility resources, and pre-established transfer agreements. This decision is a matter of medical judgment, and evidence supports the position that trauma outcomes improve if patients who are critically injured are cared for in trauma centers.[1]

Emerging Trends

As the science and evidence of trauma care continue to evolve, tools to improve patient outcomes continue to be trialed and refined. Evidence is routinely tested and replicated, and new standards of care are transitioned into practice. This section on trauma care considerations explores some of the evidence and the potential significance to trauma patient care. Regarding the initial assessment, the use of computer-aided decision making and log rolling are discussed.

Computer-Aided Decision Making in Trauma Resuscitation

A Level I trauma center in Melbourne, Australia, studied the efficacy of evidence-based trauma management algorithms in the initial 30 minutes of trauma resuscitation. Computer-generated prompts for critical decision-making points were created every 72 seconds. A computer-assisted video monitored compliance with the algorithms, and error rates were measured per patient. The researchers found that compliance with protocols increased and that the computer-prompted decision making decreased morbidity and errors in trauma management.[72]

Log Rolling the Patient

Log rolling is the most commonly used maneuver to inspect a patient's posterior surface. This procedure can cause excess movement in traumatically injured patients.[63,64,67] Alternative patient handling methods are available that produce less movement, pain, and anxiety. These methods include the lift-and-slide, 6-plus lift-and-slide, and straddle lift-and-slide, or applying assistive devices such as mechanical continuous rotation therapy, slide boards, slide sheets, roller boards, scoop stretcher, and air-assisted devices.[66,67] Incorporating these alternative patient handling methods may require assistance from other departments. See the ENA Topic Brief, "Avoiding the Log Roll Maneuver," for more information.[67]

Use of Spine Boards

Much discussion regarding the use of spine boards for immobilization and stabilization of the cervical spine and the concomitant complications of their use (the development of pressure injuries) has occurred in recent years. Spine boards are intended for use as a transport device only, and patients are placed on them only when absolutely necessary to facilitate transport and are removed from spine boards as quickly as possible. Although long backboards may be used in certain instances, it is believed that proper placement of a correctly fitted semi-rigid cervical collar is adequate to maintain cervical spine stabilization until CSI can be definitively ruled out.[73,74]

Pharmacologic Treatment to Create a Pro-Survival Phenotype

Valproic acid (VAP) has been shown to cause reversible acetylation of proteins (which creates an anti-inflammatory and pro-survival phenotype), thereby decreasing the organ damage seen as the result of hemorrhage, polytrauma, and ischemia–reperfusion injury.[75-79] Studies are ongoing regarding the use of VAP to mitigate cellular damage in trauma patients and thereby decrease morbidity and mortality.[80]

Therapeutic Hypothermia

The use of therapeutic hypothermia has been demonstrated to be effective after cardiac arrest in a process termed emergency preservation and resuscitation. Animal studies are under way to test the effectiveness of this approach when used in cases of exsanguinating cardiac arrest.[81] This technique may soon be a viable option for trauma patients to improve their survival rates.[75,81-83]

Summary

The initial assessment approach for injured patients is the essence of trauma nursing care. Initial assessment of the trauma patient is achieved through the use of a systematic, standardized approach to assessment, interventions, evaluation, and definitive care of the patient. Essential components include:

- Preparation and triage
- Primary survey (A, B, C, D, and E)
- Full set of vital signs and family support with resuscitation and use of continuous monitoring devices (F and G)
- Reevaluation (consideration of the need to transfer patient to a higher level of care)
- Secondary survey (H and I) and performance of additional tests/diagnostics as indicated/required
- Reevaluation and post-resuscitation care (J)
- Definitive care and transfer

By using this systematic and standardized approach in the care of the trauma patient, emergency and trauma nurses can be more aware of the body's pathophysiologic response to injury and proactively intervene with lifesaving, goal-directed therapies and current management strategies to promote optimal outcomes for the trauma patient.

References

1. American College of Surgeons. (2018). Initial assessment and management. In *Advanced trauma life support: Student course manual* (10th ed., pp. 2–21). Chicago, IL: Author.
2. Emergency Nurses Association. (2012). Family presence during invasive procedures and resuscitation in the emergency department [Clinical practice guideline]. Retrieved from https://www.ena.org/docs/default-source/resource-library/practice-resources/cpg/familypresencecpg3eaabb7cf0414584ac2291feba3be481.pdf?sfvrsn=9c167fc6_12
3. Newgard, C., Zive, D., Holmes, J., Bulger, E., Staudenmayer, K., Liao, M., . . . Bulger, E. M. (2011). A multisite assessment of the American College of Surgeons Committee on Trauma field triage decision scheme for identifying seriously injured children and adults. *Journal of the American College of Surgeons, 213*(6), 709–721. https://doi.org/10.1016/j.jamcollsurg.2011.09.012012
4. Prehospital Trauma Life Support Committee of the National Association of Emergency Medical Technicians & Committee on Trauma of the American College of Surgeons Committee on Trauma. (2016). Golden principles of prehospital trauma care. In *Prehospital trauma life support* (8th ed., pp. 475–486). Burlington, MA: Jones & Bartlett Learning.

5. Sasser, S. M., Hunt, R. C., Faul, M., Sugerman, D., Pearson, W., Dulski, T., . . . Galli, R. L. L. (2012). Guidelines for field triage of injured patients: Recommendations of the National Expert Panel on Field Triage, 2011. *MMWR Recommendations and Reports, 61*(RR-1), 1–20. Retrieved from https://www.cdc.gov/mmwr/preview/mmwrhtml/rr6101a1.htm
6. Cherkas, D. (2011). Traumatic hemorrhagic shock: Advances in fluid management. *EB Medicine, 13*(11), 1–20. Retrieved from https://www.ebmedicine.net/topics.php?paction=showTopic&topic_id=282
7. Chatrath, V., Khetarpal, R., & Ahuja, J. (2015). Fluid management in patients with trauma: Restrictive versus liberal approach. *Journal of Anaesthesiology Clinical Pharmacology, 31*(3), 308–316. https://doi.org/10.4103/0970-9185.161664
8. Oyeniyi, B. T., Fox., E. E., Scerbo, M., Tomasek, J. S., Wade, C. E., & Holcomb, J. B. (2017). Trends in 1029 trauma deaths at a Level 1 trauma center: Impact of a bleeding control bundle of care. *Injury, 48*(1), 5–12. https://doi.org/10.1016/j.injury.2016.10.037
9. Hodgetts, T. J., Mahoney, P. F., Russell, M. Q., & Byers, M. (2006). ABC to ABC: Redefining the military trauma paradigm. *Emergency Medicine Journal, 23*(10), 745–746. https://doi.org/10.1136%2Femj.2006.039610
10. Military Health System. (2015, April). Tactical combat casualty care. Retrieved from https://health.mil/Reference-Center/Training-Booklets-and-Toolkits?page=2#pagingAnchor/TCCC%20Guidelines%20150429%20(3).pdf
11. Kirkpatrick, A. W., Ball, C. G., D'Amours, S. K., & Zygun, D. (2008). Acute resuscitation of the unstable adult trauma patient: Bedside diagnosis and therapy. *Canadian Journal of Surgery, 5*(1), 57–69. Retrieved from http://canjsurg.ca/wp-content/uploads/2014/03/51-1-57.pdf
12. Blackham, J., & Benger, J. (2009). "Clearing" the cervical spine in conscious trauma patients. *Trauma, 11* (2), 93–109. https://doi.org/10.1177%2F1460408608101856
13. Paykin, G., O'Reilly, G., Ackland, H. M., & Mitra, B. (2017). The NEXUS criteria are insufficient to exclude cervical spine fractures in older blunt trauma patients. *Injury, 4*(5), 1020–1024. https://doi.org/10.1016/j.injury.2017.02.013
14. Kleinman, M. E., Brennan, E. E., Goldberg, Z. D., Swor, R. A., Terry, M., Bobrow, B. J., Rea, T. (2015). Part 5: Adult basic life support and cardiopulmonary resuscitation quality: 2015 American Heart Association guidelines update for cardiopulmonary resuscitation and emergency cardiovascular care. *Circulation, 132,* S414–S435. https://doi.org/10.1161/CIR.0000000000000259
15. Sulton, C. D., & Taylor, T. R. (2017). The pediatric airway and rapid sequence intubation in trauma [Monograph]. *Relias Media.* Retrieved from https://www.ahcmedia.com/articles/141562-the-pediatric-airway-and-rapid-sequence-intubation-in-trauma
16. Brown, C. A., III, & Walls, R. M. (2017). The decision to intubate. In C. A. Brown III, J. C. Skales, & N. W. Mick (Eds.), *The Walls manual of emergency airway management* (5th ed., pp. 1–43). Philadelphia, PA: Wolters Kluwer.
17. American College of Surgeons. (2018). Airway and ventilatory management. In *Advanced trauma life support: Student course manual* (10th ed., pp. 22–41). Chicago, IL: Author.
18. Graves, C. (2018). Cardiovascular system. In T. M. Hartjes (Ed.), *AACN core curriculum for high acuity, progressive and critical care nursing* (7th ed., pp. 142–199). St. Louis, MO: Saunders Elsevier.
19. Wilkinson, J. M., Trease, L. S., Barnett, K. L., & Smith, Mable H. (2015). *Fundamentals of nursing* (3rd ed.). Philadelphia, PA: F. A. Davis Company.
20. Russell, D. W., Janz, D. R., Emerson, W. L., Kay, A. K., Bernard, G.R., Zhao, Z., . . . Ware, L. B. (2017). Early exposure to hyperoxia and mortality in critically ill patients with severe traumatic injuries. *BMC Pulmonary Medicine, 17*(29), 1–7. https://doi.org/10.1186/s12890-017-0370-1
21. Vincent, J. L., Taccone, F. S., & He, X. (2017). Harmful effects of hyperoxia in postcardiac arrest, sepsis, traumatic brain injury, or stroke: The importance of individualized oxygen therapy in critically ill patients. *Canadian Respiratory Journal, 2017*, 1–7. https://doi.org/10.1155/2017/2834956
22. Helmerhorst, H. J. F., Roos-Blom, M.-J., vanWesterloo, D. J., & de Jong, E. (2015). Association between arterial hyperoxia and outcome in subsets of critical illness: A systemic review, meta-analysis, and meta-regression of cohort studies. *Critical Care Medicine, 24*(7), 1508–1519. https://doi.org/10.1097/CCM.0000000000000998
23. Taccone, F. S., Crippa, I. A., & Vincent, J.-L. (2017). Normobaric hyperoxia after stroke: A word of caution. *Expert Review of Neurotherapeutics, 18*(2), 92–93. https://doi.org/10.1080/14737175.2018.1414600
24. Long, B., Koyfman, A., & Vivirito, M. A. (2017). Capnography in the emergency department: A review of uses, waveforms, and limitations. *Journal of Emergency Medicine, 53*(6). 829–842. https://doi.org/10.1016/n.nemermed.2017.08.026
25. American Heart Association. (2016). *Basic life support for healthcare providers student manual.* Dallas, TX: Author.
26. Wernick, B., Hon, H. H., Mubang, R. N., Cipriano, A., Hughes, R., Rankin, D. D., . . . Riestenberg, M. S. (2015). Complications of needle thoracostomy: A comprehensive clinical review. *International Journal of Critical Illness & Injury Science, 5*(3), 160–169. https://doi.org/10.4103/2229-5151.164939
27. Akoglu, H., Celik, O. F., Celik, A., Ergelen, R., Onur, O., & Denizbasi, A. (2017). Diagnostic accuracy of the Extended Focused Abdominal Sonography for Trauma (E-FAST) performed by emergency physicians compared to computed tomography. *American Journal of Emergency Medicine, 36*(6), 1014–1017. https://doi.org/10.1016/j.ajem.2017.11.019
28. Verma, N., Robinson, J. D., & Gunn, M. L. (2018). Cardiac: Pericardial rupture and cardiac herniation in blunt trauma. *Radiology Case Reports, 13*(3), 573–575. https://doi.org/10.1016/j.radcr.2018.02.013
29. Hoseinikhah, H., Alizadeh, B., Shamloo, A. S., Imani, N., Sharifian, A., & Moeinipour, A. (2015). Right atrium laceration with pericardial tamponade: A rare presentation of blunt cardiac trauma. *Journal of Cardio-Thoracic Medicine, 3*(4), 384–386. http://doi.org/10.22038/jctm.2015.5849
30. Roth, M., Vaidya, R., Swartz, J., Zarling, B., Zhang, S., Walsh, C., & Macsuga, J. (2016). Application of circumferential compression device (binder) in pelvic injuries: Room for improvement. *Western Journal of Emergency Medicine: Integrating*

Emergency Care with Population Health, 17(6), 766–774. https://doi.org/10.5811/westjem.2016.7.30057

31. Milošević, D., Golić, D., Rakanović, D., Vujanović, V., & Janičić, D. (2014). Blunt chest trauma and pericardial tamponade. *Medical Journal, 20*(3), 203–204. Retrieved from http://www.kcus.ba/updf/Med%20Journal%202014%20br%203.pdf
32. Cohen, M. J., & Christie, S. A. (2016). New understanding of post injury coagulation and resuscitation. *International Journal of Surgery, 33*(Part B), 242–245. https://doi.org/10.1016/j.ijsu.2016.05.037
33. Mitra, B., Tullio, F., Cameron, P. A., & Fitzgerald, M. (2012). Trauma patients with the "triad of death." *Emergency Medicine Journal, 29*(8), 622–625. http://doi.org/10.1136/emj.2011.113167
34. Murphy, P., Colwell, C., & Pineda, G. (2012). Understand the trauma triad of death. *EMS World, 41*(20), 44–51. Retrieved from https://www.emsworld.com/article/10565011/understand-trauma-triad-death
35. Mizobata, Y. (2017).). Damage control resuscitation: A practical approach for severely hemorrhagic patients and its effects on trauma surgery. *Journal of Intensive Care, 5*(4). https://doi.org/10.1186/s40560-016-0197-5
36. Nosanov, L., Inaba, K., Okoye, O., Resnick., S., Upperman, J., Shulman, I., . . . Demetriades, D. (2016). Association of Women Surgeons: The impact of blood product rations in massively transfused pediatric trauma patients. *American Journal of Surgery, 206*(5), 655–660. https://doi.org/10.1016/j.amsurg.2013.07.009
37. Green, S. M., Haukoos, J. S., & Schringer, D. L. (2017). How to measure the Glasgow Coma Scale. *Annals of Emergency Medicine, 70*(2), 158–160. https://doi.org/10.1016/j.annemergmed.2016.12.016
38. American Association of Critical Care Nurses. (2017). Glasgow Coma Scale stands the test of time. *AACN Bold Voices, 9*(8), 18. Retrieved from http://www.nxtbook.com/nxtbooks/aacn/boldvoices_201708/index.php#/18
39. Hansen, B., Quick, J., Sinkovits, R., & Smith, J. C. (2014). Glasgow Coma Scale: How to improve and enhance documentation. *Journal of Trauma Nursing, 21*(3), 122–124. https://doi.org/10.1097/JTN.0000000000000044 10.1097/JTN.0000000000000044
40. Chen, B., Grothe, C., & Schaller, K. (2013). Validation of a new neurological score (FOUR Score) in the assessment of neurosurgical patients with severely impaired consciousness. *Acta Neurochirurgica, 155*(11), 2133–2139. https://doi.org/10.1007/s00701-013-1854-2
41. Smith, E. R., & Amin-Hanjani, S. (2017, June 21). Evaluation and management of elevated intracranial pressure in adults. *UpToDate*. Retrieved from https://www.uptodate.com/contents/evaluation-and-management-of-elevated-intracranial-pressure-in-adults
42. Bradley, C. (2017). Perceptions of adult hospitalized patients on family presence during cardiopulmonary resuscitation. *American Journal of Critical Care, 26*(2), 103–110. https://doi.org/10.4037/ajcc2017550
43. Powers, K. A. (2017). Barriers to family presence during resuscitation and strategies for improving nurses' invitation to families. *Applied Nursing Research, 38*, 22–28. https://doi.org/10.1016/j.apnr.2017.08.007
44. Bloos, F., Zhang, Z., & Boulain, T. (2016). Lactate-guided resuscitation saves lives: Yes. *Intensive Care Medicine, 42*(3), 466–469. https://doi.org/10.1007/s00134-015-4196-0
45. Mitchell, C. (2016). Tissue oxygenation/monitoring as a guide for trauma resuscitation. *Critical Care Medicine, 36*(3), 12–70. https://doi.org/10.4037/ccn2016206
46. Yousef, R., & Carr, J. A. (2014). Blunt cardiac trauma: A review of the current knowledge and management. *Annals of Thoracic Surgery, 98*(3), 1134–1140. https://doi.org/10.1016/j.athoracsur.2014.04.043
47. Kalbitz, M., Pressmar, J., Stecher, J., Weber, B., Weiss, M., Schwartz, S., . . . Huber-Lang, M. (2017). The role of troponin in blunt cardiac injury after multiple trauma in humans. *World Journal of Surgery, 41*(1), 162–169. https://doi.org/10.1007/s00268-016-3650-7
48. Huai-min, L., Qiu-lin, C., Er-yong, A., & Jai, H. (2016). Sternal fractures and delayed cardiac tamponade due to a severe blunt chest trauma. *American Journal of Emergency Medicine, 34*(4), 758.e1–758.e3. https://doi.org/10.1016/j.ajem.2015.07.075
49. American College of Surgeons. (2018). Thoracic trauma. In *Advanced trauma life support: Student course manual* (10th ed., pp. 62–81). Chicago, IL: Author.
50. Ehieli, E., Yalamuri, S., Brudney, C. S., & Pyati, S. (2017). Analgesia in the surgical intensive care unit. *Postgraduate Medical Journal, 93*, 38–45. https://doi.org/10.1136/postgradmedj-2016-134047
51. Häske, D., Böttiger, B. W., Bouillon, B., Fischer, M., Gaier, G., Gliwitzky, B., . . . Bernhard, M. (2017). Analgesia in patients with trauma in emergency medicine: A systematic review and meta-analysis. *Deutsches Ärzteblatt International, 114*(46), 785–792. https://doi.org/10.3238/arztebl.2017.0785
52. Polomano, R. C., Fillman, M., Giordano, N. A., Vallerand, A. H., Nicely, K. L., & Jungquist, C. R. (2017). Multimodal analgesia for acute postoperative and trauma-related pain. *American Journal of Nursing, 117*(3), S12–S26. https://doi.org/10.1097/01.NAJ.0000513527.71934.73
53. Montgomery, K., Hall, A. B., & Keriazes, G. (2015). Pharmacist's impact on acute pain management during trauma resuscitation. *Journal of Trauma Nursing, 22*(2), 87–90. https://doi.org/10.1097/JTN.0000000000000112
54. Oyler, D., Bernard, A. C., VanHoose, J. D., Parli, S. E., Ellis, C. S., Li, D., . . . Chang, P. K. (2018). Minimizing opioid use after acute major trauma. *American Journal of Health-System Pharmacy, 75*(3), 105–110. https://doi.org/10.2146/ajhp161021
55. Griggs, R. C., Jozefowicz, R. F., & Aminoff, M. J. (2016). Approach to the patient with neurologic disease. In L. Goldman & A. I. Schafer (Eds.), *Goldman-Cecil medicine* (25th ed., pp. 2338–2346). Philadelphia, PA: Elsevier Saunders.
56. Heegaard, W. G. (2017, July 26). Skull fractures in adults. *UpToDate*. Retrieved from https://www.uptodate.com/contents/skull-fractures-in-adults
57. Sunder, R., & Tyler, K. (2013). Basal skull fracture and the halo sign. *Canadian Medical Association Journal, 185*(5), 416. https://doi.org/10.1503/cmaj.120055
58. Welch, K. C. (2018, April 24). CSF rhinorrhea. *Medscape*. Retrieved from http://emedicine.medscape.com/article/861126-overview

59. Savage, A. R. (2014). Evidence-based practice in relation to indwelling urinary catheters. *Africa Health, 36*(1), 25–28. Retrieved from http://africa-health.com/wp-content/uploads/2015/10/10.-Catheters.pdf
60. Lam, T. B., Omar, M. I., Fisher, E., Gillies, K., & MacLennan, S. (2014). Types of indwelling urethral catheters for short-term catheterisation in hospitalised adults. *Cochrane Database of Systematic Reviews*, 9. https://doi.org/10.1002/14651858.CD004013.pub4
61. Conway, L. J., & Larson E. L. (2012). Guidelines to prevent catheter-associated urinary tract infection: 1980 to 2010. *Heart & Lung, 41*(3), 271–283. https://doi.org/10.1016/j.hrtlng.2011.08.001
62. Runyon, M. S. (2018, March 1). Blunt genitourinary trauma: Initial evaluation and Management. *UpToDate*. Retrieved from https://www.uptodate.com/contents/blunt-genitourinary-trauma-initial-evaluation-and-management
63. Conrad, B. P., Del Rossi, G., Horodyski, M. B., Prasarn, M. L., Alemi, Y., & Rechtine, G. R. (2012). Eliminating log rolling as a spine trauma order. *Surgical Neurology International, 3*(Suppl. S3), S188–S197. https://doi.org/10.4103%2F2152-7806.98584
64. Leech, C., Porter, K., & Bosanko, C. (2014). Log-rolling a blunt major trauma patient is inappropriate in the primary survey. *Emergency Medicine Journal, 31*(1), 86. https://doi.org/10.1136/emermed-2013-203283
65. Rodrigues, I. F. (2017). To log-roll or not to log-roll—that is the question! A review of the use of the log-roll for patients with pelvic fractures. *International Journal of Orthopaedic and Trauma Nursing, 27*, 36–40. https://doi.org/10.1016/j.ijotn.2017.05.001
66. Horodyski, M., Conrad, B. P., Del Rossi, G., DiPaola, C. P., & Rechtine, G. R. (2011). Removing a patient from the spine board: Is the lift and slide safer than the log roll? *Journal of Trauma-Injury Infection and Critical Care, 70*(5), 1282–1285. https://doi.org/10.1097/TA.0b013e31820ff2bc
67. Emergency Nurses Association. (2016). *ENA Topic Brief: Avoiding the log roll maneuver: Alternative methods for safe patient handling*. Des Plaines, IL: Author. Retrieved from https://www.ena.org/docs/default-source/resource-library/practice-resources/topic-briefs/avoiding-the-log-roll-maneuver.pdf?sfvrsn=78887c44_8
68. Conrad, B. P., Marchese, D. L., Rechtine, G. R., & Horodyski, M. (2012). Motion in the unstable thoracolumbar spine when spine boarding a prone patient. *Journal of Spinal Cord Medicine, 35*(1), 53–57. https://doi.org/10.1179/2045772311Y.0000000045
69. Kornhall, D. K., Jørgensen, J. J., Brommeland, T., Hyldmo, P. K., Asbjørnsen, H., Dolven, T., . . . Jeppesen, E. (2017). The Norwegian guidelines for the prehospital management of adult trauma patients with potential spinal injury. *Scandinavian Journal of Trauma, Resuscitation, and Emergency Medicine*, 25(2). https://doi.org/10.1186/s13049-016-0345-x
70. National Institute for Health and Care Excellence. (2017). Fractures (complex): Assessment and management. Retrieved from https://www.nice.org.uk/guidance/ng37
71. Docimo, S., Diggs, L., Crankshaw, L., Lee, Y., & Vinces, F. (2015). No evidence supporting the routine use of digital rectal examinations in trauma patients. *Indian Journal of Surgery, 77*(4), 265–269. https:/doi.org/10.1007/s12262-015-1283-y
72. Fitzgerald, M., Cameron, P., Mackenzie, C., Farrow, N., Scicuna, P., Gocentas, R., . . . Rosenfeld, J. V. (2011). Trauma resuscitation errors and computer-assisted decision support. *Archives of Surgery, 146*(2), 218–225. https:/doi.org/10.1001/archsurg.2010.333
73. Fischer, P. E., Perina, D. G., Delbridge, T. R., Fallat, M. E., Salamone, J. P., Dodd, J., Bulger, E. L. M., & Gestring, M. L. (2018). Spinal motion restriction in the trauma patient: A joint position statement. Prehospital Emergency Care. https://doi.org/10.1080/10903127.2018.1481476
74. Sundstrem, T., Asbjornsen, H., Habiba, S., Sunde, G. A., & Wester, K. (2014). Prehospital use of cervical collars in trauma patients: A critical review. *Journal of Neurotrauma, 31*(6), 531–540. https://doi.org/10.1089%2Fneu.2013.3094
75. Alam, H. B. (2017). Trauma care: Finding a better way. *Plos Medicine, 14*(7), e1002350. https://doi.org/10.1371/journal.pmed.1002350
76. Li, Y., & Alam, H. B. (2012). Creating a pro-survival and anti-inflammatory phenotype by modulation of acetylation in models of hemorrhagic and septic shock. *Advances in Experimental Medicine and Biology, 710*, 107–133. https://doi.org/10.1007/978-1-4419-5638-5_11
77. Halaweish, I., Nikolian, V., Georgoff, P., Li, Y., & Alam, H. B. (2015). Creating a "prosurvival phenotype" through histone deacetylase inhibition: Past, present, and future. *Shock, 44*(Suppl. 1), 6–16. https://doi.org/10.1097/SHK.0000000000000319
78. Shults, C., Sailhamer, E. A., Li, Y., Liu, B., Tabbara, M., Butt M. U., . . . Alam, H. B. (2008). Surviving blood loss without fluid resuscitation. *Journal of Trauma, 64*(3), 629–640. https://doi.org/10.1097/TA.0b013e3181650ff3
79. Alam, H. B., Shuja, F., Butt, M. U., Duggan, M., Li, Y., Zacharias N., & Velmahos, G. C. (2009). Surviving blood loss without blood transfusion in a swine poly-trauma model. *Surgery, 146*(2), 325–333. https://doi.org/10.1016/j.surg. 2009.04.007
80. Kim, K., Li, Y., Jin, G., Chong, W., Liu, B., Lu, J., . . . Alam, H. B. (2012). Effect of valproic acid on acute lung injury in a rodent model of intestinal ischemia reperfusion. *Resuscitation, 83*(2), 243–248. https://doi.org/10.1016/j. resuscitation.2011.07.029
81. Behringer, W., Safar, P., Wu, X., Kentner, R., Radovsky, A., Kochanek, P. M., . . . Tisherman, S. A. (2003). Survival without brain damage after clinical death of 60–120 minutes in dogs using suspended animation by profound hypothermia. *Critical Care Medicine, 31*(5), 1523–1531. https://doi.org/10.1097/01.CCM.0000063450.73967.40
82. Taylor, M. J., Bailes, J. E., Elrifai, A. M., Shih, S. R., Teeple, E., Leavitt, M. L., . . . Maroon, J. C. (1995). A new solution for life without blood: Asanguineous low-flow perfusion of a whole body perfusate during 3 hours of cardiac arrest and profound hypothermia. *Circulation, 91*(2), 431–444. https://doi.org/10.1161/01.cir.91.2.431
83. Alam, H. B., Bowyer, M. W., Koustova, E., Gushchin, V., Anderson, D., Stanton, K., . . . Rhee, P. (2002). Learning and memory is preserved following induced asanguineous hyperkalemic hypothermic arrest in a swine model of traumatic exsanguination. *Surgery, 132*(2), 278–288. https://doi.org/10.1067/msy.2002.125787

CHAPTER 4

Airway and Ventilation

Meghan L. McDonald, MSN, RN

OBJECTIVES

Upon completion of this chapter, the learner will be able to:

1. Describe pathophysiologic changes as a basis for assessment of the trauma patient with actual or potential airway and ventilation complications.
2. Demonstrate the nursing airway assessment of the trauma patient.
3. Plan appropriate interventions for the trauma patient with actual or potential airway and ventilation complications.
4. Evaluate the effectiveness of nursing interventions for the trauma patient with actual or potential airway and ventilation complications.

Knowledge of normal anatomy and physiology serves as a foundation for understanding anatomic derangements and pathophysiologic processes that may result from trauma. Before reading this chapter, it is strongly suggested that the learner review the following material. The anatomy material is not emphasized in the classroom but may be the basis of skill evaluation assessments and the basis of questions for testing purposes.

Anatomy and Physiology of the Airway

The pulmonary system consists of both the conducting and respiratory airways. The conducting structures—commonly referred to as the "upper airway"—include the nose, mouth, pharynx, larynx, epiglottis, and trachea (**Figure 4-1**). These structures serve to humidify, filter, and transport inhaled air from the atmosphere to the alveoli. The respiratory airway—that is, the lower airway—is composed of the bronchi, lungs, and alveoli. The alveoli cover a large surface area and are the main functional unit of the pulmonary system, responsible for circulatory gas exchange.[1]

Upper Airway

In the upper airway, the nasal passages are the primary entryway for air into the lungs.[2] Coarse hairs line the outer nasal passages and filter out dust and other particles. A mucous membrane within the nasal cavity contains small blood vessels and provides warmth and moisture.

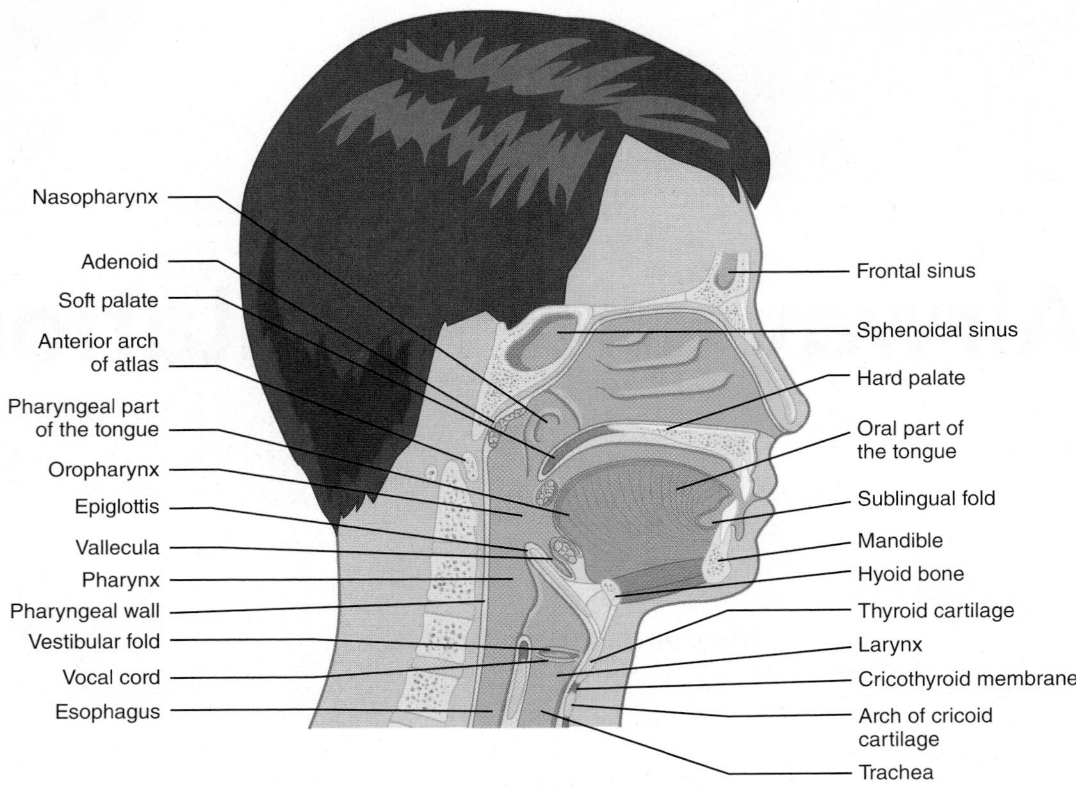

Figure 4-1 *Upper airway structures.*

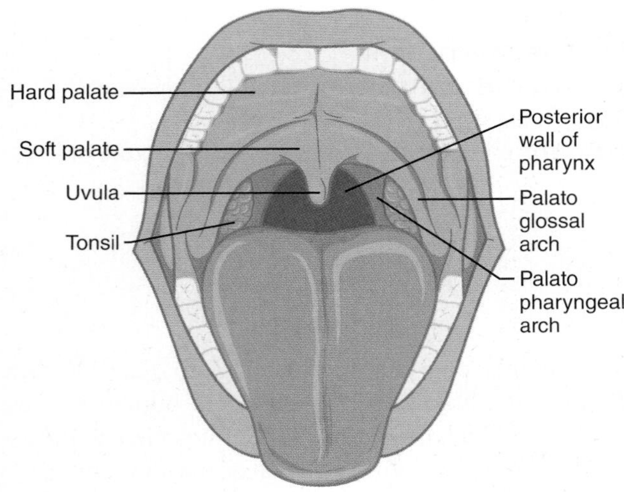

Figure 4-2 *Structures in the mouth.*

The mouth is the secondary passageway for inhaled air (**Figure 4-2**). Presence of swelling, blood, vomitus, or foreign objects in the mouth may cause a mechanical upper airway obstruction and prevent adequate ventilation. In patients who are unconscious, airway obstruction caused by the tongue is of particular concern.

The nasopharynx and oropharynx meet at the base of the skull and extend to the lower border of the cricoid cartilage. The structures within the nasopharynx and oropharynx serve as guides to locate the trachea during the intubation process.

The epiglottis is a cartilaginous structure that lies on top of the larynx. This structure serves to route air into the lungs and route liquids and foods into the esophagus, diverting them from the larynx during swallowing.

The larynx is a tubular structure composed of cartilage that connects the oropharynx to the trachea. Its primary function is to allow air into the trachea. The larynx is the most heavily innervated sensory structure in the body (**Figure 4-3**). The vagus nerve (cranial nerve X) serves as the primary parasympathetic nerve. Stimulation of the vagus nerve during intubation may activate the parasympathetic nervous system, leading to a vagal response, particularly in infants and young children.[3]

Below the larynx is the cricothyroid membrane, which extends from the upper surface of the cricoid cartilage to the inferior border of the thyroid cartilage (Adam's apple). The cricothyroid membrane is approximately 2 mm in height and 3 mm in width.[4] In women, the neck is relatively smaller and the cricoid cartilage is located slightly higher than in men.

The trachea begins just below the larynx and ends at the carina; it has an average length of 10 to 12 cm in an adult. The average tracheal diameter is 15 to 25 mm in an adult male, and 10 to 21 mm in an adult female.[5] The trachea

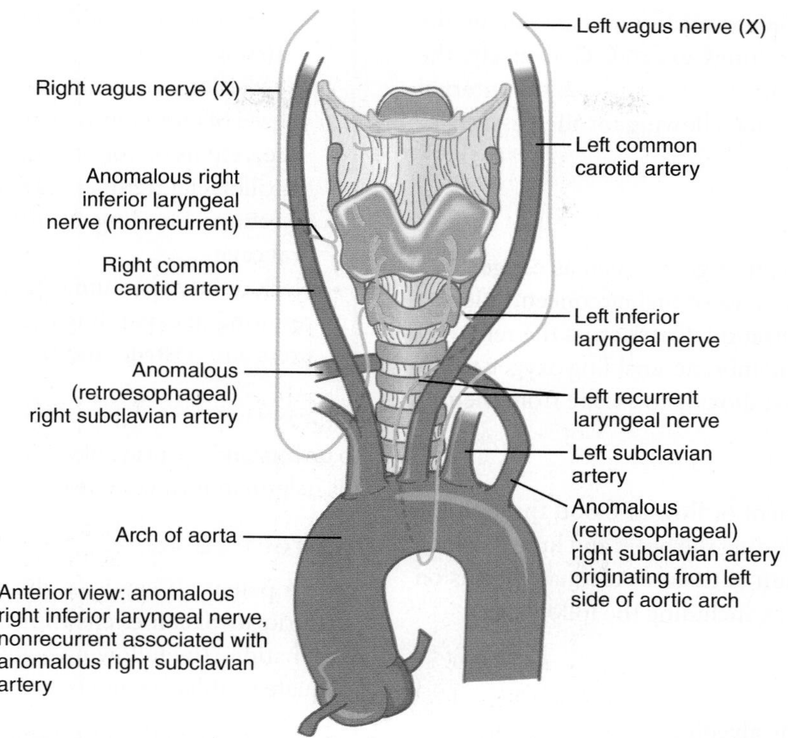

Figure 4-3 *Innervation of the larynx by the vagus nerve.*

is significantly shorter in infants and children, leading to easy displacement of this structure with head movement.[6]

Lower Airway

The lower airway is located within the thoracic cage, and includes the lungs and the bronchial tree (where the right bronchus and the left bronchus branch off from the trachea).[1] The carina, located where the two primary bronchial branches meet, is composed mostly of nerves. When stimulated, such as by suctioning, bronchospasm or severe coughing may result.

The bronchi and the bronchioles, composed mostly of epithelial tissue and smooth muscle, conduct atmospheric air to the alveoli, where gas exchange takes place. Certain anatomic features of the bronchi are clinically significant and worth noting. Specifically, the right main bronchus is shorter and wider than the left main bronchus and branches off from the carina at an almost straight angle. These structural characteristics enable easy introduction of an endotracheal tube, resulting in a right main stem intubation.

The mediastinum is bordered anteriorly by the sternum, posteriorly by the 12 thoracic vertebrae, and inferiorly by the diaphragm. The diaphragm serves the critical respiratory function of controlling the rate and volume of inspiration. The base of each lung rests against the diaphragm; the apex of each lung extends approximately 2 to 3 cm above where the clavicle meets the sternum.[7]

Physiology

Three processes transfer oxygen from the air to the lungs and bloodstream[1]:

- *Ventilation:* The active, mechanical movement of air into and out of the lungs
- *Diffusion:* The passive movement of gases from an area of higher concentration to an area of lower concentration
- *Perfusion:* The movement of blood to and from the lungs as a delivery medium of oxygen to the entire body

Ventilation

Ventilation, or breathing, begins with inhalation of air through the upper airway.[1] It is the mechanical process of air movement into and throughout the lungs. Ventilation relies heavily on signals from the nervous system in conjunction with properly functioning lungs. Signals from the brain stem direct the pharyngeal muscles to open the pharynx during inhalation. During inspiration, the diaphragm contracts and flattens, thereby increasing the size of the thorax, and extending it into the tenth or twelfth intercostal space. During expiration, the diaphragm relaxes and the lungs recoil, decreasing the size of the pleural cavity to the fourth intercostal space. The external intercostal muscles raise the rib cage and increase the anterior-to-posterior diameter of the thoracic cavity, and the lungs expand. Conversely, the anterior-to-posterior diameter decreases as the internal intercostal muscles contract, allowing for the passive exhalation of the lungs.

Diffusion

Diffusion is the movement of gases (such as oxygen and carbon dioxide) from an area of higher concentration to an area of lower concentration. Gases cross the relatively thin alveolar–capillary membrane, enabling oxygen to enter the alveoli and carbon dioxide to escape from them.[1]

Perfusion

Perfusion is the movement or flow of blood through the circulatory system (including the heart and lungs), which results in the oxygenation of tissues. Adequate perfusion depends on many factors, including the following:

- Airway patency
- Ventilatory effort
- Gas exchange in the alveoli
- Hemoglobin's oxygen-carrying capacity
- Cardiac output

Introduction

A priority objective in managing a trauma patient—after control of obvious life-threatening external hemorrhage—is airway assessment and the establishment of a patent, protected airway. Knowledge of airway and ventilatory management provides the trauma nurse with the understanding and skill set necessary to effectively manage a trauma patient's airway and ventilation so as to support the delivery of oxygenated blood to the brain and other vital organs.[8]

Pathophysiology as a Basis for Assessment Findings

Airway pathophysiology may involve airway obstruction, oxygenation, ventilation, and ineffective ventilation.

Airway Obstruction

The trauma patient's airway may become obstructed in many ways and due to certain circumstances[9]:

- Altered level of consciousness:
  - The tongue: This is a common cause of obstruction in patients who are not alert.
  - Alcohol or other substances: Patients who are under the influence may have an altered level of consciousness and be unable maintain a patent airway.
  - Secretions or vomit: Patients who have an altered level of consciousness may lack the ability to clear secretions or vomitus by swallowing or coughing.
- Maxillofacial trauma: May cause edema, increased secretions, bleeding, or dislodged teeth within the oral cavity
- Neck or larynx trauma: May cause vascular injuries resulting in expanding hematomas that can compress and obstruct the airway

Oxygenation and Ventilation

To understand the principles of oxygenation and ventilation it is helpful to review some terminology (**Table 4-1**).[8,10-14]

Ineffective Ventilation

Once a patent airway is established and confirmed, the next priority becomes ensuring adequate ventilation and oxygenation. The following factors may contribute to inadequate ventilation and oxygenation:

- Altered mental status: From brain injury, prolonged loss of consciousness, increased intracranial pressure, hypoxia, medications, substance abuse, or alcohol use.
- High cervical spine trauma or spinal cord injury: May cause disruption of the sympathetic pathways.
- Blunt thoracic trauma: May result in chest wall instability and ineffective ventilation.
- Penetrating thoracic trauma: May result in a hemothorax or a pneumothorax.
- Underlying pulmonary comorbidities: Conditions such as chronic obstructive pulmonary disease, severe asthma, community-acquired pneumonia, obesity hypoventilation syndrome, or chronic respiratory failure may lead to hypercapnic respiratory failure.[15]
- Advanced age: Older patients may have decreased pulmonary reserve.
- Tachypnea: A sign of compensation for diminished oxygenation and perfusion.

Nursing Care of the Trauma Patient with Airway and Ventilation Problems

Refer to Chapter 3, "Initial Assessment," for the systematic approach to care of the trauma patient. The following assessment parameters are specific to airway and ventilation.

TABLE 4-1 Oxygenation and Ventilation Terminology

Component	Definition	Measurement	Normal Range
Oxygenation			
SaO_2	Percentage of red cells with hemoglobin bound to oxygen	Arterial blood gas (ABG)	> 94%
SpO_2	Peripheral oxygen saturation	Pulse oximeter	> 94%
PaO_2	Amount of oxygen dissolved in plasma	ABG	80–100 mm Hg
Ventilation			
$PaCO_2$	Partial pressure of carbon dioxide (CO_2) in arterial blood	ABG	35–45 mm Hg
$ETCO_2$	Maximum concentration of CO_2 at the end of each breath	Colorimetric	2–5% $ETCO_2$ (15–38 mm Hg)
		Capnometer or capnography	35–45 mm Hg
Delivery			
FiO_2	Fraction of inspired oxygen	—	21–100%
Room air	Ambient air oxygen concentration	—	0.21 FiO_2 (21%)
Condition			
Hypoxemia	Insufficient level of oxygen in the blood	PaO_2	80–100 mm Hg
Hypoxia	Inadequate oxygen supply to tissue	PaO_2	80–100 mm Hg
Hyperoxia	Excess of supplemental oxygen in blood	PaO_2	100 mm Hg

Data from Feller-Kopman, D., & Schwartzstein, R. (2017, September 8). Mechanisms, causes, and effects of hypercapnia. *UpToDate*. Retrieved from https://www.uptodate.com/contents/mechanisms-causes-and-effects-of-hypercapnia; Hyzy, R. C., & McSparron, J. (2018, May 8). Overview of mechanical ventilation. *UpToDate*. Retrieved from https://www.uptodate.com/contents/overview-of-mechanical-ventilation; Krauss, B., & Falk, J. (2018, January 19). Carbon dioxide monitoring (capnography). *UpToDate*. Retrieved from https://www.uptodate.com/contents/carbon-dioxide-monitoring-capnography; Mechem, C. C. (2017, December 13). Pulse oximetry. *UpToDate*. Retrieved from https://www.uptodate.com/contents/pulse-oximetry; Theodore, A. C. (2017, March 16). Arterial blood gases. *UpToDate*. Retrieved from https://www.uptodate.com/contents/arterial-blood-gases; Theodore, A. C. (2017, November 7). Oxygenation and mechanisms of hypoxemia. *UpToDate*. Retrieved from https://www.uptodate.com/contents/oxygenation-and-mechanisms-of-hypoxemia.

Preparation

Preparation includes safe practice and triage.

Safe Practice, Safe Care

Effective oxygenation and ventilation are essential components for an optimal outcome in the trauma patient. Preparation for the arrival of the trauma patient with potential airway or ventilation compromise includes the following measures:

- Equipment: Assure availability and working order of equipment and supplies in various sizes to accommodate all patients.
- Education: Trauma education includes a review of airway and ventilation as well as hands-on practice in management of the airway, early identification of changes or deterioration in patient condition, and proficiency with utilizing and troubleshooting relevant equipment.
- Communication: Determine whether the appropriately trained personnel are all present, whether anyone else needs to be paged to the trauma resuscitation, who will function in which roles, and who will perform identified tasks.

Triage

The prehospital report may provide clues to the patient's potential risks for airway and ventilation problems:

- Mechanism of injury
- Injuries sustained

- Facial, neck, or thoracic trauma
- Inhalation injury and/or thermal or chemical burns
- Signs and symptoms
  - Altered mental status
  - Complaints of dyspnea, dysphagia, or dysphonia
  - Indications of substance use
  - Nausea or vomiting

Primary Survey

The primary survey begins with assessing the patient's alertness and airway.

A: Alertness and Airway

In the trauma patient population, failure to adequately assess the airway and recognize the need for an airway intervention can result in a preventable death.[9] After recognition of and intervention for life-threatening external hemorrhage, recognition of an airway problem is an essential first step. Once the problem has been identified, lifesaving interventions can be implemented.

Assess for Alertness

Use the AVPU mnemonic to determine the patient's level of alertness (**Table 4-2**). If the patient is not alert, the ability to protect his or her airway may be lost.

Open the Airway

Until injury to the cervical spine has been ruled out, maintain the spine in proper alignment. While maintaining cervical spinal motion restriction, assess for airway patency:

- Talk to the patient. Asking for the patient's name, current location ("Do you know where you are?"), and ability to open his or her mouth is a simple technique to determine whether a patient is alert.
- If the patient is unable to open his or her mouth, responds only to pain, or is unresponsive, use the jaw-thrust maneuver (**Figure 4-4**) to open the airway and assess for obstruction.
  - Stand at the head of the bed, place the index fingers under the angle of the lower jaw on each side, with the thumbs on each cheekbone for stabilization, and move the mandible forward and upward.[12]
  - In any patient in whom cervical spine (c-spine) injury is suspected, c-spine stabilization must be maintained to minimize the risk of further injury. This is best achieved with two operators performing the jaw-thrust procedure. While one operator maintains manual inline stabilization, the second operator performs the jaw thrust procedure previously described.[16]

Once the airway is open, continue with the airway assessment:

- Inspect for the following:
  - Tongue obstruction
  - Loose or missing teeth
  - Foreign objects
  - Blood, vomitus, or secretions
  - Edema
  - Facial burns or evidence of inhalation injury (e.g., soot, singed facial hairs, blistering to the face)
- Listen for the following:
  - Obstructive airway sounds such as snoring, gurgling, stridor, or hoarse voice
- Palpate for the following:
  - Bony deformity (from fractures)
  - Subcutaneous emphysema (from pneumothorax, tracheal or esophageal laceration)

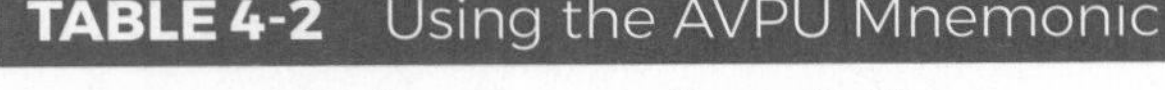

TABLE 4-2 Using the AVPU Mnemonic

Letter	Level	Description
A	Alert	The patient is alert and responsive
V	Verbal	The patient responds to verbal stimulation
P	Pain	The patient responds only to painful stimulation
U	Unresponsive	The patient is unresponsive

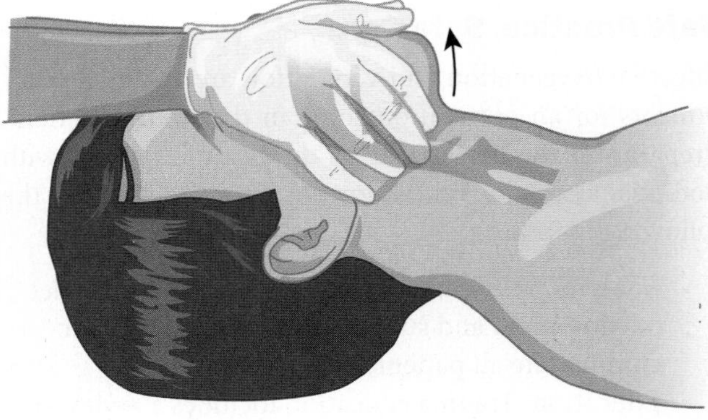

Figure 4-4 *Jaw-thrust maneuver.*

If the patient has a definitive airway in place, assess for proper placement by using the following techniques:

- Inspect for equal and adequate rise and fall of the chest.
- Auscultate for gurgling over the epigastrium.
- Auscultate for bilateral breath sounds.
- Use capnometry to assess for presence of exhaled carbon dioxide. (See Appendix 4-3 for more information.)

Airway Interventions

If the airway is patent, proceed with the following in mind:

- An airway that is currently patent is not guaranteed to stay that way.
  - Note any potential risks for airway obstruction—injury to the mouth, active bleeding, blistering of the oral mucosa, decreased level of consciousness.
- Continually monitor airway patency while the trauma patient assessment continues.

If the airway is *not* patent, then do the following:

- Use the two-person jaw-thrust maneuver to open the airway and maintain cervical spine stabilization.
- Suction for blood, vomitus, or secretions, using care not to stimulate the gag reflex, which may cause vomiting and aspiration.
- Reassess the airway:
  - If suctioning does not relieve the airway obstruction, the tongue may be the cause.
- Insert an airway adjunct (see "Airway Adjuncts"):
  - Oral and nasal airways may be used to support spontaneous ventilation.
  - Keep in mind that airway adjuncts are temporary measures, to be used until a definitive airway is established.
  - Airway adjuncts facilitate bag-mask ventilations.
- Consider the need for a definitive airway (see "Definitive Airways").
- Reassess the effectiveness of all interventions.

B: Breathing and Ventilation

To assess breathing, expose the patient's chest and complete the following steps:

- Inspect for the following:
  - Spontaneous breathing
  - Symmetric and adequate rise and fall of the chest
  - Depth, pattern, and rate of respirations
  - Work of breathing, including:
    - Use of accessory muscles, including diaphragmatic or abdominal breathing in adult patients
    - Suprasternal, substernal, or intercostal retractions in the pediatric patient
    - Nasal flaring, grunting, or head bobbing
    - Skin color
      - Observe for pallor, duskiness, or cyanosis
    - Jugular venous distention (JVD) and position of the trachea
      - Tracheal deviation and JVD are late signs that may indicate a tension pneumothorax
    - Signs of inhalation injury
      - Singed nasal hairs
      - Blistering of the oral mucosa
      - Facial burns
    - Sucking chest wounds or open pneumothoraces
- Auscultate for the following:
  - Diminished or absent breath sounds, which may be the result of airway obstruction, inadequate ventilation as a response to pain, pneumothorax, or hemothorax.
  - When auscultating lung sounds, listen bilaterally at the second intercostal space midclavicular line and at the fifth intercostal space at the anterior axillary line.
- Palpate for the following:
  - Tenderness and swelling
  - Jugular venous pulsations at the suprasternal notch or in the supraclavicular area
  - Bony deformities or crepitus (from sternal or rib fractures)
  - Subcutaneous emphysema—may be a sign of a pneumothorax or pneumomediastinum
  - Soft-tissue injury (e.g., contusions and lacerations)

Breathing Interventions

If breathing is present, assess the patient for ventilation effectiveness, including skin color and respiratory effort.

If breathing is absent, then do the following:

- Open the airway and reassess breathing.
- Insert an airway adjunct (see "Airway Adjuncts").
- Use a bag-mask device connected to an oxygen source to administer 10 to 12 normal breaths per minute or one breath every 5 to 6 seconds.[17]
- Reassess the effectiveness of the interventions.
- Prepare for insertion of a definitive airway.

If ventilation is effective, consider the following points:

- Oxygenation in the trauma patient is an essential resuscitative priority.[8]
- Initially, deliver oxygen with a flow rate of 10 to 15 L/minute via a nonrebreather mask.
- To prevent hyperoxia and its deleterious effects, rapid weaning of oxygen (maintaining pulse oximetry [SpO_2] at 94% or greater) should begin as soon as the patient is stabilized and arterial oxygenation can be assessed.[13]
- Reassess ventilation effectiveness.

If ventilation is ineffective, do the following:

- Use a bag-mask device connected to an oxygen source at 15 L/minute to support breathing and ventilation. Bag-mask ventilation is an essential skill of airway management and can require practice to master.[16] Form a tight seal between the mask and the patient's face using the "E-C" technique:
  - Cover the patient's nose and mouth with the mask. The mask should not extend beyond the chin. (The mask size may need to be changed to ensure a proper fit.)
  - Position the fingers so the pinky, ring, and middle fingers spread along the mandible (forming the letter "E"). The pinky finger should be placed by the angle of the jaw with the middle finger under the chin, lifting the jaw upward.
  - Place the thumb and index finger on top of the mask so that they form the letter "C" around the neck of the mask, pressing the mask into the patient's face.
  - Squeeze the bag just enough to produce visible chest rise every 5 to 6 seconds (10 to 12 breaths per minute).[17]
  - Excessive volume delivered with the bag-mask and rapid rates have been associated with gastric distention, which can cause vomiting and aspiration, as well as barotrauma.[18]
- Anticipate the need for a definitive airway.
- Life-threatening injuries require rapid identification and immediate intervention before proceeding to the next step in the primary survey. These injuries include the following (see Chapter 7, "Thoracic and Neck Trauma," for more information):
  - Tension pneumothorax
  - Flail chest
  - Hemothorax
  - Open pneumothorax
- Consider other conditions as a source of inadequate ventilations:
  - Preexisting pulmonary disease
  - Circumferential burns to the chest
  - Pain
  - Spinal cord injury, which may cause diaphragmatic breathing and inadequate ventilation and/or paralysis of the intercostal muscles
  - Multiple rib fractures
  - Blunt thoracic trauma

Airway Adjuncts

Airway adjuncts include nasopharyngeal and oropharyngeal airways.

Nasopharyngeal Airway

A nasopharyngeal airway (NPA), also known as a nasal trumpet, is a hollow soft tube that is inserted into the naris and down into the posterior pharynx. Use of an NPA is contraindicated in patients with facial trauma or a suspected basilar skull fracture. When inserting an NPA, consider the following points[16]:

- Use the largest diameter that can be easily inserted into the patient's naris.
- Select the correct length by measuring from the tip of the patient's nose to the tip of the patient's earlobe.
- Apply a water-soluble lubricant to the NPA before insertion, then:
  - Insert the NPA with the bevel facing the nasal septum.
  - Direct the airway toward the posterior pharynx until the flange rests against the naris.
  - If resistance is met, rotate the NPA slightly.
  - Most commercially available NPAs are made to be inserted into the right naris.
  - If inserting an NPA into the left naris, rotate the NPA upside down so the bevel faces the septum before inserting.
- Reassess airway patency and determine the need for a definitive airway.
- Reassess for adequate ventilation and oxygenation. If inadequate, consider the use of bag-mask ventilation to support the patient.

Oropharyngeal Airway

An oropharyngeal airway (OPA) is used in the unresponsive patient as a temporary measure to facilitate ventilation with a bag-mask device or spontaneous ventilation until the patient can be intubated. When using an OPA, it is important to measure for the correct fit. If the airway adjunct is too large, it may occlude the patient's airway, hinder the use of a face mask, or damage laryngeal structures. If it is too small, it may occlude the airway by pushing the tongue back. A correctly sized OPA will hold the tongue in the normal anatomic position and follows its natural curvature. When inserting an OPA, consider the following points[8]:

- An OPA should be considered only in a patient who is unresponsive and unable to maintain their airway.
- Insertion of an OPA in a responsive patient could result in vomiting and aspiration.
- Measure the correct size airway by placing the proximal end (or flange) of the airway adjunct at the corner of the mouth. If the distal end reaches the tip of the mandibular angle,[16] it is a correct fit.
- Depress the tongue using a tongue blade or rigid suction and insert the OPA straight over the tongue, or at a 90 degree angle, and then turn to avoid injuring the palate. Be careful not to push the tongue backward so that it blocks the airway.[19]

Definitive Airways

A definitive protective airway is a tube that has been securely placed in the trachea with the cuff inflated. In an emergency or trauma situation, there are three indications for immediate definitive airway management[20]:

- Failure to maintain or protect the airway
- Failure to maintain oxygenation or ventilation
- A specific anticipated clinical course

Indications for urgently or emergently securing an airway in the trauma patient include the following:

- Severe facial trauma
- Cardiac arrest
- Hemorrhagic shock
- Respiratory distress
- Hypoxia
- Glasgow Coma Scale ≤ 8
- Expanding hematoma in or around the airway
- Mucosal edema caused by smoke, burns, or inhalation of chemical or biological agents[21]

Definitive airways are placed by licensed practitioners with demonstrated competency and whose practice standards include the performance of these interventions. Trauma nurses help prepare the patient and equipment, assist during the procedure, and continuously reassess the patient post procedure. Refer to **Appendix 4-1** and **Appendix 4-2** for more details regarding the preparations and procedure for placing a definitive airway.

Types of Definitive Airways

An endotracheal tube (ETT) is the most commonly placed definitive airway, but alternatives are available for management of patients with difficult airways.

Endotracheal Tubes

ETTs are semi-rigid, slightly curved, opaque tubes designed for passage into the upper airway. Most have an inflatable cuff on the distal end that occludes the space between the tube and the trachea, thereby preventing aspiration and enabling consistent tidal volumes.[1] Other points related to ETTs include the following:

- ETTs can be inserted via the nasal or oral route.
- Nasotracheal intubation (NTI) is performed blindly and requires that the patient is breathing on his or her own. It has a relatively high failure rate and has largely been replaced with alternative techniques.
    - NTI is not recommended in the pregnant trauma patient because of the fragility of the nasal mucosa and risk for bleeding.
    - NTI is rarely utilized to secure the airway in an acute trauma setting due to the risks associated with facial and basilar skull fractures.[1]

Surgical Airways

In situations where a clinician is unable to intubate or oxygenate a patient, an emergency surgical cricothyrotomy is considered a last resort in establishing an airway.[22] In surgical cricothyrotomy, the provider makes an incision through the cricothyroid membrane (**Figure 4-5**), with an ETT or tracheostomy tube then being inserted through the incision.[1] Possible complications include the following[1]:

- Hemorrhage
- Pneumomediastinum
- Laceration of the cricoid ring
- Tracheal trauma
- Subglottic stenosis
- Vocal cord damage

In recent years, several commercial percutaneous cricothyrotomy devices have gained popularity, enabling providers without surgical experience to perform this emergency airway rescue technique. However, only

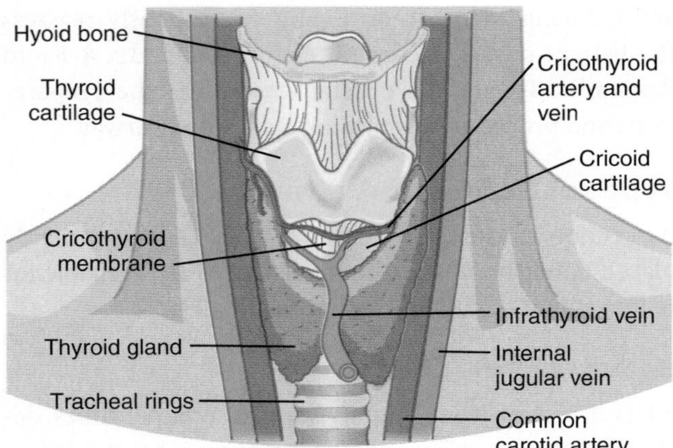

Figure 4-5 *Anterior cervical anatomy of the larynx and trachea.*

limited data are available regarding the effectiveness of ventilating and oxygenating patients with the use of these products.[22]

Difficult Airways

It is crucial to identify, in advance, any patient characteristics or factors that may result in a failed intubation and potential adverse outcome. Signs of a potentially difficult airway include the presence of any of the following:

- Cervical spine injury or severe arthritis
- Mandibular trauma
- Obesity
- Signs of swelling or inflammation (stridor)
- Signs of inhalation injury
- Anatomic variations (short neck)

The LEMON mnemonic is a helpful tool in physically assessing for a difficult airway (**Table 4-3**).[23]

An increasing trend in assuring a successful intubation is the use of a video laryngoscope. This type of laryngoscopy should be performed by an experienced provider after assessment of the airway.

TABLE 4-3 The LEMON Mnemonic for Assessing a Difficult Airway

Letter	Step	Description
L	Look externally	Assess the patient for facial trauma, deformity, or abnormal anatomy.
E	Evaluate	3-3-2 rule. A patient who will not be a difficult intubation will be able to open the mouth wide enough to allow three fingers. There will be a three-finger width between the chin and the neck. Finally, there will be two finger breadths between the neck/mandible junction and the hyoid.
M	Mallampti score	This score relates mouth opening to the size of the tongue. It ranges from I (easy) to IV (extreme difficulty).
O	Obstruction/obesity	Assess for presence of hematoma, upper airway injury, or other obstruction that might obstruct tube passage. Obese patients have an excess of glottic tissue, which may make intubation difficult.
N	Neck mobility	Most, if not all, trauma patients require inline cervical spine stabilization during intubation, limiting the ability to visibly inspect the glottis.

Data from Brown, C. A., III, & Walls, R.M. (2018). Identification of the difficult and failed airway. In C. A. Brown III, J. C. Sakles, & N. W. Mick (Eds.), *The Walls manual of emergency airway management* (5th ed., pp. 10–16). Philadelphia, PA: Wolters Kluwer.

Extraglottic Rescue Airways

Extraglottic airway (EGA) devices can be used for airway management in trauma patients with failed airways and in situations when unsuccessful intubation is anticipated. They are blindly positioned above or posterior to the larynx to facilitate immediate ventilation and oxygenation. EGA devices can be divided into two categories: (1) supraglottic, which are placed above and seal the glottis, and (2) retroglottic, which enter the esophagus and isolate the glottic opening.

- Supraglottic airways do not provide protection against aspiration. One example of a supraglottic airway is the laryngeal mask airway (LMA; **Figure 4-6**). Certain LMAs afford the practitioner the ability to intubate through the LMA, which is advantageous in emergency airway situations.
- Retroglottic airways (such as the King Tube; **Figure 4-7**) sit in the upper esophagus. These tubes

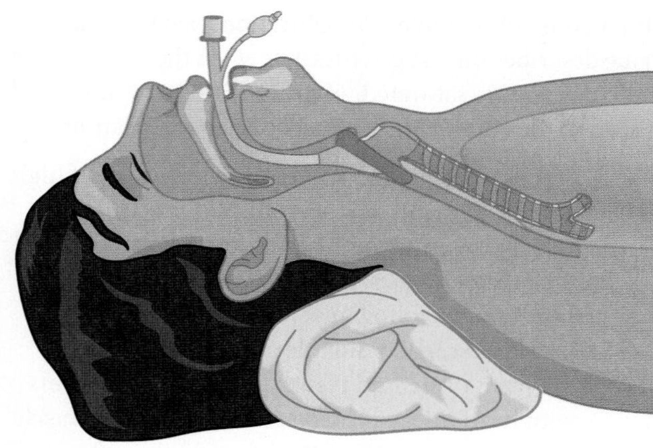

Figure 4-6 *Laryngeal mask airway.*

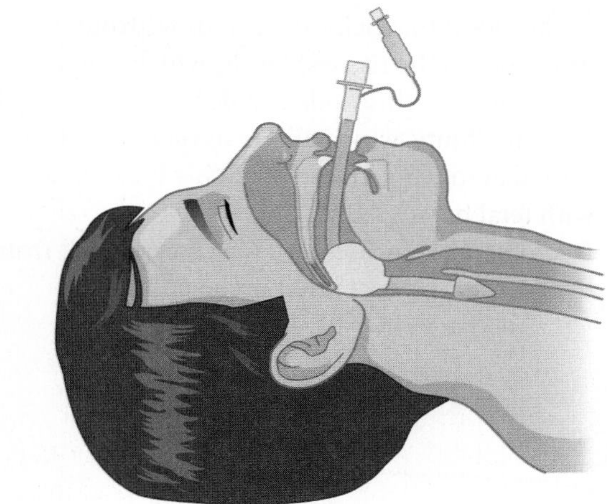

Figure 4-7 *Retroglottic airway.*

have two balloon cuffs with ventilation fenestrations located between the balloons. One balloon sits in the posterior pharynx while the other seals off the esophagus; this design forces air into the lungs while preventing gastric distention. In addition to being used subsequent to a failed airway or unsuccessful intubation attempt, retroglottic airways may be useful in patients with upper gastrointestinal bleeding, upper airway bleeding, or severe facial burns.

Breathing Intervention Reassessment

After intubation, the cuff is inflated and placement is confirmed using the following:

- Attach a carbon dioxide (CO_2) detection device or monitoring sensor and begin assisted ventilations.
- Watch for symmetric rise and fall of the chest; at the same time, listen for the presence of gurgling over the epigastrium, which may indicate the tube is in the esophagus.
- Listen for the presence of bilateral breath sounds at the midaxillary and midclavicular lines.
    - If breath sounds are absent, there is no rise and fall of the chest, gurgling is heard at the epigastrium and there is no evidence of exhaled CO_2, remove the ETT and oxygenate the patient before making another intubation attempt.
    - If breath sounds are heard only on the right side, the ETT is likely in the right mainstem bronchus and has been inserted too far. It should be pulled back until equal breath sounds are heard bilaterally.
    - If breath sounds are heard bilaterally, assess for positive indications of exhaled carbon dioxide from the CO_2 device or monitor after six breaths have been delivered.
- Secure the ETT: Note the measurement at the teeth or gums for positioning, and document it.
- Prepare for mechanical ventilation.
- Monitor the patient's skin color for improvement; the patient's color is likely to improve once ventilations are assisted and the patient is oxygenated.
- Obtain a chest radiograph for verification of ETT depth, after the secondary survey.

G: Get Monitoring Devices and Give Comfort

Pulse oximetry and capnography are used in conjunction with the primary survey to assess for adequacy of oxygenation and effectiveness of ventilation.

L: Laboratory Studies

Laboratory studies include the following:

- Arterial blood gases (ABGs) provide information regarding oxygenation and ventilation through analysis of acid–base balance, lactic acid, and base excess.
    - A base deficit can serve as an endpoint measurement of the adequacy of cellular perfusion, and be useful in guiding resuscitations when used in conjunction with serum lactate.[24]
- Serum lactate serves as an indicator of end-organ perfusion and tissue hypoxia, and can also serve as a guide to resuscitation. A lactate level that normalizes within 24 hours of injury due to resuscitation and supportive care correlates with improved outcomes and mortality rates.[25]

O: Oxygenation and Ventilation

Several methods and indicators are used to measure oxygenation during ventilation. Oxygen is weaned based on clinical condition and these indicators to avoid hyperoxia.

Pulse Oximetry

Pulse oximetry is a noninvasive method of providing oxygenation information and detecting changes in oxygenation that cannot be readily observed with visual assessment.[1] Unreliable readings are especially likely to occur in the following circumstances[1]:

- Poor peripheral perfusion caused by vasoconstriction, hypotension, or hypothermia
- A blood pressure cuff inflated above the sensor
- Carbon monoxide (CO) poisoning (carboxyhemoglobin)
- Methemoglobinemia
- Severe dehydration

Pulse oximetry reflects oxygen saturation (SpO_2). It does not reflect the amount of oxygen dissolved in plasma, which is measured in blood gases as the PaO_2. The nonlinear relationship between the two measurements is reflected in the oxyhemoglobin dissociation curve (**Figure 4-8**).

Oxyhemoglobin Dissociation Curve

The oxyhemoglobin dissociation curve (Figure 4-8) indicates the correlation between tissue oxygenation (PaO_2) and hemoglobin molecule saturation (SaO_2). The P50 value describes the oxygen pressure when the hemoglobin molecule is 50% saturated. Normal P50 is 26.7 mm Hg.[1] A shift in the curve indicates a change in this relationship:

- *A shift to the right* occurs in an environment of high metabolic demand. Hemoglobin's affinity for oxygen decreases, making it easier to release the bound oxygen to the tissues. A shift to the right occurs in response to the following conditions[1]:
  - Increased carbon dioxide (hypercapnia) resulting from decreased respiratory drive in patients with head injury or decreased respiratory muscle function as a result of spinal cord injury.[26]
  - Increased temperature (hyperthermia).
  - Increased 2,3-diphosphoglycerate (a substance in the blood that helps oxygen move from hemoglobin to the tissues) levels, which can occur in pregnancy. This leads to a decreased maternal oxygen affinity, which allows oxygen to be transported across the placenta, so that it can bind with fetal hemoglobin.[27]
  - Decreased pH (acidemia), which can result from hypercapnia or decreased tissue perfusion.

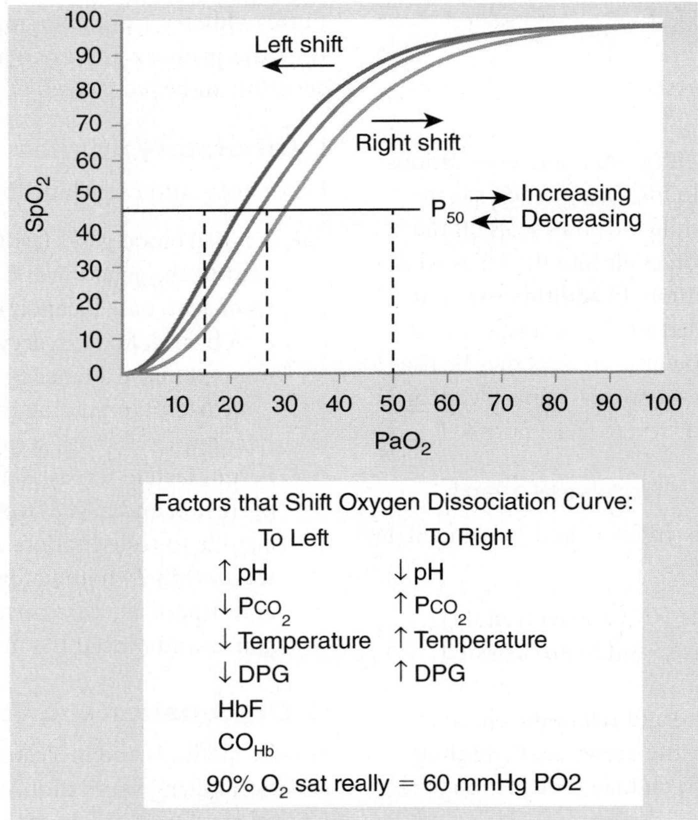

Figure 4-8 *Oxyhemoglobin dissociation curve.*

- *A shift to the left* occurs in an environment of low metabolic demand. Hemoglobin's affinity for oxygen increases, making it harder to release bound oxygen to the tissues. A shift to the left occurs in response to the following conditions[1]:
  - Decreased carbon dioxide (hypocapnia).
  - Decreased temperature (hypothermia), which can result from administration of large volumes of unwarmed blood and/or exposure in the trauma bay. Active and passive warming techniques should always be utilized to assist the patient in maintaining normothermia.
  - Decreased 2,3-diphosphoglycerate levels.
  - Elevated pH (alkalosis).
  - Carbon monoxide, methemoglobinemia, and cyanide poisoning.
  - A shift to the left will be present in patients with carbon monoxide poisoning, as carboxyhemoglobin prevents the release of oxygen to tissues, thereby causing hypoxia. Until ruled out by a normal carboxyhemoglobin serum level, carbon monoxide poisoning should be suspected in patients involved in house fires and/or with inhalation injury.[28]

Pulse oximetry alone does not indicate how effectively oxygen is diffusing into the cells. Considerations for the trauma nurse are to attempt to maintain normothermia and normocarbia, both of which decrease the risk of hypothermia, acidosis, or coagulopathy (also known as the "trauma triad of death").

Carbon Dioxide Monitoring

Carbon dioxide is the end product of ventilation; it is a reflection of metabolism and pulmonary function. Capnometry monitors gauge the partial pressure of CO_2. If the measurement is taken at the end of a breath, it is referred to as the end-tidal CO_2 ($ETCO_2$); this level is similar to the CO_2 level in the alveoli. Presence of exhaled CO_2 can help to confirm correct ETT positioning. Ongoing monitoring can provide insight into the effectiveness of mechanical ventilation. Capnometry devices provide quantitative and/or qualitative measurements (**Appendix 4-3**).[1] See **Figure 4-9**.

Capnography monitors provide a numeric value as well as a continuous waveform, indicating both real-time measurements and trends over time.[1] Capnometers only provide a numeric value of the $ETCO_2$ after each breath; there is no associated waveform.[1] They can be useful in obtaining a snapshot measurement for confirmation of ETT placement or after movement or repositioning.[1]

Colorimetric CO_2 detectors provide information about the presence or absence of CO_2.[1] With these devices, a chemically treated indicator strip changes color to reveal the presence or absence of exhaled CO_2.

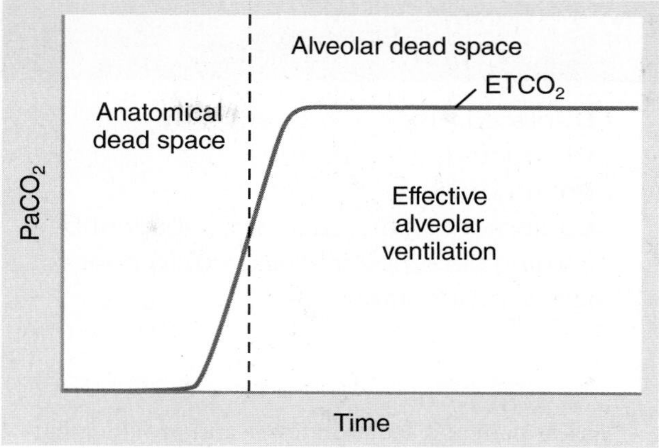

Figure 4-9 *$ETCO_2$ values may be five points lower than the $PaCO_2$ from the ABG due to the alveolar dead space.*

Please refer to Appendix 4-3 for further demonstration as to the importance of $ETCO_2$, capnography, and adjuncts in the assessment of ETT placement.

Diagnostics and Interventions for Airway and Ventilation Problems

A chest radiograph can determine the presence of a hemothorax, pneumothorax, or rib fractures and can help to confirm the position of the ETT. If the trauma patient is hemodynamically stable, a computed tomography scan may be ordered to further evaluate for intrathoracic and intra-abdominal injury.

Reevaluation and Post-Resuscitation Care

Frequent reevaluation of airway patency and adequacy of ventilation is essential. Reassessment includes the following elements:

- Alertness or level of consciousness to determine the patient's ability to protect the airway.
- Respiratory rate and pattern, work of breathing, and breath sounds.
- Vital signs, including pulse oximetry and capnography.
- Arterial blood gases.
- Response to interventions.
- Tolerance for and effectiveness of mechanical ventilation.
- Reevaluation of ETT placement and the effectiveness of ventilation. Use the DOPE mnemonic to troubleshoot ventilator or capnography alarms (**Box 4-1**).[29]

BOX 4-1 Troubleshooting Alarms: DOPE Mnemonic

- **D**isplaced tube
- **O**bstructed or kinked tube
- **P**neumothorax
- **E**quipment failure, such as the patient becoming detached from the equipment or loss of capnography

- Assess pain and sedation levels and provide pharmacologic and nonpharmacologic interventions to facilitate effective breathing and ventilation.

Definitive Care or Transport

Patients with airway or ventilation considerations may require the following transports:

- Transfer to an alternative level of care (designated trauma center)
- Admission to an inpatient unit
- Transfer to the operating room/suite

Emerging Trends

As the science and evidence of trauma care continues to evolve, tools to improve patient outcomes continue to be trialed and refined. Until the evidence has been tested and replicated, controversies remain. Considerations related to the care of patients involving airway and ventilation interventions include hyperoxia, visualizing the vocal cords, and drug-assisted intubation medications (Appendix 4-2).

Hyperoxia

Several studies have reported their findings regarding hyperoxia and patient outcomes:

- A 2016 observational cohort study of patients intubated in the emergency department at a tertiary academic medical center concluded that hyperoxia (defined as $PaO_2 > 120$ mm Hg) in the immediate post-intubation period, despite normalization of PaO_2 within 24 hours, was associated with an increased mortality rate. The researchers felt that hyperoxia likely contributed to free radical production as well as vasoconstriction and subsequent contradictory decrease in oxygenation of vital organs including the heart, brain, and kidneys.[30]
- The evidence-based 2015 American Heart Association (AHA) guidelines support administration of high oxygen concentrations until the patient's arterial oxygenation can be measured. It is recommended that oxygen be titrated to maintain saturations of greater than or equal to 94%.[17]
- A multicenter, prospective cohort study examined adult, mechanically ventilated patients with cardiac arrest who experienced return of spontaneous circulation and had undergone targeted temperature management. It was concluded that early hyperoxia (defined as $PaO_2 > 300$ mm Hg) in the post-resuscitative phase was independently associated with higher risk of death as well as poor neurologic function at discharge.[31]
- Another retrospective study examined 653 consecutive patients who were mechanically ventilated and suffering from traumatic injuries. All ABGs from the first 24 hours of patient admission were analyzed, comparing survivors to nonsurvivors. This study concluded that in this patient population, there was no association between hyperoxia and an increased mortality rate or worse neurologic function at discharge.[32]

Laryngeal Manipulation to Visualize the Cords

Laryngeal manipulation of the thyroid cartilage can be used to help visualize the cords as an alternative to cricoid pressure. One commonly used method of laryngeal manipulation is BURP: **b**ackward, **u**pward, and **r**ightward **p**ressure.[33] **Figure 4-10** illustrates this method.

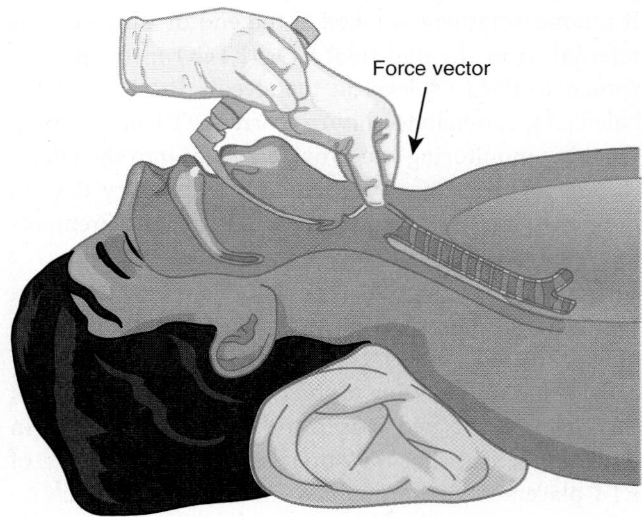

Figure 4-10 *The BURP maneuver.*

Summary

Maintenance of an adequate airway is paramount for achieving optimal outcomes in the trauma patient. Assessment is the most important step in the identification of any airway problem that the trauma patient may experience; therefore, it is important for trauma nurses to learn this important skill. Recognition of the problem and anticipation of an impending problem are the primary focus of trauma care assessment. If an airway problem is not identified during the assessment, the results can be catastrophic for the patient. It is essential for trauma nurses to be able to quickly and accurately assess and recognize/identify certain life-threatening presentations and to intervene quickly. Familiarity with multiple types of airway adjuncts and their use is essential for nurses who care for trauma patients. A thorough understanding of the pathophysiology underlying adequate airway and ventilation will assist the trauma nurse to implement lifesaving interventions expediently.

References

1. Wagner, K., & Hardin-Pierce, M. (2014). Determinants and assessment of pulmonary function. In *High acuity nursing* (6th ed., pp. 266–295). Boston, MA: Pearson.
2. Schuman, L. L. (2019). Respiratory function and alterations in gas exchange. In J. L Banasik & L. E. Copstead (Eds.). *Pathophysiology* (6th ed., pp. 451–477). St. Louis, MO: Saunders Elsevier.
3. Nagler, J. (2017, May 9). Emergency endotracheal intubation in children. *UpToDate*. Retrieved from https://www.uptodate.com/contents/emergency-endotracheal-intubation-in-children
4. Mittal, M. (2017, October, 8). Needle cricothyroidotomy and percutaneous transtracheal ventilation. *UpToDate*. Retrieved from https://www.uptodate.com/contents/needle-cricothyroidotomy-with-percutaneous-transtracheal-ventilation
5. Stark, P. (2017, June 15). Radiology of the trachea. *UpToDate*. Retrieved from https://www.uptodate.com/contents/radiology-of-the-trachea
6. Nagler, J. (2018, January 15). Emergency airway management in children: Unique pediatric considerations. *UpToDate*. Retrieved from https://www.uptodate.com/contents/emergency-airway-management-in-children-unique-pediatric-considerations
7. Stranding, S. (2015). Pleura, lungs, trachea, and bronchi. In S. Stranding (Ed.), *Gray's anatomy: The anatomical basis of clinical practice* (41st ed., pp. 953–969). St. Louis, MO: Saunders Elsevier.
8. Theodore, A. C. (2017, November 7). Oxygenation and mechanisms of hypoxemia. *UpToDate*. Retrieved from https://www.uptodate.com/contents/oxygenation-and-mechanisms-of-hypoxemia
9. American College of Surgeons. (2018). Airway and ventilatory management. In *Advanced trauma life support student manual* (10th ed., pp. 22–41). Chicago, IL: Author.
10. Mechem, C. C. (2017, December 13). Pulse oximetry. *UpToDate*. Retrieved from https://www.uptodate.com/contents/pulse-oximetry
11. Feller-Kopman, D., & Schwartzstein, R. (2017, September 8). Mechanisms, causes, and effects of hypercapnia. *UpToDate*. Retrieved from https://www.uptodate.com/contents/mechanisms-causes-and-effects-of-hypercapnia
12. Krauss, B., & Falk, J. (2018, January 19). Carbon dioxide monitoring (capnography). *UpToDate*. Retrieved from https://www.uptodate.com/contents/carbon-dioxide-monitoring-capnography
13. Hyzy, R. C., & McSparron, J. (2018, May 8). Overview of mechanical ventilation. *UpToDate*. Retrieved from https://www.uptodate.com/contents/overview-of-mechanical-ventilation
14. Theodore, A. C. (2017, March 16). Arterial blood gases. *UpToDate*. Retrieved from https://www.uptodate.com/contents/arterial-blood-gases
15. Nickson, C. (2017, March 22). Oxygen and carbon dioxide retention in CPOD. *Life in the Fastlane*. Retrieved from https://lifeinthefastlane.com/ccc/oxygen-and-co2-retention-in-copd/
16. Wittels, K. (2018, April 4). Basic airway management in adults. *UpToDate*. Retrieved from https://www.uptodate.com/contents/basic-airway-management-in-adults
17. Callaway, C. W., Donnino, M. W., Fink, E. L., Romergryko, G. G., Golan, E., Kern, K. B., . . . Zimmerman, J. L. (2015). Part 8: Post-cardiac arrest care. *2015 American Heart Association Guidelines Update for Cardiopulmonary Resuscitation and Emergency Cardiovascular Care, 132*(18 Suppl. 3), S465–S482. https://doi.org/10.1161/CIR.0000000000000262
18. Bucher, J., & Cooper, J. (2017). Bag mask ventilation. *StatPearls*. Retrieved from https://www.ncbi.nlm.nih.gov/books/NBK441924/
19. Malamed, S. F. (2018). Emergency drugs and equipment. In *Sedation: A guide to patient management* (6th ed., pp. 442–445). St. Louis, MO: Elsevier.
20. Mills, T., & DeBlieux, P. (2017, May 2). Emergency airway management in the adult with direct airway trauma. *UpToDate*. Retrieved from https://www.uptodate.com/contents/emergency-airway-management-in-the-adult-with-direct-airway-trauma
21. Jain, U., McCunn, M., Smith, C., & Pittet, J. (2016). Management of the traumatized airway. *Anesthesiology, 124*(1), 199–206. https://doi.org/10.1097/ALN.0000000000000903
22. Warner, M., Smith, H., & Zielinski, M. (2016). Impaired ventilation and oxygenation after emergency cricothyrotomy: Recommendations for the management of suboptimal invasive airway access. *Anesthesia and Analgesia Case Reports, 7*(10), 212–214. https://doi.org/10.1213/XAA.0000000000000388
23. Brown, C. A., III, & Walls, R.M. (2018). Identification of the difficult and failed airway. In C. A. Brown III, J. C. Sakles, & N. W. Mick (Eds.),*The Walls manual of emergency airway management* (5th ed., pp. 10–16). Philadelphia, PA: Wolters Kluwer.

24. Raja, A., & Zane, R.D. (2018, May 30). Initial management of trauma in adults. *UpToDate*. Retrieved from https://www.uptodate.com/contents/initial-management-of-trauma-in-adults
25. Johnson, M. C., Alarhayem, A., Convertino, V., Carter, R., Chung, K., Stewart, R., . . . Eastridge, B. J. (2017). Comparison of compensatory reserve and arterial lactate as markers of shock and resuscitation. *Journal of Trauma and Acute Care Surgery, 83*(4), 603–608. https://doi.org/10.1097/TA.0000000000001595
26. Feller-Kopman, D. J., & Schwartzstein, R. M. (2017, September 8). Mechanisms, causes, and effects of hypercapnia. *UpToDate*. Retrieved from https://www.uptodate.com/contents/mechanisms-causes-and-effects-of-hypercapnia
27. Bauer, K. (2018, July 23). Maternal adaptations to pregnancy: Hematologic changes. *UpToDate*. Retrieved from https://www.uptodate.com/contents/maternal-adaptations-to-pregnancy-hematologic-changes
28. Mlcak, P. (2018, February 28). Inhalation injury from heat, smoke, or chemical irritants. *UpToDate*. Retrieved from https://www.uptodate.com/contents/inhalation-injury-from-heat-smoke-or-chemical-irritants
29. Ridell, A. (2017). The effect of apneic oxygenation on reducing hypoxemia during rapid sequence induction and intubation in the acutely ill or injured. *Advanced Emergency Nursing Journal, 39*(4), 309–317. https://doi.org/10.1097/TME.0000000000000168
30. Page, D., Ablordeppey, E., Wessman, B. T., Mohr, N. M., Trzeciak, S., Kollef, M. H., Roberts, B. W., & Fuller, B. M. (2018). Emergency department hyperoxia is associated with increased mortality in mechanically ventilated patients: A cohort study. *Critical Care, 22*(1), 9. https://doi.org/10.1186/s13054-017-1926-4
31. Roberts, B. W., Kilgannon, J. H., Hunter, B. R., Puskarich, M. A., Pierce, L., Donnino, M., . . . Trzeciak, S. (2018). Association between early hyperoxia exposure after resuscitation from cardiac arrest and neurological disability: A prospective multi-center protocol-directed cohort study. *Circulation, 137*(20), 2114–2124. https://doi.org/10.1161/CIRCULATIONAHA.117.032054
32. Russell, D. W., Janz, D. R., Emerson, W. L., May, A. K., Bernard, G. R., Zhao, Z., Koyama, T., & Ware, L. B. (2017). Early exposure to hyperoxia and mortality in critically ill patients with severe traumatic injuries. *BMC Pulmonary Medicine, 17*(1), 29. https://doi.org/10.1186/s12890-017-0370-1
33. Brown, C. A., III, & Walls, R. M. (2018). Rapid sequence intubation. In C. A. Brown III, J. C. Sakles, & N. W. Mick (Eds.), *The Walls manual of emergency airway management* (5th ed., pp. 235–249). Philadelphia, PA: Wolters Kluwer.

APPENDIX 4-1

Seven P's of Rapid-Sequence Intubation

Phase	Description[1-3]
Preparation	› Ensure all necessary equipment and personnel are assembled at the bedside. › Ensure all equipment is in working order and the patient's cardiac monitor, blood pressure cuff, pulse oximetry, and end-tidal capnography are placed on the patient and functioning correctly. › Verify patent intravenous access. › Draw up and label DAI medications (Appendix 4-2) at the bedside.
Preoxygenation	› Patients requiring emergent intubation should be preoxygenated with the highest possible oxygen concentration via high-flow delivery for a minimum of 3 minutes. · For patients not on spinal precautions, the position to preoxygenate is with the head of the bed elevated 20 degrees. · If the patient is on spinal precautions, place the bed in reverse Trendelenburg position at 30 degrees. › Consider apneic oxygenation in all other intubations to reduce the risk of hypoxemia. · Oxygen is administered via a nasal cannula placed underneath the standard preoxygenation device (nonrebreathing mask or bag-mask) with a flow rate from 10 to 15 L/minute in a conscious patient and at least 15 L/minute in an unconscious patient. · To optimize oxygen flow past the upper airway, the jaw-thrust maneuver should be utilized to maintain airway patency.
Pre-intubation optimization	› During this phase, medications can be administered to mitigate the adverse effects associated with endotracheal intubation (Appendix 4-2). › If possible, patients should be hemodynamically optimized prior to DAI with blood products, IV fluid, vasopressors, and decompression of tension pneumothorax/release of hemothorax.
Paralysis with induction	› The goal during DAI is to produce deep sedation and muscular relaxation quickly. › Refer to Appendix 4-2 for further induction and neuromuscular blocking agents.
Protection	› After the neuromuscular blocking agent is administered, the priorities are to protect the airway from aspiration by avoiding bag-mask ventilation. › Use of a bag-mask device after induction but before tube placement can result in regurgitation and aspiration. › If the patient has been properly preoxygenated, there should be no role for bag-mask device use between induction and tube placement.

(continues)

Phase	Description[1-3]
Placement with proof	› Once intubation is completed, inflate the ETT cuff and secure the tube. › Use end-tidal CO_2 (colorimetric or quantitative) to confirm tube placement.
Post-intubation management	› Secure the ETT per institutional protocol and note the measurement at the teeth/gums. › A post-intubation chest radiograph may be useful for determining evidence of complications.

Abbreviations: DAI, drug-assisted intubation; ETT, endotracheal tube.

Data from Brown, C. A., & Sakles, J. C. (2017, November 16). Rapid sequence intubation for adults outside the operating room. *UpToDate*. Retrieved from https://www.uptodate.com/contents/rapid-sequence-intubation-for-adults-outside-the-operating-room; Pourmand, A., Robinson, C., Dorwart, K., O'Connell, F. (2017). Pre-oxygenation: Implications in emergency airway management. *American Journal of Emergency Medicine, 35*(8), 1177–1183. https://doi.org/10.1016/j.ajem.2017.06.006; Reardon, R. F., Driver, B. E, & Carleton, S. C. (2018). Principles of preparatory oxygenation. In C. A. Brown III, J. C. Sakles, & N. W. Mick (Eds.), *The Walls manual of emergency airway management* (5th ed., pp. 49–65). Philadelphia, PA: Wolters Kluwer.

Drug-Assisted Intubation

Drug-assisted intubation (DAI) uses a strong sedative (or "induction agent") to render the patient unconscious immediately, followed by a neuromuscular blocking agent (or "paralytic") to facilitate the insertion of an ETT. This technique presumes the patient to be at risk for aspiration and was designed to mitigate that risk and increase the chance of a successful emergency intubation.[4]

Administration of the induction agent and the paralytic will render the patient apneic. Therefore, preoxygenation is an important component in preparation for DAI, as it prolongs the time to hypoxia. Due to the risk of aspiration, assisted ventilation with a bag-mask device is not recommended. To prepare the patient for this apneic phase, high-flow oxygen is administered at the maximum concentration for at least 3 minutes prior to intubation attempts. This high concentration of oxygen replaces other mixed gases ("denitrogenation") in the lungs and creates a reserve of oxygen. This reserve allows the patient to maintain the oxygen saturation during the apneic phase of intubation (also known as apneic oxygenation).[5]

It is important for the trauma nurse to understand how to optimize the DAI process to be able to anticipate the needs of the team.

References

1. Brown, C. A., & Sakles, J. C. (2017, November 16). Rapid sequence intubation for adults outside the operating room. *UpToDate*. Retrieved from https://www.uptodate.com/contents/rapid-sequence-intubation-for-adults-outside-the-operating-room
2. Pourmand, A., Robinson, C., Dorwart, K., O'Connell, F. (2017). Pre-oxygenation: Implications in emergency airway management. *American Journal of Emergency Medicine, 35*(8), 1177–1183. https://doi.org/10.1016/j.ajem.2017.06.006
3. Reardon, R. F., Driver, B. E, & Carleton, S. C. (2018). Principles of preparatory oxygenation. In C. A. Brown III, J. C. Sakles, & N. W. Mick (Eds.), *The Walls manual of emergency airway management* (5th ed., pp. 49–65). Philadelphia, PA: Wolters Kluwer.
4. Brown, C. A., III, & Walls, R. M. (2018). Rapid sequence intubation. In C. A. Brown III, J. C. Sakles, & N. W. Mick (Eds.), *The Walls manual of emergency airway management* (5th ed., pp. 235–249). Philadelphia, PA: Wolters Kluwer.
5. Ridell, A. (2017). The effect of apneic oxygenation on reducing hypoxemia during rapid sequence induction and intubation in the acutely ill or injured. *Advanced Emergency Nursing Journal, 39*(4), 309–317. https://doi.org/10.1097/TME.0000000000000168

APPENDIX 4-2

Drug-Assisted Intubation Medications

Medication	Indication/Action	Dose	Onset	Duration	Clinical Pearls
Pretreatment					
Lidocaine	May reduce risk of rise in intracranial pressure during intubation	1.5 mg/kg	45–90 seconds	20 minutes	Contraindicated in patients with known lidocaine allergy or Mobitz II/third-degree heart block
Fentanyl	Mitigates sympathetic response (increased BP and HR) during intubation	3 mcg/kg	2–3 minutes	30–60 minutes	Last pretreatment medication given Administer over 60 seconds to prevent "wooden chest" syndrome
Induction					
Etomidate	Acts on GABA receptors to block neuroexcitation and produce anesthesia	0.3 mg/kg	15–45 seconds	3–12 minutes	Does not affect hemodynamic stability Can cause temporary 24-hour decrease in circulating cortisol levels
Ketamine	Acts on GABA receptors, causing neuroinhibition and anesthesia; antagonizes opioid receptors, causing analgesia	1–2 mg/kg	45–60 seconds	10–20 minutes	Does not decrease respiratory drive; induction agent of choice for awake intubation Unique in that it provides analgesia
Midazolam	Acts on GABA receptor complex to produce sedation and amnesia	0.2 mg/kg	30–60 seconds	15–30 minutes	Causes 10% to 25% decrease in MAP Use with caution in hypovolemic and/or hypotensive patients
Propofol	Sedative amnestic agent; suppresses brain activity and inhibits long-term memory creation	1.5–3 mg/kg	15–45 seconds	5–10 minutes	Causes vasodilation and decrease in MAP Can be used for long-term sedation, procedural sedation, and anesthesia induction Use with caution in patients with egg/soy allergies

(*continues*)

Medication	Indication/Action	Dose	Onset	Duration	Clinical Pearls
Paralysis					
Succinylcholine	Depolarizing agent that stimulates all cholinergic receptors (sympathetic and parasympathetic), causing muscular paralysis	1.5 mg/kg	45–60 seconds	6–10 minutes	Absolute contraindication in patients with family history or past history of malignant hyperthermia, stroke, or burn that occurred greater than 72 hours prior, rhabdomyolysis, or significant hyperkalemia
Rocuronium	Nondepolarizing agent that inhibits neuromuscular receptors, causing muscular paralysis	1 mg/kg	45–60 seconds	45 minutes	Drug of choice when succinylcholine is contraindicated
Vecuronium	Nondepolarizing agent that inhibits neuromuscular receptors, causing muscular paralysis	0.15 mg/kg	75–90 seconds	25–40 minutes	Alternative to rocuronium

Abbreviations: BP, blood pressure; GABA, gamma-aminobutyric acid; HR, heart rate; MAP, mean arterial pressure.

Data from Caro, D. (2017, March 29). Induction agents for rapid sequence intubation in adults outside the operating room. *UpToDate*. Retrieved from https://www.uptodate.com/contents/induction-agents-for-rapid-sequence-intubation-in-adults-outside-the-operating-room; Caro, D. (2018, July 11). Neuromuscular blocking agents (NMBAs) for rapid sequence intubation in adults outside the operating room. *UpToDate*. Retrieved from https://www.uptodate.com/contents/neuromuscular-blocking-agents-nmbas-for-rapid-sequence-intubation-in-adults-outside-of-the-operating-room; Caro, D. (2018, August 14). Pretreatment medications for rapid sequence intubation in adults outside the operating room. *UpToDate*. Retrieved from https://www.uptodate.com/contents/pretreatment-medications-for-rapid-sequence-intubation-in-adults-outside-the-operating-room

APPENDIX 4-3

Capnometry Measurements

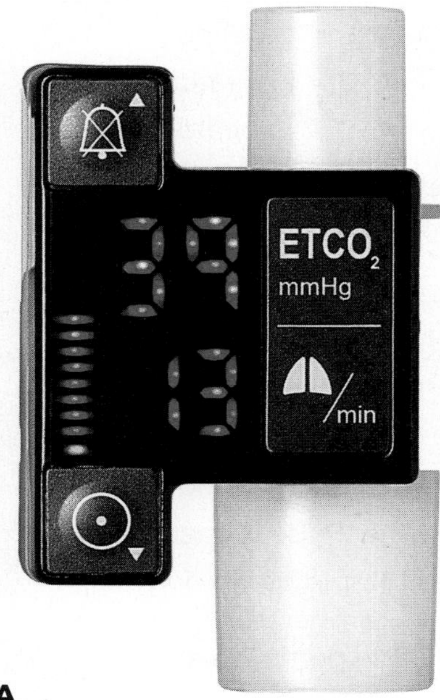

A

Capnometry devices: Measure and display $ETCO_2$ as a number on a digital or analogue monitor

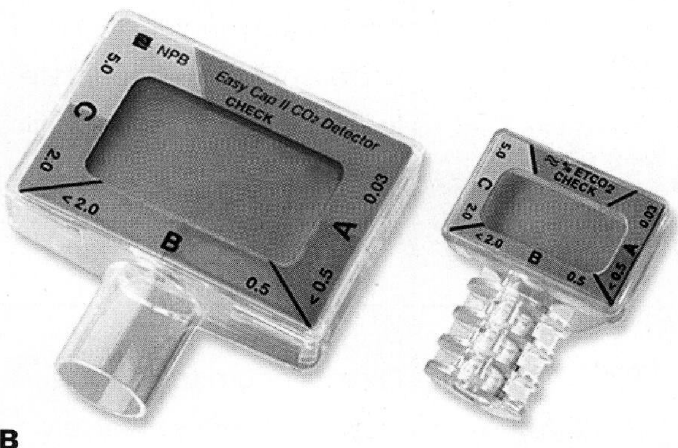

B

Colorimetric devices: Use chemically treated indicator to detect exhaled carbon dioxide ($ETCO_2$)

- Evaluate the color change after 5–6 full breaths
- Effective up to 2 hours, then discard
- Review manufacturer instructions/color code key

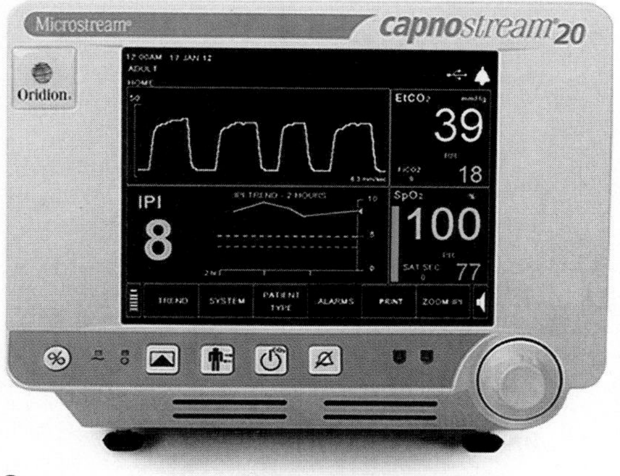

C

Capnography devices: Provide a graphic/waveform display of the $ETCO_2$ instantaneously

Ways to measure end-tidal carbon dioxide. ***A.*** *Capnometer.* ***B.*** *Colorimetric detector.* ***C.*** *Capnography monitor.*

Capnography Waveforms and Their Meanings

Normal Capnography Waveform

Normal (35–45 mm Hg)

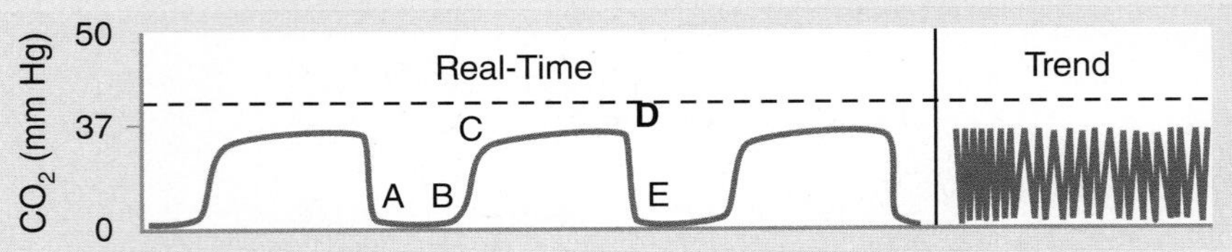

- A–B = Baseline
- B–C = Expiratory upstroke
- C–D = Expiratory plateau
- **D = $ETCO_2$ value**
- D–E = Inspiration begins

Breathing Variations

Hypercarbia ($ETCO_2 > 45$ mm Hg)

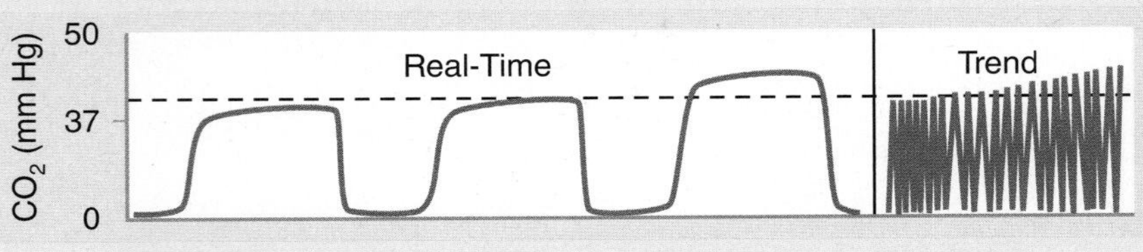

Possible causes include:

- Decrease in respiratory rate
- Decrease in tidal volume
- Increase in metabolic rate
- Rapid rise in body temperature (hyperthermia)

Hypocarbia ($ETCO_2 < 35$ mm Hg)

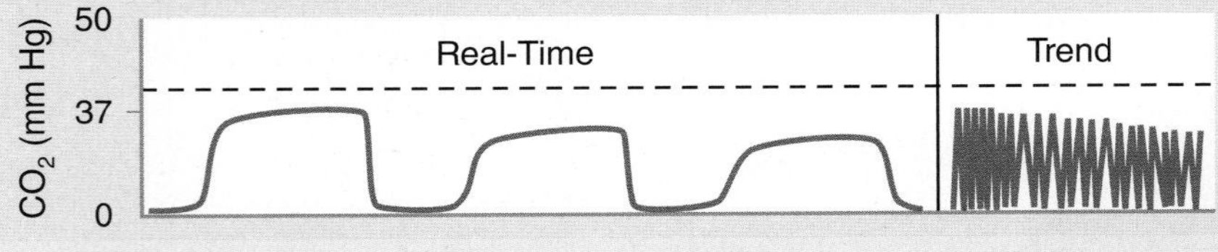

Possible causes include:

- Increase in respiratory rate
- Increase in tidal volume
- Decrease in metabolic rate
- Fall in body temperature

Muscle Relaxants Wearing Off

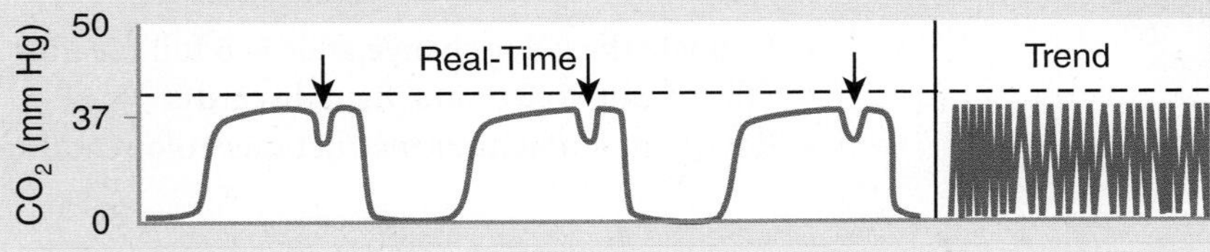

- Appear when muscle relaxants begin to subside
- Depth of cleft is inversely proportional to degree of drug activity

Apnea

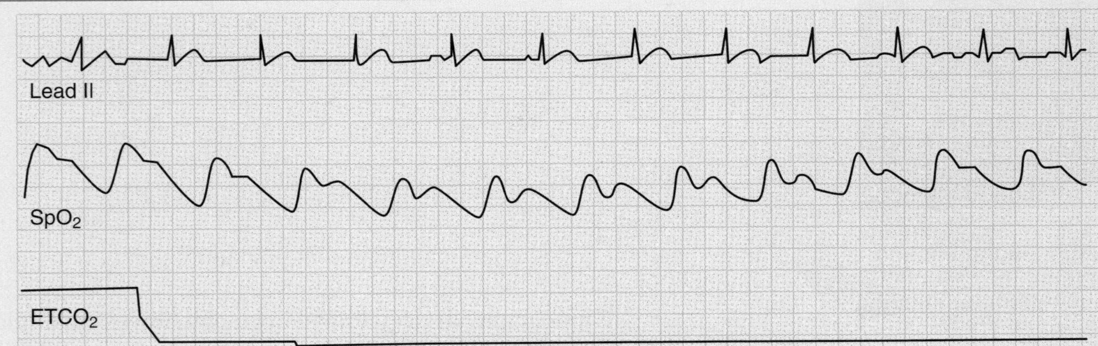

Note how in this example, the SpO_2 waveform (middle waveform) continues to show an adequate oxygenation status after the patient has gone apneic, but the $ETCO_2$ waveform (bottom waveform) abruptly drops to zero.

Intubation Waveforms

Right Main Stem Intubation

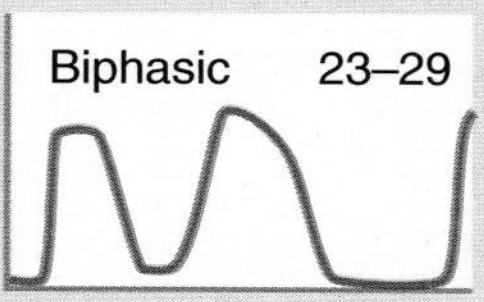

Biphasic waveform as a result of ETT in the right main bronchus

Esophageal Intubation

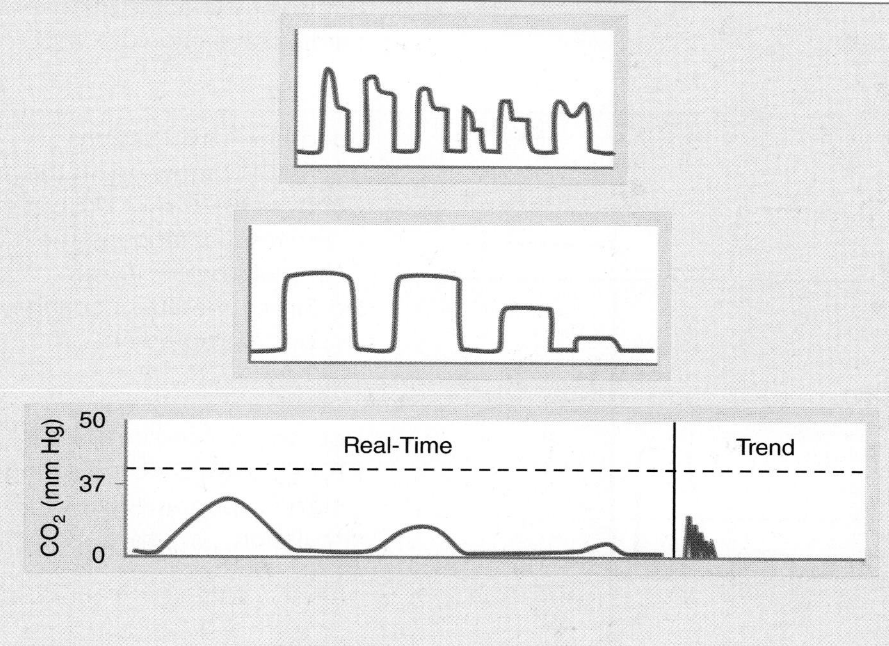

Base line fluctuation
0–2

Possible causes include:

- Missed intubation; ETT in the esophagus, little or no CO_2 is present
- ETT disconnected, kinked, or obstructed
- Loss of circulatory function

Obstructed Airway or Breathing Circuit

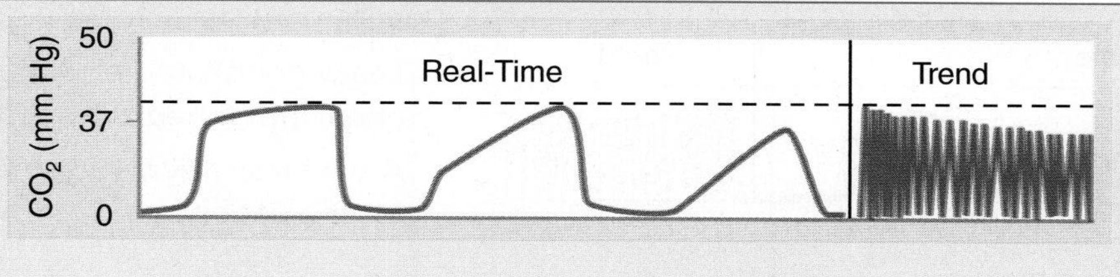

Possible causes include:

- Partially kinked or occluded artificial airway
- Presence of foreign body in the airway
- Obstruction in expiratory limb of breathing circuit
- Bronchospasm

Perfusion Waveforms

$ETCO_2$ Below Normal

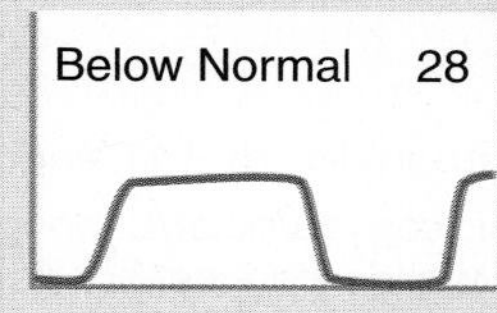

$ETCO_2$ well below normal may be due to:

- Low cardiac output
- Pulmonary embolus
- Hypothermia, etc

(continues)

Capnography Waveforms and Their Meanings (*continued*)

Perfusion Waveforms (*continued*)

Decreasing Cardiac Output

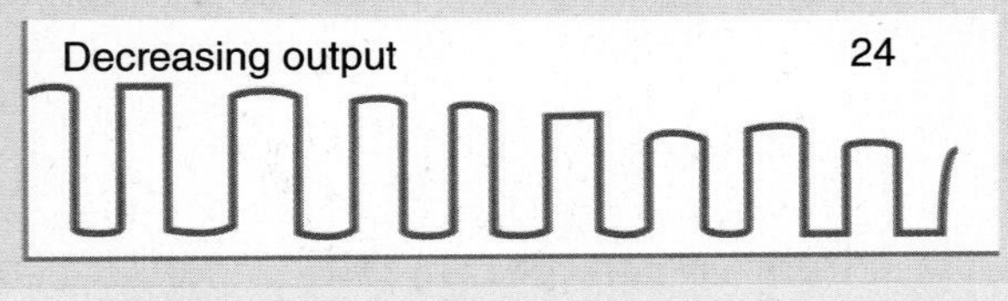

Low cardiac output and a low perfusion state will show up as a decreasing $ETCO_2$

A decreasing $ETCO_2$ waveform may also indicate a cuff leak, ETT in the hypopharynx, or a partial obstruction of the ETT

CPR Performance: Tired Rescuer

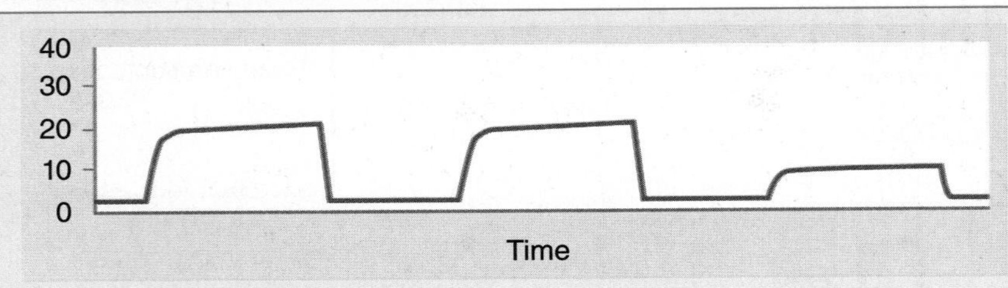

Adequate compressions during CPR show up on the $ETCO_2$ as 15–20 mm Hg, but as the rescuer fatigues, the $ETCO_2$ falls below 10 mm Hg. Time to rotate or change rescuers/compressors

Return of Spontaneous Circulation

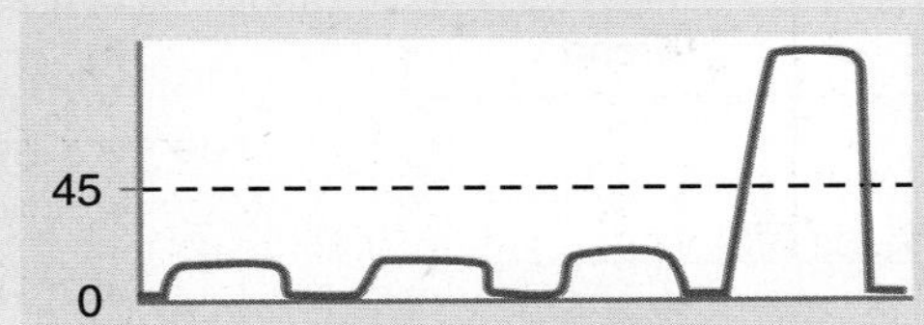

Note the sudden increase in $ETCO_2$ during CPR, indicating return of spontaneous circulation

Equipment Malfunction

Inadequate Seal around ETT

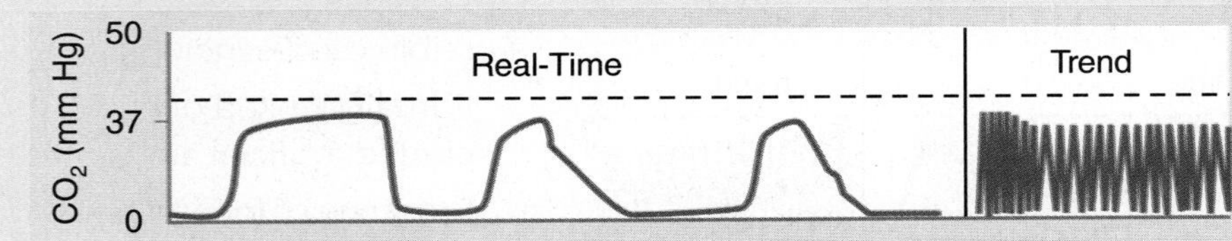

Possible causes include:

- Leaky or deflated endotracheal or tracheotomy cuff
- Artificial airway is too small for the patient

Rebreathing

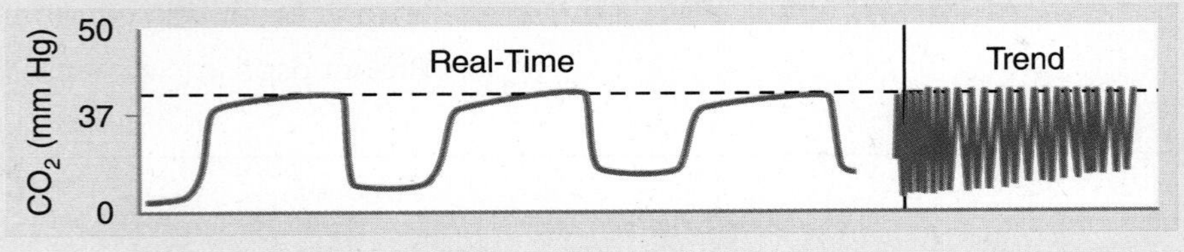

Possible causes include:

- Faulty expiratory valve
- Inadequate inspiratory flow
- Insufficient expiratory time
- Malfunction of CO_2 absorber system

Abbreviations: CPR, cardiopulmonary resuscitation; ETCO2, end-tidal carbon dioxide; ETT, endotracheal tube.

Data from Acuclinic. (2015). Capnography. Retrieved from http://acuclinic.com.au/pocit/Capnography.htm; Chaturvedi, S. (2014). Oxygenation & ventilation monitoring. Retrieved from https://www.slideshare.net/subodhchaturvedi1/oxygenation-and-ventilation-monitoring; DiCorpo, J. E., Schwester, D., Dudley, L. S., & Merlin, M. A. (2015). Capnography provides bigger physiological picture to maximize patient care (Blog post). Retrieved from http://midtownblogger.blogspot.com/2015/12/jems_4.html; Fire Engineering. (2007). Capnography: A versatile life-saving tool. Retrieved from http://www.fireengineering.com/articles/print/volume-160/issue-4/features/capnography-a-versatile-life-saving-tool.html; Medicscribe. (2009). Capnography. Retrieved from http://www.medicscribe.com/capnography/.

CHAPTER 5

Shock

Justin J. Milici, MSN, RN, CEN, CPEN, TCRN, CCRN, FAEN

OBJECTIVES

Upon completion of this chapter, the learner will be able to:

1. Identify causes and characteristics of shock in the trauma patient.
2. Describe pathophysiologic changes as a basis for assessment of the trauma patient in shock.
3. Demonstrate nursing assessment priorities for the trauma patient in shock.
4. Plan appropriate interventions for the trauma patient in shock.
5. Evaluate the effectiveness of nursing interventions for the trauma patient in shock.

Introduction

Shock is a syndrome of inadequate tissue perfusion, which results from insufficient oxygen delivery, uptake, and utilization to meet the metabolic demands of cells and organs. This ultimately results in cellular and tissue hypoxia. Shock is a dynamic process that begins when cells are hypoperfused, setting off a series of responses to preserve homeostasis and producing far-reaching effects on all systems and organs.

Shock is a complex state; thus, "[t]he first step in the initial management of shock is to recognize its presence."[1(p43)] In its early stages, the presence of shock is likely to be subtle. If this condition goes unrecognized and untreated, the hypoperfused cells shift from aerobic to anaerobic metabolism, leading to life-threatening acidosis, tissue ischemia, and cellular death when coupled with the incomplete removal of metabolic waste products. A basic understanding of the concepts, types, and stages of shock as well as the body's response to inadequate tissue perfusion is essential for early recognition, early goal-directed interventions, and optimal care of the trauma patient in shock.

Pathophysiology as a Basis for the Body's Response to Shock

Shock begins at the cellular level. For cells to perform basic metabolic functions and maintain their cellular integrity, they require the production of adenosine triphosphate (ATP; **Figure 5-1**).[2] In the presence of oxygen, aerobic metabolism produces ATP through the

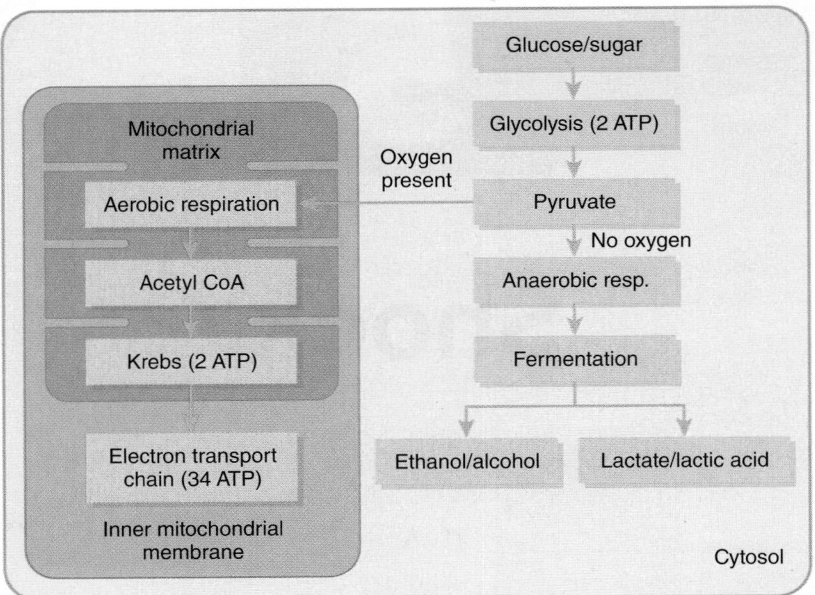

Figure 5-1 *Anaerobic and aerobic cellular metabolism.*

breakdown of fats, carbohydrates, and proteins. This efficient process has a high ATP yield that supports energy production[3] and the maintenance of the electrical gradient, known as the sodium–potassium pump.

Hypoperfusion deprives the cell of oxygen. In an effort to maintain homeostasis, compensation occurs in which the body shifts to anaerobic metabolism. ATP production occurs at a less efficient rate, with this process resulting in lactic acid formation and metabolic acidosis. If shock is prolonged and ATP production does not meet the body's energy demands, the cellular membrane loses the ability to maintain its integrity. In addition, the normal electrical gradient of the sodium–potassium pump is lost, causing sodium to remain within the cell and potassium outside of the cell. This results in cellular swelling and ultimately cellular death and destruction (**Figure 5-2**).

Basic cardiac function is key to maintaining cellular perfusion. Shock has many causes, classifications, and stages. Regardless of the cause, shock can be linked to one or more components of cardiac output. Cardiac output is the volume of blood pumped by the heart per minute; it is determined by the product of heart rate and stroke volume (**Figure 5-3**).[1] Stroke volume is the amount of blood pumped with each cardiac contraction; it is affected by preload, afterload, and myocardial contractility. Preload reflects the central venous pressure or the volume of blood returning to the heart at the end of diastole. Afterload reflects the pressure that the heart must overcome to pump blood into the circulation, also known as systemic and pulmonary arterial pressures or vascular resistance. Contractility is the ability of the ventricles to contract, forcefully ejecting blood. Different injuries can affect this contractility *and* any of the components of cardiac output.[1]

Stages of Shock

In the early stages of shock, delivery of cellular nutrients and oxygen is inadequate to meet the body's metabolic needs. To protect and maintain perfusion to essential organs, the body reacts by activating various compensatory mechanisms. In the short term, these compensatory mechanisms may improve tissue perfusion to vital organs; however, that feat is accomplished by shunting perfusion away from other organs.[3] Blood pressure alone is not an indication of cardiac output and adequate perfusion: Several other endpoints of resuscitation can be monitored proactively to identify early stages of shock.

If the shock state is unrecognized, untreated, or prolonged or if the protective mechanisms fail to restore perfusion, profound effects on microcirculation and vascular permeability will ensue and the patient will progress to irreversible shock. The cellular membrane loses its ability to maintain integrity, leading to cellular destruction and death, followed by a systemic inflammatory response, organ ischemia, end-organ damage, multiple organ dysfunction, and ultimately death. Early recognition and management are crucial, as failure to intervene will allow progression to the terminal stage of shock, in which morbidity and mortality are inevitable.

There are three stages of shock: Stage I (compensated), Stage II (decompensated or progressive), and Stage III (irreversible).[4] These stages are illustrated in **Figure 5-4**.[5]

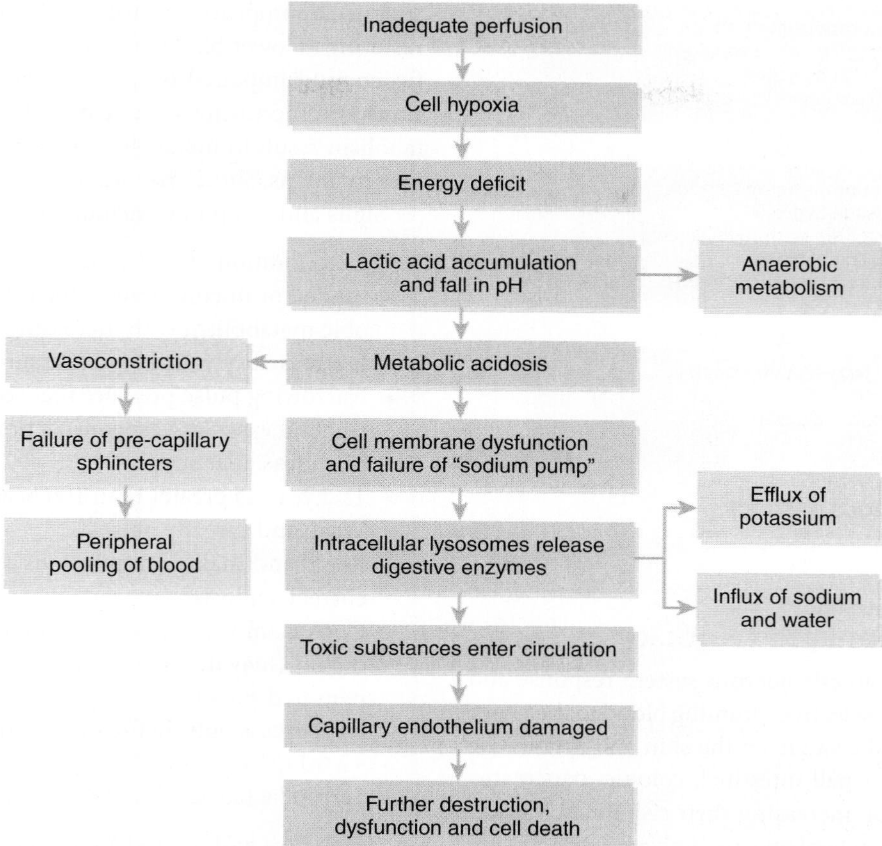

Figure 5-2 *Cellular response to shock.*

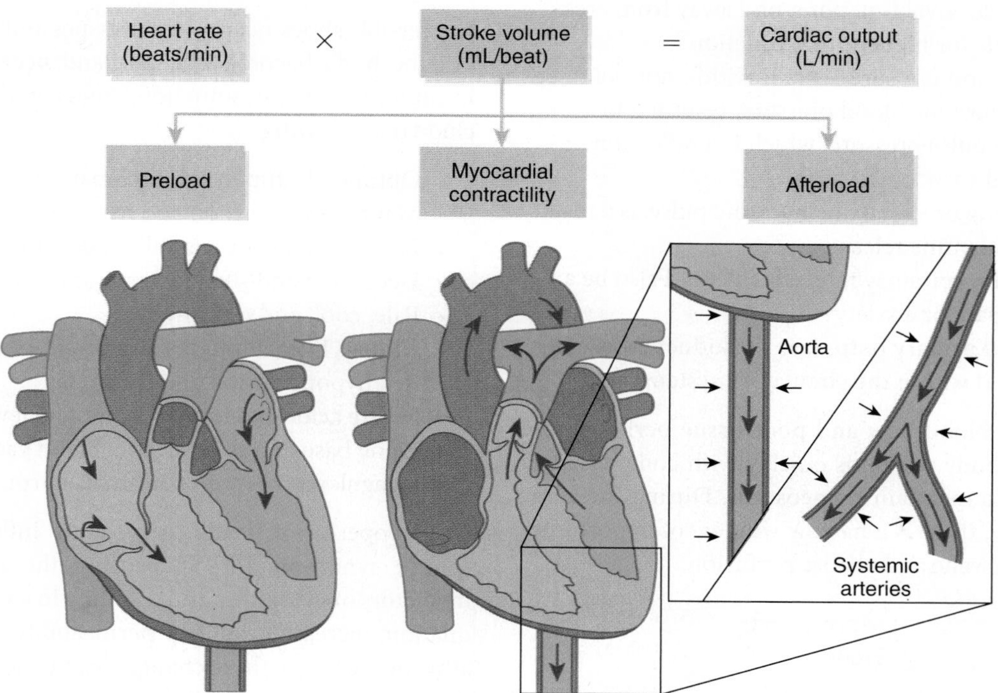

Figure 5-3 *Cardiac output is the product of stroke volume and heart rate.*

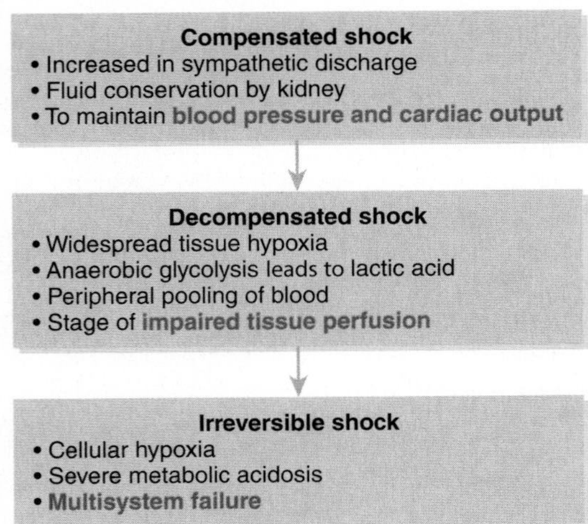

Figure 5-4 *The stages of shock.*

Stage I: Compensated Shock

In Stage I, the sympathetic nervous system response and vasoconstriction are selective, shunting blood to the heart, brain, and lungs and away from the skin and splanchnic circulation (gastric, small intestinal, colonic, pancreatic, hepatic, and splenic), increasing their risk for ischemia.[3] As compensatory mechanisms are activated, the patient may begin to exhibit subtle changes in level of consciousness (LOC) and vital signs, including the following:

- Anxiety, lethargy, confusion, and restlessness from oxygen being shunted to the brain stem, so as to maintain survival functions, and away from areas responsible for higher brain function
- Systolic blood pressure, usually within normal range
- A rising diastolic blood pressure, resulting in a narrowed pulse pressure, which is a reflection of peripheral vasoconstriction
- A bounding or slightly tachycardic pulse as a result of catecholamine release
- Increased respiratory rate, which could also be a result of pain or anxiety
- Decreased urinary output, as the kidney works to retain fluid within the circulatory system

When low blood flow and poor tissue perfusion are detected, the body responds quickly with compensatory mechanisms to maintain homeostasis. During the compensated stage, there is a narrow window of opportunity to rapidly intervene and restore perfusion.

Stage II: Decompensated or Progressive Shock

Decompensated or progressive shock occurs when compensatory mechanisms begin to fail and are unable to support or improve perfusion.[4] Blood flow is reduced, resulting in lower blood pressure, reduction in organ perfusion, and impaired oxygen and carbon dioxide (CO_2) transport. Increasing lactic acid levels from anaerobic metabolism result in metabolic acidosis, causing further injury to organs. Shock may still be reversible at this stage.[6]

Signs and symptoms include the following:

- Deterioration of LOC; the patient becomes obtunded or unconscious as the cells switch to anaerobic metabolism with increasing levels of lactic acid
- Decreased systolic blood pressure, hypotension
- Narrowing pulse pressure that continues until peripheral vascular vasoconstriction fails to provide cardiovascular support
- Tachycardia greater than 100 beats/min
- Weak and thready pulses
- Rapid and shallow respirations as the lungs try to correct acidosis
- Cool, clammy, cyanotic skin as blood shunts to vital organs (may develop toward the end of the decompensated stage)
- Base excess outside the normal range (−2 mEq/L to +2 mEq/L)
- Serum lactate levels greater than 2 to 4 mmol/L[7]

Aggressive and immediate interventions must be implemented as the patient develops acidosis and decompensation, both of which result in tissue death and organ dysfunction.

Stage III: Irreversible Shock

Irreversible shock occurs when tissues and cells throughout the body become ischemic and necrotic, resulting in multiple organ dysfunction.[7] Signs and symptoms include the following:

- Obtunded, stuporous, or comatose state
- Marked hypotension and heart failure
- Bradycardia with possible dysrhythmias
- Decreased and shallow respiratory rate
- Pale, cool, and clammy skin
- Kidney, liver, and other organ failure due to continued hypoperfusion and ischemia
- Severe acidosis, elevated lactic acid levels, and worsening base excess on arterial blood gases (ABGs)
- Coagulopathies with petechiae, purpura, or bleeding

Hypoperfusion leads to systemic inflammatory response syndrome (SIRS), causing the release of cell mediators or cytokines, and resulting in a wholesale vasodilation, increased capillary permeability, and coagulopathy. In the lungs, these changes lead to acute respiratory distress syndrome (ARDS). Increased permeability of the pulmonary capillaries results in noncardiogenic pulmonary edema, alveolar collapse, and ventilation–perfusion mismatch.[3] Other vital organ systems begin to fail, leading to multiple organ dysfunction syndrome (MODS). The lungs, heart, and kidneys are often the first organs to be affected. Liver failure may occur later due to that organ's compensatory capacity.[3]

Despite aggressive resuscitation at this level, it becomes increasingly difficult to restore tissue perfusion, correct the coagulopathies, and minimize organ damage. Interventions in this stage of shock have minimal ability to reverse morbidity and mortality.

The Body's Compensatory Response to Shock

The human compensatory response includes a vascular component. As blood flow decreases and the arterial pressure falls below 80 mm Hg, oxygen delivery becomes impaired, resulting in decreased oxygen levels and increased CO_2 levels.[3] As a result of the lower blood pressure, a cascading response is set into motion to preserve tissue perfusion. The vascular response can be activated along two different pathways.

- *Baroreceptor activation:* Baroreceptors, found in the carotid sinus and along the aortic arch, are sensitive to the degree of stretch within the arterial wall. When the baroreceptors sense a decrease in stretch, they stimulate the sympathetic nervous system to release epinephrine and norepinephrine, causing stimulation of cardiac activity and constriction of blood vessels, which triggers a rise in heart rate and diastolic blood pressure.[3]
- *Chemoreceptor activation:* Peripheral chemoreceptors consist of carotid and aortic bodies, whereas central chemoreceptors are located in the medulla of the brain stem. Peripheral chemoreceptors detect changes in blood oxygen levels, whereas central chemoreceptors respond to changes in CO_2 and pH.[3] When CO_2 rises or the oxygen level or pH falls, these receptors are activated and information is relayed to the central nervous system and to the cardiorespiratory centers in the medulla, which increases respiratory rate and depth and blood pressure.

Adrenal Gland Response

Activation of the sympathetic nervous system triggers the "fight or flight" response, which causes the adrenal glands to release the two catecholamines—epinephrine and norepinephrine:

- High levels of *epinephrine* produce smooth muscle relaxation in the airways and cause arteriole smooth muscle contractility (potentiating inotropic effect). Epinephrine also increases heart rate (positive chronotropic effect), peripheral vasoconstriction, and glycogenolysis (breakdown of glycogen stores in the liver into glucose for cellular use).
- Peripheral vasoconstriction manifests as a narrowed pulse pressure.

NOTE

As diastolic pressure rises, systemic and peripheral vascular resistance (afterload) increases. A narrowing pulse pressure may be one of the first concrete measurements signaling that the patient's circulatory status is compromised and that the body is trying to compensate.

- *Norepinephrine* increases heart rate, vascular tone through alpha-adrenergic receptor activation, and blood flow to skeletal muscle. It also triggers the release of glucose from energy stores.

These changes in vital signs may have a subtle presentation, so the trauma nurse must be observant and alert to their presence. Recognizing this early shock response can be essential to preventing further tissue injury and progression of the shock state.

In addition to the release of catecholamines, the adrenal glands stimulate the release of cortisol and aldosterone to raise blood glucose and promote renal retention of water and sodium.

Pulmonary Response

During shock, the pulmonary system responds to both hypoperfusion and acidosis. The respiratory rate increases in an attempt to improve oxygen delivery to the tissues as well as to decrease the CO_2 level in an effort to maintain acid–base balance. Metabolic acidosis stemming from anaerobic metabolism results in the compensatory response of tachypnea and is one of the earliest responses to inadequately perfused tissue. If shock is left untreated, the pulmonary response may become ineffective, weaken, and fail, necessitating assisted ventilations.

Cerebral Response

As shock progresses, the primary goal of the body is to maintain perfusion to the vital organs—the midbrain, heart, lungs and kidneys—by shunting blood away from liver, bowel, skin, and muscle. Sympathetic stimulation has little effect on the cerebral and coronary vessels since they are capable of autoregulation.[1] Cerebral autoregulation maintains a constant cerebral vascular blood flow as long as the mean arterial pressure is maintained in the range of 50 to 150 mm Hg.[1] When autoregulation in the brain fails, perfusion becomes dependent solely on systemic blood pressure.[1] Chapter 6, "Head Trauma," provides additional information on this response.

Renal Response

Hypoperfusion of the kidneys triggers a complex compensatory mechanism in the adrenal glands in an attempt to improve tissue perfusion. This mechanism includes the following steps[6]:

- Renal ischemia causes the kidneys to secrete renin.
- Renin accelerates the production of angiotensin I.
- Angiotensin I is converted into angiotensin II in the lungs by angiotensin-converting enzyme, which is produced by the vascular endothelium.
- Angiotensin II effects include the following:
    - Potent vasoconstriction, which increases vascular resistance and arterial pressure
    - Release of aldosterone, which increases reabsorption of sodium and water in the distal tubules to increase intravascular volume
    - Stimulation of arginine vasopressin, also known as vasopressin, argipressin, or antidiuretic hormone, which further increases retention of water

Decreased urinary output may be noted, which can be an indication of poor renal perfusion and progression of the shock state. If shock is left untreated, it will progress to oliguria and renal failure.

Systemic Inflammatory Response Syndrome

The initial post-traumatic inflammatory response is both protective and essential for survival. Tissue hypoxia activates a systemic inflammatory response, and neutrophils are sent to the injury sites, engaging signaling pathways that mobilize inflammatory cells. Tissue hypoxia also stimulates the secretion of multiple inflammatory mediators or biomarkers.[6]

An exaggerated immune inflammatory response can result from massive tissue injury and hemorrhage or a prolonged and untreated shock state. It can induce a generalized, acute inflammatory response that affects multiple organ systems and sets in motion a cycle of inflammation–tissue damage–inflammation that is driven by cytokines, chemokines, and products of damaged, dysfunctional, or stressed tissue.

Apoptosis (programmed cell death) of neutrophils may be inhibited, leading to an accumulation of neutrophils that stimulates the release of inflammatory mediators. In other cells, apoptosis may be magnified, increasing cell death and worsening organ function. The neutrophils change and move from the capillaries into the interstitial space and trigger further release of free oxygen radicals and tissue-destructive enzymes, leading to additional tissue injury.[4] This process may start when hypoperfusion begins or during resuscitation. If hypoxia is not corrected early, the inflammatory response becomes destructive, leading to organ failure and death.[4]

Trauma Triad of Death

Resuscitation-associated coagulopathy is associated with the *trauma triad of death* (**Figure 5-5**).[8] It includes the following elements:

- *Hypothermia:* Impairs thrombin production and platelet function. Activated protein C inhibits factors V and VIII, reducing thrombin formation, and decreases inhibition of tissue plasminogen activator, accelerating fibrinolysis and bleeding.[9]
- *Acidosis:* Impairs thrombin production and other coagulation factors due to a reduced pH, elevated lactate production, and increasing base deficit. Laboratory values of pH less than 7.4, elevated serum lactate, and base deficits reaching −10 mmol/L reduce the activity of various coagulation factors by as much as 40%.[9] Metabolic acidosis also contributes to prolonged clotting times and reduced clot strength.[10]
- *Coagulopathy:* With whole-blood loss, clotting factors are depleted. "Coagulopathy is present at the time of admission to the emergency department in up to 25–35% of trauma patients."[10(p1)] Replacement with packed red blood cells (RBCs) and hemodilution with saline without transfusing platelets and plasma further dilutes the blood's ability to clot.[1]

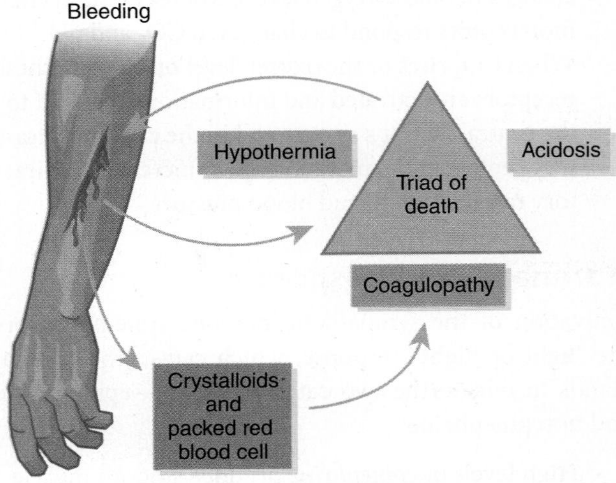

Figure 5-5 *Trauma triad of death.*

Hypoperfusion leads to increased levels of thrombomodulin, which inhibits thrombin and activates activated protein C. Activated protein C impairs clot formation and increases existing clot dissolution.[9]

Recent studies have shown that acute endogenous coagulopathy often occurs within minutes following injury, before and independent of iatrogenic causes such as hypothermia and metabolic acidosis, making this a primary cause of coagulopathy after injury. The result is disseminated intravascular coagulopathy, MODS, and death.

Classification and Etiology of Shock

Whether the cause of shock is a volume problem (hypovolemic), a pump problem (cardiogenic), a problem with the pipes (distributive), or a mechanical problem (obstructive), the common denominator is the same: inadequate tissue perfusion and cellular oxygenation. The etiology of the different types of shock can be traced back to an issue with one of these four components (**Figure 5-6**).[11] **Table 5-1** provides a summary of shock etiology; each type is discussed in the following subsections.[12]

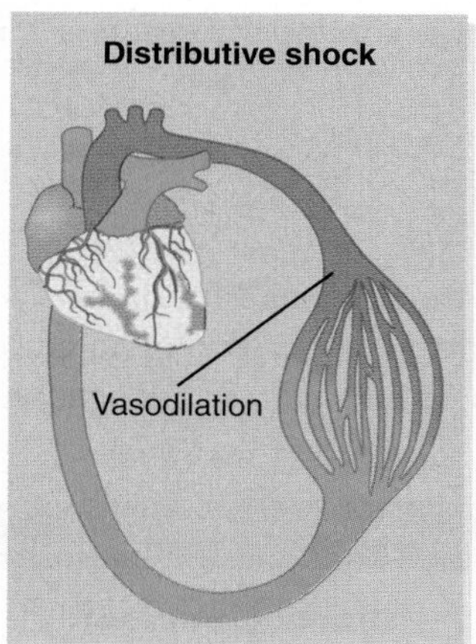

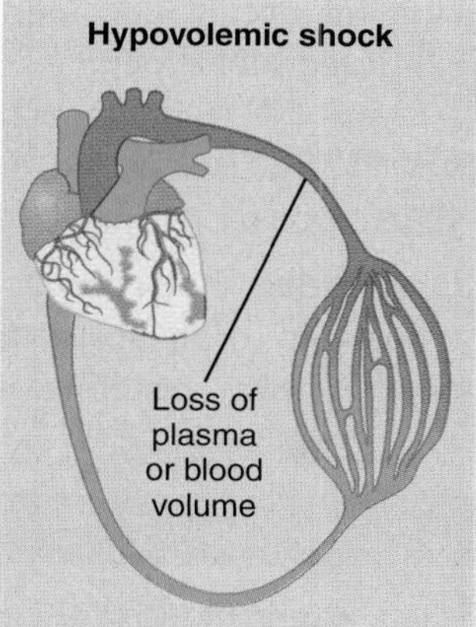

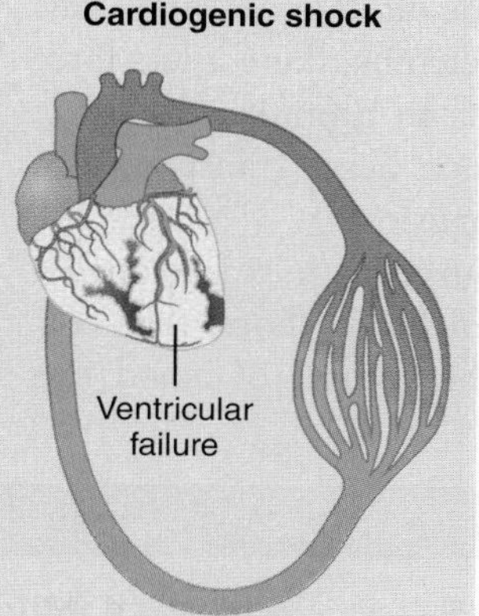

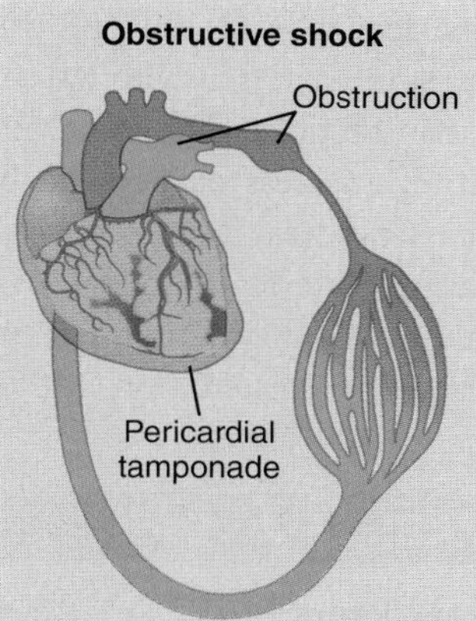

Figure 5-6 *Types of shock.*

TABLE 5-1 Classification of Shock Etiology and Underlying Defects

Classification	Etiology	Underlying Pathology
Hypovolemic	Hemorrhage	Whole-blood loss
	Burns	Plasma loss, fluid shifts
Cardiogenic	Myocardial infarction	Loss of cardiac contractility
	Dysrhythmias	Reduced cardiac output
	Blunt cardiac trauma	Loss of cardiac contractility and dysrhythmias
Obstructive	Cardiac tamponade	Compression of heart with obstruction to atrial filling
	Tension pneumothorax	Mediastinal shift with obstruction to atrial filling
	Tension hemothorax	Combination of compression of the heart and mediastinal shift
Distributive	Neurogenic shock	Loss of vasomotor tone due to decreases in sympathetic control
	Anaphylactic shock	Vasodilation of vessels due to immune reaction to allergens (release of histamine)
	Septic shock	Mediated by systemic inflammatory response syndrome with hypotension and perfusion abnormalities

Reproduced from Jacobs, B. B. (Ed.). (2000). *Trauma nursing core course* (5th ed.). Des Plaines, IL: Emergency Nurses Association.

Hypovolemic Shock (Volume Problem)

Hypovolemia is caused by a decrease in the amount of circulating volume. In trauma, this typically results from hemorrhage but could result from a condition that leads to a precipitous loss of volume, such as vomiting, diarrhea, or burn trauma. Hemorrhage is the most common cause of shock in the trauma patient and the leading cause of preventable deaths. "Victims can quickly die from uncontrolled bleeding, within five to 10 minutes."[13(par3)] Thus, hemorrhage control is a first-line intervention, followed by restoration of circulating volume.[1]

In hypovolemic shock, decreased circulating volume results in decreased venous return and decreased preload. With less filling of the ventricles, heart muscle fibers stretch less at the end of the diastole. Starling's Law states, in part, that with less stretching, there is less force of contraction; this effect leads to diminished cardiac output and less oxygenated blood being transported to the tissues, resulting in hypoperfusion.[4]

The American College of Surgeons has developed a classification system for hemorrhagic shock that correlates its presentation with the volume of blood loss (**Table 5-2**).[1] This classification system is a useful tool for estimating percentage of acute blood loss. Patient presentations may vary, however, and may not match these classifications precisely.

Goal-directed therapy for hypovolemic shock is aimed at replacing the type of volume the patient has lost in an effort to restore physiologic homeostasis (electrolytes with precipitous nonhemorrhagic losses or blood products with blood loss).[13] Not all hemorrhage involves obvious external bleeding. When solid organs (liver, spleen), and large bone structures (pelvis, femur) are injured, concealed major blood loss may occur internally, so it becomes imperative to consider the mechanism of injury, maintain a high index of suspicion for occult bleeding, and continually reassess for subtle signs of shock.

Obstructive Shock (Mechanical Problem)

Obstructive shock results from hypoperfusion of the tissue due to an obstruction in either the vasculature or the heart, resulting in decreased cardiac output.

TABLE 5-2 Estimated Blood Loss in a 70-kg Man Based on Initial Presentation

Parameter	Class I	Class II (Mild)	Class III (Moderate)	Class IV (Severe)
Blood loss (mL)	Up to 750	750–1,500	1,500–2,000	> 2,000
Blood loss (% blood volume)	Up to 15%	15–30%	31–40%	> 40%
Pulse rate (beats/minute)	< 100	100–120	120–140	> 140
Systolic blood pressure	Normal	Normal	Decreased	Decreased
Pulse pressure	Normal or increased	Decreased	Decreased	Decreased
Respiratory rate (breaths/minute)	14–20	20–30	30–40	> 35
Urine output (mL/h)	> 30	20–30	5–15	Negligible
Central nervous system/mental status	Slightly anxious	Mildly anxious	Anxious, confused	Confused, lethargic
Base deficit	0 to −2 mEq/L	−2 to −6 mEq/L	−6 to −10 mEq/L	−10 mEq/L or more
Initial fluid replacement	Crystalloid	Crystalloid or blood	Blood	Massive transfusion protocol

Data from American College of Surgeons. (2018). Shock. In *Advanced trauma life support: Student course manual* (10th ed., pp. 42–61). Chicago, IL: Author.

Goal-directed therapy is aimed at relieving the obstruction and improving perfusion. Examples of obstructive shock include the following:

- With tension pneumothorax, the increase in intrathoracic pressure leads to displacement of the vena cava (kinked), obstruction to atrial filling, decreased preload, and decreased cardiac output. See Chapter 7, "Thoracic and Neck Trauma," for additional information.
- With cardiac tamponade, an accumulation of blood within the inflexible pericardial sac impedes diastolic expansion and filling, which in turn leads to decreases in preload, stroke volume, and cardiac output. See Chapter 7 for additional information.
- A venous air embolism can occur on the right side of the heart during systole in the pulmonary artery. If it is severe enough, this embolism in the right ventricular outflow tract may precipitate an obstruction, causing a decrease in cardiac output.

Cardiogenic Shock (Pump Problem)

Cardiogenic shock results from pump failure in the presence of adequate intravascular volume. A lack of cardiac output and end-organ perfusion occurs secondary to a decrease in myocardial contractility and/or valvular insufficiency (aortic and/or mitral). The most common cause of trauma-related cardiogenic shock is blunt cardiac injury. Any injury or ischemia to myocardial tissue or the conduction system could cause a dysrhythmia and affect cardiac output.

Cardiogenic shock may be either chronic or acute in origin. Common acute etiologies include myocardial infarction (MI), dysrhythmias, cardiomyopathy, and toxicologic pathologies. While trauma rarely causes cardiogenic shock, one of these more common etiologies may have been the precursor to a traumatic injury. Heart failure is an example of a chronic cause of cardiogenic shock.

When presented with a decreased cardiac output without volume loss in the context of trauma, assess the patient for signs of an MI, dysrhythmia, or heart failure, as these are more common reasons for cardiogenic shock. Goal-directed therapy includes inotropic support, antidysrhythmic medications, and correction or treatment of the underlying cause.[6]

Excessive volume administration or an increase in afterload can result in pulmonary edema and increased myocardial ischemia. Successful emergent stabilization includes administering controlled fluid boluses to improve preload and inotropic support to improve contractility. If signs of fluid overload are present, afterload reduction may be indicated.[6]

Distributive Shock (Pipe Problem)

Distributive shock occurs as a result of maldistribution of an adequate circulating blood volume with the loss of vascular tone or increased permeability. Diffuse vasodilation lowers the systemic vascular resistance, creating a relative hypovolemia, reduction of the mean systemic volume and venous return to the heart, or drop in preload, resulting in distributive shock. Causative factors include[6]:

- *Anaphylactic shock*, typically resulting from a release of inflammatory mediators such as histamine, which contracts bronchial smooth muscle and increases vascular permeability and vasodilation. Treatment includes immediate removal of the allergen (if known), airway management, and early administration of epinephrine followed by intravenous (IV) fluid administration. Epinephrine's therapeutic effects will cause vasoconstriction, increase peripheral vascular resistance and bronchodilation, and decrease release of inflammatory mediators.
- *Septic shock*, which is caused by the systemic release of bacterial endotoxins, resulting in an increased vascular permeability and vasodilation. Treatment for septic shock includes the early administration of antibiotics, IV fluid administration, and potential need for norepinephrine to vasoconstrict the peripheral vasculature, increase blood volume return to the heart, and improve cardiac output.[3]
- *Neurogenic shock*, which occurs with spinal cord injury (SCI) that results in the loss of sympathetic nervous system control of vascular tone, leading to venous and arterial vasodilation. Under normal homeostatic conditions, the sympathetic and parasympathetic systems oppose each other, allowing vasoconstriction and dilation to accommodate changing vascular volumes. With the loss of sympathetic nervous system input owing to SCI, unopposed (parasympathetic) vagal activity may result in decreased cardiac output through bradycardia. See Chapter 9, "Spinal Trauma," for additional information.

Close monitoring of volume status and medications, such as norepinephrine, dopamine, epinephrine, phenylephrine, and vasopressin, are interventions that can be used to produce vasoconstriction and increase peripheral vascular resistance. In some cases, atropine or transcutaneous pacing may be added to counteract parasympathetic bradycardia described.

Current Management Strategies

Current strategies for managing shock are discussed in this section.

Tourniquet Use

Extensive military experience and research has reinforced the effectiveness of tourniquet use for limb injuries with uncontrolled hemorrhage. Increased use of tourniquets in civilian trauma systems has grown as prehospital providers, first responders, and hospital providers have identified the tourniquet as a beneficial tool in controlling isolated limb exsanguination.[14] Direct pressure and pneumatic splinting devices are hemorrhage-control methods used in addition to tourniquets. Commercial versions of the tourniquets, such as the C-A-T and SOFTT, as well as improvised devices using a swathe and windlass are effective types of tourniquets so as long as they can quickly and reliably stop venous and arterial bleeding. Early application of the tourniquet on an actively bleeding limb will minimize the likelihood of mortality from hemorrhagic shock.[15] There is a low rate of complications, typically related to prolonged use, such as nerve palsy, muscle necrosis, vascular thrombosis, acute kidney injury, compartment syndrome, soft-tissue damage, and amputation. However, a life saved outweighs the risk of a limb injury.

Damage Control Resuscitation

Damage control resuscitation (DCR) is a principle that focuses on prevention of shock rather than intervention after shock develops. Early recognition of the patient at risk for shock facilitates the use of goal-directed therapies. DCR involves two strategies: hypotensive and hemostatic resuscitation.

Hypotensive Resuscitation

The use of large volumes of crystalloid solution is associated with increased bleeding and decreased survival rates, often as a result of hemodilution and decreased clotting factors.[1] "Persistent infusion of large volumes of fluid and blood in an attempt to achieve a normal blood pressure is not a substitute for definitive control of bleeding."[1(p52)] Several studies have posited that delayed and restrictive administration of isotonic crystalloid solution in trauma patients (without head injury) may lead to better outcomes and lower mortality, by allowing the clotting cascade to work. This approach of permissive hypotension might limit the complications that lead to increased bleeding and rebleeding, informally known as "popping the clot."[1] Plasma and blood products are the primary fluids administered to correct blood loss and inadequate coagulation. The goal is not to achieve hypotension, but rather to ensure adequate resuscitation without producing hypertension.[1]

Hemostatic Resuscitation

The key to early goal-directed therapy is to optimize tissue and cellular oxygenation and perfusion by preventing further losses through hemodilutional coagulopathy.[1] When hemorrhage occurs, clotting factors and platelets are lost along with RBCs. Excessive use of isotonic crystalloids alone or replacing whole-blood loss with only packed RBCs can produce a hemodilutional coagulopathy in which the effective concentrations of both platelets and clotting factors are significantly reduced.[1] It can also lead to a worsening acidosis (due to anaerobic metabolism), dilution of coagulation factors, increased inflammatory response (due to large volumes of crystalloid), and potentially ARDS, abdominal compartment syndrome, and increased mortality.

- Hemorrhage control is optimized by giving component therapy, using the transfusion of both packed RBCs and fresh frozen plasma in a 1:1 ratio.[1] Platelets are added at a 1:1:1 ratio in the presence of actual or anticipated thrombocytopenia.[1]
- Balanced fluid resuscitation is an approach to resuscitation that addresses all components that are lost with hemorrhage, including fluid, packed RBCs, and fresh frozen plasma, while surgically controlling the source of bleeding.[1] It is crucial that hemorrhage control and balanced fluid resuscitation be initiated early.[1]

Fluid Resuscitation

Current recommendations suggest administration of a lesser volume of crystalloid solutions[16] and use of boluses to follow the principle of permissive hypotension.[1] Initial fluid management for the adult trauma patient in hemorrhagic shock consists of 500-mL boluses of isotonic crystalloid solution given as rapidly as possible until blood products are available or a systolic blood pressure (SBP) of 90 mm Hg is achieved, with a maximum of 1 liter of crystalloid solution being administered. Fluids given by prehospital providers must also be taken into account.[1] Fluid warmer/rapid infuser devices should be used to administer warmed fluid and blood products rapidly. These devices typically require the insertion of a large-caliber IV catheter (16 or 14 gauge) or intraosseous (IO) needle to facilitate rapid administration.

In pediatric patients, fluid management is weight based, with 20 mL/kg of warmed isotonic fluid being given to pediatric patients weighing less than 40 kg.[1] Large-caliber IVs or IOs are acceptable forms of vascular access. Rapid infusers are not recommended in pediatric patients weighing less than 40 kg, due to the use of smaller IV catheters (24 or 22 gauge) and specific weight-based fluid boluses. However, rapid infusion can be accomplished using the push/pull technique. See Chapter 12, "Special Populations: The Pediatric Trauma Patient," for more information.

Massive Transfusion

The U.S. military first demonstrated that providing a balanced resuscitation (limited use of crystalloid solution) and following a massive transfusion protocol (MTP) with a defined blood-to-plasma ratio results in hemostasis and decreased mortality in hemorrhaging patients. Similar findings have been achieved in civilian settings, and the U.S. Department of Defense is continuing research to determine the optimal ratio of blood-to-blood products. Recognizing that a predefined MTP leads to early blood, plasma, and platelet transfusions with improved outcomes, the American College of Surgeons (ACS) delineated use of MTP as a critical criterion for trauma centers in its *Resources for Optimal Care of the Injured Patient.*[17] Success of MTP is dependent on early recognition and implementation, using a defined ratio of one part RBCs to one part thawed plasma to one part platelets (1:1:1 ratio) and providing a detailed process for implementation. Limitations associated with MTP include the timing and immediacy of implementing the protocol and the availability of thawed plasma and platelets. For more information on this protocol, refer to the ACS's Trauma Quality Improvement Program best practice guidelines.[18]

Calcium Chloride Replacement

Hypocalcemia is a concern with massive transfusion because citrate is added as a preservative to banked blood to prevent coagulation. Citrate chelates (binds with) calcium, rendering it inactive. Because calcium is a vital part of the clotting cascade, hypocalcemia, as a result of massive transfusion, can actually worsen hypovolemic shock by permitting continued bleeding. Signs of hypocalcemia include cardiac dysrhythmias, muscle tremors, and seizures.[6] If calcium administration is indicated, this therapy should be guided by the patient's serum ionized calcium levels. Excessive supplemental calcium can be harmful as well.

If the trauma patient requires more than one unit of blood every 5 minutes, anticipate citrate toxicity and hypocalcemia and prepare to replace losses with calcium gluconate or calcium chloride. If calcium chloride is used, monitor closely for infiltration, as this infusion can cause tissue necrosis. Patients taking calcium-channel blockers (diltiazem) may be predisposed to cardiac dysrhythmias. Monitoring of calcium levels may be indicated earlier for these patients.

Autotransfusion

Autotransfusion, or administration of the patient's own blood from the chest tube collection chamber, may be an option when transfusion is needed, often for a massive hemothorax.[1] Follow the package recommendations, which usually suggest administration within 6 hours. Benefits include the following:

- The patient is transfused with his or her own fresh whole blood, eliminating the risk of transfusion reaction.
- Blood is warmer than room temperature, with no waiting for blood products to warm.
- RBCs in autotransfused blood may have better oxygen-carrying capacity, as older, banked blood may have RBCs that have begun to degrade.
- Autotransfusion has a lower cost than transfusion of banked blood.
- The transfusion carries a lower risk of communicable disease.
- The transfused blood has a lower potassium level than banked blood.
- Patients do not require anticoagulation (fibrinogen and other clotting factors adhere to the pleura; without fibrinogen, blood cannot clot).[1]

Disadvantages of autotransfusion include the following:

- There is a risk of contamination from a microorganism within the patient's chest.
- Use is limited to patients with an isolated hemothorax without diaphragmatic perforation.
- RBCs may become hemolyzed during hemorrhage.
- Coagulation factors, including platelets and cryoprecipitate may be destroyed, increasing the D-dimer in the collected blood.
- Patients may develop an enhanced inflammatory response, contributing to multiple-organ failure.

Damage Control Surgeries

Damage control surgery is a shift from rapid definitive surgery and complete repair to surgery that is intended to stop the bleeding, restore normothermia, and treat coagulopathy and acidosis; in other words, it is geared toward providing resuscitation from the trauma triad (Figure 5-5).[19] Damage control surgery is recommended to last no longer than 90 minutes due to the high morbidity and mortality rate from this type of procedure.[19] Definitive injury repair is accomplished later during planned or staged operations after the patient has been further resuscitated, stabilized, and warmed in the intensive care unit (ICU).

Tranexamic Acid

Tranexamic acid (TXA) is a synthetic version of the amino acid lysine. This antifibrinolytic agent inhibits activation of plasminogen, a substance that is responsible for dissolving clots. TXA has been safely used to reduce intraoperative bleeding in elective medical and dental surgery and for the control of heavy menstrual bleeding.

Some jurisdictions are giving TXA in the prehospital setting in response to a study that showed increased survival rates if this medication is given within 3 hours of the injury. The first dose is typically given over 10 minutes in the prehospital setting, with a follow-up dose of 1 g given over 8 hours.[1] The U.S. Food and Drug Administration has not approved TXA for use in trauma, but given its promising research results, approval and widespread use are likely to occur in the near future.[20]

Nursing Care of the Patient in Shock

Nursing care of the patient in shock begins with preparation and triage.

Preparation and Triage

The American College of Surgeons Committee on Trauma (ACS-COT) considers an SBP of 90 mm Hg or less in the prehospital setting to be a criterion for trauma team activation at the highest level.[17] One study found that a single SBP reading of less than 105 mm Hg was associated with severe injuries that often required operative or endovascular treatment and admission to the ICU. In light of this risk, an isolated hypotensive blood pressure measurement in a prehospital setting is considered to be significant.[1]

Safe Practice, Safe Care

In the patient at risk for or experiencing traumatic shock, it is essential that assessment and intervention occur simultaneously and systematically. The primary survey is performed; life-threatening problems are treated and reassessed prior to moving to the next step and prior to moving to the secondary survey. Integrated ongoing assessments, history, physical examination, imaging and laboratory studies, and serial assessments are crucial to optimizing patient outcomes by anticipating potential blood loss from suspected or actual injuries and having a proactive management plan that anticipates the patient's potential course.

Primary Survey and Resuscitation Adjuncts

Refer to Chapter 3, "Initial Assessment," for the systematic approach to the nursing care of the trauma patient. The following assessment parameters are specific to patients with signs of shock.

A: Alertness and Airway

Considerations for assessing alertness and airway of patients with signs of shock include the following:

- Unresponsiveness in the trauma patient may be due to hypovolemia, not head trauma.
- A patient may experience uncompensated shock with a blood volume loss of 30% to 40% before becoming unresponsive.[1]
- Use of alcohol and other substances may mask shock-induced changes in LOC in early shock, and contribute to the inability to protect the airway.

B: Breathing and Ventilation

Inspect for the following:

- Increased work of breathing may indicate compensation for early hypovolemic shock and respiratory correction of metabolic acidosis.
- Administer supplemental oxygen via nonrebreather mask to achieve optimal oxygenation if not already completed as indicated in the assessment of the airway and breathing. Administer oxygen to maintain oxygen saturation (SpO_2) between 94% and 98%.[6]

C: Circulation and Control of Hemorrhage

Inspect for the following:

- Active external bleeding
- Skin color, temperature, and moisture
- Bruised, swollen, and deformed extremities, particularly long bone fractures
- A distended abdomen, which may indicate occult blood loss
- An unstable pelvis

Auscultate for the following:

- Diminished breath sounds (possible pneumothorax or hemothorax)
- Muffled heart tones (possible pericardial tamponade)

Palpate for the following:

- Central and peripheral pulses
  - Increased or bounding central pulses may indicate increased cardiac output, which can be the result of the release of catecholamines from the sympathetic nervous system in an effort to increase cardiac output.
  - Peripheral pulses do not demonstrate a similar effect in the presence of hypovolemia due to vasoconstriction. Thus, strong central pulses combined with weak peripheral pulses may be indicative of shock.
- Tenderness and rigidity in the abdomen and instability in the pelvis may be signs of occult hemorrhage.

Interventions

Interventions include the following:

- Control external hemorrhage with direct pressure. Tourniquets are indicated if bleeding in the extremities is not controlled with direct pressure.[1]
- A pelvic binder or sheet is recommended for stabilization for confirmed unstable pelvic fracture. See Chapter 8, "Abdominal and Pelvic Trauma," for more information.
- Insert two large-caliber peripheral IV catheters.
  - If IV access cannot be rapidly obtained, default to IO access. IO and peripheral IV access allow for a more rapid infusion because the catheter length is shorter than a central line.[1]
  - Use a rapid infuser that warms the blood with blood tubing adequate to transfuse blood components.
    - Infuse blood products maintaining the 1:1:1 ratio.
    - Once hemostasis is achieved, it is estimated that one unit of packed RBCs will increase hemoglobin by 1 g/dL and hematocrit by 3%.[4]
    - Use Rh-negative blood whenever possible. If O-negative blood is limited, O-positive blood can be administered to men and postmenopausal women. If O-positive blood is administered to premenopausal women, they may become sensitized to the Rh factor, which may impact future pregnancies.
    - Consider activation of the MTP (unmatched type O blood, thawed fresh frozen plasma, and platelets). If blood is not available, infuse a 500-mL bolus of warmed isotonic crystalloid solution and reassess the patient's fluid status after each bolus.[21]
    - Vasopressors are contraindicated in early shock because they can worsen tissue perfusion.[1] However, studies have recently shown that controlled use of vasopressors may be beneficial in persistent hemorrhagic shock that does not respond to fluids and blood products. Further research is required.[21]

D: Disability (Neurologic Status)

Assess for loss of consciousness. A decrease may be indicative of hypoxemia and uncontrolled internal bleeding.

E: Exposure and Environmental Control

Address exposure and environmental control concerns by doing the following:

- Remove clothing to inspect for additional injuries and bleeding.
- Prevent hypothermia by warming resuscitation fluids to maintain the patient's temperature at 37°C (98.6°F).

Other warming measures include warm blankets, warmed IV fluids, convective temperature management systems, and intravascular temperature management systems.

F: Full Set of Vital Signs

Obtain a full set of vital signs.

Blood Pressure Measurements

SBP does not directly reflect cardiac output, although trending vital signs may offer useful information regarding improved blood flow to the organs and tissue oxygenation to guide continued care. Additional measurements include the following:

- Frequent and serial blood pressure measurements to determine narrowing pulse pressure changes and monitor for signs of vascular compensatory mechanisms
- Blood pressure differences between the right and left arm, which may be a sign of thoracic aorta injury

Obtain the patient's temperature because hypothermia causes decreased tissue oxygenation, acidosis, and increased coagulopathy, resulting in increased morbidity and mortality.

Heart Rate

Heart rate may indicate the following:

- Tachycardia is one of the first signs of compensated shock in adults and especially in pediatric patients.
- Bradycardia and hypotension in combination with an SCI can reflect neurogenic shock.

Respirations

Respiration may indicate the following:

- Tachypnea is an early indicator of compensated shock.
- Bradypnea may reflect the irreversible stage of shock.

G: Get Monitoring Devices and Give Comfort

Resuscitation adjuncts include laboratory studies, monitoring, and oxygenation.

L: Laboratory Studies

Laboratory studies used to guide resuscitative efforts in shock include the following:

- Platelet count and clotting studies, including prothrombin time-international normalized ratio (PT-INR), partial thromboplastin time (PTT), fibrinogen and D-dimer.
- Serum lactate, anion gap, base deficit, and ABGs to assess the degree of acidosis and oxygen debt.
- Toxicology screen to help assess mental status and differentiate shock from head injury.
- Calcium level when rapidly infusing large volumes of blood products.
- Additional blood specimens including those for a type and cross-match, hemoglobin and hematocrit, electrolytes, serum osmolarity, blood urea nitrogen, creatinine, amylase, and liver enzymes. These tests may be directly correlated to the shock pathophysiology and injuries; however, unlike serum lactate, platelets, and clotting factors, they are less useful in the initial treatment and more useful in ongoing reevaluation.

M: Monitor

Place the patient on the monitor in case of a blunt cardiac injury or a trauma-related cardiac mechanism of injury.

O: Oxygenation

Oxygenation resuscitation adjuncts include pulse oximetry and end-tidal carbon dioxide ($ETCO_2$) monitoring.

- *Pulse oximetry:* The goal is to maintain an SpO_2 reading of 94% to 98%.[4] As many variables may potentially skew pulse oximeter readings, including hemodilution, carbon monoxide exposure, hypothermia, and peripheral vasoconstriction, it is essential that patient management decisions not be made on pulse oximetry values alone.
- *$ETCO_2$ monitoring:* $ETCO_2$ monitoring can be used to rapidly assess endotracheal tube placement, symptomatic pneumothoraces, or other pulmonary pathologies. It may also be used to indirectly assess cardiac output as a function of pulmonary perfusion. Continuous waveform capnography will provide a breath-to-breath analysis of both ventilation and perfusion and serve as a valuable adjunct during resuscitation and ongoing monitoring. Capnography also indirectly measures cardiac output and can be used to monitor effectiveness of cardiopulmonary resuscitation (CPR) and the return of spontaneous circulation.[22]

J: Just Keep Reevaluating

Determine whether there is an early need for transport to a trauma center or to surgery.

Focused Assessment with Sonography for Trauma

Following the primary survey, a focused assessment with sonography for trauma (FAST) examination may be used to rapidly and noninvasively assess for bleeding resulting from damage to the heart, liver, bladder, pelvis, kidneys, and spleen. The FAST examination is also increasingly used to detect pneumothorax, especially tension pneumothorax.[1]

Portable Radiograph

If the trauma patient is suspected of having or being at risk for internal hemorrhage, chest and pelvic imaging can be performed in the resuscitation room to expedite early goal-directed management. This is true for patients who may have a sequestering hemorrhage in the highly vascular pelvis.

Secondary Survey

The secondary survey is concerned with additional history.

H: History

Additional history to be collected when the patient is at risk for shock includes the following:

- What was the estimated blood loss at the scene?
- Was there any episode of SBP less than 90 mm Hg during prehospital care?
- Does the patient have changes to LOC or other symptoms that might indicate the onset of shock?
- Does the patient have complaints of chest or abdominal pain?

Additional history also includes past medical history:

- Is there a history of hypertension? Does the patient take any antihypertensive medication?
- Is there a history of anticoagulant therapy?
- Is there a history of anemia or other blood dyscrasia (hemophilia)?

Positive responses may provide clues regarding acute blood loss, and careful inspection with close monitoring can lead to early detection of shock.

Diagnostics and Interventions

Reevaluation adjuncts include diagnostic studies and other types of studies.

Diagnostic Studies

Diagnostic studies include diagnostic peritoneal aspiration (DPA) and lavage as well as computed tomography (CT).

Diagnostic Peritoneal Aspiration and Lavage

Diagnostic peritoneal lavage is not used frequently but continues to be an option when FAST examination or CT is not available or when the patient is too unstable to move for a CT scan. One of the benefits to this procedure over a FAST exam is its high sensitivity for bleeding within the abdominal cavity; it may also reveal free enteric contents.[1] DPA may be an alternative to quickly identify intraperitoneal bleeding and lessen the delay if operative intervention is indicated.[23]

Computed Tomography

After stabilization and completion of the primary survey, CT is used to explore possible findings not seen on initial chest and abdominal radiography. An important caveat is that CT images are not required for transfer and should not delay transfer of the patient to a higher level of care if needed. Hemodynamically unstable trauma patients are high risk for deterioration during transport to radiology and imaging.

Other Studies

Subsequent to achieving hemodynamic stability, echocardiography and a 12-lead electrocardiogram will provide additional cardiac assessment data.

Consider insertion of a urinary catheter to monitor urine output:

- Urine output is an important indicator of fluid volume status and organ perfusion and needs to be monitored hourly.
- Adequate urinary output is 0.5 mL/kg per hour (for the 70-kg adult patient).[6]
- Output of less than 0.5 mL/kg per hour for 2 consecutive hours indicates oliguria.

Reevaluation and Post-Resuscitation Care

Reevaluation specific to shock includes the following measures:

- Continued assessments of the primary survey are performed to monitor for rebleeding and previously unnoticed injuries and to ensure sources of hemorrhage are controlled. Ongoing monitoring of hemoglobin, hematocrit, platelets, and clotting times may help to identify coagulopathy due to continued blood loss or hemodilutional effects of massive volume resuscitation.
- SpO_2 via pulse oximetry, $ETCO_2$ monitoring, and serial ABGs provide ongoing indicators of improved oxygenation, ventilation, and perfusion, including the following:
  - Normal serum pH
  - Decreasing serum lactate
  - Improved base excess
  - Signs of adequate perfusion to periphery
  - Adequate SpO_2
- Monitoring of urine output hourly is needed to assess effective resuscitation and renal perfusion and function. Oliguria and an elevated blood urea nitrogen-to-creatinine ratio are signs of possible hypoperfusion.
- Continued frequent monitoring of vital signs for the following:
  - Normothermia
  - Normotension
  - Stable heart and respiratory rates

Definitive Care and Transport

Prepare the patient for surgical interventions to explore body cavities for occult blood loss, such as thoracotomy or laparotomy for the patient with continued hypotension despite ongoing resuscitation or uncontrollable hemorrhage from the torso.

Emerging Trends

As the science and evidence of trauma care continue to evolve, tools to improve patient outcomes continue to be trialed and refined. Evidence is tested and replicated, and new standards of care are transitioned into practice. This section on care considerations for patients with shock explores some of the evidence and the potential significance to trauma patient care.

Thromboelastometry and Rotational Thromboelastometry

Thromboelastography (TEG) is a point-of-care testing method to evaluate the efficiency of blood clotting in the actively bleeding patient.[24] Unlike the standard coagulation assays, such as PT-INR and PTT, which measure only clotting factor function, TEG can also evaluate platelet function, clot strength, and fibrinolysis. Rotational thromboelastometry (ROTEM) is similar to TEG but uses a rotational technology. Both tests are used to guide transfusion strategies (including MTP) in the actively bleeding patient as well as to reduce the need for unnecessary transfusions.[24] Limitations include the following: The tests have varying sensitivity for diagnosing hyperfibrinolysis; body temperature of 37°C (98.6°F) is required for accuracy; the definitions of fibrinolysis as determined by TEG/ROTEM vary; and additional time is required to perform and read the test.[24]

Resuscitative Endovascular Balloon Occlusion of the Aorta

Resuscitative endovascular balloon occlusion of the aorta (REBOA) is an emerging technique used in trauma patients to stop life-threatening hemorrhage within the chest, abdomen, and pelvis (**Figure 5-7**).[25] In this procedure, a balloon is inserted in the aorta, occluding blood flow below the balloon and stopping the bleeding. REBOA can temporarily restore blood pressure to within normal physiological values by increasing cardiac afterload, thereby increasing cerebral and myocardial perfusion long enough until the patient can be taken to the operating room for definitive hemorrhage control.[26]

REBOA has emerged as a viable alternative to open aortic occlusion via open thoracotomy in trauma centers that have developed this capability, but further research is required to clarify its utility.[26] One study found that complications from REBOA were uncommon but included pseudoaneurysm, embolism, and limb ischemia.[26] Other

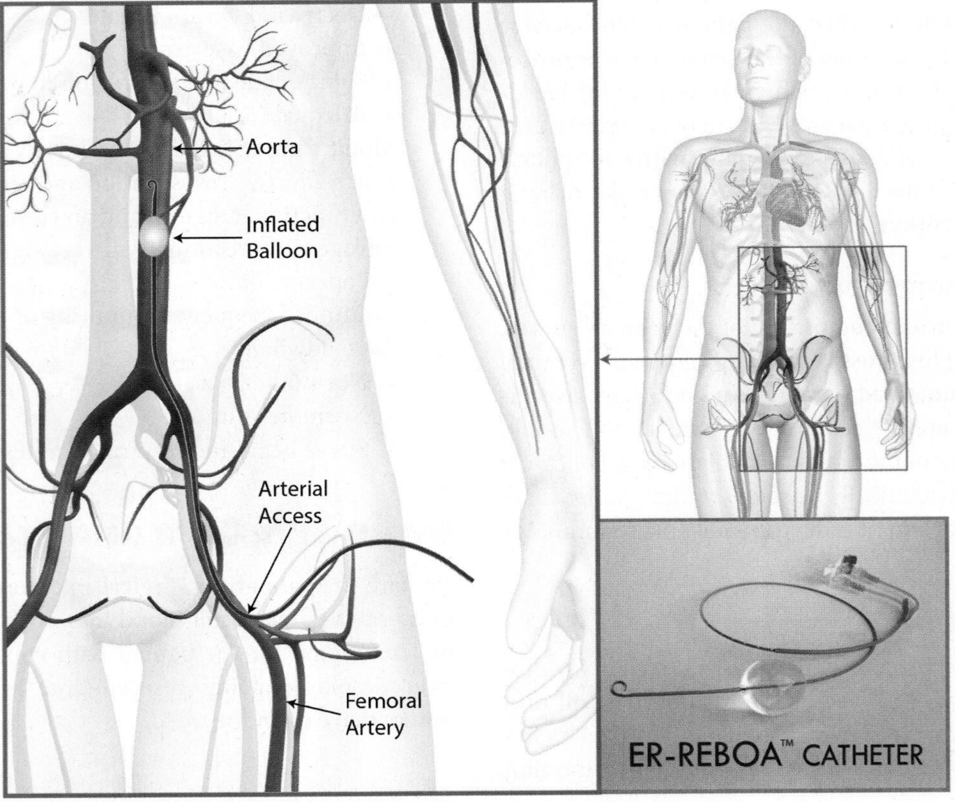

Figure 5-7 *Resuscitative endovascular balloon occlusion of the aorta.*

Reproduced from Trauma Ready. (n.d.). REBOA: Resuscitative endovascular balloon occlusion of the aorta. Retrieved from http://www.traumaready.com/reboa/.

limitations include limited data regarding outcomes, poorly defined indications, and limited provider training.

Whole Blood

Transfusion of whole blood, commonly used by the military and in austere environments, may be more beneficial than use of individual blood components in treating hemorrhagic shock. According to Murdock et al., the use of whole blood, compared to individual blood components, may result in faster resolution of shock and coagulopathy, reduced transfusion requirements, and decreased donor exposure to the recipient.[27] In addition, the rapid treatment of shock and coagulopathy with whole blood may improve patient outcomes by reducing the risk of organ failure and death, decreasing complications, and reducing care costs.[27]

Freeze-Dried Plasma

The use of freeze-dried plasma has been adopted by the military in France and is being trialed by U.S. Army Special Forces. The advantage of this product is that it can remain effective in its freeze-dried form for up to two years, until it is reconstituted with sterile water and administered to a patient. Further research into this product continues.[28]

Hemostatic Dressings

Hemostatic dressings such as CELOX and QuickClot have been used by the military for patients with active bleeding since the war in Afghanistan and have been shown to be effective in conjunction with tourniquet use, especially on wounds where a tourniquet would be difficult to use.[29] These dressings contain a hemostatic agent that hastens clotting until definitive hemorrhage control can be initiated. The ACS-COT has released an evidence-based guideline on the use of these agents.[29]

Bleeding Control Education and Training for the Community

Evidence continues to show that trauma victims can die from uncontrolled bleeding within 5 to 10 minutes.[13] Just as the general public and lay community learn and perform CPR, education on bleeding control techniques using hands, dressings, and tourniquets is being offered in a new program available to the community that can also save a life. The ACS-COT and the Hartford Consensus have developed education and training for the general public on bleeding control. The "STOP the Bleed" course continues to be offered nationwide with the goal being to help prevent death from uncontrolled bleeding.[13] See Chapter 10, "Musculoskeletal Trauma," for more information on the "Stop the Bleed" campaign.

Summary

Shock is a syndrome of impaired tissue perfusion and oxygenation. Mismatch between the supply and demand of oxygen and nutrients leads to ischemia at the cellular level, a transition to anaerobic metabolism and acidosis, and ultimately organ death. Shock may be classified into four broad categories: hypovolemic, obstructive, cardiogenic, and distributive. Hypovolemic shock and depletion of circulating volume secondary to hemorrhage is the most common and primary shock state observed in trauma and the leading cause of preventable death in trauma. Regardless of the shock's etiology, it is essential for the trauma nurse to rapidly recognize and intervene to optimize oxygen transport and tissue perfusion. Primary contributors to mortality in hemorrhagic shock include failure to recognize and failure to intervene early.[1] This leads to a shock state progressing and leading to the resuscitation complications of hypothermia, acidosis, and coagulopathy. Early recognition and management of these concomitant variables is essential to ultimately optimizing patient outcomes in traumatic shock.

References

1. American College of Surgeons. (2018). Shock. In *Advanced trauma life support: Student course manual* (10th ed., pp. 42–61). Chicago, IL: Author.
2. Wyzant. (n.d.). Cellular respiration. Retrieved from https://www.wyzant.com/resources/lessons/science/biology/cellular-respiration
3. Von Rueden, K. T., Des Champs, E. S., & Johnson, K. L. (2013). Shock, systemic inflammatory response syndrome, and multiple organ dysfunction syndrome. In P. G. Morton & D. K. Fontaine (Eds.), *Critical care nursing: A holistic approach* (10th ed., pp. 1209–1233). Philadelphia, PA: Lippincott Williams & Wilkins.
4. Holleran, R. S. (2010). Shock emergencies. In P. K. Howard & R. A. Steinmann (Eds.), *Sheehy's emergency nursing principles and practice* (6th ed., pp. 445–456). Philadelphia, PA: Elsevier.
5. Othman, F. (2014). Shock (Blog post). Retrieved from http://thesternkey.blogspot.com/2014/12/i-was-shocked.html
6. Holleran, R. S. (2018). Shock emergencies. In V. Sweet (Ed.), *Emergency nursing core curriculum* (7th ed., pp. 473–482). St. Louis, MO: Elsevier.
7. Carlson, B., & Fitzsimmons, L. (2018). Shock, sepsis, and multiple organ dysfunction syndrome. In L. D. Urden, K. M. Stacy, & M. E. Lough (Eds.), *Critical care nursing: Diagnosis and management* (8th ed., pp. 801–839). St. Louis, MO: Elsevier Mosby.
8. Gerecht, R. (2014). Trauma's lethal triad of hypothermia, acidosis & coagulopathy create a deadly cycle for trauma patients.

Journal of Emergency Medical Services. Retrieved from http://www.jems.com/articles/print/volume-39/issue-4/features/trauma-s-lethal-triad-hypothermia-acidos.html

9. Katrancha, E. D., & Gonzalez, L. S. (2014). Trauma-induced coagulopathy. *Critical Care Nurse, 34*(4), 54–63. https://doi.org/10.4037/ccn2014133
10. Kushimoto, S., Kudo, D., & Kawazoe, Y. (2017). Acute traumatic coagulopathy and trauma-induced coagulopathy: An overview. *Journal of Intensive Care, 5*. https://doi.org/10.1186/s40560-016-0196-6
11. Vincent, J., & De Backer, D. (2013). Circulatory shock. *The New England Journal of Medicine, 369*, 1726–1734. https://doi.org/10.1056/NEJMra1208943
12. Jacobs, B. B. (Ed.). (2000). *Trauma nursing core course* (5th ed.). Des Plaines, IL: Emergency Nurses Association.
13. American College of Surgeons Committee on Trauma. (2018). Stop the bleed. Retrieved from https://www.bleedingcontrol.org/about-bc
14. Bulger, E. M., Snyder, D., Schoelles, K., Gotschall, C., Dawson, D., Lang E., . . . McSwain, N., Jr. (2014). An evidence-based prehospital guideline for external hemorrhage control: American College of Surgeons Committee on Trauma. *Prehospital Emergency Care, 18*(2), 163–173. https://doi.org/10.3109/10903127.2014.896962
15. American College of Surgeons Committee on Trauma. (2017). Hartford Consensus. Hemorrhage control devices: Tourniquets and hemostatic dressings. Retrieved from https://www.bleedingcontrol.org/~/media/bleedingcontrol/files/hartford%20consensus%20compendium.ashx
16. Chatrath, V., Khetarpal, R., & Ahuja, J. (2015). Fluid management in patients with trauma: Restrictive versus liberal approach. *Journal of Anaesthesiology Clinical Pharmacology, 31*(3), 308–316. https://doi.org/10.4103/0970-9185.161664
17. American College of Surgeons Committee on Trauma. (2014). *Resources for optimal care of the injured patient.* Chicago, IL: Author. Retrieved from https://www.facs.org/~/media/files/quality%20programs/trauma/vrc%20resources/resources%20for%20optimal%20care.ashx
18. American College of Surgeons Committee on Trauma. (2013). Trauma Quality Improvement Program best practice guidelines: Massive transfusion in trauma. Retrieved from https://www.facs.org/~/media/files/quality%20programs/trauma/tqip/massive%20transfusion%20in%20trauma%20guildelines.ashx
19. Gupta, A., Kumar, S., Sagar, S., Sharma, P., Mishra, B., Singhal, M., & Misra, M. C. (2017). Damage control surgery: 6 years of experience at a Level I trauma center. *Turkish Journal of Trauma and Emergency Surgery, 23*(4), 322–327. https://doi.org/10.5505/tjtes.2016.03693
20. Huebner, B. R., Dorlac, W. C., & Cribari, C. (2017). Tranexamic acid use in prehospital uncontrolled hemorrhage. *Wilderness & Environmental Medicine, 28*(2 Suppl.), S50–S60. https://doi.org/10.1016/j.wem.2016.12.006
21. Gupta, B., Garg, N., & Ramachandran, R. (2017). Vasopressors: Do they have any role in hemorrhagic shock? *Journal of Anaesthesiology Clinical Pharmacology, 33*(1), 3–8. https://doi.org/10.4103/0970-9185.202185
22. American Heart Association. (2016). Part 5: The ACLS cases: Cardiac arrest: VF/Pulseless VT. In *Advanced cardiovascular life support provider manual* (pp. 92–109). Dallas, TX: Author.
23. Kuncir, E. J., & Velmahos, G. C. (2007). Diagnostic peritoneal aspiration: The foster child of DPL: A prospective observational study. *International Journal of Surgery, 5*(3), 167–171. https://doi.org/10.1016/j.ijsu.2006.06.013
24. Walsh, M., Fritz, S., Hake, D., Son, M., Greve, S., Jbara, M., . . . Castellino, F. J. (2016). Targeted thromboelastographic (TEG) blood component and pharmacologic hemostatic therapy in traumatic and acquired coagulopathy. *Current Drug Targets, 17*(8), 954–970. http://doi.org/10.2174/1389450117666160310153211
25. Trauma Ready. (n.d.). REBOA: Resuscitative endovascular balloon occlusion of the aorta. Retrieved from http://www.traumaready.com/reboa/
26. DuBose, J. J., Scalea, T. M., Brenner, M., Skiada, D., Inaba, K., Cannon, J., . . . AAST AORTA Study Group (2016). The AAST prospective Aortic Occlusion for Resuscitation in Trauma and Acute Care Surgery (AORTA) registry: Data on contemporary utilization and outcomes of aortic occlusion and resuscitative balloon occlusion of the aorta (REBOA). *Journal of Trauma and Acute Care Surgery, 81*(3), 409–419. https://doi.org/10.1097/TA.0000000000001079
27. Murdock, A. D., Berséus, O., Hervig, T., Strandenes, G., & Lunde, T. H. (2014). Whole blood: The future of traumatic hemorrhagic shock resuscitation. *Shock, 41*, 62–69. https://doi.org/10.1097/SHK.0000000000000134
28. Soares, J. M. (2017). Saving lives with freeze-dried plasma. U.S. Army. Retrieved from https://www.army.mil/article/197409/saving_lives_with_freeze_dried_plasma
29. Sigal, A., Martin, A., & Ong, A. (2017). Availability and use of hemostatic agents in prehospital trauma patients in Pennsylvania translation from the military to the civilian setting. *Open Access Emergency Medicine, 9*, 47–52. https://doi.org/10.2147/OAEM.S134657

CHAPTER 6

Head Trauma

Melody R. Campbell, DNP, APRN-CNS, CEN, CCNS, CCRN, TCRN

OBJECTIVES

Upon completion of this chapter, the learner will be able to:

1. Describe the mechanisms of injury associated with brain, cranial, and maxillofacial trauma.
2. Describe pathophysiologic changes as a basis for assessment of the trauma patient with brain, cranial, and maxillofacial injuries.
3. Demonstrate the nursing assessment of the trauma patient with brain, cranial, and maxillofacial injuries.
4. Plan appropriate interventions for the trauma patient with brain, cranial, and maxillofacial injuries.
5. Evaluate the effectiveness of nursing interventions for the trauma patient with brain, cranial, and maxillofacial injuries.

Knowledge of normal anatomy and physiology serves as a foundation for understanding anatomic derangements and pathophysiologic processes that may result from trauma. Before reading this chapter, it is strongly suggested that the learner review the following material. The anatomy material is not emphasized in the classroom but may be the basis of skill evaluation assessments and the basis of questions for testing purposes.

Anatomy and Physiology of the Brain, Cranium, and Face

This section provides a review of the anatomy and physiology of the brain, cranium, and face.

Scalp

The scalp consists of five layers of tissue. These layers can be remembered by using the mnemonic **SCALP**: **s**kin, **c**onnective tissue, **a**poneurosis (galea aponeurotica), **l**oose areolar tissue, and **p**ericranium.[1] The scalp provides a protective covering and absorbs some energy transferred during an injury event. Since the scalp is highly vascular, lacerations or tears of it can result in profuse bleeding.[2]

Skull

The skull, which is formed by the cranial bones (frontal, ethmoid, sphenoid, occipital, parietal, and temporal) and the facial bones, provides protection to the contents within the cranial vault (**Figure 6-1**).[3] The cranial

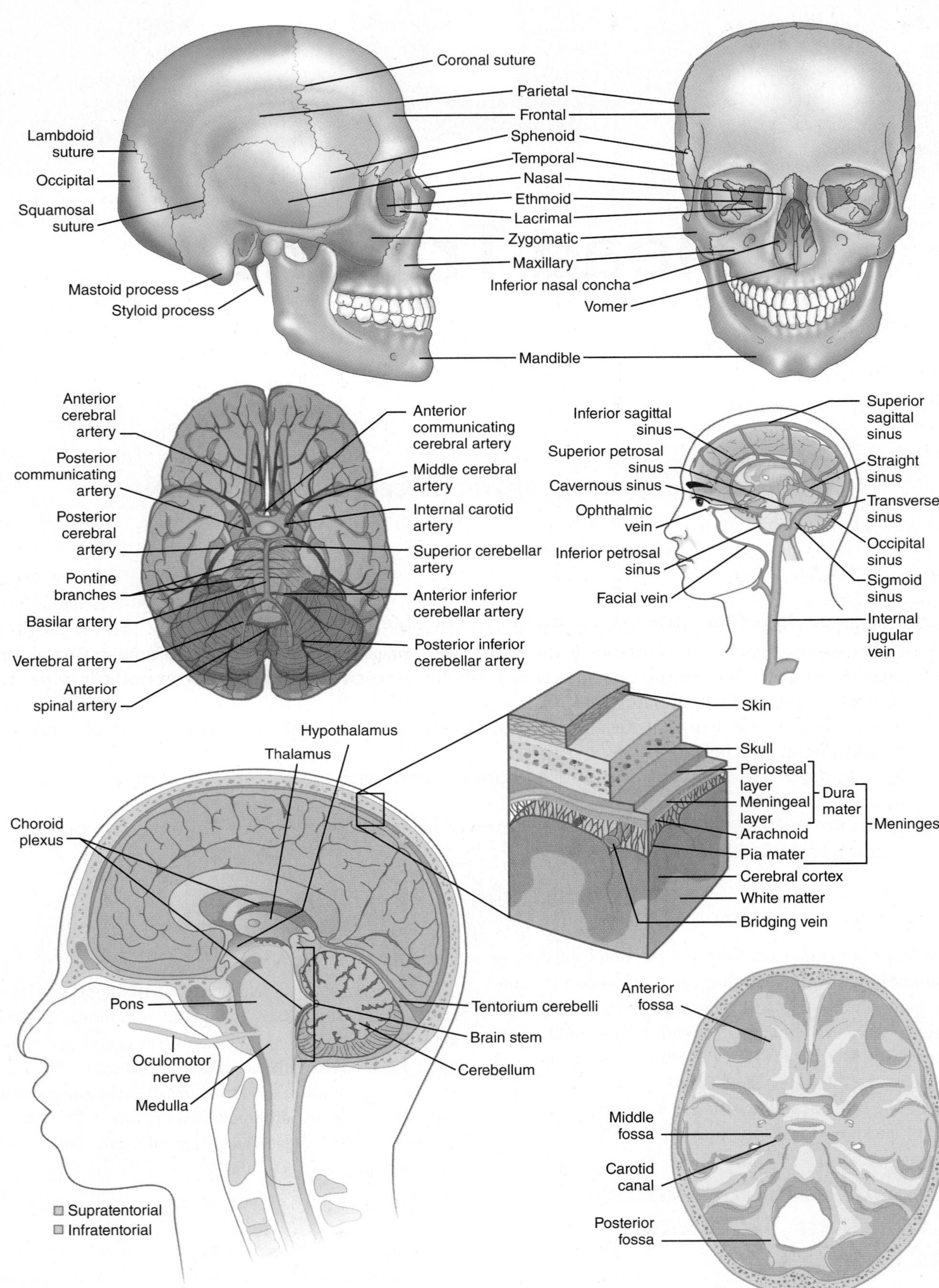

Figure 6-1 *Anatomy of the skull.*

bones are relatively thick (up to 6 mm), with the exception of the temporal bone. Because of the thickness of the cranium, the skull may not fracture when struck by excessive force. However, its lack of flexibility prevents absorption of energy, such that the force is transmitted to the parenchyma and vascular structures of the brain, causing injury without skull fracture. The base of the skull forms three depressions: the anterior, middle, and posterior fossae. The internal surface of the skull base is rough and irregular. As a result of acceleration and deceleration, the brain moves across these rough inner surfaces, resulting in contusions, lacerations, and shearing injuries.[2]

Meninges

The meninges consist of three layers of protective coverings—the **p**ia mater, **a**rachnoid membrane, and **d**ura mater—that **PAD** the brain and spinal cord. The pia mater, the innermost layer, firmly attaches to the brain and spinal cord. The arachnoid membrane is thin and transparent. The dura mater, the outermost layer, is a tough, fibrous membrane that adheres to the internal surface of the skull.[4]

The choroid plexus in the ventricles of the brain produces cerebrospinal fluid (CSF), which circulates around the brain beneath the arachnoid membrane (subarachnoid space) and through the central canal of the spinal cord.[5] The CSF cushions and protects the brain and spinal cord. Arteries, including the middle meningeal arteries, are located above the dura mater. Small bridging veins lie beneath the dura mater. Potential spaces may expand following injury due to bleeding and swelling that occurs above the dura (epidural) or below the dura (subdural).[2]

Tentorium

The tentorium cerebelli, which is part of the dura mater, extends from the occipital bone to the center of the cranium. The tentorium divides the cranial vault into two compartments—supratentorial and infratentorial. The supratentorial compartment contains the cerebral hemispheres in the anterior and middle fossae. The infratentorial compartment contains the lower parts of the brainstem (pons and medulla) and the cerebellum in the posterior fossa. The upper part of the brain stem (midbrain) and the oculomotor nerve (cranial nerve [CN] III) pass through a gap in the tentorium. Injury or edema near the tentorium gap may cause compression and shifting of the brain stem structures and the oculomotor nerve against the tentorium.[5,6]

Brain

The two cerebral hemispheres of the brain are divided into the frontal, parietal, temporal, and occipital lobes (**Figure 6-2**). The lobes are responsible for judgment, reasoning, social restraint, and voluntary motor functions (frontal); sensory functions and spatial orientation (parietal); speech, auditory, and memory functions (temporal); and vision (occipital).[3,6]

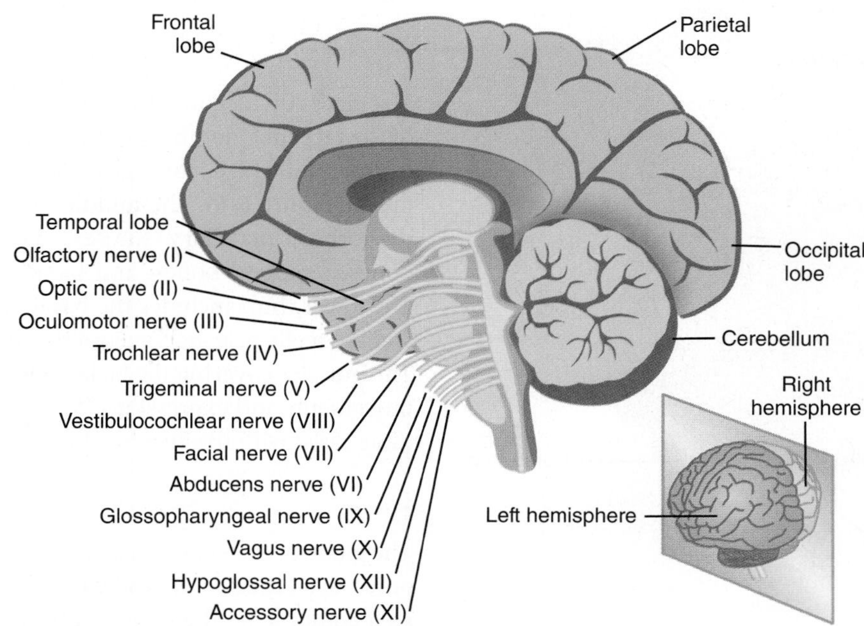

Figure 6-2 *Lobes of the brain.*

The diencephalon (**Figure 6-3**) connects the two cerebral hemispheres with the midbrain; it includes the thalamus, hypothalamus, optic chiasma, and pineal gland. These subcortical structures play major roles in hormonal regulation and metabolic functions, including the following:

- Sensation of pain and temperature regulation
- Motor control
- Release of hormones from the pituitary gland and adrenal cortex
- Activation of the sympathetic and parasympathetic nervous systems[7]

The three divisions of the brain stem are the midbrain, pons, and medulla (**Figure 6-4**). The reticular activating system (RAS) is composed of clusters of specialized neural tissue that originate in the midbrain and pons. The RAS is primarily responsible for wakefulness or consciousness, while the medulla and the pons are responsible for vital functions such as cardiovascular function and respiration. Injury to the brain stem is associated with changes in consciousness and impairment in vital functions—specifically, blood pressure (BP), heart rate, and respiration.[5]

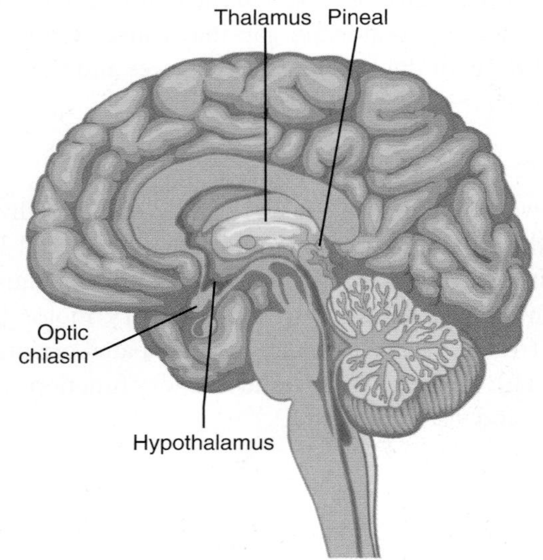

Figure 6-3 *Diencephalon.*

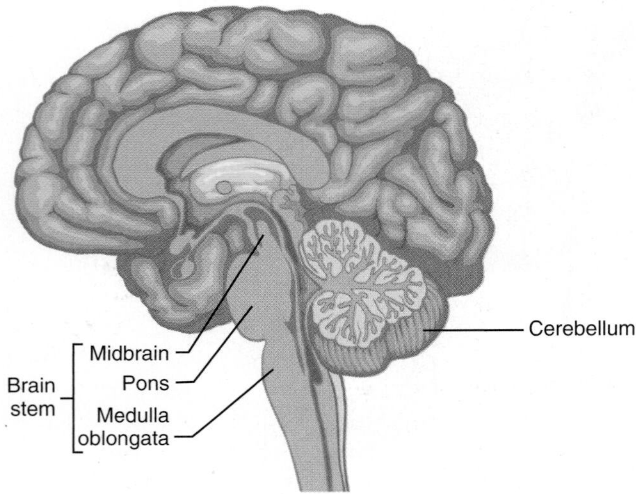

Figure 6-4 *Brainstem.*

The cerebellum is located in the posterior fossa and lies behind the brain stem and beneath the cerebral hemispheres. It has extensive neural connections with the spinal cord, midbrain, and cerebral hemispheres.[3,5] Primary functions of the cerebellum include voluntary and involuntary muscle coordination, movement, balance, and posture.

Cranial Nerves

There are 12 pairs of CNs (**Figure 6-5**).[6] The olfactory nerve (CN I) consists of a group of nerves located within a fiber tract that connect the nasal mucosa to the olfactory bulb. The optic nerve (CN II) originates in the retina and is considered a fiber tract once it leaves the optic chiasm. Millions of optic fibers then branch out to the occipital and temporal lobes. The brain stem is the point of origin for CNs III through X and XII, all of which exit via the skull foramina, leaving the cranial vault through the base of the lower brain. This shared exit pathway increases the risk for compression injury to the nerve tissue with subsequent swelling and tissue damage.[3] The accessory nerves (CN XI) have both a cranial component and a spinal component.[8]

Face

The face is divided into functional thirds. The upper third of the face includes the lower portion of the frontal bone, supraorbital ridge, nasal glabellar region, and frontal sinuses (**Figure 6-6**). The middle third (midface) includes the orbits, maxillary sinuses, nasal bone, zygomatic bones, temporal bones, and basal bone of the maxilla. The lower third includes the basal bone of the mandible and the teeth-bearing bones of the maxilla and mandible. The muscles covering the facial bones contribute to facial movements and expressions. Muscles covering the mandible assist with mastication and jaw movement.

Eyes

The globe of the eye consists of multiple layers. The white outer layer, the *sclera*, can be easily seen without specialized equipment. The *cornea*, a transparent, multilayered convex structure, covers the iris and pupil. The globe

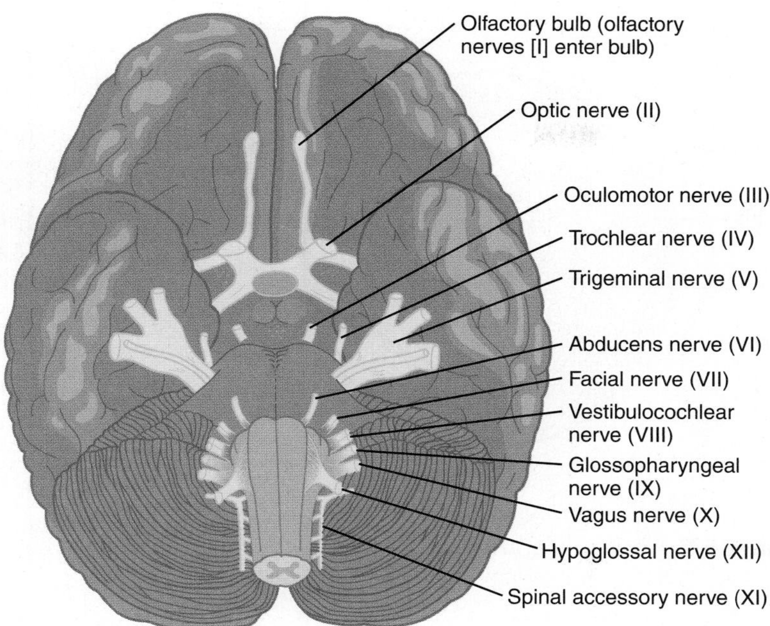

Figure 6-5 *Cranial nerves.*

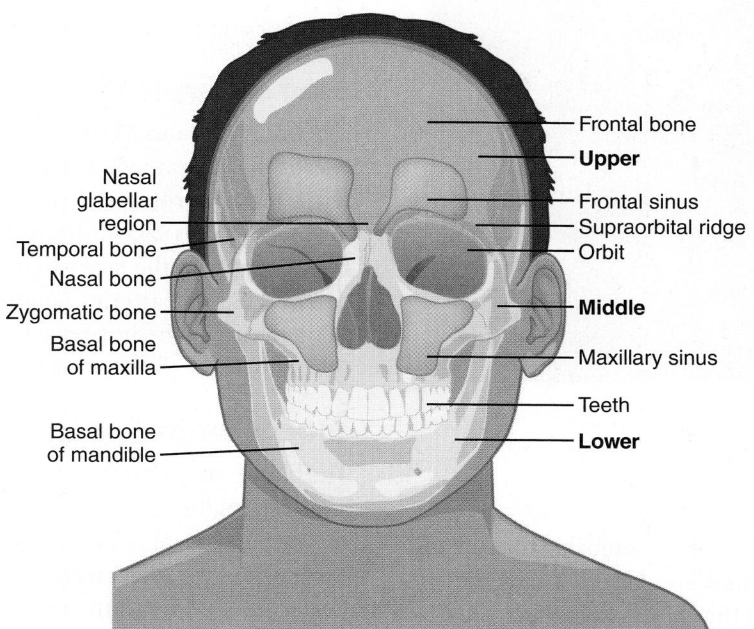

Figure 6-6 *Anatomy of the face.*

consists of the anterior and posterior chamber and the vitreous chamber (**Figure 6-7**).

The *conjunctiva*, which is a mucous membrane, covers the sclera and inner surface of the eyelid. Tears are secreted from the lacrimal glands in the upper eyelids and lubricate and protect the eye. These tears drain through the punctum located at the inner canthus of the eye.

The *vitreous humor* is located behind the lens and fills most of the eye. The anterior chamber is located between the cornea and iris and is filled with aqueous humor. *Aqueous humor* is a watery substance that supports the cornea and lens. The cornea is an avascular layer of tissue that covers the iris and pupil. The iris is the colored portion of the eye and is positioned between the cornea and

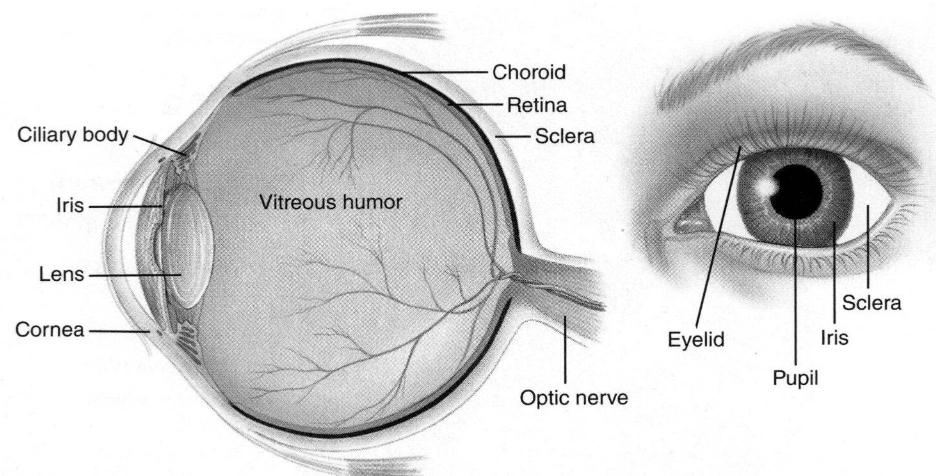

Figure 6-7 *Anatomy of the eye.*

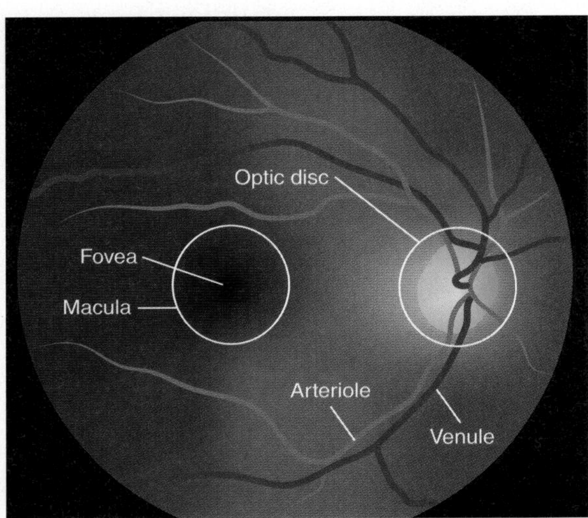

Figure 6-8 *Fundus of the eye.*

the lens; it contains the muscles responsible for constriction and dilation of the pupil.[9]

The retina is located at the back of the globe. The macula and fovea are located within the retina. The macula is the dark spot on the fundus of the eye that provides for clear and distinct vision, whereas the fovea is where vision is the sharpest. The optic disc exits the back of the eye to form the optic nerve; it appears as a pale round area with a large number of blood vessels (**Figure 6-8**).

The movement of the eye is controlled by four rectus muscles and two oblique muscles. The eye is innervated by CNs II, III, IV, V, and VI. Eye movement is controlled by CNs III, IV, and VI. CN VII innervates the eyelids to close, and CN III innervates them to open. Ptosis (eyelid drooping) occurs due to oculomotor nerve (CN III) palsy. The blood supply to the eye comes from the ophthalmic artery, which branches off to form the central retinal artery. The majority of venous drainage occurs through the superior and inferior ophthalmic veins.

Blood Supply for the Head

The brain contains a large vascular supply. Arterial blood travels to the brain via two pairs of arteries: the right and left internal carotid and the right and left vertebral arteries.[10] Venous blood drains via the jugular veins. The blood supply to the face originates from the internal and external carotid arteries (**Figure 6-9**).[11] Injury resulting in uncontrolled hemorrhage from any of these blood vessels may be life threatening.[9]

Blood–Brain Barrier

The blood–brain barrier (BBB) is a network of capillaries and cells tightly surrounding the brain that act as a filter for the central nervous system. The BBB controls the exchange of oxygen, carbon dioxide, and metabolites between the blood and the brain. This barrier makes brain capillaries less permeable, preventing some substances from crossing into the brain tissue.[6] Traumatic brain injury causes the BBB to become dysfunctional, ultimately contributing to the edema, increased intracranial pressure (ICP), and decreased perfusion pressure.[12]

Cerebral Blood Flow

The brain uses approximately 20% of the body's total oxygen supply and is heavily dependent upon glucose metabolism for energy.[10] The brain does not have the ability to store essential nutrients; therefore, it requires

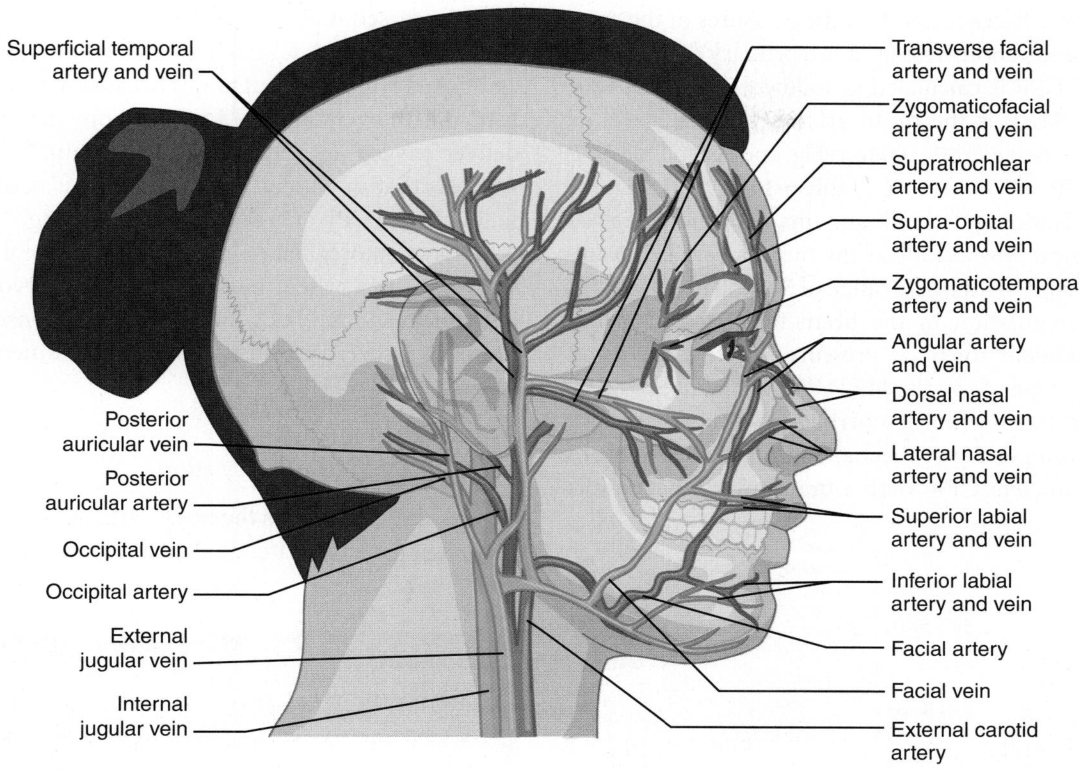

Figure 6-9 *Blood supply for the head.*

a continuous supply of both oxygen and glucose through the cerebral blood flow (CBF). The brain can self-regulate to maintain CBF through a process that is both complex and multifaceted. Cerebral vessels change their diameter in response to physiologic changes in the body. Hypotension, hypercarbia, and acidosis will result in cerebral vasodilation, whereas cerebral vasoconstriction results from hypertension, hypocarbia, and alkalosis. Normal CBF can be maintained with mean arterial BPs in the range of 50–150 mm Hg.[3] Outside of these parameters, cerebral autoregulation will fail, resulting in further injury to the brain. Carbon dioxide (CO_2) is a primary regulator of blood flow to the brain as well as a strong vasodilator. At higher than normal levels (e.g., when a trauma patient has slow, shallow respirations), the increased partial pressure of carbon dioxide ($PaCO_2$) causes cerebral vasodilation, which increases cerebral blood volume and perfusion.[8,13,14] Conversely, if the level of $PaCO_2$ decreases (e.g., as a result of aggressive bag-mask ventilation/hyperventilation), cerebral vasoconstriction occurs, reducing blood volume and perfusion, subsequently decreasing ICP. Initially, the brain responds to the hypoxemia by increasing oxygen extraction from blood. When hypoxia becomes acute (PaO_2 less than 50 mm Hg), cerebral vasodilation occurs and blood flow increases.[10]

Intracranial Pressure

The cranial vault contains three main components:

- The brain, which occupies about 80%
- Blood (arterial and venous), which occupies about 10%
- Cerebral spinal fluid, which occupies about 10%

These volumes are relatively fixed, and together they create a normal ICP of 0–15 mm Hg. Small changes in individual volumes can occur without affecting ICP or changing the constant total volume. Sustained ICP greater than 20 mm Hg is considered abnormal.[8,15] According to the Monro–Kellie doctrine, as the volume of one component of the cranial vault triad expands, the volume of one or both of the other components must decrease to maintain a constant ICP (**Figure 6-10**).[8] The potential for intracranial compensation is limited because the cranial vault is inflexible. Thus, even small increases in total volume may cause significant increases in ICP, resulting in a decrease in CBF and a decrease in cerebral perfusion pressure (CPP).

Cerebral Perfusion Pressure

Adequate perfusion of oxygen and supply of nutrients (glucose) to the brain tissue is dependent on the CPP and CBF. CPP is defined as the pressure gradient across the brain tissue, or the difference between the pressures of the cerebral artery and venous vessels. It is a primary determinant of CBF.[5,8,12] CPP is calculated as follows: CPP = MAP – ICP, where MAP is the mean arterial pressure. Normal CPP is in the range of 60–100 mm Hg, and acceptable CPP is between 50 and 70 mm Hg (**Table 6-1**).[10,14,16-18]

Cerebral autoregulation maintains a constant cerebral vascular blood flow as long as the mean arterial pressure (MAP) is maintained in the range of 50–150 mm Hg.[3,10,14] When autoregulation in the brain fails, perfusion becomes dependent solely on pressure—that is, perfusion of the brain depends on the MAP. If maintenance of MAP is disrupted (such as in hemorrhage and hypovolemia), the body's compensatory mechanisms may not be able to sustain a sufficient CPP. With a brain injury that results in an increased ICP, a normal MAP may not be sufficient to maintain CPP. A CPP of less than 60 mm Hg has been associated with poor outcomes because arterial pressure is unable to overcome the increased pressure gradient to deliver oxygen and nutrients to the brain.[14] One report suggests that in patients with ischemia, it is advisable to maintain the CPP at greater than 70 mm Hg.[14]

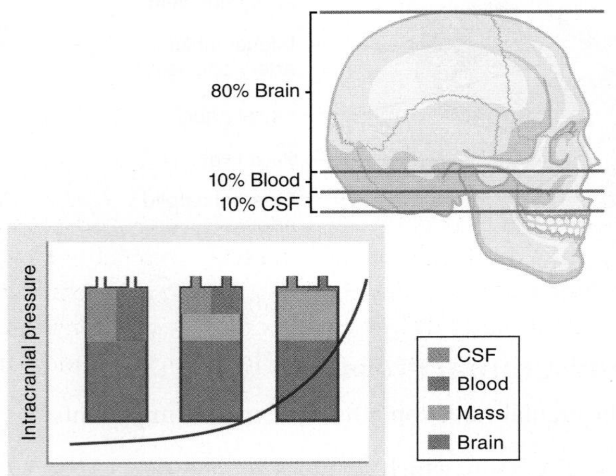

Figure 6-10 *Monro-Kellie doctrine.*

Loss of autoregulation can result in cerebral and brain stem ischemia, which initiates a central nervous system ischemic response, known as Cushing response. Cushing response is characterized by a triad of assessment findings:

- Widening pulse pressure
- Reflex bradycardia
- Decreased respiratory effort

Cushing response is the body's attempt to increase the MAP against an elevated ICP, so as to raise the CPP.[8]

CLINICAL PEARL

Maintain Adequate Cerebral Perfusion Pressure in the Head Trauma Patient

A CPP of less than 60 mm Hg has been associated with poor outcomes because such a low arterial pressure is unable to overcome the increased pressure gradient to deliver oxygen and nutrients to the brain. It is advisable to maintain the CPP at greater than 60 mm Hg. Monitoring and supporting the BP and MAP are important methods to ensure that CPP will be adequate.[2,13]

TABLE 6-1 Definitions of Terms

Term	Range	Definition
Cerebral perfusion pressure (CPP)	Normal = 60–100 mm Hg Acceptable = 50–70 mm Hg	The pressure gradient across the brain tissue; a measure of the adequacy of cerebral blood flow[16] determined by the difference between MAP and ICP.
Hypercarbia	$PaCO_2 > 45$ mm Hg	An excess of carbon dioxide in the blood, indicated by an elevated $PaCO_2$ as determined by blood gas analysis.[17]
Intracranial pressure (ICP)	0–15 mm Hg	The pressure of the cerebrospinal fluid in the subarachnoid space.
Mean arterial pressure (MAP)	50–150 mm Hg	The average blood pressure in a single cardiac cycle, roughly calculated as the systolic blood pressure + 2 × the diastolic blood pressure divided by 3.

Data from Carney, N., Totten, A. M., O'Reilly, C., Ullman, J. S., Hawryluk, G. W., Bell, M. J., . . . Ghajar, J. (2016). *Guidelines for the management of severe traumatic brain injury* (4th ed.). Retrieved from https://braintrauma.org/uploads/03/12/Guidelines_for_Management_of_Severe_TBI_4th_Edition.pdf; Cerebral perfusion pressure. (n.d.). *The Free Dictionary*. Retrieved from https://medical-dictionary.thefreedictionary.com/cerebral+perfusion+pressure; Hypercarbia. (n.d.). *The Free Dictionary*. Retrieved from https://medical-dictionary.thefreedictionary.com/hypercarbia.

Introduction

Traumatic brain injury (TBI) is a significant public health problem. According to recent U.S. data, 1.7 million individuals sustain a TBI annually.[2] Altogether, 2.5 million emergency department visits and hospitalizations are related to TBI. About 75% of 1.7 million TBI patients are classified as having minor trauma, 15% are considered moderately injured, and 10% are severely injured.[2,13] TBI contributes to one-third of the injury-related deaths in the United States.[14,19] Penetrating trauma has increased over the course of the last two decades, and is responsible for approximately 12% of all TBIs.[15] The most common cause of facial fractures is motor vehicle collisions (MVCs).[20] Approximately 2.4 million ocular injuries occur annually in the United States.[21] Motor vehicle collisions, and assaults are common mechanisms for ocular injuries in middle-aged males, while falls remain the most common cause for geriatric patients.[2,21-23]

Mechanism of Injury

Injuries are classified as blunt, penetrating, or burns.

- Blunt injuries result from the following causes:
  - Falls (the most frequent cause of TBI)[14,24]
  - Motor vehicle collisions
  - Sports-related injuries
  - Recreation- and recreational vehicle–related injuries
- Penetrating injuries may occur from the following causes (see Chapter 2, "Biomechanics, Kinematics, and Mechanisms of Injury," for more information)[15]:
  - Firearms
  - Exploding objects
  - Projectiles
- Ocular burns may occur from thermal, chemical, and radiation injury.

Primary injury to brain tissue may result from several factors, including the following:

- Compressive or direct-impact force with injury to the tissue under the point of impact on the skull
- Acceleration/deceleration forces creating a pressure wave, resulting in energy transfer to several sites within the brain
- Severe rotation or spinning that causes shearing or tensile force, resulting in tearing of cellular structures and bleeding
- A blast from an explosive device, creating a pressure wave and contused tissue
- Penetrating injury from a sharp object or firearm, causing severe, irreparable damage to brain cells, blood vessels, and protective tissues around the brain
- Lacerations as the brain moves across the irregular, rough base of the skull
- Fractures of the skull and facial bones

Risk Factors

Certain risk factors contribute to sustaining a brain injury. These include the following:

- Age: Children age 0 to 4 years, young adults age 15 to 24 years, and adults older than 75 years are at high risk.[17,24]
- Anticoagulant therapy.
- Use of substances that may cause dizziness, imbalance, or delayed response times, such as the following:
  - Alcohol
  - Medications
  - Illicit substances
- Previous head injury.

Usual Concurrent Injuries

Individuals with brain or craniofacial injuries are at risk for concurrent injuries to the cervical spinal cord and vertebral column.[2] Facial injuries may be associated with severe bleeding due to vascular disruption. Bony injuries may entrap nerves, causing injury to the underlying structures and presenting as ocular trauma.

Types of Injury

Brain injury is classified as primary or secondary injury. Primary injuries result from a direct transfer of energy and include the following:

- Skull and craniofacial fractures
- Intracranial lesions:
  - Diffuse injuries (concussion or diffuse axonal injury)
  - Focal injuries (epidural, subdural, intracerebral hematomas or contusions)[2]
- Secondary injury is caused by complex pathophysiologic changes that include the following:
  - Hypotension
  - Hypoxemia
  - Hypercarbia
  - Cerebral edema
  - Increased ICP
  - Decreased CPP
  - Cerebral ischemia

Secondary injury increases the extent of the actual injury and damage. The goal of caring for the patient who has experienced head trauma is to prevent or limit secondary injury and the catastrophic cascade of events that result from those conditions, including death.[2,14,19]

Pathophysiology as a Basis for Assessment Findings

Pathophysiologic concepts that affect the patient with brain, cranial, or maxillofacial injuries include problems related to the following:

- Hypoxia
- Hypercarbia
- Hypotension and CBF
- Increase or decrease in ICP

Hypoxia and Hypercarbia

Signs and symptoms of hypoxia may initially be obscured by the brain's ability to compensate by extracting more oxygen from the blood. Early changes in mental status may be subtle, so it is crucial to be aware of the potential for deterioration. A single episode of hypoxemia (apnea or PaO_2 < 60 mm Hg) can be detrimental to the patient's outcome.[2]

Carbon dioxide causes vasodilation, which can have a powerful, but reversible effect on CBF. Hypercapnia causes significant dilation of cerebral arterial vasculature and increased blood flow to the brain. Conversely, hypocapnia causes vasoconstriction and decreased blood flow.[10] This factor is important as it relates to assisted bag-mask ventilation and ventilator settings for the intubated patient. Hyperventilation decreases $PaCO_2$, causing cerebral vasoconstriction and hypoperfusion and may result in cerebral ischemia.[18] Hypercarbia ($PaCO_2$ > 45 mm Hg) promotes vasodilation and increases ICP, so it is also to be avoided.[13,25]

A brief period of hyperventilation may be indicated if the patient demonstrates signs of impending herniation (unilateral or bilateral pupillary dilation, asymmetric pupillary reactivity, or abnormal posturing). This is a temporizing measure, however, and should be maintained only until definitive interventions are implemented.[2,18] Hypocapnia may cause harm and is limited to emergency management of life-threatening intracranial hypertension awaiting definitive measures.[2,18]

CLINICAL PEARL 

Avoid Hypoxemia in the Patient with Head Trauma

A single episode of hypoxemia (PaO_2 < 60 mm Hg) can be detrimental to the patient's outcome. Maintain pulse oximetry at 95% or greater and obtain an arterial blood gas (ABG) measurement as soon as possible for patients with severe TBI.[2,13]

Hypotension and Cerebral Blood Flow

If injury causes the CPP to fall outside the normal range, the brain loses its ability to autoregulate and CBF becomes directly dependent on MAP for maintaining perfusion.[5] If the trauma patient is bleeding and becomes hypotensive, changes in the MAP are unable to produce a perfusing CPP, so that the brain tissue becomes hypoxic. The hypoperfused brain becomes ischemic and suffers irreversible damage, leading to symptoms such as dizziness and confusion, with the patient eventually becoming unresponsive and comatose. A single episode of hypotension (systolic blood pressure [SBP] < 90 mm Hg) can be harmful to patient outcomes.[2] In the context of severe head injuries, hypotension has been linked to more than double the mortality rate experienced by normotensive patients.[2,25]

If autoregulation fails and the MAP becomes elevated, cerebral edema may result, which can be disastrous for the patient with TBI. Therefore, it is important to maintain BP and MAP within normal limits.

CLINICAL PEARL 

Avoid Hypotension in the Patient with Head Trauma

A single episode of hypotension can be harmful to patient outcomes. Maintain SBP at or greater than 100 mm Hg.[2,13]

Intracranial Pressure

As ICP rises, CPP decreases, resulting in cerebral ischemia, hypoxemia, and secondary injury.[25] Small elevations in BP and MAP represent attempts by the body to protect against brain ischemia in a patient with elevated ICP. Intricate physiologic alterations result in a decreased PaO_2 and increased $PaCO_2$, both of which act to dilate cerebral blood vessels, increasing CBF. ICP sustained at greater than 22 mm Hg and unresponsive to treatment is associated with poor outcomes.[2,13,18] Increased ICP produces signs and symptoms that are both predictable and sequential (**Table 6-2**). Ultimately, increased ICP combined with an expanding hematoma, inflammation, or edema can result in brain stem herniation.[5]

TABLE 6-2 Assessment Findings of Increased Intracranial Pressure

Early
Headache
Nausea and vomiting
Amnesia
Behavior changes (impaired judgment, restlessness, drowsiness)
Altered level of consciousness (hypoarousability and hyperarousability)
Late
Dilated, nonreactive pupils
Unresponsiveness to verbal or painful stimuli
Abnormal motor posturing (flexion, extension, flaccidity)
Cushing response: › Widening pulse pressure · Pulse pressure is the difference between the systolic and diastolic pressures–normal is 40–60 mm Hg[26] › Reflex bradycardia › Decreased respiratory effort

CLINICAL PEARL 

Manage Intracranial Pressure in the Patient with Head Trauma

An ICP sustained at greater than 22 mm Hg and unresponsive to treatment is associated with poor outcomes.[13,18]

Nursing Care of the Patient with Head Trauma

Refer to Chapter 3, "Initial Assessment," for information on the systematic approach to the nursing care of the trauma patient. The following assessment parameters are specific to patients with head trauma.

Preparation and Triage

The Centers for Disease Control and Prevention's Field Triage Criteria suggest including the presence/use of anticoagulation medication as a triage parameter.[27] As part of the prehospital report, ask if the patient takes anticoagulation medications. These medications have the capability to cause uncontrolled hemorrhage in the trauma patient, so it becomes essential to identify the possible need for treating this condition in the primary survey as part of controlling hemorrhage. Data indicate that trauma patients taking medications such as warfarin, aspirin, or clopidogrel have a higher potential for injury and death compared to those trauma patients who are not taking anticoagulants or antiplatelet medications.[28]

Primary Survey and Resuscitation Adjuncts

The primary survey elements and resuscitation adjuncts specific to the patient with head trauma follow.

A: Alertness and Airway

Alertness and airway concerns include the following:

- Assess the patient using the AVPU mnemonic: A patient response other than "alert" may be associated with a brain injury.
- Be prepared to assist with early endotracheal intubation for patients who are unable to protect their airway, especially those with facial injuries and bleeding.
    - Obtain and document a brief neurologic exam before administering sedating/paralyzing medications for intubation.[2]
- Rigid cervical collars may contribute to an increase in ICP, as these devices can interfere with venous outflow and cause increased pain and discomfort to the patient.
    - The fit of the rigid collar may need to be adjusted.

B: Breathing and Ventilation

Breathing and ventilation concerns include the following:

- If the patient is alert, administer oxygen at 10–15 L/minute via nonrebreather mask with a tight-fitting seal and reservoir bag.
- Obtain an ABG measurement as soon as possible.
    - Titrate the oxygen for normoxia and maintain SpO_2 at 95% or greater (see Chapter 4, "Airway and Ventilation," for additional information).[3,13]

CLINICAL PEARL 

Maintain Adequate Oxygenation and Ventilation in the Patient with Head Trauma

- Maintain $SpO_2 \geq 95\%$.
- Maintain $ETCO_2$ between 35 mm Hg and 45 mm Hg.[3,13]

TABLE 6-3 Goals of Treatment for Severe Traumatic Brain Injury

Pulse oximetry ≥ 95%	ICP < 15 mm Hg	Serum sodium 135–145
PaO_2 ≥ 100 mm Hg	$PbtO_2$ ≥ 15 mm Hg	INR ≤ 1.4
$PaCO_2$ 35–45 mm Hg	CPP ≥ 60 mm Hg[a]	Platelets ≥ 75 x $10^3/mm^3$
SBP ≥ 100 mm Hg[b]	Temperature 36.0–38.0°C (96.8–100.4°F)	Hemoglobin ≥ 7 g/dL
pH 7.35–7.45	Glucose 80–100 mg/dL	

Abbreviations: CPP, cerebral perfusion pressure; ICP, intracranial pressure; INR, international normalized ratio; PaO_2, partial pressure of oxygen; $PaCO_2$, partial pressure of carbon dioxide; $PbtO_2$, brain tissue oxygen tension; SBP, systolic blood pressure.

[a] Depending on the status of cerebral autoregulation.

[b] See Clinical Pearl *Avoid Hypotension in the Patient with Head Trauma* and section *C: Circulation and Control of Hemorrhage* for age-specific blood pressure goals.

Reproduced from ACS Trauma Quality Improvement Program. (2015). *ACS TQIP best practices in the management of traumatic brain injury*. Chicago, IL: American College of Surgeons Committee on Trauma.

Table 6-3 presents the goals for treatment in the care of the patient with severe TBI.[13]

C: Circulation and Control of Hemorrhage

Concerns related to circulation and control of hemorrhage include the following:

- If applying direct pressure to bleeding sites, avoid placing pressure in the area over a depressed skull fracture.
- Avoid hypotension in patients with head trauma. Hypotension has been associated with an increased mortality rate in adults.[2,25]
  - The goal of fluid support is to restore euvolemia. Blood products and isotonic intravenous fluid should be utilized to achieve SBP at or greater than 100 mm Hg or greater in patients 50–69 years or 110 mm Hg.[2,13]
  - Hypotension in the trauma patient is usually caused by bleeding. The source of bleeding should be identified and treated immediately.[2]
  - Vasopressors may be indicated to maintain CPP once bleeding is controlled and the patient adequately resuscitated.

D: Disability (Neurologic Status)

Disability or neurologic status concerns include the following:

- Assess pupillary size and response to light.
  - A unilaterally fixed and dilated pupil may indicate compression of the oculomotor nerve (CN III) from increased ICP and indicate impending herniation syndrome.
  - Bilaterally fixed and pinpoint pupils may indicate an injury at the pons or the effects of opioids.
  - A moderately dilated pupil with sluggish response may be an early sign of herniation syndrome.
  - Bilateral pupillary constriction may be caused by sedatives such as opiates.
  - Bilateral pupillary dilation may be caused by stimulants such as epinephrine or cocaine.
- Assess the Glasgow Coma Scale (GCS) score or FOUR (Full Outline of UnResponsiveness) score (**Table 6-4** and **Figure 6-11**).[2,29-32]
  - Intubation is recommended if the GCS score is less than 8 or the level of consciousness decreases acutely.[2,13,19]
  - Obtain an ABG measurement to determine and ensure adequate oxygenation and ventilation.
  - Obtain a blood glucose measurement, as hypoglycemia may present as lethargy or unresponsiveness.[2,13,19]

Glasgow Coma Scale

The GCS score ranges from 3 to 15 and provides a measure of the patient's level of consciousness as well as a predictor of morbidity and mortality after brain injury.[13] The patient's total score derives from the patient's response to three aspects that are independently measured:

- *Best* eye opening
- *Best* verbal response
- *Best* motor response

The initial GCS score provides a baseline score, and repeated assessments determine whether the patient's neurologic status is improving or deteriorating. The motor component of the GCS score is the most sensitive subscore for identifying patients with severe brain injury.[2,13] An updated GCS has not been widely adopted into

TABLE 6-4 Comparison of the Glasgow Coma Scale and the FOUR Score

Glasgow Coma Scale

Eye Opening	
4	Spontaneous
3	To speech
2	To pain
1	None
Best Verbal Response	
5	Oriented
4	Confused conversation
3	Inappropriate words
2	Incomprehensible words
1	None
Best Motor Response	
6	Obeys commands
5	Localizes to pain
4	Withdrawal (normal flexion)
3	Abnormal flexion (decorticate)
2	Extension (decerebrate)
1	None

FOUR Score

Eye Response	
4	Eyelids open or opened, tracking, or blinking to command
3	Eyelids open but not tracking
2	Eyelids closed but open to loud voice
1	Eyelids closed but open to pain
0	Eyelids remain closed with pain
Motor Response	
4	Thumbs up, fist, or peace sign
3	Localizing to pain
2	Flexion response to pain
1	Extension response to pain
0	No response to pain or generalized myoclonus status
Brain Stem Reflexes	
4	Pupil and corneal reflexes present
3	One pupil wide and fixed
2	Pupil or corneal reflexes absent
1	Pupil and corneal reflexes absent
0	Absent pupil, corneal, and cough reflex
Respiration	
4	Not intubated, regular breathing pattern
3	Not intubated, Cheyne-Stokes breathing pattern
2	Not intubated, irregular breathing
1	Breathes above ventilator rate
0	Breathes at ventilator rate or apnea

Data from Jagoda, A. S., Bazarian, J. J., Bruns, J. J., Cantrill, S. V., Gean, A. D., Howard, P. K., . . . Whitson, R. R. (2008). Clinical policy: Neuroimaging and decision making in adult mild traumatic brain injury in the acute setting. *Annals of Emergency Medicine, 52*(6), 714–748; Wijdicks, E. F., Bamlet, W. R., Maramottom, B. V., Manno, E. M., & McClelland, R. L. (2005). Validation of a new coma scale: The FOUR score. *Annals of Neurology, 58*, 585–593. https://doi.org/10.1002/ana.20611.

practice at this time, but information is available online (www.glasgowcomascale.org).

One or more of the patient's limbs may sometimes be immobilized due to the effects of sedation, pharmacologic paralysis, fractures, brain or spinal cord injury, or other circumstances. Avoid misinterpreting a grasp reflex or postural adjustment as a response to a command. Remember the *best* response is to be measured. This is particularly important when one limb's response is better than the others, or the patient moves the eyelids purposefully yet has paralysis from the neck down. If one component is not able to be tested, the reason should be documented; a score of 1 should not be assigned. This enables the assessment to be more reliable over time.[13] The severity of brain injury is classified by the GCS as in **Table 6-5**; this classification guides management of the patient with head trauma.[2]

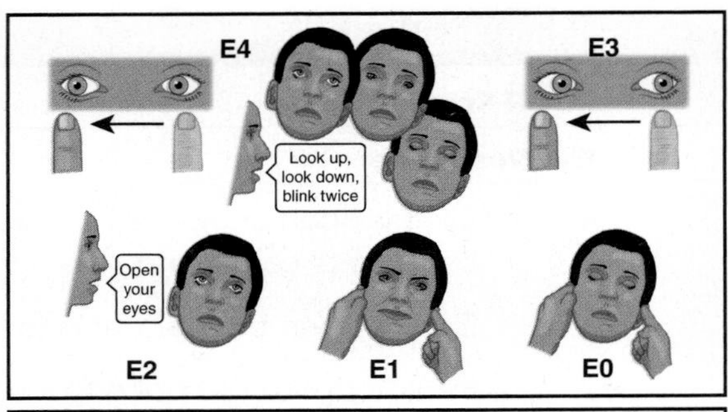

Eye response

4 = Eyelids open or opened, tracking or blinking to command

3 = Eyelids open but not to tracking

2 = Eyelids closed but opens to loud voice

1 = Eyelids closed but opens to pain

0 = Eyelids remain closed with pain stimuli

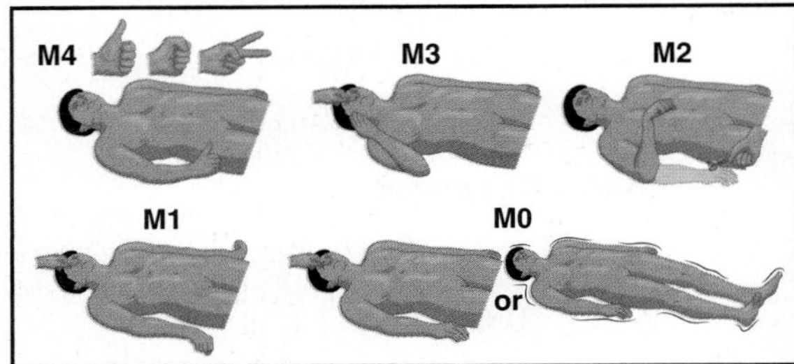

Motor response

4 = Thumbs up, fist, or peace sign

3 = Localizing to pain

2 = Flexion response to pain

1 = Extension response

0 = No response to pain or generalized Myoclonus status

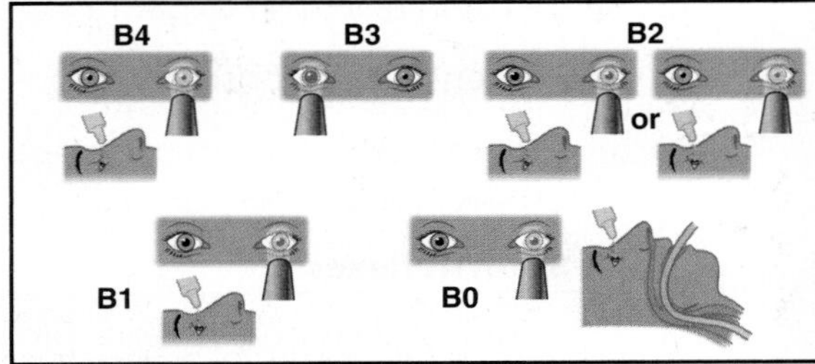

Brainstem reflexes

4 = Pupil and corneal reflexes present

3 = One pupil wide and fixed

2 = Pupil or corneal reflexes absent

1 = Pupil and corneal reflexes absent

0 = Absent pupil, corneal, or cough reflex

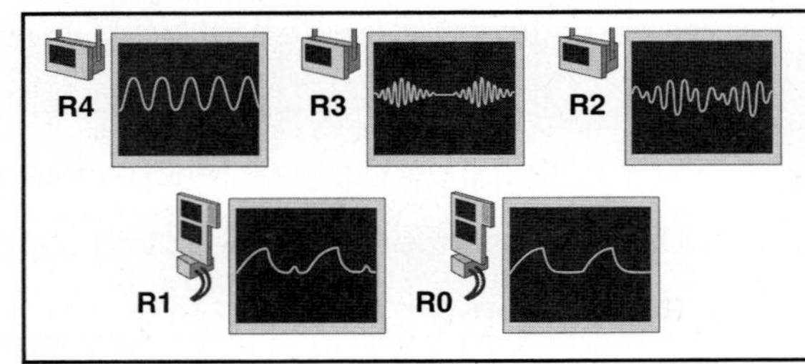

Respiration

4 = Regular breathing pattern

3 = Cheyne-Stokes breathing pattern

2 = Irregular breathing

1 = Triggers ventilator or breathes above ventilator rate

0 = Apnea or breathes at ventilator rate

Figure 6-11 *The FOUR Score.*

Reproduced from Mayo Foundation for Medical Education and Research. For complete rationale and instructions for using the FOUR Score scale, contact the Mayo Clinic at www.mayo.edu.

NOTE

GCS versus GCS 40: What's the Difference?

- Original GCS was developed in 1974; 40 years later, it was time for a tweak or two
- Two small terminology changes
  - Eye opening response to *pressure*, not pain and *speech*, not sound
  - Verbal changed incomprehensible to *sounds* and inappropriate to *words*
- When eye opening or verbal response cannot be tested (swelling, intubation), previously scored as 1, now scored as non-testable, "NT" and total score cannot be calculated. (GCS: E1 V1T M2 = 4T, GCS 40: E1 V NT M2 (no total)
- Pupillary response, nonreactive to light: Both 2, One 1, Neither 0
  - Subtracted from GCS 40, changing possible score from 1–15 instead of 3–15[33]

TABLE 6-5 Classification of Severity of Traumatic Brain Injury by Glasgow Coma Scale Score

TBI Classification	GCS Score
Mild	13–15
Moderate	9–12
Severe	3–8

FOUR Score

The FOUR score (Figure 6-11) ranges from 0 to 16, with each category score ranging from best (4) to worst (0). The FOUR score provides greater neurologic detail compared to the GCS score (Table 6-4).[29-31] The patient's total score results from a summative score of four components of response:

- Eye response (E)
- Motor response (M)
- Brain stem reflexes (B)
- Respiration (R)

All components of the FOUR score can be rated in patients with or without an endotracheal tube. Therefore, this score may have advantages in the critical care setting. Early research on the FOUR score's predictive reliability and validity is promising.[29-31] The scores R2–R4 are reserved for non-intubated patients.

In patients who are mechanically ventilated, assessment is done preferably when $PaCO_2$ is within normal limits and no adjustments are being made to the ventilator. Assess the pressure waveform on spontaneous respiration or when the patient triggers the ventilator. A score of R1 is given to a patient who breathes at greater than the ventilator rate. A score of R0 is given to a patient who breathes only at the ventilator rate or is apneic. A standard apnea test may be needed for patients with a score of R0.[31]

E: Exposure and Environmental Control

Hypothermia in combination with shock can have a deleterious effect on oxygenation of brain tissue (see Chapter 5, "Shock," for more information). However, currently there remains controversy about whether prophylactic or therapeutic hypothermia in patients with severe brain injury is beneficial, or is effective in reducing morbidity and mortality.[18] See "Emerging Trends" for more information.

F: Full Set of Vital Signs and Facilitate Family Presence

As previously mentioned, monitoring and supporting BP and oxygenation are key components to improve outcomes for the patient with a TBI. It can be distressing for family members to see patients with altered levels of consciousness and exhibiting repetitive questioning. Providing psychosocial support is challenging, as it can be months before it is known what the patient's functional status will be. The nurse can provide simple, realistic explanations while acknowledging the unknown to support the patient and family.

G: Get Monitoring Devices and Give Comfort (LMNOP)

Be alert for bradycardia, alterations in respirations, MAP, hypo- or hypertension, hypoxia, and hypercapnia with continuous monitoring. Any changes may indicate the body's attempt to compensate for increased ICP or herniation. Nasogastric tubes are contraindicated in facial trauma, as some facial fractures may provide a route for the tube to pass directly into the brain. Pain management is not to be withheld, but shorter acting pain and sedation medications may be used to allow more frequent assessments of mental status.

Reevaluation for Transfer

Determine whether the patient is a candidate for immediate surgery or meets the criteria for transport to a trauma center. Any head-injured patient with evidence of neurologic deficits meets the criteria for transport if the services and expertise are not available.[2,13,19]

The patient's BP is a determinant for further interventions[2]:

- Hypotension: Rarely will intracranial hemorrhage in an adult patient produce a volume of blood loss large enough to produce hypotension.
  - If hypotension is present, the priority is to determine the cause of bleeding.[2]
- Normotension: With a neurologic deficit (unequal pupils or asymmetric motor examination), the priority is to obtain a computed tomography (CT) scan of the head.
- Hypertension: Hypertension should be managed as well. Ensuring effective pain management is the first step.

Secondary Survey and Diagnostics and Therapeutics for Head Trauma

H: History

History-taking questions specific to patients with suspected head trauma include the following:

- If the patient is conscious, what are the patient's complaints?

- Headache, nausea and vomiting, and amnesia may be early signs of increased ICP.
- If the patient's level of consciousness is altered, does the history suggest head trauma?
  - Impact to the head or face.
  - Post-injury lucid interval (rule out an epidural hematoma).
- Was there any vomiting or other signs and symptoms of a brain or cranial injury?
- Was there any loss of consciousness (LOC)? For how long?
- Does the patient have amnesia from the injury event?
- Does the patient take anticoagulant or antiplatelet medications? When was the last dose taken?[14,34] (Such medications could lead to increased bleeding into the brain.)

Specific to Ocular Trauma

History-taking questions specific to ocular trauma include the following:

- Was the patient wearing protective eyewear or corrective eyewear? Has it been removed?
- If a penetrating injury occurred, what was the material that caused the injury (metallic or organic)?
  - Organic material carries a high incidence of infection.
  - Metallic foreign objects can cause permanent staining.
- Did the trauma cause a change in vision? What are those changes—blurring, double vision, or loss of vision?
- Was there a chemical exposure? What type of chemical (acid or alkali)? Was any type of treatment or decontamination performed prior to patient arrival?

H: Head-to-Toe Assessment

Inspect for the following:

- Inspect the craniofacial area for ecchymosis or contusion.
  - Basilar skull fractures can produce bleeding that may not become evident until several hours after the injury. These collections of blood under the tissue may become apparent in one of three areas (**Figure 6-12**):
    - Periorbital ecchymoses, also known as raccoon eyes, indicate an anterior fossa fracture.
    - Mastoid process ecchymoses, also known as Battle sign, indicate a middle fossa fracture.
    - Hemotympanum, blood behind the tympanic membrane, may indicate a middle fossa fracture.
- Inspect the craniofacial area for symmetry, flattening of the face, or malocclusion.

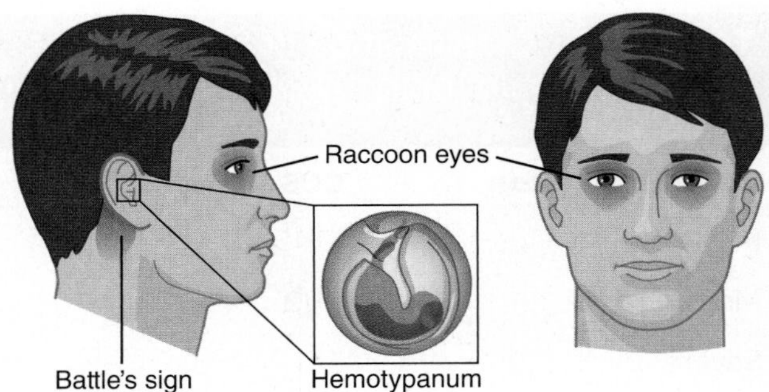

Figure 6-12 *Signs of a basilar skull fracture.*

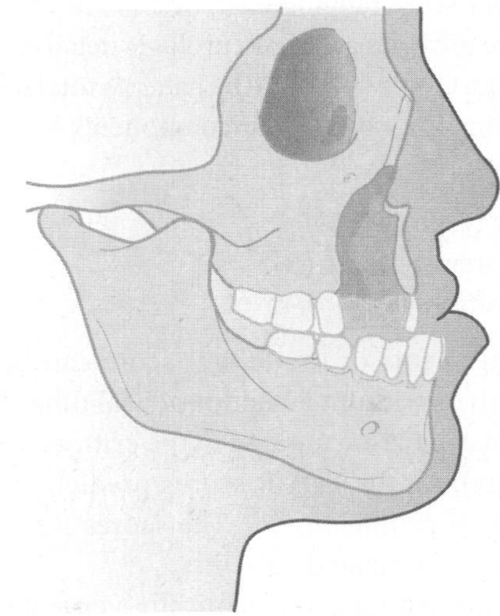

Figure 6-13 *Flattening of face due to facial fracture.*

  - Asymmetrical facial appearance can indicate soft-tissue injury or facial fracture.
  - Flattening of the face or a dish-like appearance is consistent with Le Fort fractures (**Figure 6-13**).
  - Malocclusion may be a sign of mandibular fracture.
  - Evert the upper eyelid and inspect for any potential foreign body, if needed.
- Palpate for tenderness or step-offs, which may indicate a fracture.

Visual Acuity

Visual acuity is a fundamental part of the ocular examination.[35] Key elements to assess while performing the examination include the following:

- Ask about the patient's vision.
- What can the patient see? Ask the patient to describe his or her vision (blurry, decreased, or normal).[36]
- Use a standard-distance Snellen chart to assess visual acuity, positioning the chart 20 feet away from the patient[36] (**Figure 6-14**).

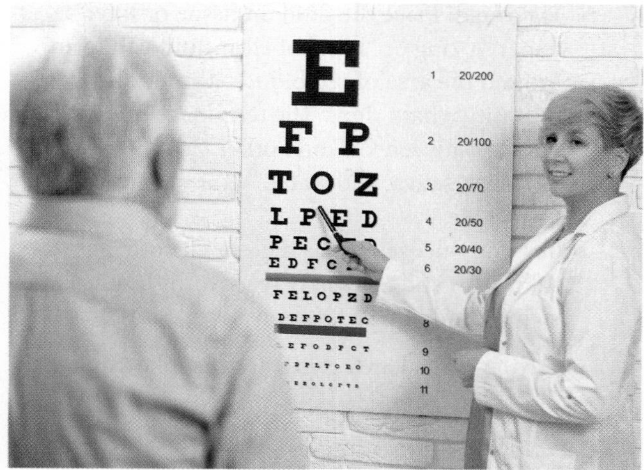

Figure 6-14 *Visual acuity exam.*

- If the patient is unable to stand, use a handheld near-vision card held 14 inches away from the patient's face.[37]
- If the patient cannot read the chart, ask the patient what he or she can see: fingers, objects, light or shadows.[37]
- Assess extraocular eye movements (EOMs) to test the function of CNs III, IV, and VI (**Figure 6-15**).
    - Assess ability to perform, looking at smoothness of movement, symmetry, and speed. If nystagmus is present, determine if the presence of nystagmus is the patient's baseline or if it began after the traumatic incident.
    - In the presence of facial fractures, the inability to perform EOMs may indicate extraocular muscle entrapment.

Pupil Examination

Assess pupils for shape, size, reactivity, and symmetry. As much as 10% of the general population has unequal pupils (anisocoria), which is a benign physiologic condition.[38] Causes of abnormal anisocoria include trauma, uncal herniation, oculomotor nerve (CN III) palsy, medications, and some nebulizers (ipratropium). Pupils are normally round; an oval pupil may indicate a tumor, retinal detachment, or prior injury. A teardrop-shaped pupil suggests a globe rupture.

Pupils are tested using a penlight in a darkened room. The normal pupillary response is a brisk constriction, with both pupils constricting to the same size.

Ophthalmoscope Examination

The ophthalmoscope is used to look at the fundus, optic nerve, disc, and the major blood vessels. If possible, dim the lights to allow the patient's pupil to dilate; alternatively, the provider may dilate the pupil with medication. If the patient is having a difficult time keeping his or her eyes open, topical anesthetics may be used. Note that these medications are *not* sent home with the patient—their use without medical supervision puts the patient at risk for inhibited corneal healing. Additionally, the use of medications to dilate the pupil may blur vision for up to 2 hours and make it unsafe for the patient to drive. This factor should be considered in preparing for patient discharge.[39]

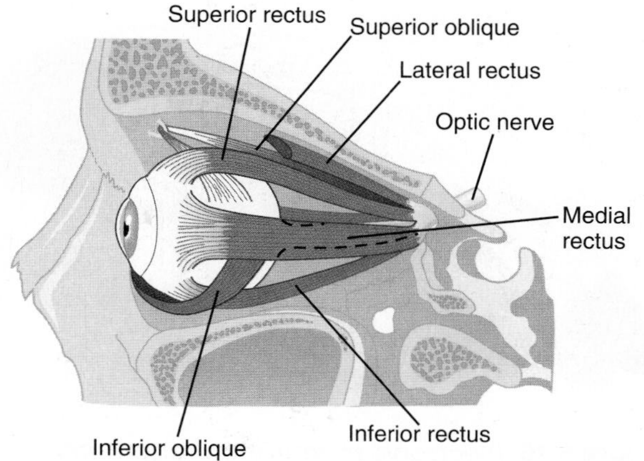

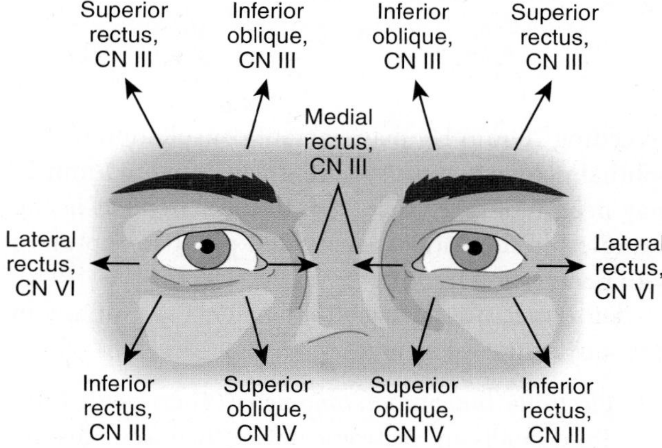

Figure 6-15 *Innervation and movement of extraocular muscles.*

Intraocular Pressure Measurement

Intraocular pressure (IOP) is fairly stable; however, if the production of aqueous humor exceeds the outflow in cases such as glaucoma or hyphema, IOP is increased. The opposite condition, decreased IOP, results from a decrease in the production of fluid, severe dehydration, or a disruption in the globe.[39] IOP measurement is routinely performed in patients who have loss of vision, suspected glaucoma, or blunt trauma. Normal pressure readings are between 10 and 20 mm Hg.[38] IOPs

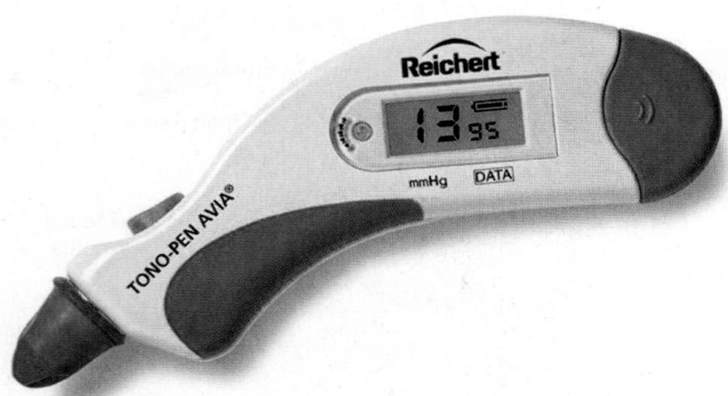

Figure 6-16 *Electronic indentation tonometry (Tono-pen).*

Courtesy of Reichert Technologies.

exceeding 20 mm Hg may warrant consultation with an ophthalmologist, and pressure greater than 30 mm Hg may need rapid treatment.[38] IOP measurement is contraindicated for patients suspected of globe rupture or with penetrating trauma.

IOP is measured using a tonometer. Types of tonometry include the following:

- *Electronic indentation tonometry* (Tono-pen): The Tono-pen is an electronic device that uses a disposable cover (**Figure 6-16**). This device, which can be difficult to use, is touched to the cornea three to four times, with the findings then being averaged. Prior to the procedure, anesthetic drops are administered as prescribed.[37]
- *Applanation tonometry* (Goldmann applanation): This procedure is used by most ophthalmologists and optometrists and is usually found on the slit lamp.[37]

Inspect the nose and ears for drainage. CSF drainage from the nose or ear is due to a tear in the dura.[40] To test otorrhea/rhinorrhea for CSF, consider the following:

- β_2-Transferrin is a test that requires fluid to be sent to the laboratory and is considered the gold standard for identifying CSF in otorrhea or rhinorrhea. Beta-trace protein is found in high concentrations in CSF and can help in distinguishing the cause of otorrhea. These tests may not be available in some hospitals.
- Two other tests have historically been performed rapidly to suggest a general suspicion of CSF leak but have high rates of false positives and are considered unreliable.
  - Halo sign: Place the fluid on tissue or filter paper. A ring or "halo" of clear fluid will form around the area of red blood—this constitutes a "positive halo sign." The test does not differentiate between CSF and other clear fluids such as saline, saliva, and water.[41] It is considered unreliable.
  - Test for glucose: CSF is high in glucose, but nasal mucus and tears may react with the glucose strips, producing a false-positive result.[42]

Palpate the cranial area gently for the following:

- Point tenderness
- Depressions or deformities
- Hematomas

Assess all four extremities bilaterally for the following:

- Motor function
- Muscle strength
- Sensory function
- Abnormal motor posturing (abnormal flexion, abnormal extension) or flaccidity (sign of head injury)

Selected Head Injuries

Selected head injuries discussed in this section include coup/contrecoup injury, focal brain injuries, diffuse injuries, penetrating injuries, and craniofacial fractures.

Coup/Contrecoup Injury

When the head strikes a solid object, the sudden deceleration force may result in bony deformity and injury to cranial contents. Within the cranial vault, a pressure wave is generated at the point of impact, which may tear tissue and cause injury at the site of impact (coup injury). As the pressure wave travels across the cranial contents and dissipates, injury may occur on the side opposite the impact (contrecoup injury). **Figure 6-17** shows both types of injury. It is possible to suffer this type of head injury without experiencing a direct blow to the head.[10] Assessment findings include the following:

- Altered level of consciousness
- Behavioral, motor, or speech deficits
- Abnormal motor posturing
- Signs of increased ICP

Focal Brain Injuries

Focal brain injuries occur in a localized area with grossly observable and identifiable brain lesions. These lesions may expand, causing damage to other areas of the brain or resulting in secondary brain injury from increased ICP. Focal brain injuries include cerebral contusion,

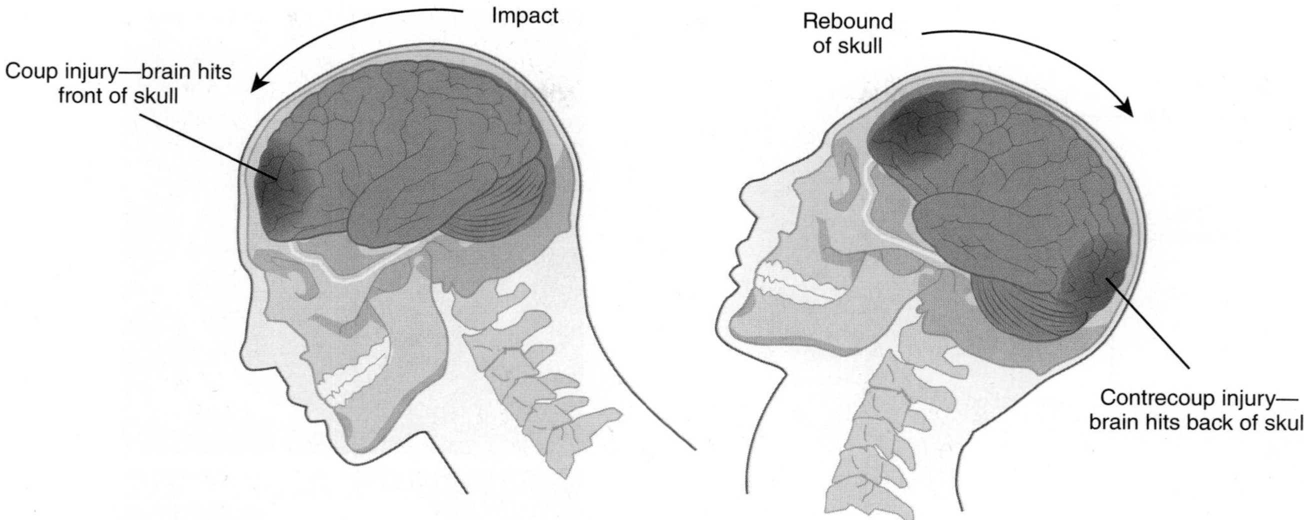

Figure 6-17 *Coup/contrecoup brain injury.*

intracerebral hematoma, epidural hematoma, subdural hematoma, and herniation syndromes.

Cerebral Contusion

A cerebral contusion is damaged brain tissue, usually caused by blunt trauma. Most cerebral contusions are located in the frontal and temporal lobes, but they may also occur in tissue beneath a depressed skull fracture.[43] Contusions begin when the capillaries within the brain tissue are damaged, resulting in hemorrhage, infarction, necrosis, and edema. Significant contusions with swelling may cause a midline shift within the cranial vault. The maximum effects of contusion and edema formation usually peak 18 to 36 hours after injury. Delayed hemorrhage or formation of intracranial hematomas may occur.

Intracerebral Hematoma

Intracerebral hematomas occur deep within the brain tissue, may be single or multiple, and may be associated with skull fractures and cerebral contusions.[43] Similar to cerebral contusions, most intracerebral hematomas are located in the frontal and temporal lobes. They may create a significant mass effect, increase ICP, and result in neurologic deterioration. Assessment findings include the following:

- Progressive and often rapid decline in level of consciousness
- Headache
- Signs of increasing ICP (see Table 6-2)
- Pupil abnormalities
- Contralateral hemiparesis, hemiplegia, or abnormal motor posturing

Epidural Hematoma

An epidural hematoma occurs when a collection of blood forms between the dura mater and the skull. Such hematomas are frequently (90%) associated with fractures of the temporal or parietal bone that lacerate the middle meningeal artery (**Figure 6-18**).[43] Since the source of bleeding is arterial, blood can accumulate rapidly, and the expanding hematoma may cause compression of underlying brain tissue, a rapid rise in ICP, decreased CBF, and secondary brain injury. Significant epidural hematomas require immediate surgical intervention. The most common causes of epidural hematoma are MVCs and falls, but they can also result from sports-related injuries. Assessment findings include the following[5]:

- Transient LOC followed by a lucid period lasting minutes to hours, then rapid deterioration in neurologic status. Although this is considered the "classic" presentation of a patient with an epidural hematoma, most patients do not present with this history or symptomatology.[43]
- Headache and dizziness.
- Nausea and vomiting.
- Contralateral hemiparesis, hemiplegia, or abnormal motor posturing (flexion or extension).
  - Extension is associated with brain stem herniation and poor outcomes.
  - Ipsilateral unilateral fixed and dilated pupil may occur.[43]

Subdural Hematoma

A subdural hematoma occurs when a collection of blood forms immediately beneath the dura mater, usually

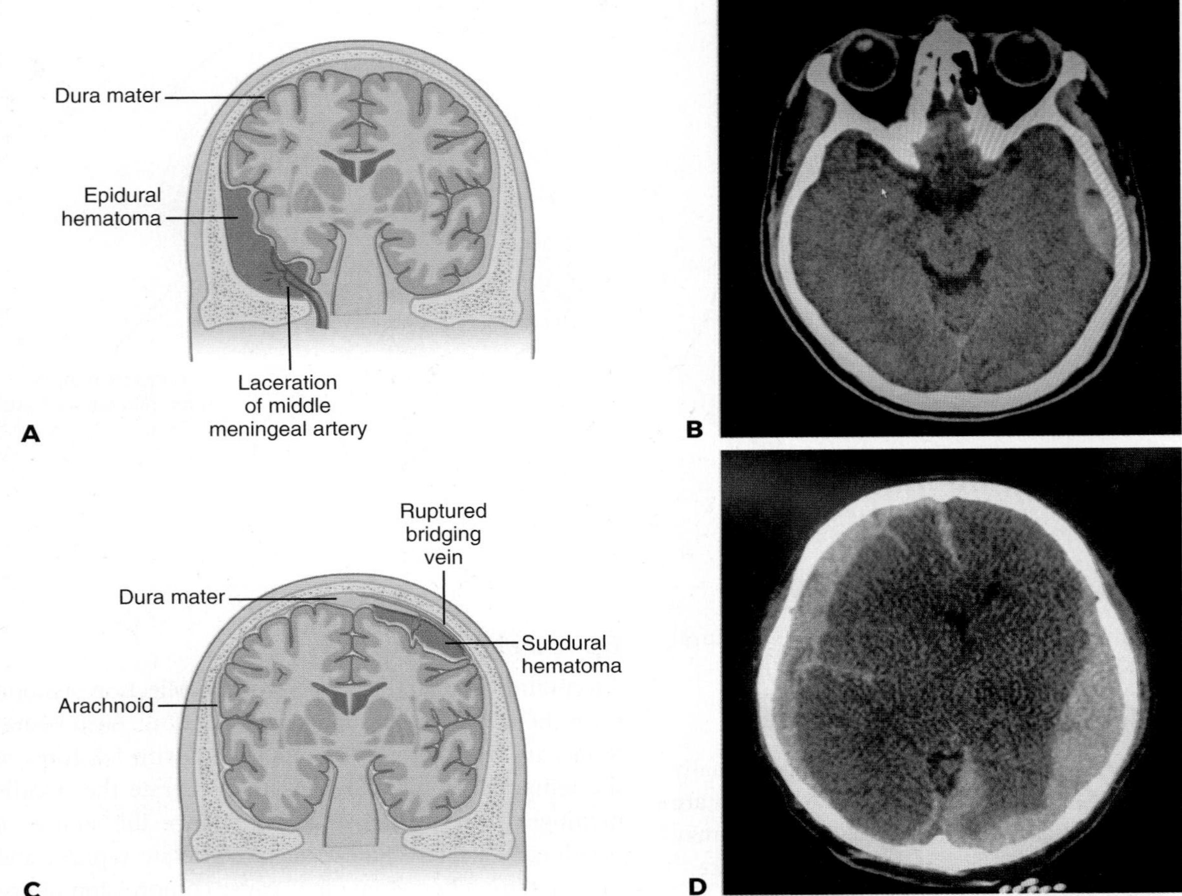

Figure 6-18 *Epidural and subdural hematomas.* ***A.*** *Diagram of epidural hematoma.* ***B.*** *Scan showing epidural hematoma.* ***C.*** *Diagram of subdural hematoma.* ***D.*** *Scan showing subdural hematoma.*

following impact involving acceleration, deceleration, or combination forces. Subdural hematomas are usually caused by tearing of the bridging veins and associated direct injury to the underlying brain tissue (Figure 6-18). They may be acute, subacute, or chronic.

Acute Subdural Hematoma

Patients with acute subdural hematomas generally manifest signs and symptoms within 72 hours of the injury event.[24] The hematoma can cause a reduction in CBF. This is commonly the type of bleed sustained from a fall or assault, with a smaller percentage of acute subdural hematomas being caused by MVCs. Assessment findings in patients with such hematomas include the following:

- Nausea, vomiting, and headache
- Changes in level of consciousness
- Ipsilateral dilated or nonreactive pupil
- Unilateral weakness or hemiparesis[44]

Chronic Subdural Hematoma

Chronic subdural hematomas are frequently associated with minor injury in older adults, patients taking anticoagulation medications, and patients with chronic alcohol use. This increased incidence is due to brain atrophy, fragility of the bridging veins, and coagulation alterations. The onset of signs and symptoms and effect on neurologic function vary depending on the size and rapidity of the hematoma formation. The assessment findings in patients with chronic subdural hematomas develop over time and may not be evident until as long as 2 weeks after the injury event. Symptoms may be intermittent and be confused with transient ischemic attacks. The symptoms may include the following:

- Alterations in cognitive abilities, or altered or steady decline in level of consciousness
- Headache—the most common symptom[45]
- Loss of memory or altered reasoning

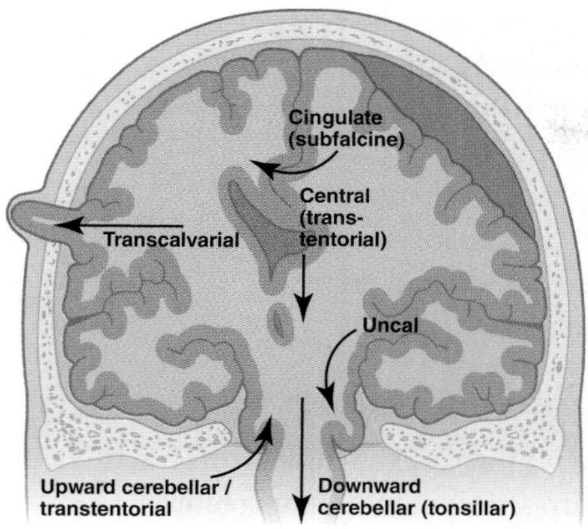

Figure 6-19 *Herniation syndrome.*

- Motor deficit—contralateral hemiparesis, hemiplegia, or abnormal motor posturing or ataxia
- Slurred speech, difficulty with word finding
- Ipsilateral unilateral fixed and dilated pupil
- Incontinence
- Seizures

Herniation Syndrome

Herniation is a shifting of brain tissue with displacement into another compartment as the result of bleeding or edema (**Figure 6-19**). This shift compresses, tears, or shears the vasculature, decreasing perfusion. The most common trauma herniation syndrome is uncal herniation. Assessment findings may include the following[44]:

- Asymmetric pupillary reactivity
- Unilateral or bilateral pupillary dilation
- Abnormal motor posturing
- Other evidence of neurologic deterioration (loss of normal reflexes, paralysis, or change in level of consciousness)

The two major types of supratentorial herniation are named by the site of herniation:

- Uncal transtentorial herniation: The uncus of the temporal lobe is displaced unilaterally over the tentorium into the posterior fossa, causing a shift of the midbrain to the opposite side.[8]
- Central or transtentorial herniation: The cerebral hemispheres are pushed downward through the tentorial notch, directly compressing the brain stem.[8]

Diffuse Injuries

Diffuse TBIs occur over a widespread area. They may not always be identifiable on radiograph or CT imaging because the damage involves contusions or shearing and stretching of the axons, rather than a localized hematoma, contusion, or laceration.[43] These injuries commonly follow a direct blow to the head and very often are sports related. Patients who sustain these injuries may have varying degrees of symptoms that last from minutes to days. Assessment findings include the following:

- Transient loss of consciousness
- Headache and dizziness
- Nausea and vomiting
- Confusion and disorientation
- Memory loss and concentration difficulty
- Irritability and fatigue

Concussion

A mild form of diffuse injury is concussion, often called a mild TBI. The injury to the brain is caused by blunt injury to the head or neck, or on a different part of the body that causes forces to be transmitted to the brain.[46] Most concussions have no findings on CT.[47] Changes in neurologic status last for a very brief period (i.e., LOC $<$ 30 minutes).[46,47] Patients may not have or notice TBI symptoms for several hours or days after injury. Approximately 20% of patients diagnosed with concussion are younger than 19 years, with sports- or recreation-related injuries.[48] Assessment findings include the following:

- GCS score of 13–15 (at least 30 minutes post injury)
- Confusion and disorientation
- Headache and fatigue
- Poor concentration, anxiety, and irritability
- Post-traumatic amnesia for less than 24 hours
- Photophobia/phonophobia[46]

Postconcussive Syndrome

Patients who sustain a mild TBI may develop postconcussive syndrome. Typically, postconcussive syndrome manifests several days or months after the head trauma. Signs and symptoms usually resolve but may persist for long periods of time. These patients may require ongoing evaluation, treatment, and extended rehabilitation before they are able to return to their previous level of activities or athletic participation. As it cannot be determined who will develop postconcussive syndrome, education related to this condition is included in patient discharge instructions, along with information regarding when to return for care. Assessment findings may include the following[46,48]:

- Nausea
- Dizziness and persistent headache
- Memory and judgment impairment, as well as attention deficits
- Insomnia and sleep disturbance

- Loss of libido
- Anxiety, irritability, depression, and emotional lability
- Noise and light oversensitivity
- Attention or concentration problems[46,48,49]

Diffuse Axonal Injury

Diffuse axonal injury (DAI) is widespread microscopic damage, primarily to the axons, from diffuse shearing, tearing, or compressive stresses from a rotational or acceleration/deceleration mechanism of injury (MOI).[43] Such damage may also occur following hypoxic or ischemic insults from the initial trauma.[2] DAI presents as diffuse, microscopic, hemorrhagic lesions, and cerebral edema, which may be detected on magnetic resonance imaging (MRI). Deeper brain structures, the brain stem, and the RAS (responsible for regulating wakefulness and sleep) are most at risk for injury, which commonly results in prolonged coma. The DAI is graded as Grades I through III based on the location of the lesion and severity of the injury.[4] Severe DAI has significant morbidity and mortality.[50] Assessment findings may include the following:

- Unconsciousness
- Increased ICP
- Abnormal motor posturing
- Hypertension (SBP between 140 and 160 mm Hg)
- Hyperthermia with temperature between 40°C and 40.5°C (104°F and 105°F)
- Excessive sweating
- Mild to severe memory loss; cognitive, behavioral, and intellectual deficits

Penetrating Injuries

Penetrating injuries to the brain can be life-threatening, and it is essential to discover the site and extent of the injury. The most common cause of penetrating injuries of the brain are gunshot injuries.[15] The decision to operate is based on CT and GCS. The presence of a large contusion, hemorrhage, or hematoma, especially when both hemispheres are involved, is associated with increased mortality.[15] Keep the following points in mind when dealing with penetrating injuries to the brain:

- Leave any protruding penetrating objects in place and stabilize them.
- Prepare for emergent surgery or transfer to a trauma center with neurosurgical capabilities.

Consider limiting resuscitation efforts in the presence of devastating injuries. The following variables are associated with increased mortality rate[51]:

- Age greater than 50 years
- Self-inflicted injury
- Hypotension
- Coagulopathy
- Respiratory distress
- Low GCS score
- Fixed and dilated pupils
- High ICP

Craniofacial Fractures

Craniofacial fractures include skull fractures, maxillofacial fractures, and mandibular fractures.

Skull Fractures

The significance of a skull fracture is related to the force it takes to cause the injury. Injuries may occur to the skull vault or the base. Types of skull fractures include the following:

- Linear skull fracture
  - A non-displaced fracture goes through the entire thickness of the skull.[52]
  - Assessment findings may include:
    - Headache
    - Surrounding soft-tissue injury
    - Possible decreased level of consciousness
- Depressed skull fracture
  - Pieces of the fractured bone extend below the surface of the skull and may cause dura mater laceration and brain tissue injury.[44]
  - Assessment findings may include the following:
    - Headache
    - Surrounding soft-tissue injury
    - Palpable depression of the skull over the fracture site (assess with care)
    - Possible open fracture
    - Possible decreased level of consciousness
- Basilar skull fracture (**Figure 6-20**)

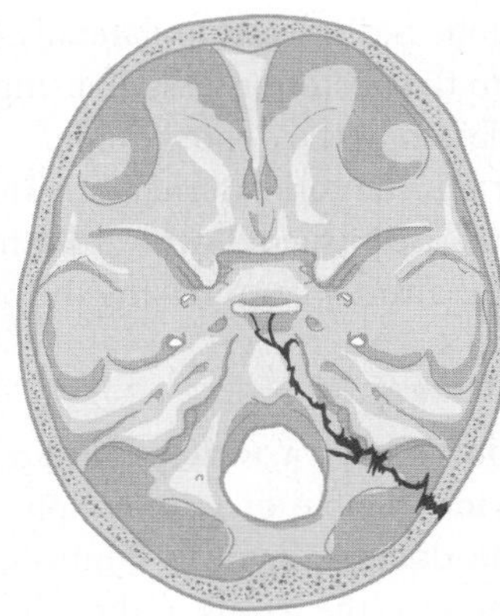

Figure 6-20 *Basilar skull fracture.*

- Fracture of any of the five bones in the base of the skull is associated with a considerable amount of force that caused the injury.[44]
- The injury can result in punctures or lacerations to brain tissue or CNs and CSF leakage.
- It may also result in laceration of the dura mater, creating an open passage for CSF, which places the patient at risk for infections (meningitis, encephalitis, brain abscess).[52]
- Basilar skull fracture occurs concurrently with facial fractures.
- Fractures may cross the carotid canals and injure the carotid arteries. Cerebral arteriography or CT angiography may be used to identify and manage the bleeding.[2]
- Assessment findings may include the following[2,44]:
  - Headache and dizziness
  - Hearing loss
  - Altered level of consciousness
  - CSF in rhinorrhea or otorrhea
  - Periorbital ecchymoses (raccoon eyes)
  - Mastoid ecchymoses (Battle sign)
  - Bleeding behind the tympanic membrane (hemotympanum)
  - Facial nerve palsy (CN VII injury)

Maxillary Fractures

The Le Fort classification system provides precise definitions of maxillary fractures (**Figure 6-21**).[44] Le Fort I is a transverse maxillary bone fracture that occurs above the level of the teeth and results in a separation of the teeth from the maxilla. Assessment findings include the following[53]:

- Independent movement of the maxilla from the rest of the face
- Slight swelling of the maxillary area
- Lip laceration or fractured teeth
- Malocclusion

A Le Fort II fracture is a pyramidal maxillary bone fracture involving the mid-face area.[44] The apex of the fracture transverses the bridge of the nose. The two lateral fractures of the pyramid extend through the lacrimal bone of the face and ethmoid bone of the skull into the median portion of both orbits. The base of the fracture extends above the level of the upper teeth into the maxilla. Assessment findings include the following[54]:

- Massive facial edema
- Nasal swelling with obvious fracture of the nasal bones
- Epistaxis
- Malocclusion
- Possible CSF rhinorrhea

A Le Fort III fracture is a complete craniofacial separation involving the maxilla, zygoma, orbits, and bones of the cranial base.[54] Assessment findings include the following[54]:

- Massive facial edema
- Mobility and depression of zygomatic bones
- Periorbital ecchymoses (racoon eyes)
- Diplopia

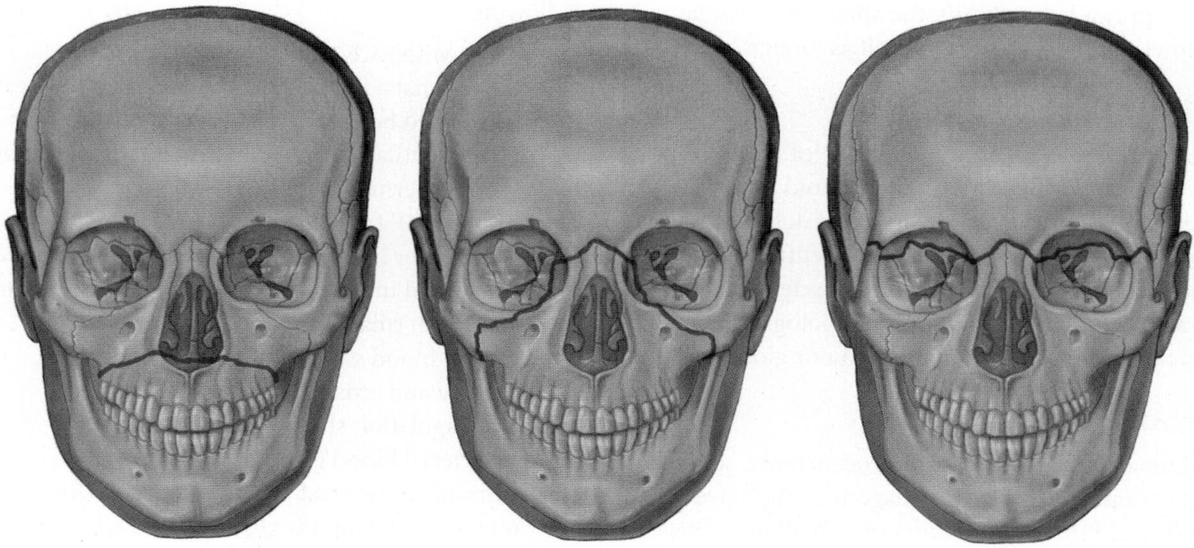

Figure 6-21 *Le Fort classification system.*

Reproduced from Solheim, J. (2013). Facial, ocular, ENT, and dental trauma. In B. B. Hammond & P. G. Zimmerman (Eds.), *Sheehy's manual of emergency care* (7th ed., 439–452). St. Louis, MO: Mosby Elsevier. Reprinted with permission.

- Open bite or malocclusion
- CSF in rhinorrhea or otorrhea

Mandibular Fractures

Mandibular fractures occur to the horseshoe-shaped lower jawbone that attaches to the cranium at the temporomandibular joints. The common fracture sites are at the canine and third molar tooth and the angle of the mandible and the condyles. Mandibular fractures may be open or closed, have multiple breaks on the same bone, or be impacted (one fragment pushed into another).[55] Assessment findings include the following[55]:

- Malocclusion
- Inability to open the mouth (trismus)
- Drooling
- Lacerations or bleeding between the teeth
- Pain and tenderness, especially on movement
- Facial asymmetry and a palpable step-off deformity
- Edema or hematoma formation at the fracture site
- Blood behind the tympanic membrane or ruptured tympanic membrane
- Anesthesia of the lower lip

Selected Eye Injuries

Corneal Injury

Traumatic injury to the cornea can result from abrasion, laceration, or foreign bodies. Corneal abrasions are commonly caused by fingernail injury or contact lens use. The corneal epithelium is highly innervated, so injury to it results in a great deal of pain. Staining of the eye with fluorescein can help identify the abrasion. A slit lamp is used to visualize lacerations as well as foreign bodies.[56]

Orbital Fracture

Orbital fractures are usually a result of a direct blow to the eye. The orbital floor and ethmoid bones are the weakest parts of the orbit and at high risk for fracture. A complication of this type of fracture is entrapment of the inferior rectus or inferior oblique muscle. Orbital fractures are not considered an ophthalmologic emergency unless the patient has impaired vision or globe rupture.

Retrobulbar Hematoma

Retrobulbar hematoma is a rare occurrence secondary to blunt trauma. This hemorrhage into the retrobulbar space (behind the globe) occurs in a small percentage of patients with non-displaced orbital fractures. Bleeding causes increased pressure behind the globe, which causes an elevation in IOP that compresses the optic nerve and blood vessels. Early recognition is imperative to save vision. This is a true ophthalmologic emergency.[56]

Globe Rupture

When a full-thickness injury occurs to the cornea or sclera, or both, it is termed a *globe rupture*. This condition is considered a genuine emergency. Once the diagnosis is confirmed, it is important to protect the area from further injury.[56] The most common area of rupture is at the limbus, where the sclera is the thinnest.

Ocular Burns

Ocular burns can result from contact with chemical, thermal, or radiant sources. Chemical burns are considered a true emergency. Saving the eyesight in such a case requires immediate irrigation of the eye[57]—taking precedence over completion of a history, testing the pH of the eye, and thorough assessment. Alkaline products cause liquefaction necrosis and produce burns that are deeper than acid burns.[9] In general, acidic burns are less severe, causing immediate damage through coagulation necrosis, which ultimately forms a barrier to deeper penetration. The exceptions to this pattern are burns caused by hydrofluoric and sulfuric acids, which cause the same severity of burn as alkali substances.[9]

Assessment findings, treatment, and follow-up for these eye injuries are summarized in **Table 6-6**.[9,35,38,56-58]

Interventions for the Patient with Head Trauma

For the patient with severe TBI (GCS score of 3–8) do the following[2,13,18,19]:

- Assist with early intubation and ventilation.
- Ensure that a focused neurologic exam has been performed before giving sedating medications.
- Hyperventilation may be utilized temporarily for signs of herniation only.
- Monitor BP frequently.
- Administer blood products or warmed isotonic crystalloid intravenous fluid as ordered to treat hypotension (maintain SBP $\geq$ 100 mm Hg[2,13]).
- Obtain blood sample for laboratory testing.
  - Type and cross-match
  - Coagulation studies
  - Arterial blood gas
- Administer reversal agents as ordered (for patients on anticoagulant/antiplatelet medications).
- Evaluate for other injuries.
- Accompany the patient to CT imaging and monitor vital signs closely during the transport.

TABLE 6-6 Summary of Assessment Findings, Treatment, and Follow-Up for Selected Eye Injuries

Eye Injury	Assessment Findings	Treatment	Follow-Up
Corneal injury	Photophobia Pain Eye redness Lid swelling Foreign body sensation in the eye	Topical anesthesia Topical ophthalmic nonsteroidal anti-inflammatory drugs No eye patch For laceration, may need topical antibiotic prophylaxis Remove foreign body	Follow-up with ophthalmologist in 24–48 hours Ophthalmology consultation for deep and large foreign bodies
Orbital fracture	Periorbital ecchymosis Facial swelling Double vision Enophthalmos (posterior displacement of eyeball within the orbit) Ptosis	Nasal decongestant Ice packs to the orbit for 48 hours Oral antibiotics	Large fractures of orbital floor may require urgent surgery Follow-up with ophthalmology within 1–2 weeks Discharge instructions: Avoid blowing nose, sneezing, and/or performing Valsalva maneuver
Retrobulbar hematoma	Severe pain Decreased vision or loss of vision Reduced eye movement Double vision IOP greater than 40 mm Hg	Administer medications to decrease IOP Emergency decompression via lateral canthotomy	Emergent consultation with ophthalmology
Globe rupture	Irregular or teardrop-shaped pupils Periorbital ecchymosis Decreased visual acuity and EOM Severe subconjunctival hemorrhage Deep eye pain Nausea	Avoid any pressure on the globe Apply a rigid shield to protect the affected eye Consider tetanus vaccine Keep patient NPO Assess and treat pain Administer antiemetics to decrease risk of vomiting (which may increase IOP) Elevate the head of bed (to decrease IOP) Avoid ophthalmic drops or medications Administer systemic antibiotics	Emergent consultation with ophthalmology Prepare patient for CT scan, operating room

(*continues*)

TABLE 6-6 Summary of Assessment Findings, Treatment, and Follow-Up for Selected Eye Injuries (*continued*)

Eye Injury	Assessment Findings	Treatment	Follow-Up
Ocular burns	Swelling of the sclera Conjunctival irritation Corneal clouding (may be indicative of severe burn) Pain	Determine baseline pH of the eye Topical anesthesia Immediate copious irrigation until the pH returns to normal range (pH = 7.4); this may require more than 2 L of irrigating solution Visual acuity reassessment	Ophthalmology consultation and close follow-up

Abbreviations: EOM, extraocular eye movement; IOP, intraocular pressure; NPO, nothing by mouth.

Data from Bowling, B. (2016). Trauma. In *Kanski's clinical ophthalmology* (8th ed., pp. 861–885). Philadelphia, PA: Elsevier; Desai, U., Roeder, R., Lemelman, B. T., & Thaller, S. R. (2016). Maxillofacial trauma. In J. A. Asensio & D. D. Trunkey (Eds.), *Current therapy of trauma and surgical critical care* (2nd ed., pp. 153–161). Philadelphia, PA: Elsevier; Dupre, A. A., & Wightman, J. M. (2018). Red and painful eye. In R. M. Walls, R. S. Hockberger, & M. Gaushe-Hill (Eds.), *Rosen's emergency medicine: Concepts and clinical practice* (9th ed., pp. 169–183). Philadelphia, PA: Elsevier; Guluma, K., & Lee, J. E. (2018). Ophthalmology. In R. M. Walls, R. S. Hockberger, & M. Gaushe-Hill (Eds.), *Rosen's emergency medicine: Concepts and clinical practice* (9th ed., pp. 790–819). Philadelphia, PA: Elsevier; Pargament, J. A., Armenia, J., & Nerad, J. A. (2015). Physical and chemical injuries to eyes and eyelids. *Clinics in Dermatology, 33*(2), 234–237. https://doi.org/10.1016/j.clindermatol.2014.10.015; Sharma, N., Kaur, M., Agarwal, T., Sangwan, V. S., & Vajpayee, R. B. (2017). Treatment of acute ocular chemical burns. *Survey of Ophthalmology, 63*(2), 214–235. https://doi.org/10.1016/j.survophthal.2017.09.005.

- Assist with communication to neurosurgery or with emergent transfer to a trauma center with neurosurgical capabilities as needed.
- Elevation of the patient's head of bed by 30 degrees is recommended to decrease ICP.[8,19] Position the head midline to facilitate venous drainage. Rotation of the head can compress the neck veins and result in venous engorgement and decreased venous drainage.[8]
- Prepare for insertion of an ICP monitoring device, and then monitor the ICP according to institutional protocols. A brain tissue oxygenation monitoring device can be inserted at the same time as ICP monitor placement. ICP monitoring should be considered for the following patients[13]:
  - Patients with severe TBI (GCS score of 3–8) with an abnormal CT scan
  - Patients with GCS score greater than 8 with abnormal CT scan with high risk of progression (large hematomas or coagulopathy)
  - Patients requiring anesthesia or mechanical ventilation where analgesia/sedation makes neurologic assessment more difficult
  - Patients who have worsening CT results or deterioration on neurologic exam[13]
- Administer mannitol, as prescribed:
  - Rule out other injuries before administering this medication.
  - Administer mannitol via bolus rather than via continuous infusion with a dosage of 1 g/kg rapidly over 5 minutes (20% solution). Other dosage amounts may be used to control elevated ICP.[2,13,18]
  - Indications for mannitol include acute neurologic deterioration indicated by:
    - Dilated pupils
    - Loss of consciousness
    - Hemiparesis while the patient is being monitored[2]
  - Mannitol is not used in patients with active intracranial bleeding.
    - Mannitol is *not for use in hypotensive patients* since it will not lower ICP in hypovolemia and is a potent osmotic diuretic.[2]
- Administer hypertonic saline, as prescribed.[2,13]
  - This treatment may be used to decrease ICP, and can be used in hypotensive patients as it does not have a diuretic effect.[2]
- Administer anticonvulsant medication, as prescribed.
- Early post-traumatic seizures (PTS), defined as those that occur within the first 7 days after injury, occur in 12% to 15% of patients with severe head injuries.[2,18] Prolonged seizures can contribute

to secondary brain injury.[2] Seizure activity is associated with higher incidence of pneumonia and acute respiratory distress syndrome as well. Seizure prophylaxis is usually administered to those patients at risk for early PTS. Patients at risk for early PTS include those with the following conditions[59]:
  - Linear or depressed skull fracture
  - Seizure at the time of injury
  - History of seizures
  - Penetrating brain injury
  - Severe head injury
  - Acute subdural hematoma
  - Acute epidural hematoma
  - Age 65 years or older
  - Chronic alcoholism[44]
- Treating fever in patients with head trauma includes the following considerations:
  - Lowered temperature is a result of a change in the thermoregulatory set point, while an elevated temperature from brain injury stems from a disruption in thermoregulation.
  - Antipyretics are not effective at treating hyperthermia related to acute brain injury.
  - A cooling blanket or ice packs may be used.
  - If fever is present as a result of an inflammatory process, antipyretics may be useful.
  - Hyperthermia increases ICP and the cerebral metabolic rate.[43]
  - Avoid causing shivering with the cooling process; shivering increases the cerebral metabolic rate and may precipitate a rise in ICP.
- Do not pack the ears or nose if a CSF leak is suspected.
- Administer tetanus prophylaxis, as needed.
- Assist with wound repair as indicated.
- Administer other medications, as prescribed.
  - Analgesics or sedatives may be indicated for pain or agitation.
- If the change in mental status is suspected to be the result of an overdose, naloxone may be given for opioid use, and flumazenil for benzodiazepine use. Use caution when giving either of these medications, as abrupt withdrawal from long-term opioid use or reversal of benzodiazepine use as an anticonvulsant may precipitate seizures or vomiting, causing further deterioration.
- Administer antibiotics, as prescribed.

Diagnostics and Interventions for Head Trauma

Reevaluation adjuncts include radiographic and laboratory studies.

Radiographic Studies

Radiographic studies include the following:

- CT scans[2]
  - Patient movement may produce artifact and result in an inaccurate CT reading. Patient movement may be a result of seizures, inability to cooperate based on mental status changes, or inappropriate flexion or extension.
  - Sedation may be administered as prescribed.
    - Closely monitor patients who have received sedation or neuromuscular blocking medications during a CT procedure.
    - Be judicious with the use of sedation because of the changes in ability to do neurologic assessments.
- Magnetic resonance imaging
  - MRI is not typically used in the acute resuscitation phase. It may be indicated to provide better delineation of a patient's injury and prognosis.
- Angiography
  - Angiography may be indicated if vascular injury is known or suspected.
  - CT angiography is becoming more common in the initial evaluation of the patient with suspected vascular injury and can be done much more quickly (less than 5 minutes) utilizing less contrast than traditional angiography.[60]
- Skull series
  - Radiographs of the skull are generally not needed, and have largely been replaced by CT of the head.

If the patient is being emergently transferred, the transfer should not be delayed to perform radiologic testing.[2] If there is time while awaiting helicopter or ground transport, CT imaging can be obtained. Ensure that images are sent with the patient, or can be retrieved by the tertiary center.

Laboratory Studies

Laboratory studies include the following:

- Coagulation studies
  - Analysis of coagulation status may be helpful in directing the management for those patients taking anticoagulants or antiplatelet medications.[2]
- Blood alcohol and urine toxicology screens
  - These studies may be helpful to determine the presence or absence of alcohol or other substances that may contribute to an altered mental status.

Reevaluation and Post-Resuscitation Care

Reevaluation of the patient with head trauma includes the following steps:

- Serial scoring of the GCS or FOUR score—this is crucial for early detection of patient deterioriation[2,13]
- Frequent reassessment of pupils
- ABG trending, plus ensuring appropriate adjustments are made to prevent hypoxia[2,13,19]
- Trends in vital signs, especially BP, respiratory rate and pattern, temperature, SpO_2, and end-tidal carbon dioxide
- Reevaluation for the development of the following:
  - Headache
  - Nausea
  - Vomiting
  - Seizure activity
  - Changes in motor or sensory function
  - Response to interventions such as fluid administration and diuretic therapy

Continuous ICP Monitoring

Continuous ICP monitoring is important for assessing brain injury and the response of the patient to treatment. The addition of a brain tissue oxygenation monitoring device can provide for early detection of secondary brain injury, such as cerebral hypoxia and possible ischemia. Such an oxygenation device determines the level of oxygen delivery to the cerebral tissues as well as monitors the temperature of the brain tissue. Any change in brain tissue can alter cerebral metabolism and affect CBF and ICP. The monitoring system detects poor oxygenation to the brain tissue before ICP changes can be detected. In combination with this early detection, early intervention and management can result in a better patient outcome.[61]

Definitive Care or Transport

Consider the need to transport the patient to a trauma center and/or prepare the patient for operative intervention, hospital admission, or transfer, as indicated.

Emerging Trends

As the science and evidence of trauma care continue to evolve, tools to improve patient outcomes continue to be trialed and refined. Evidence is tested and replicated, and new standards of care are transitioned into practice. This section on trauma care considerations explores some of the evidence and the potential significance to trauma patient care. Regarding the care of patients with head trauma, the use of the GCS, FOUR score, and therapeutic hypothermia are discussed. The use of bedside ocular ultrasound is also reviewed.

Validity and Reliability of the Glasgow Coma Scale

The GCS has long been considered the gold standard by which other scoring systems are evaluated.[13,30] Recently, however, the GCS has come under question with regard to inter-rater reliability and lack of prognostic utility. In addition, there is no standard approach regarding what should be done when one component cannot be assessed (e.g., with intubated or aphasic patients). There is a need for continued education to aid in improving reliability.[62,63] A revised GCS is just beginning to emerge into practice and can be found online (www.glasgowcomascale.org).

The FOUR score was developed in 2005 and assesses four variables, as noted earlier. Since all components of the FOUR score can be rated even when patients are intubated, this scoring system may have advantages for use in trauma patients especially in critical care (Table 6-4). It is beginning to be translated into other languages and validated in other countries.[64-67] Initial studies have demonstrated that FOUR score has similar effectiveness to the GCS in predicting mortality in patients with TBI.[29,30,66]

Therapeutic Hypothermia for Traumatic Brain Injury

Many studies have demonstrated the benefit of therapeutic hypothermia for the patient who has return of spontaneous circulation following out-of-hospital cardiac arrest, causing this intervention to become the standard of care.[68] Because of its favorable impact on outcomes, additional research has examined the benefits of prophylactic hypothermia (initiated before a rise in ICP) as well as therapeutic hypothermia (implemented when other measures to decrease ICP have failed) for patients with TBI. Two studies in children related to therapeutic hypothermia demonstrated worse outcomes with hypothermia.[69,70] A recent Cochrane review compared mild hypothermia with normothermia in regard to mortality and unfavorable outcomes; the review included 37 trials with more than 3,000 patients.[70] At present, there is still not enough high-quality evidence to support the intervention of hypothermia in the care of the patient with TBI.[25,47,71]

Bedside Ocular Ultrasound

Bedside ocular ultrasound is being applied to assist in the diagnosis of ocular trauma. This technology can facilitate the evaluation of altered vision, pain, trauma to the eye, and head injury. It is not used in cases involving globe rupture due to the risk of vitreous extrusion.[37] Certain foreign bodies, such as wood, glass, or organic foreign matter, can be better visualized with ultrasound.[58]

Summary

Approximately 1.7 million individuals sustain a TBI each year.[2] Early intervention and appropriate resuscitation are crucial to prevent or minimize the effects of secondary brain injury. Secondary brain injury may result from a hypoxic event, cerebral edema, hypotension, or increased ICP. Facilitating oxygenation and ventilation and maintaining BP are priorities in treating patients with TBI. Frequently reassessing the patient's neurologic status will minimize the effects of any neurologic deterioration.

References

1. Pribaz, J. J., & Ceterson, E. J. (2018). Scalp and forehead reconstruction. In P. C. Neligan & E. D. Rodriguez (Eds.), *Plastic surgery: Volume 3: Craniofacial, head and neck surgery and pediatric plastic surgery* (4th ed., pp. 92–125). St. Louis, MO: Elsevier.
2. American College of Surgeons. (2018). Head trauma. In *Advanced trauma life support: Student course manual* (10th ed., pp. 103–126). Chicago, IL: Author.
3. Patton, K. T., & Thibodeau, G. A. (2018). Nervous system. In *The human body in health and disease* (7th ed., pp. 248–289). St. Louis, MO: Elsevier.
4. Mtui, E., Gruener, G., & Dockery, P. (2016). Hypothalamus. In *Fitzgerald's clinical neuroanatomy and neuroscience* (7th ed., pp. 253–259). Philadelphia, PA: Elsevier.
5. Patton, K. T., & Thibodeau, G. A. (2016). Central nervous system. In *Anatomy and physiology* (9th ed., pp. 436–478). St. Louis, MO: Elsevier.
6. Scanlon, V. C., & Sanders, T. (2015). The nervous system. In *Essentials of anatomy and physiology* (7th ed., pp. 185–221). Philadelphia, PA: F. A. Davis Company.
7. Ransom, B. R. (2017). Organization of the nervous system. In E. L. Boulpaep & W. F. Boron (Eds.), *Medical physiology* (3rd ed., pp. 254–274). Philadelphia, PA: Elsevier.
8. Shier, D., Butler, J., & Lewis, R. (2015) Nervous system. In *Hole's essentials of human anatomy and physiology* (12th ed., pp. 223–272). New York, NY: McGraw-Hill.
9. Pargament, J. A., Armenia, J., & Nerad, J. A. (2015). Physical and chemical injuries to eyes and eyelids. *Clinics in Dermatology, 33*(2), 234–237. https://doi.org/10.1016/j.clindermatol.2014.10.015
10. Hall, J. E. (2016). Cerebral blood flow, cerebrospinal fluid, and brain metabolism. In *Guyton and Hall textbook of medical physiology* (13th ed., pp. 787–794). Philadelphia, PA: Elsevier.
11. Shier, D., Butler, J., & Lewis, R. (2015). Cardiovascular systems. In *Hole's essentials of human anatomy and physiology* (12th ed., pp. 349–385). New York, NY: McGraw-Hill.
12. Alluri, H., Wiggins-Dohlvik, K., Davis, M. L., Huang, J. H., & Tharakan, B. (2015). Blood–brain barrier dysfunction following traumatic brain injury. *Metabolic Brain Disease, 30*(5), 1093–1104. https://doi.org/10.1007/s11011-015-9651-7
13. ACS Trauma Quality Improvement Program. (2015). *ACS TQIP best practices in the management of traumatic brain injury*. Chicago, IL: American College of Surgeons Committee on Trauma.
14. Marehbian, J. S. M., Edlow, B. L., Hinson, H. E., & Hwang, D. Y. (2017). Medical management of the severe traumatic brain injury patient. *Neurocritical Care, 27*, 430–446. https://doi.org/10.1007/s12028-017-0408-5
15. Vakil, M. T., & Singh, A. K. (2017). A review of penetrating brain trauma: Epidemiology, pathophysiology, imaging assessment, complications and treatment. *Emergency Radiology, 24*, 301–309. https://doi.org/10.1007/s10140-016-1477-z
16. Cerebral perfusion pressure. (n.d.). *The Free Dictionary*. Retrieved from https://medical-dictionary.thefreedictionary.com/cerebral+perfusion+pressure
17. Hypercarbia. (n.d.). *The Free Dictionary*. Retrieved from https://medical-dictionary.thefreedictionary.com/hypercarbia
18. Carney, N., Totten, A. M., O'Reilly, C., Ullman, J. S., Hawryluk, G. W., Bell, M. J., . . . Ghajar, J. (2016). *Guidelines for the management of severe traumatic brain injury* (4th ed.). Retrieved from https://braintrauma.org/uploads/03/12/Guidelines_for_Management_of_Severe_TBI_4th_Edition.pdf
19. Garvin, R., & Mangat, H. S. (2017). Emergency neurological life support: Severe traumatic brain injury. *Neurocritical Care, 27* (Suppl. 1), 159–169. https://doi.org/10.1007/s12028-017-0461-0
20. Motamedi, M. H., Dadgar, E., Ebrahimi, A., Shirani, G., Haghighat, A., & Jamalpouru, M. R. (2014). Pattern of maxillofacial fractures: AAA 5-year analysis of 8,818 patients. *Journal of Trauma and Acute Care Surgery, 77*(4), 630–634. https://doi.org/10.1097/TA.0000000000000369
21. Cheung, C. A., Rogers-Martel, M., Golas, L., Chepurny, A., Martel, J. B., & Martel, J. R. (2014). Hospital-based ocular emergencies: Epidemiology, treatment, and visual outcomes. *American Journal of Emergency Medicine, 32*(3), 221–224. https://doi.org/10.1016/j.ajem.2013.11.015
22. Toivari, M., Suominen, A. L., Apajalahti, S., Lindqvist, C., Snall, J., & Thoren, H. (2018). Isolated orbital fractures are severe among geriatric patients. *Journal of Oral Maxillofacial Surgery, 76*(2), 388–395. https://doi.org/10.1016/j.joms.2017.09.019
23. Chang, S. L., Patel, V., Giltner, J., Lee, R., & Marco, C. A. (2017). The relationship between ocular trauma and substance abuse in emergency department patients. *American Journal of Emergency Medicine, 35*, 1734–1737. https://doi.org/10.1016/j.ajem.2017.07.015
24. Centers for Disease Control and Prevention. (2017). Traumatic brain injury & concussion. Retrieved from https://www.cdc.gov/traumaticbraininjury/get_the_facts.html#risk
25. March, K. (2018). Head injury and dysfunction. In V. Good & P. Kirkwood (Eds.), *Advanced critical care nursing* (2nd ed., pp. 218–252). St Louis, MO: Elsevier.

26. Stephens, C. (2018). Pulse pressure calculation explained. *Healthline Media*. https://www.healthline.com/health/pulse-pressure
27. Sasser, S. M., Hunt, R. C., Faul, M., Sugarman, D., Pearson, W. S., Dulski, T., . . . Lerner, E. B. (2012). Guidelines for field triage of injured patients: Recommendations of the National Expert Panel on Field Triage, 2011. *MMWR Recommendations and Reports, 61*(RR-1), 1–20. Retrieved from https://www.cdc.gov/mmwr/preview/mmwrhtml/rr6101a1.htm
28. Watson, V. L., Louis, N., Seminara, B. V., Muizelaar, J. P., & Alberico, A. (2017). Proposal for the rapid reversal of coagulopathy in patients with non-operative head injuries on anticoagulant and/or antiplatelet agents: A case study and literature review. *Neurosurgery, 81*(6), 899–909. https://doi.org/10.1093/neuros/nyx072
29. Okasha, A. S., Fayed, A. M., & Saleh, A. S. (2014). The FOUR score predicts mortality, endotracheal intubation and ICU length of stay after traumatic brain injury. *Neurocritical Care, 21*(3), 496–504. https://doi.org/10.1007/s12028-014-9995-6
30. Nyam, T. E., Hung, S., Shen, M., Yu, T., & Kuo, J. (2017). FOUR score predicts early outcome in patients after traumatic brain injury. *Neurocritical Care, 26*(2), 225–231. https://doi.org/10.1007/s12028-016-0326-y
31. Wijdicks, E. F., Bamlet, W. R., Maramottom, B. V., Manno, E. M., & McClelland, R. L. (2005). Validation of a new coma scale: The FOUR score. *Annals of Neurology, 58*, 585–593. https://doi.org/10.1002/ana.20611
32. Jagoda, A. S., Bazarian, J. J., Bruns, J. J., Cantrill, S. V., Gean, A. D., Howard, P. K., . . . Whitson, R. R. (2008). Clinical policy: Neuroimaging and decision making in adult mild traumatic brain injury in the acute setting. *Annals of Emergency Medicine, 52*(6), 714–748.
33. Teasdale, G., Maas, A., Lecky, F., Manle G., Stocchetti, N., & Murray, G. (2014). The Glasgow Coma Scale at 40 years: Standing the test of time. *The Lancet Neurology, 13*(8), 844–854. https://doi.org/10.1016/S1474-4422(14)70120-6
34. Brophy, G. M., & Human, T. (2017). Pharmacotherapy pearls for emergency neurological life support. *Neurocritical Care, 27*(Suppl. 1), 51–73. https://doi.org/10.1007/s12028-017-0456-x
35. Bowling, B. (2016). Trauma. In *Kanski's clinical ophthalmology* (8th ed., pp. 861–885). Philadelphia, PA: Elsevier.
36. Pflipsen, M., Massaquoi, M., & Wolf, S. (2016). Evaluation of the painful eye. *American Family Physician, 93*(12), 991–998. Retrieved from https://www.aafp.org/afp/2016/0615/p991.html
37. Knoop, K. J., & Dennis, W. R. (2019). Ophthalmologic procedures. In J. R. Roberts (Ed.), *Roberts and Hedges' clinical procedures in emergency medicine and acute care* (7th ed., pp. 1295–1337). Philadelphia, PA: Elsevier.
38. Dupre, A. A., & Wightman, J. M. (2018). Red and painful eye. In R. M. Walls, R. S. Hockberger, & M. Gaushe-Hill (Eds.), *Rosen's emergency medicine: Concepts and clinical practice* (9th ed., pp. 169–183). Philadelphia, PA: Elsevier.
39. Coombes, A. (2018). Eyes. In M. Glynn & W. M. Drake (Eds.), *Hutchison's clinical methods* (24th ed., pp. 419–437). Philadelphia, PA: Elsevier.
40. Lupo, J. E., & Jenkins, H. A. (2016). Traumatic facial paralysis. In D. E. Brackmann, C. Shelton, & M. A. Arriaga (Eds.), *Otologic surgery* (4th ed., pp. 299–313). Philadelphia, PA: Elsevier.
41. Heegaard, W. G., & Biros, M. H. (2017, July 26). Skull fractures in adults. *UpToDate*. Retrieved from https://www.uptodate.com/contents/skull-fractures-in-adults
42. Citardi, M. J., & Fakhri, S. (2015). Cerebrospinal fluid rhinorrhea. In P. W. Flint, B. H. Haughey, V. Lund, J. K. Niparko, K. T. Robbins, J. R. Thomas, & M. M. Lesperance (Eds.), *Cummings otolaryngology* (6th ed., pp. 803–815). Philadelphia, PA: Elsevier Saunders.
43. Shalaie, K., Zwienenberg-Lee, M., & Muizelaar, J. P. (2017). Clinical pathophysiology of traumatic brain injury. In H. Richard Winn (Ed.), *Youmans and Winn neurological surgery* (7th ed., pp. 2843–2859). Philadelphia, PA: Elsevier.
44. Papa, L., & Goldberg, S. A. (2018). Head trauma. In R. M. Walls, R. S. Hockberger, & M. Gaushe-Hill (Eds.), *Rosen's emergency medicine: Concepts and clinical practice.* (9th ed., pp. 301–329). Philadelphia, PA: Elsevier.
45. Garza, I., Schwedt, T. J., Robertson, C. E., & Smith, J. H. (2016). Headache and other craniofacial pain. In R. B. Daroff, J. Jankovic, J. C. Mazzotta, & S. L. Pomeroy (Eds.), *Bradley's neurology in clinical practice* (7th ed., pp. 1686–1719). Philadelphia, PA: Elsevier.
46. Dashnaw, L., Petraglia, A. L., Patel, V., & Bailes, J. E. (2017). Mild traumatic brain injury in adults and concussion in sports. In H. Richard Winn (Ed.), *Youmans and Winn neurological surgery* (7th ed., pp. 2860–2867). Philadelphia, PA: Elsevier.
47. Kamins, J., & Giza, C. C. (2016). Concussion—mild traumatic brain injury: Recoverable injury with potential for serious sequelae. *Neurosurgery Clinics of North America, 27*(4), 441–452. https://doi.org/10.1016/j.nec.2016.05.005
48. Maegele, M. (2018). Traumatic brain injury in 2017: Exploring the secrets of concussion. *Lancet Neurology, 17*(1), 13–15. https://doi.org/10.1016/S1474-4422(17)30419-2
49. Kerr, Z. Y., Zuckerman, S. L., Wasserman, E. B., Vander Vegt, C. B., Yengo-Khan, A., Buckley, T. A., . . . Dompier, T. P. (2017). Factors associated with post-concussion syndrome in high school student-athletes. *Journal of Science and Medicine in Sport, 21*(5), 447–452. https://doi.org/10.1016/j.jsams.2017.08.025
50. Van Eijck, M. M., Schoonman, G. G., Van der Naalt, J., De Vries, J., & Roks, G. (2018). Diffuse axonal injury after traumatic brain injury is a prognostic factor for functional outcome: A systematic review and meta-analysis. *Brain Injury, 30*(4). https://doi.org/10.1080/02699052.2018.1429018
51. Mueller, K., Cirivello, M. J., Bell, R. S., & Armonda, R. A. (2018). Penetrating brain injury. In R. G. Ellenbogen, L. N. Sekhar, & N. D. Kitchen (Eds.), *Principles of neurological surgery* (4th ed., pp. 420–444). Philadelphia, PA: Elsevier.
52. Stippler, M. (2016). Craniocerebral trauma. In R. B. Daroff, J. Jankovic, J. C. Mazzotta, & S. L. Pomeroy (Eds.), *Bradley's neurology in clinical practice* (7th ed., pp. 867–880). Philadelphia, PA: Elsevier.
53. Rosenbloom, L., Delman, B. N., Stein, E. G., & Som, P. M. (2015). Imaging of facial and skull trauma. In T. L. Pope, H. L. Bloem, J. Beltran, W. B. Morrison, & D. J. Wilson (Eds.), *Musculoskeletal imaging* (2nd ed., pp. 21–31). Philadelphia, PA: Saunders.

54. Park, C. M., Shook, E., & Indresano, A. T. (2018). Maxillofacial trauma. In A. H. Harken & E. E. Moore (Eds.), *Abernathy's surgical secrets* (7th ed., pp. 158–160). Philadelphia, PA: Elsevier.
55. Rodriguez, E. D., Dorafshar, A. H., & Manson, P. N. (2018). Facial injuries. In P. C. Neligan (Ed.), *Craniofacial, head and neck surgery and pediatric plastic surgery* (4th ed., Vol. 3, pp. 47–81). Philadelphia, PA: Elsevier.
56. Guluma, K., & Lee, J. E. (2018). Ophthalmology. In R. M. Walls, R. S. Hockberger, & M. Gaushe-Hill (Eds.), *Rosen's emergency medicine: Concepts and clinical practice* (9th ed., pp. 790–819). Philadelphia, PA: Elsevier.
57. Sharma, N., Kaur, M., Agarwal, T., Sangwan, V. S., & Vajpayee, R. B. (2017). Treatment of acute ocular chemical burns. *Survey of Ophthalmology, 63*(2), 214–235. https://doi.org/10.1016/j.survophthal.2017.09.005
58. Desai, U., Roeder, R., Lemelman, B. T., & Thaller, S. R. (2016). Maxillofacial trauma. In J. A. Asensio & D. D. Trunkey (Eds.), *Current therapy of trauma and surgical critical care* (2nd ed., pp. 153–161). Philadelphia, PA: Elsevier.
59. Majidi, S., Makke, Y., Ewida, A., Sianati, B., Qureshi, A. I., & Koubeissi, M. Z. (2017). Prevalence and risk factors for early seizure in patients with traumatic brain injury: Analysis from National Trauma Data Bank. *Neurocritical Care, 27*(1), 90–95. https://doi.org/10.1007/s12028-016-0363-6
60. Starnes, B. W., & Arthurs, Z. M. (2019). Vascular trauma: Head and neck. In A. N. Sidawy & B. A. Perler (Eds.), *Vascular surgery and endovascular therapy* (9th ed., pp. 2365–2377). Philadelphia, PA: Elsevier.
61. Rosenthal, G., & Le Roux, P. D. (2017). Physiologic monitoring for traumatic brain injury. In H. R. Winn (Ed.), *Youmans and Winn neurological surgery* (7th ed., pp. 2898–2090). Philadelphia, PA: Elsevier.
62. Reith, F. C., Brennan, P. M., Maas, A. I., & Teasdale, G. M. (2016). Lack of standardization in the use of the Glasgow Coma Scale: Results of international surveys. *Journal of Neurotrauma, 33*(1), 89–94. https://doi.org/10.1089/neu.2014.3843
63. Teasdale, G. (2014). Forty years on: Updating the Glasgow Coma Scale. *Nursing Times, 110*(42), 12–16.
64. Sivula, A., Luoto, T., Heinila, J., Karlsson, S., Yli-Hankala, A., & Langsjo, J. (2017). FOUR score in monitoring the level of consciousness of an intensive care patient: First experience of the use of the Finnish language version. *Duodecim, 133*(11), 1081–1091.
65. Momenyan, S., Mousavi, S. M., Dadkhahtehrani, T., Sarvi, F., Heidarifar, R., Kabiri, F., . . . Koohbor, M. (2017). Predictive validity and inter-rater reliability of the Persian version of full outline of unresponsiveness among unconscious patients with traumatic brain injury in an intensive care unit. *Neurocritical Care, 27*(2), 229–236. https://doi.org/10.1007/s12028-016-0324-0
66. Nyam, T. E., Ao, K. H., Hung, S. Y., Shen, M. L., Yu, T. C., & Kuo, J. R. (2017). FOUR score predicts early outcome in patients after traumatic brain injury. *Neurocritical Care, 26*(2), 225–231. https://doi.org/10.1007/s12028-016-0326-y
67. Hickisch, A., & Holmefur, M. (2016). Swedish translation and reliability of the full outline of unresponsive score. *Journal of Neuroscience Nursing, 48*(4), 195–205. https://doi.org/10.1097/JNN.0000000000000205
68. Donnino, M. W., Andersen, L. W., Berg, K. M., Reynolds, J. C., Nolan, J. P., Morley, P. T., . . . ILCOR ALS Task Force. (2015). Temperature management after cardiac arrest: An advisory statement by the Advanced Life Support Task Force of the International Liaison Committee on Resuscitation and the American Heart Association Emergency Cardiovascular Care Committee and the Council on Cardiopulmonary, Critical Care, Perioperative and Resuscitation. *Circulation, 132*(25), 2448–2456. Retrieved from https://www.ahajournals.org/doi/10.1161/CIR.0000000000000313
69. Crompton, E. M., Lubomirova, I., Cotlarciuc, I., Han, T. S., Sharma, S. D., & Sharma, P. (2017). Meta-analysis of therapeutic hypothermia for traumatic brain injury in adult and pediatric patients. *Critical Care Medicine, 45*(4), 575–583. https://doi.org/10.1097/CCM.0000000000002205
70. Beca, J., McSharry, B., Erickson, S., Yung, M., Schibler, A., Slater, A., & Pediatric Study Group of the Australia and New Zealand Intensive Care Society Clinical Trials Group. (2015). Hypothermia for traumatic brain injury in children: A Phase II randomized controlled trial. *Critical Care Medicine, 43*(7), 1458–1466. https://doi.org/10.1097/CCM.0000000000000947
71. Lewis, S. R., Evans, D. J., Butler, A. R., Schofield-Robinson, O. J., & Alderson, P. (2017, September). Hypothermia for traumatic brain injury. *Cochrane Database of Systematic Reviews*. https://doi.org/10.1002/14651858.CD001048.pub5

Design credits: Clipboard designed by Vectors Market from Flaticon.

CHAPTER 7

Thoracic and Neck Trauma

Roger M. Casey, MSN, RN, CEN, TCRN, FAEN

OBJECTIVES

Upon completion of this chapter, the learner will be able to:

1. Describe the mechanisms of injury associated with thoracic and neck trauma.
2. Describe pathophysiologic changes as a basis for assessment of the trauma patient with thoracic and neck injuries.
3. Demonstrate the nursing assessment of the trauma patient with thoracic and neck injuries.
4. Plan appropriate interventions for the trauma patient with thoracic and neck injuries.
5. Evaluate the effectiveness of nursing interventions for the trauma patient with thoracic and neck injuries.

Knowledge of normal anatomy and physiology serves as a foundation for understanding anatomic derangements and pathophysiologic processes that may result from trauma. Before reading this chapter, it is strongly suggested that the learner review the following material. The anatomy material is not emphasized in the classroom but may be the basis of skill evaluation assessments and the basis of questions for testing purposes.

Anatomy and Physiology of the Thoracic Cavity and Neck

The anatomy and physiology of the thoracic cavity and neck involves a number of systems and structures, including the respiratory system, heart and thoracic great vessels, and the neck.

Respiratory System

Three processes transfer oxygen from the atmosphere to the lungs and bloodstream: ventilation, diffusion, and perfusion. See Chapter 4, "Airway and Ventilation," for a detailed description of the physiology of ventilation.

The upper airway consists of the nose, oropharynx, larynx, and trachea. The lower airway consists of the bronchi, bronchioles, and alveoli with its associated capillaries found within the lungs.[1]

The thoracic cavity extends from the top of the sternum to the diaphragm and is enclosed by the sternum, ribs, and costal cartilage. The main thoracic structures are the lungs and the mediastinum. The mediastinum is the space between the sternum, thoracic vertebrae, and diaphragm. The heart, pericardium, thoracic aorta, superior and inferior vena cava, phrenic and vagus nerves, and other vascular structures are found within the mediastinum.[1]

The correlation of thoracic surface landmarks and the underlying structures are important in the physical assessment of the chest (**Figure 7-1**).

Heart and Thoracic Great Vessels

The heart is enclosed within the mediastinum, with the right ventricle located behind the sternum and the left ventricle anterior to the thoracic vertebrae. The heart is surrounded by the pericardium. The two layers of the pericardium consist of a tough, outer layer and a thinner, serous layer closely adhering to the heart. The space between the two layers contains approximately 25 mL of lubricating pericardial fluid, which allows the heart to expand and contract without causing friction against surrounding structures.

Cardiac output (CO) is a product of heart rate (HR) and stroke volume (SV): CO = HR × SV. CO is defined as the volume of blood ejected from the heart in 1 minute.[1] (See Chapter 5, "Shock," for more information.) Stroke volume, in turn, is affected by the factors identified in **Table 7-1**. Injury to the myocardium can affect any one of these

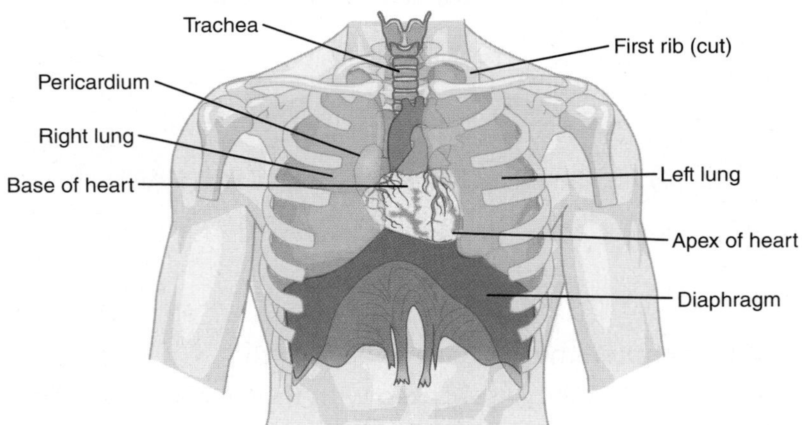

Figure 7-1 *Chest and anatomic landmarks.*

TABLE 7-1 Factors Influencing Cardiac Output

Factor	Description
Preload	› The volume of blood in the left ventricle at the end of diastole[1] • Preload is directly related to the amount of blood volume that is returned to the heart. • If there is less volume, the ventricles will not have much stretch, decreasing preload. • A bleeding trauma patient may have reduced preload as the total blood volume decreases.
Afterload	› The resistance of the system (either systemic or pulmonary) that the ventricles must overcome to eject blood[2] • Intrathoracic pressure affects right ventricular pressure as it contracts against the pulmonary system. • The patient's blood pressure and elasticity of the peripheral vasculature affect left ventricular pressure. • A hypotensive trauma patient may have reduced afterload as the pressure within the vasculature system is lower than that in the ventricles.
Contractility	› The heart's contractile strength[2] • Factors affecting myocardial contractility include preload and sympathetic nervous system stimulation.

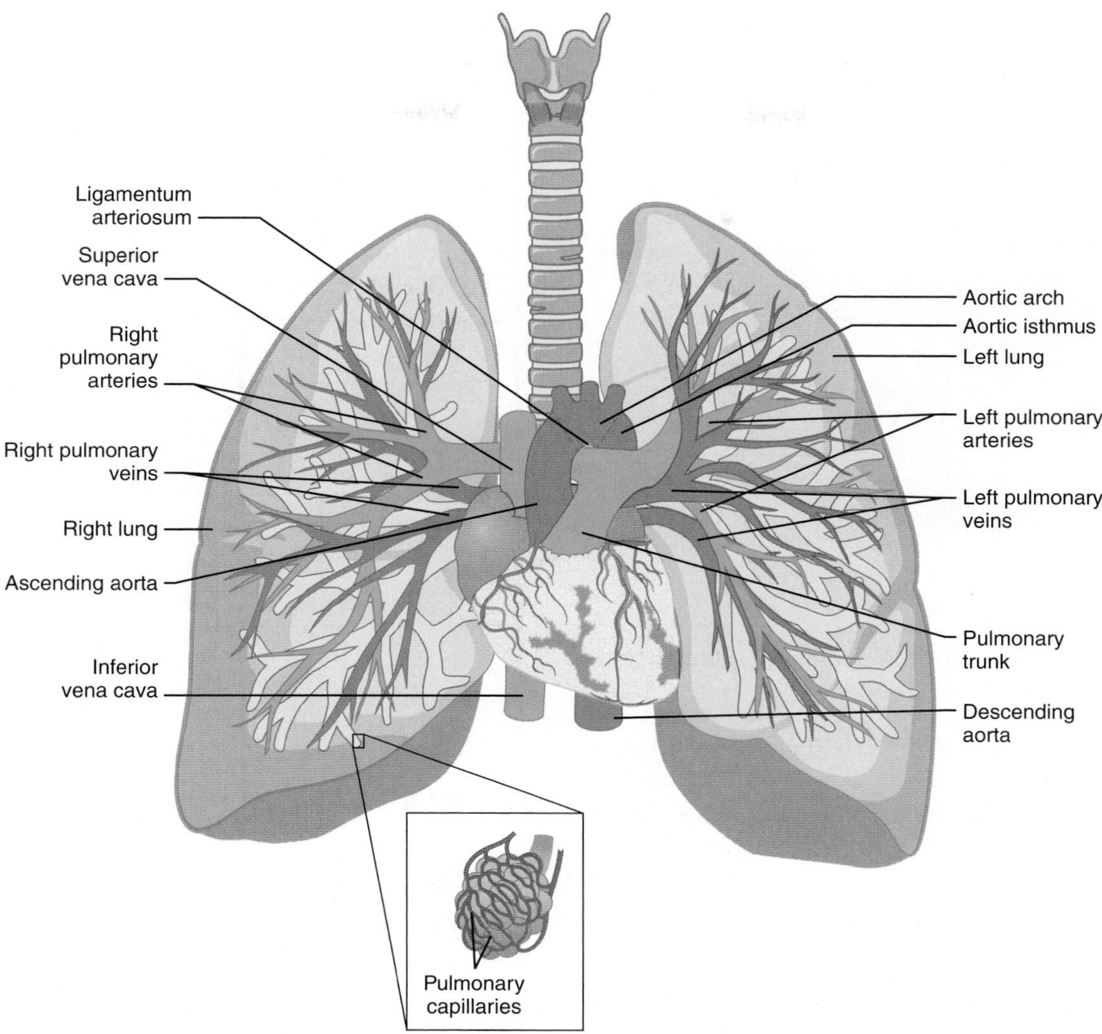

Figure 7-2 *Thoracic vasculature.*

functions, resulting in decreased cardiac output and the ability to perfuse oxygenated blood to the tissues.

The thoracic aorta carries oxygenated blood from the heart to the body and is located in the mediastinum. The three segments of the thoracic aorta are the ascending aorta, the aortic arch, and the descending aorta (**Figure 7-2**). The ascending aorta is the portion located most proximal to the heart. The aortic arch extends from the ascending thoracic aorta to the descending thoracic aorta and is the source for both the carotid and subclavian arteries. The descending aorta continues distally from the aortic arch and constricts slightly at the aortic isthmus, where it is held in place by the ligamentum arteriosum, the left mainstem bronchus, and the paired intercostal arteries. The aortic isthmus is the transition from the more mobile aortic arch to the relatively fixed descending aorta and is less able to tolerate rapid acceleration/deceleration forces. It is most often the site of aortic injury.[3]

Neck

The neck contains several important anatomic structures relative to its size (**Figure 7-3**). It is commonly divided into three zones, based on bony and superficial landmarks[4]:

- Zone I landmarks: sternal notch to the cricoid cartilage
- Zone II landmarks: the cricoid cartilage to the angle of the mandible
- Zone III landmarks: angle of the mandible to the base of the skull

The neck's anatomic structures are contained within two fascial layers. The superficial fascia contains the

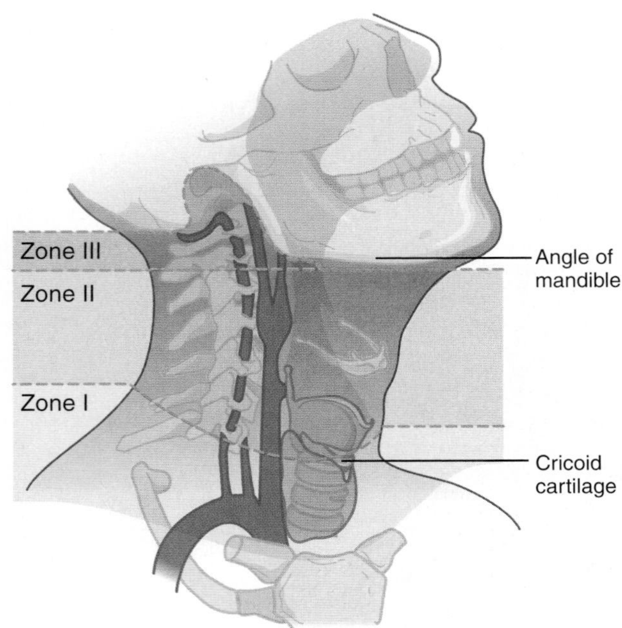

Figure 7-3 *Anatomy of the neck (including zones).*

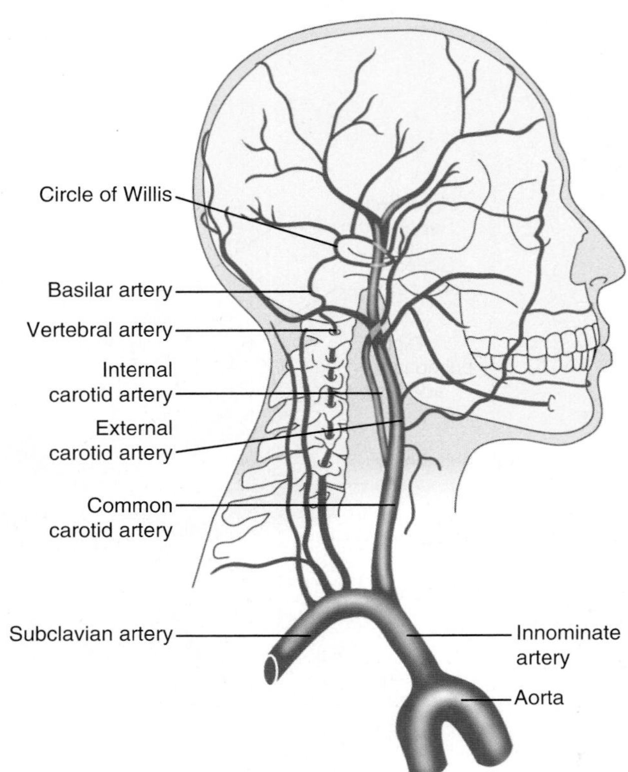

Figure 7-4 *The vascular supply to the brain.*

platysma muscle, which protects the underlying structures. If the platysma is damaged, injury to the structures beneath is suspected. The deep cervical fascia supports the muscles, vessels, and organs of the neck. The compartments formed by the fascia may limit external bleeding but may also allow a hematoma to form, which may compromise the airway.[4-7]

CLINICAL PEARL 

Mortality and Neck Injuries

Mortality is the highest with injuries to Zone I in the neck, as they typically involve major vessels, trachea, esophagus, and lungs.[4] The trauma nurse will have a high degree of suspicion of a more serious underlying injury in patients who have dysphonia, dysphagia, subcutaneous emphysema, or hematomas to the neck region, indicating vascular trauma, airway injuries, or esophageal injuries that may not be diagnosed on imaging studies.[8]

The vascular supply for the brain and the brain stem arises from the vertebral and internal carotid arteries (**Figure 7-4**).

Nerve roots from C5 through T1 merge, forming the brachial plexus (**Figure 7-5**). This structure then subdivides and merges to form the multiple nerves that are responsible for the arm and hand function, such as the axillary, musculocutaneous, median, radial, and ulnar nerves.[5]

Introduction

Thoracic and neck trauma are a significant cause of morbidity and mortality in trauma patients. Many of the injuries that occur in this anatomic region are severely life threatening if not identified and treated in a rapid manner. Motor vehicle collisions (MVCs) are the most common cause of blunt trauma to the neck and thoracic regions, while gunshot wounds and stabbings are the most common cause of penetrating trauma. Identifying these injuries through a thorough assessment process is key to increasing the chances of patient survival.[3,9-12]

Epidemiology

Thoracic and neck trauma can cause significant life-threatening injuries necessitating emergent intervention. In the United States, MVCs involving automobiles, motorcycles, and pedestrians account for more than half of all blunt injuries to the neck and chest. Penetrating injuries to the neck in adults are most commonly caused by personal assaults with firearms and stabbing instruments. However, in children, most penetrating neck trauma is

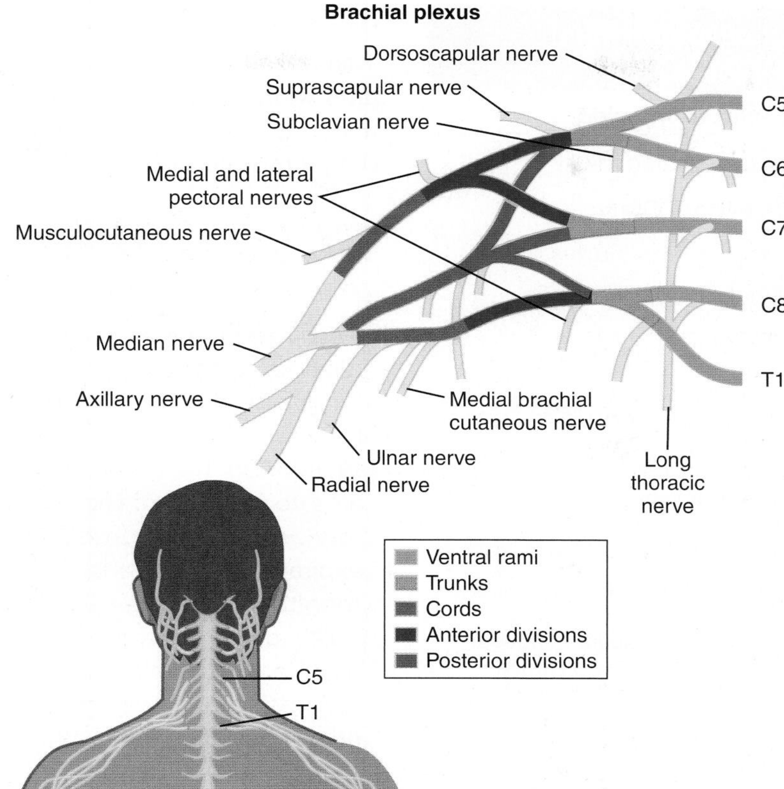

Figure 7-5 *Nerves responsible for arm and hand functions.*

unintentional—for example, when children fall on sharp objects or are involved in MVCs. Interpersonal violence is increasingly a more common cause of thoracic trauma.[3,9-11]

Biomechanics and Mechanisms of Injury

While MVCs are the most common cause of thoracic trauma, other mechanisms of injury (MOIs) include falls, crush injuries, assaults, gunshot and stabbing wounds, and pedestrian-versus-vehicle collisions.[3,9-11] Additional considerations include the following:

- The energy forces associated with acceleration and deceleration can result in devastating injury to the major vessels as the body makes impact, yet the internal organs stay in motion. The descending aorta is at increased risk of being torn, as it is fixed in place by the ligamentum arteriosum.[3]
- Mechanical energy forces applied to the thorax can cause rib fractures, pulmonary contusion, pneumothorax, hemothorax, and blunt cardiac injury (BCI). The sternum and first and second ribs are relatively more resistant to energy forces because they are protected.[3] As a result, first rib fractures are a known sign of life-threatening injuries in trauma patients.[13] As more force is required to damage these structures, there is increased risk of injury to the underlying structures, as well as death.[3]
- Direct blunt injury to the myocardium may result in ventricular perforation or rupture, and can often be fatal.
- Penetrating injury to the heart commonly injures the right ventricle due to its anterior position in the thoracic cavity.

Usual Concurrent Injuries

Thoracic injuries are often associated with life-threatening conditions such as airway disruption, impaired breathing, or impaired circulation. Thoracic trauma is most often associated with concurrent head, spine, extremity,

CLINICAL PEARL 

Penetrating Thoracic Wound Below the Fourth Intercostal Space

If a penetrating thoracic wound is found below the fourth intercostal space, penetration into the abdominal cavity is suspected until proven otherwise.[3]

TABLE 7-2 Thoracic Skeletal Fractures and Associated Injuries

Fractures	Associated Injuries
Sternal fractures	› Blunt cardiac injury › Pneumothorax
First and second rib fractures	› Great vessel injuries › Brachial plexus injuries › Head and spinal cord injuries
Multiple rib fractures and flail chest	› Pulmonary contusion › Pneumothorax › Hemothorax
Lower rib fractures (7–12)	› Liver (right-sided fractures) › Spleen (left-sided fractures)

Data from Dennis, D. M., Bellister, S. A., & Guillamondegui, O. D. (2017). Thoracic trauma. *Surgical Clinics of North America, 97*, 1047–1064. https://doi.org/10.1016/j.suc.2017.06.009; Fallouh, H., Dattani-Patel, R., & Rathinam, S. (2017). Blunt thoracic trauma. *Surgery, 35*(5), 262–268. https://doi.org/10.1016/j.mpsur.2017.02.005; Schellenberg, M., & Inaba, K. (2018). Critical decisions in the management of thoracic trauma. *Emergency Medicine Clinics of North America, 33*(1), 135–147. https://doi.org/10.1016/j.emc.2017.08.008.

and abdominal injuries. Thoracic skeletal injuries are often linked with specific injuries (**Table 7-2**).[14-16] Penetrating thoracic trauma can occur with penetrating abdominal trauma due to the movement of the diaphragm in and out of the thoracic cavity.

Neck injuries may be isolated, but may also be associated with head, cervical spine, or upper thoracic injuries. Identifying the specific zone of neck injury is helpful in identifying the structures that may potentially be injured, the need for diagnostic studies, and the approach to surgical management. Injuries to the neck may occlude the airway, interrupt blood flow to the brain, or cause cervical spinal cord injury. Because of the risk of concurrent cervical spinal injuries, the motion of patients with neck injuries is restricted and they are assessed for cervical spinal injury.[1,5]

Pathophysiology as a Basis for Assessment Findings

An understanding of the physiological processes associated with organs likely affected in certain types of injuries will help the trauma nurse anticipate potential problems, interventions, monitoring, and management for the trauma patient.

Ineffective Ventilation

Trauma to the thoracic cavity, the neck, and the structures within these areas can result in ineffective ventilation. Any loss of integrity to the lungs or diaphragm may compromise normal respiration and ventilation.[12,15]

CLINICAL PEARL 

Respiration versus Ventilation

Respiration: The exchange of oxygen and carbon dioxide, across a membrane either between the lungs and the blood or between the blood and the tissues, at the cellular level.[1]

Ventilation: The active, mechanical movement of air into and out of the lungs during the respiratory cycle, which consists of both inspiration and expiration.[1,17] End-tidal carbon dioxide ($ETCO_2$) monitoring can be used to determine whether ventilation is effective; it is more sensitive than monitoring pulse oximetry. An increase in $ETCO_2$ can indicate airway obstruction, embolism, or other clinical changes affecting ventilation.[17]

A pneumothorax, pulmonary bleeding, pulmonary contusions, and sternal or rib fractures may interfere with the mechanics of breathing, owing to both increased intrathoracic pressure and pain. Sternal and rib fractures can also result in damage to underlying organs. Pulmonary contusions may cause interstitial and alveolar edema. Lacerations to the lung allow for the accumulation of blood in the interstitial and alveolar spaces. Oxygen (O_2) and carbon dioxide (CO_2) diffusion across the alveolar membrane is impaired by interstitial and alveolar edema or blood. Damaged alveoli and capillary injuries produce abnormalities in the ventilation to perfusion ratio.[14]

Penetrating injury to the chest wall and lacerated lung tissue can cause the loss of normal negative intrapleural pressure. The collection of air or blood in the pleural space may cause lung collapse. The degree of collapse depends on the extent of the air or blood that collects in the pleural space and the severity of the underlying lung injury.[3]

The airway can be easily compromised or occluded due to neck trauma. Edema or hematomas from disrupted blood vessels following a neck injury may narrow or completely obstruct the upper airway. Tears or lacerations of the tracheobronchial tree can disrupt the integrity of the upper and lower airway. Patients with these injuries initially present with dramatic symptoms, including airway obstruction, hemoptysis, cyanosis, and subcutaneous emphysema from massive air leaks into the tissues of the face, neck, and chest.[3]

BOX 7-1 Beck's Triad

The three signs of acute cardiac tamponade are:

- Low arterial blood pressure
- Distant, muffled heart sounds
- Distended neck veins

Ineffective Circulation

Air or blood that continues to accumulate in the thoracic cavity can cause an increase in intrapleural pressure on the same side of the chest that is injured. If this pressure is allowed to expand without intervention, it can produce a mediastinal shift that compresses the heart and great vessels, resulting in a decrease in venous return (preload) and subsequent decrease in cardiac output. The increased pressure can also compress the opposite lung, further decreasing ventilation. In such a case, the patient usually exhibits signs of increased work of breathing, tachypnea, shortness of breath, tachycardia, hypotension, and a unilateral decrease in breath sounds on the injured side. Neck vein distention from the increased intrathoracic pressure and tracheal deviation caused by the mediastinal shift are late signs and may not be clearly evident upon initial presentation.[3,12,14,15]

Injury to the heart or great vessels can be fatal from an immediate uncontrolled hemorrhage. Direct injury to the heart may cause damage to the tissue, reduce myocardial contractility, and ultimately lead to a reduction in cardiac output. The rapid accumulation of even small amounts of blood in the pericardial sac (pericardial tamponade) may result in compression of the heart, making it difficult for the heart to fill during diastole, and in turn resulting in decreased cardiac output. Assessment findings include hypotension, tachycardia, muffled heart sounds, and neck vein distention.[3,12,14,15] See **Box 7-1**. Jugular venous distention may not be evident in significantly hypovolemic patients.

Injury to the arteries in the neck may cause decreased blood flow to the brain, subsequently producing cerebral hypoxia and neurologic deficits. Penetrating injuries to certain neck vessels (carotid or vertebral arteries or vertebral, brachiocephalic, and jugular veins) may cause rapid exsanguination.[5]

Nursing Care of the Patient with Thoracic or Neck Trauma

Refer to Chapter 3, "Initial Assessment," for a systematic approach to the nursing care of the trauma patient. The following assessment parameters are specific to patients with thoracic or neck injuries.

Primary Survey

If there is no uncontrolled, life-threatening external hemorrhage and need to reprioritze to <C>ABC, the primary survey begins with alertness and airway.

A: Alertness and Airway

Assess the patient's alertness and airway.

Assessment

Inspect for the following:

- Injuries to the neck that may indicate edema or blood in the airway
- Signs of injury that may obstruct or impede the patient's ability to maintain a patent airway:
  - Foreign objects
  - Loose or missing teeth
  - Blood, vomitus, or secretions
  - Edema
  - Burns or evidence of inhalation injury
  - Tongue swelling
- Swelling
  - Hematoma (underlying blunt trauma)
  - Subcutaneous emphysema (from a pneumothorax or a tracheal or esophageal laceration)
  - Impaled objects
  - Lacerations
  - Bleeding
  - Tracheal deviation (from a tension pneumothorax)

Auscultate for restrictive airway sounds. Hoarseness and stridor may be signs of tracheal injury and airway narrowing.

Interventions

Interventions include the following:

- Apply direct pressure to bleeding sites.
  - Take care to ensure that pressure to control bleeding does not impact airway patency.
- Stabilize any impaled objects.
- Prepare to assist with a definitive airway as indicated.

Cervical Spinal Stabilization/Spinal Motion Restriction

Neck trauma carries a risk for concurrent cervical spinal injury. Whenever trauma to the neck occurs, take care to restrict spinal motion until injury can be ruled out.[1]

B: Breathing and Ventilation

Breathing and ventilation assessment and interventions come next.

Assessment

Inspect for the following:

- Chest wall injuries that may severely impair the adequacy of breathing, such as open chest wounds or flail segments
  - Removal of debris or blood from the skin may be necessary to avoid overlooking any wounds.
- Breathing effectiveness to include rate and depth of respirations (if present) and work of breathing
- Symmetrical or paradoxical chest wall movement
- Evidence of blunt or penetrating trauma to the thorax or upper abdomen

Auscultate for the following:

- Equality of bilateral breath sounds
- Unilateral or generalized diminished breath sounds (pneumothorax or hemothorax)

Percuss for dullness or hyperresonance of the chest (presence of blood or air).

Palpate for the following:

- Tenderness (contusions, rib fractures)
- Edema (hematomas, contusions)
- Hematoma/ecchymosis (contusions, rib fractures)
- Subcutaneous emphysema (pneumothorax, tension pneumothorax, tracheal or esophageal laceration)
- Bony crepitus (possible fractured ribs or sternum)
- The trachea at the level of the suprasternal notch to assess for tracheal deviation (tension pneumothorax)

Interventions

Interventions include the following:

- Begin administering oxygen at 10–15 L/minute via a nonrebreather mask attached to an oxygen reservoir.
- As soon as the patient is stabilized, maintain SpO_2 between 94% and 98%.[3]
- Prepare to monitor and titrate oxygen delivery to maintain SpO_2 between 94% and 98%. See Chapter 4 for information regarding hyperoxia.
- Implement selected interventions based on assessment findings.

C: Circulation and Control of Hemorrhage

If there is a high degree of suspicion of cardiac injury, auscultate for muffled heart sounds or murmurs.

Palpate for the following:

- Central pulses
  - Compare the quality of pulses between the left and right and the lower and upper extremities.
- External jugular veins for distention as a potential sign of cardiac tamponade or tension pneumothorax
- Extremities for motor and sensory function
  - Lower extremity paresis or paralysis may indicate an aortic injury or thoracic spinal injury.[5]
  - Upper extremity paresis or paralysis may indicate a brachial plexus injury.

Reevaluation

If the assessment findings provoke a suspicion of uncontrolled internal bleeding, a chest radiograph or focused assessment with sonography for trauma (FAST) examination may be indicated. Determine if the patient needs immediate definitive operative intervention or transport.[3,15]

Chest Radiograph

A supine chest radiograph will likely identify any significant pneumothorax. If a hemothorax is suspected, the position of the patient during the test directly influences the reading. If the patient is supine, blood will likely spread throughout the affected side, creating general opacification. If the patient is upright, the air–fluid boundary will appear horizontally. If a potential spinal cord injury has been ruled out, an upright chest radiograph can be used to evaluate a hemothorax. Chest radiographs may suggest an aortic injury but cannot confirm or rule out the diagnosis.[15]

Focused Assessment with Sonography for Trauma

A FAST examination may be indicated to detect the presence of pericardial blood and heart wall motion (**Figure 7-6**). FAST may also indicate the presence of pneumothorax or rib fractures. See Chapter 8, "Abdominal and Pelvic Trauma," for more information on performing the FAST examination.

Resuscitative Thoracotomy

Resuscitative thoracotomy may be necessary when a patient with penetrating chest trauma arrives with unstable vital signs or impending arrest. Indications for performing this invasive procedure in the resuscitation room include:

- Relief of cardiac tamponade
- Support cardiac output (with internal massage)
- Cross-clamp the descending aorta (to preserve blood flow to the brain and thoracic organs)
- Defibrillate the heart internally (more effective than external defibrillation)
- Limit hemorrhage from the heart or great vessels

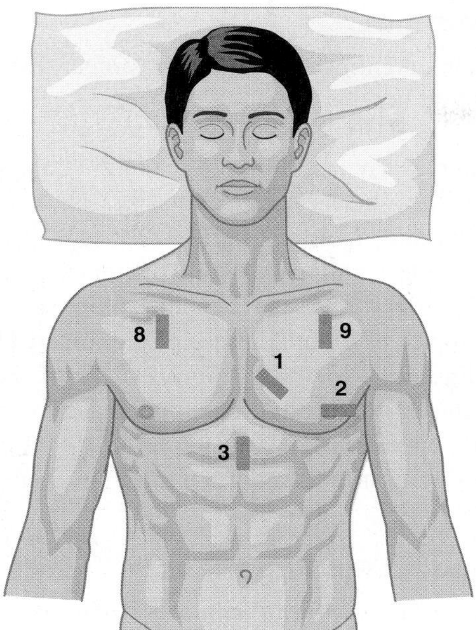

1. Parasternal Long Cardiac View
2. Apical Four-Chamber Cardiac View
3. Inferior Vena Cava View
8. Pulmonary View
9. Pulmonary View

Figure 7-6 *FAST exam in thoracic trauma.*

In regard to the need for or success of resuscitative thoracotomy in the emergency department (ED), the American College of Surgeons (ACS) notes that, "[with] the availability of a surgical team skilled in repair of such injuries, a resuscitative thoracotomy may be required if there is no return of spontaneous circulation (ROSC). If no surgeon is available to perform the thoracotomy and cardiac tamponade has been diagnosed or is highly suspected, a decompressive needle pericardiocentesis may be performed, preferably under ultrasound guidance."[3] Resuscitative thoracotomy is rarely successful in patients with blunt chest trauma and cardiac arrest.[3,12,14]

CLINICAL PEARL 

Internal Defibrillation

When defibrillation is required following a resuscitative thoracotomy, the internal paddles are placed on opposite sides of the myocardium (a saline-soaked gauze dressing may be placed between the myocardium and the paddles to improve conduction and decrease injury to the myocardium). Lower energy settings are used for internal defibrillation because the paddles are placed directly on the myocardium. For adults, 30 to 50 joules should be used. Internal paddles are programmed to deliver no more than 50 joules.[10]

Resuscitative Endovascular Balloon Occlusion of Aorta

Resuscitative thoracotomy is very invasive and has limited success rates. An emerging option is the resuscitative endovascular balloon occlusion of the aorta (REBOA). With REBOA, a catheter enters via the femoral artery into the aorta in specified zones to provide an endovascular block, not unlike cross-clamping the aorta during a thoracotomy (see Figure 5-7). REBOA may achieve occlusion more rapidly than thoracotomy in the hands of a skilled practitioner. Indications for REBOA include the following:

- Traumatic life-threatening hemorrhage below the diaphragm in the presence of hemorrhagic shock with transient responders, or non-responders to resuscitation
- Patients arriving to the ED in arrest from injury due to presumed life-threatening hemorrhage below the diaphragm
- Inflation of the balloon in the distal thoracic aorta (Zone 1) for intra-abdominal or retroperitoneal hemorrhage, or traumatic arrest; or the distal abdominal aorta (Zone 3) for severe pelvic, junctional, or proximal lower-extremity hemorrhage

Note that REBOA is an emerging procedure, so the evidence supporting its use is limited. The ACS and the American College of Emergency Physicians have provided a joint statement with recommendations for REBOA use, guidelines, and recommendations for implementation.[18]

Secondary Survey

Secondary survey begins with the history.

H: History

Questions specific to patients with thoracic or neck injuries include:

- Is the MOI blunt or penetrating?
- Is the patient complaining in a way that would indicate one or more of the following conditions is present?
    - Dyspnea
    - Dysphagia
    - Dysphonia
- Was there a cardiac event prior to the injury?
- If cardiopulmonary resuscitation (CPR) is being performed, when was it started and why?

This information is important in determining the indications for performing an emergency thoracotomy or when to consider withdrawal of support.

Selected Neck and Thoracic Injuries

This section covers selected neck and thoracic injuries.

Tracheobronchial Injury

Tracheobronchial trauma is most likely to be caused by penetrating mechanisms.[7] The majority of penetrating injuries occur in the proximal trachea. Direct blows to the neck or "clothesline"-type injuries are common mechanisms for blunt tracheobronchial trauma. Diagnosis is based on assessment findings and confirmed with bronchoscopy or computed tomography (CT) for large disruptions. Bronchoscopy can be used to help advance an endotracheal tube past the injury to assure adequate ventilation.[7]

Assessment Findings

Assessment findings include the following:

- Dyspnea or tachypnea
- Hoarseness
- Subcutaneous emphysema in the neck, face, or upper thorax
- Pneumothorax, possibly tension pneumothorax
- Hemoptysis
- Decreased or absent breath sounds
- Signs and symptoms of airway obstruction

Interventions

Attempts at endotracheal intubation may cause further injury or contribute to airway occlusion. Anesthesiology, if available, may reduce the risk of intubation injury. Other approaches that may minimize trauma to the airway include use of flexible endoscopy, a smaller endotracheal tube (ETT), or an emergent cricothyrotomy, if indicated.[3,5,7]

Blunt Esophageal Injury

Injury to the esophagus as a result of blunt trauma is rare.

Assessment Findings

Assessment findings include the following:

- Air in the mediastinum with possible widening
- Concurrent left pneumothorax or hemothorax
- Esophageal matter in a chest tube
- Subcutaneous emphysema

Interventions

The only intervention in this case is to prepare for surgery.

Neck Trauma

Neck trauma may result in injuries to the airway structures (trachea or larynx), blood vessels (subclavian, jugular, carotid, and vertebral), esophagus, endocrine glands (thyroid and parathyroid), thoracic duct, and brachial plexus. MOIs may be either blunt or penetrating. Examples of blunt trauma include direct blows or "clothesline"-type injury to the neck region. Penetrating trauma may be caused by either sharp instruments or missile injuries (gunshot wounds). Neck trauma may damage significant airway or vascular structures or the spinal column.

Assessment Findings

Assessment findings include the following:

- Dyspnea or tachypnea
- Hemoptysis
- Subcutaneous emphysema
- Decreased or absent breath sounds
- Penetrating wounds or impaled objects
- Bruits, which may indicate potential carotid artery injury[3]
- Active external bleeding
- Expanding hematoma
- Neurologic deficits (aphasia or loss of extremity movement or sensation)
- Dysphonia
- Dysphagia

Interventions

Interventions include the following:

- Stabilize any impaled objects.
- Control external bleeding with direct pressure.
- Continuously monitor for continued bleeding or expanding hematomas.
- Prepare for surgery.

Rib and Sternal Fractures

Rib fractures are found in 4% to 10% of all hospitalized trauma patients and are one of the most frequent diagnoses in trauma admissions.[19-21] More than 90% of patients with multiple rib fractures have associated injuries, most commonly involving the head, abdomen, and/or extremities. If the patient has fractures of the right lower ribs, suspect the possibility of underlying injury to the liver. In contrast, fractures of the left lower ribs are suggestive of injuries to the spleen. With any displaced rib fracture, lung contusion or laceration is possible.

Sternal fractures are usually caused by a blow to the anterior chest. Due to the force required to fracture the sternum, most of these fractures are not isolated, but rather may be associated with multiple rib or thoracic spine fractures. A severely displaced sternal fracture may indicate serious cardiac injury.[1,12,22,23]

Assessment Findings

Assessment findings include the following:

- Dyspnea
- Localized pain on movement, palpation, or inspiration
- Patient assumes a position of comfort, which splints the chest wall to reduce pain
- Paradoxical chest wall movement (flail)
- Chest wall contusions
- Bony crepitus or deformity

Interventions

Interventions include the following:

- Administer supplemental oxygen as needed.
- Administer analgesia to promote adequate chest expansion and depth of respiration.
- Prepare for intubation and ventilator support if severe respiratory distress is present.

Flail Chest

A flail chest injury is defined as the fracture of three or more sequential ribs in two or more locations that results in a flail section.[13,19,23,24] (**Figure 7-7**). This flail segment may create an unstable chest wall that moves paradoxically, drawing in with chest expansion and pushing out with exhalation.[23] In the mechanics of breathing, inspiration is generated by negative intrapleural pressure that draws air in from the outside. This type of negative pressure cannot be generated with a flail segment, owing to the paradoxical motion of the flail segment.[16] This paradoxical, or asynchronous, movement of the chest may be limited by the surrounding musculature, making it generally more easily detected with palpation than with inspection. Ineffective ventilation in flail chest is caused by several factors:

- Pain that causes the patient to splint, with rapid, shallow breathing
- Deformity of the chest wall resulting in loss of tidal volume, atelectasis, and the ability to clear secretions[23]
- Underlying injury to thoracic organs, including parenchymal laceration, pulmonary contusion, pneumothorax, or hemothorax[13,16]

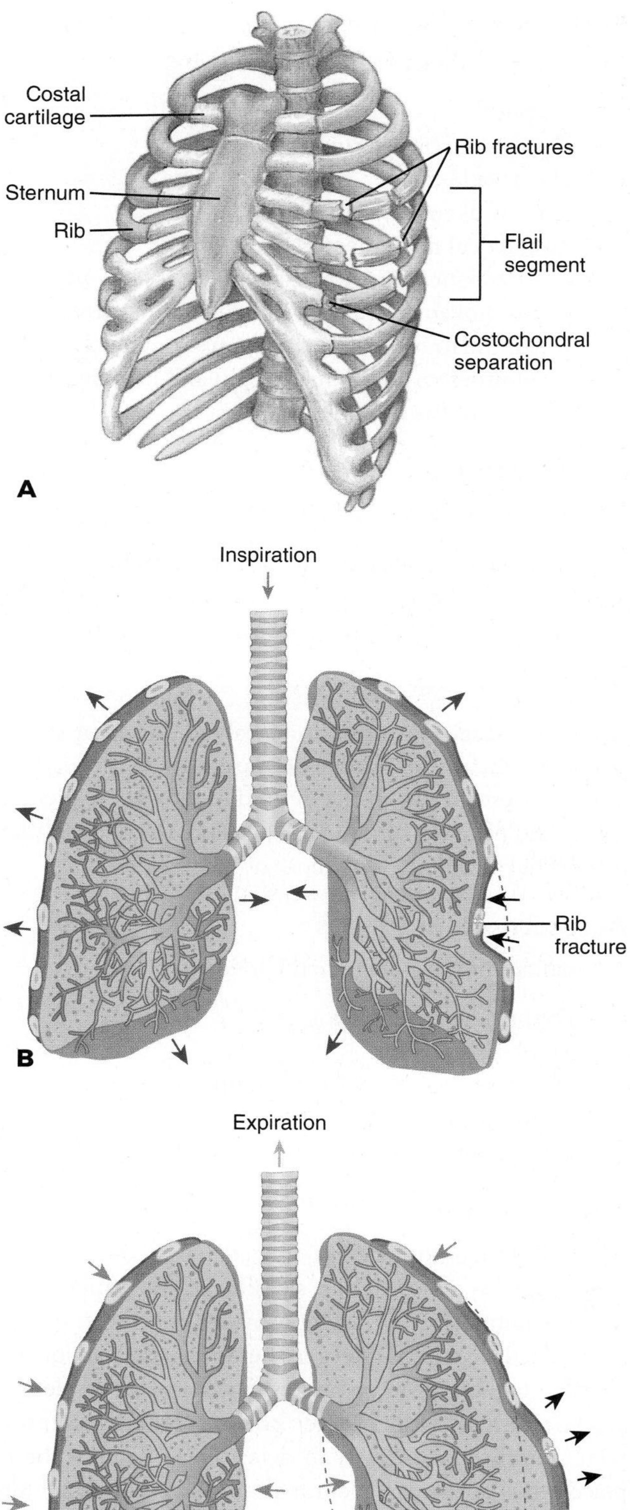

Figure 7-7 *Flail chest.* ***A.*** *Flail chest injury.* ***B.*** *Paradoxical movement inward on inspiration.* ***C.*** *Paradoxical movement outward on expiration.*

Assessment Findings

Assessment findings include the following:

- Dyspnea
- Diminished breath sounds
- Chest wall pain
- Chest wall contusions
- Paradoxical movement of the chest
  - If the patient is splinting as a response to pain, this movement may be difficult to visualize.
  - Administration of analgesia may reduce the splinting response due to pain and improve visibility of the flail chest.

Interventions

Interventions include the following:

- Support adequate oxygenation and ventilation.
- Administer analgesia to the patient.
- Prepare for intubation and mechanical ventilation.

Simple Pneumothorax

A simple (closed) pneumothorax can be caused by either blunt or penetrating trauma (**Figure 7-8**). With such an injury, air escapes from the injured lung into the pleural space, and negative intrapleural pressure is lost, resulting in a partial or complete collapse of the lung.[3,12,13]

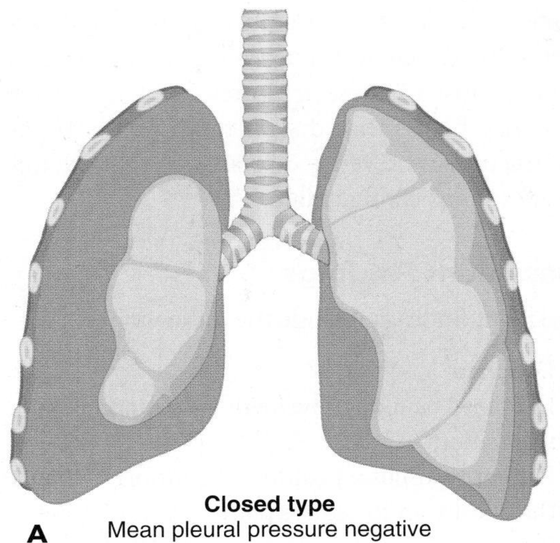

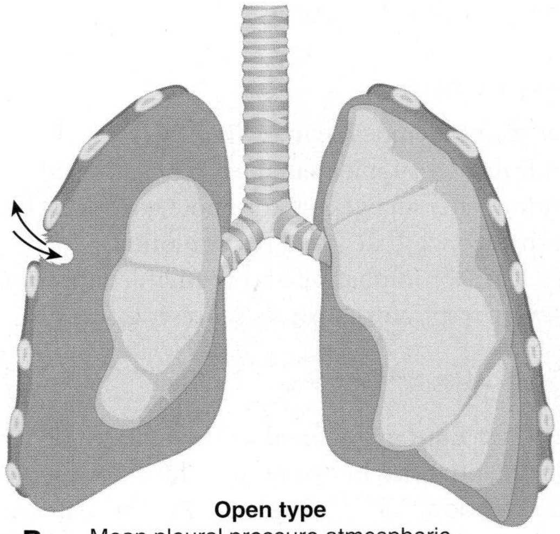

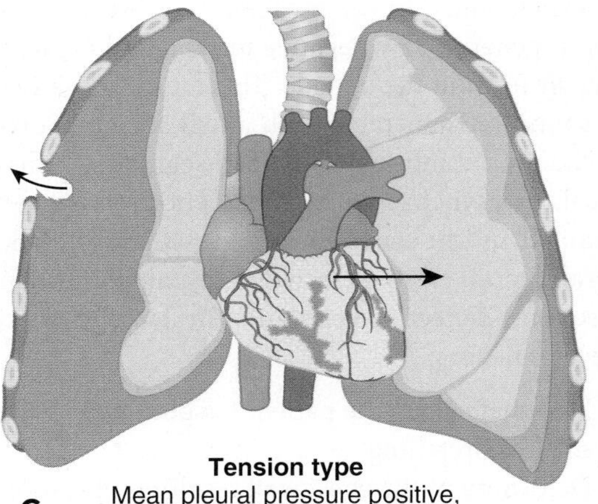

Figure 7-8 *Types of trauma-related pneumothorax.* ***A.*** *Closed type: mean pleural pressure negative.* ***B.*** *Open type: mean pleural pressure atmospheric.* ***C.*** *Tension type: mean pleural pressure positive mediastinal shift to opposite side.*

Assessment Findings

Assessment findings include the following:

- Dyspnea or tachypnea
- Tachycardia
- Decreased or absent breath sounds on the injured side
- Chest pain

Interventions

A simple pneumothorax is treated based on the size, presence of symptoms, and stability of the patient. For those patients who are asymptomatic and stable, observation, with or without oxygen therapy, is often adequate. Supplemental oxygen promotes reabsorption of pleural air. For patients with a larger pneumothorax and those who are unstable or likely to deteriorate, a chest tube is placed to evacuate the pleural air and maintain the lung expansion.[12,15]

Open Pneumothorax

An open (complex) pneumothorax can be the result of a penetrating wound through the chest wall that causes air to become trapped in the intrapleural space (Figure 7-8B). During inspiration, air enters the pleural space through the wound as well as through the trachea.

CLINICAL PEARL

Pneumothorax with Positive-Pressure Ventilation

Mechanically ventilated patients with even a relatively small pneumothorax are at a higher risk for expansion of the pneumothorax, or development of a tension pneumothorax, due to positive-pressure ventilation. Maintain a high index of suspicion for this condition with ventilated patients with a pneumothorax and no thoracostomy tube.

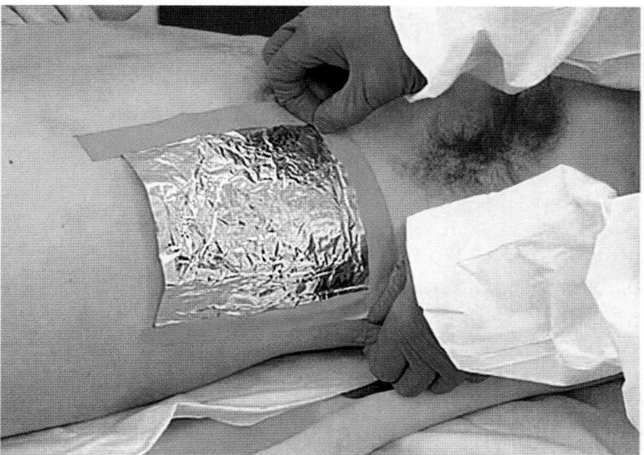

Figure 7-9 *Three-sided dressing.*

Reproduced from American College of Surgeons. (2018). Thoracic trauma. In *Advanced trauma life support: Student course manual* (10th ed., pp. 62–81). Chicago, IL: Author.

Assessment Findings

In addition to the assessment findings of a simple pneumothorax, the following may be present:

- Subcutaneous emphysema (air escaping from the lung into the subcutaneous tissue)
- Chest wound that creates a sucking sound on inspiration

Interventions

Interventions include the following:

- Completely cover open chest wounds with a nonporous dressing (plastic wrap, petroleum gauze) and tape the dressing securely on three sides (**Figure 7-9**).[3] This measure is temporary and has variable effectiveness; it is meant to prevent air from becoming trapped in the pleural space, potentially leading to a tension pneumothorax, and is more commonly applied in the prehospital setting. Definitive repair is completed as quickly as possible in the form of a chest tube and wound closure or surgical repair.[3]
- Monitor for the potential risk of tension pneumothorax if the wound is completely sealed without adequate decompression.
- If signs and symptoms of a tension pneumothorax develop after the application of the dressing, remove the dressing and reevaluate the patient.

Tension Pneumothorax

A tension pneumothorax occurs when air enters the pleural space but cannot escape on expiration. The increasing intrathoracic pressure causes the lung on the injured side to collapse (**Figure 7-10**). If the pressure is not relieved,

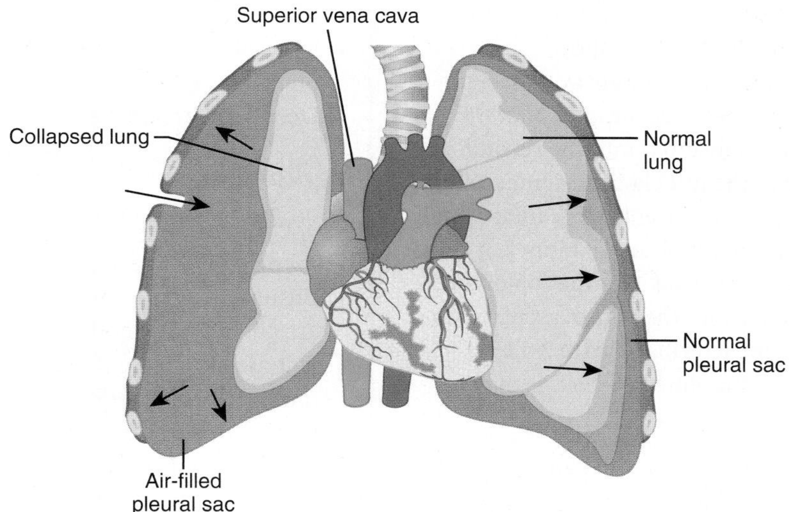

Figure 7-10 *Tension pneumothorax.*

the mediastinum can shift toward the uninjured side, compressing the heart, the great vessels, and ultimately the opposite lung. An alert, responsive patient may be able to compensate for a short time by increasing the respiratory rate, tidal volume, and chest expansion; a sedated and intubated patient may not be able to mount this response. As the intrathoracic pressure rises, venous return is hampered, cardiac output decreases, and hypotension occurs.[3,14,16]

Assessment Findings

Assessment findings include the following:

- Anxiety or severe restlessness
- Severe respiratory distress
- Significantly diminished or absent breath sounds on the injured side
- Hypotension
- Distended neck, head, and upper extremity veins (may not be evident if the patient has experienced significant blood loss)
- Tracheal deviation or a shift toward the uninjured side
  - Symptoms such as jugular venous distention, tracheal shift, and cyanosis may not be present unless the patient's condition has deteriorated; thus, they may be considered late signs of tension pneumothorax.[9,14]
- Cyanosis

Interventions

Interventions include the following:

- Immediate decompression is indicated for patients who exhibit the assessment findings of a tension pneumothorax. If the patient is relatively stable, an immediate and rapid chest radiograph may confirm the diagnosis.[15,25]
  - Do not delay interventions in the deteriorating patient to perform chest radiography.
- If chest tube placement is not readily available, immediately prepare for needle decompression.
  - A 14-gauge needle is inserted into the second intercostal space in the midclavicular line OR the fifth intercostal space at the anterior axillary line, depending on the patient's body habitus.
  - The needle should be placed over the top of the third or sixth rib to avoid the neurovascular bundle that runs under each rib. (**Figure 7-11**).[3,15]
- Prepare for chest tube placement, which is the definitive treatment.

A rush of air and improvement in the patient's condition is both diagnostic (confirming the condition) and therapeutic (removing the threat), and should be immediately noted.

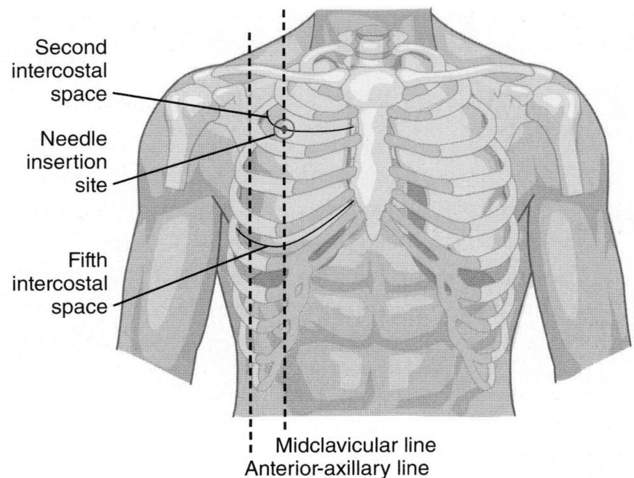

Figure 7-11 *Insertion sites for needle decompression.*

Hemothorax

A hemothorax is caused by blood accumulating in the pleural space. It results from injury to multiple structures, including the lung, costal blood vessels, great vessels, and other structures. Hemothorax may also result from laceration to the liver or spleen combined with an injury to the diaphragm. A massive hemothorax is defined as the rapid accumulation of more than 1,500 mL of blood in the pleural space.[3,14]

Assessment Findings

Assessment findings include the following:

- Anxiety or restlessness
- Dyspnea or tachypnea
- Chest pain
- Signs of shock such as tachycardia, cyanosis, diaphoresis, and hypotension
- Decreased breath sounds on the injured side

Interventions

Interventions include the following:

- Prepare for chest tube insertion.
- Ensure two large-caliber intravenous (IV) catheters are patent and blood is available so as to treat large volume blood loss if needed. If immediate open thoracotomy is performed, chest tube insertion is deferred.
- The large-bore chest tube is inserted at the fifth intercostal space at the anterior or midaxillary line

(Figure 7-11). After the chest tube is inserted, it is connected to a chest drainage system.
- Perform autotransfusion if banked blood is not readily available.[26]
- Prepare for transfer to the operating room/suite.

CLINICAL PEARL 

Hemothorax Management: Large-Bore Chest Tube

Blood is thick and has the ability to clot off smaller-diameter tubes. The largest-bore chest tube for the size of the patient should be considered to avoid unnecessary tube obstruction events.

Pulmonary Contusion

Pulmonary contusions (or lung contusions) most commonly occur as a result of absorption of energy across the pulmonary structures and chest wall from forces such as those experienced in MVCs and falls.[12] A contusion develops when capillary blood leaks into the lung parenchyma, leading to edema and inflammation. The contusion may be localized or diffuse. The degree of respiratory insufficiency is related to the size of the contusion, the severity of the injury to the alveolar–capillary membrane, and the development of subsequent atelectasis. The subtle assessment findings associated with pulmonary contusions usually develop over time rather than immediately after injury.[14] Pulmonary contusions are not always identified on a plain radiograph but may be more apparent on CT imaging; however, this rarely changes management. Potentially significant complications include pneumonia and acute respiratory distress syndrome.

Assessment Findings

Assessment findings include the following:

- Dyspnea
- Ineffective cough
- Increased work of breathing
- Hypoxia
- Chest pain
- Chest wall contusions or abrasions
- Hemoptysis

Interventions

Interventions include the following:

- Maintain SpO_2 between 94% and 98% for adequate oxygenation and to avoid hyperoxia. See Chapter 4 for additional information.
- Minimize or use IV fluids judiciously.
- Prepare for possible intubation and ventilatory support.

CLINICAL PEARL 

Pulmonary Contusion

Pulmonary contusions may produce only vague symptoms[14] and begin to progress at 4–6 hours following the trauma; they can take as long as 24–48 hours to fully develop. Care of a pulmonary contusion is generally supportive in nature—maximizing oxygenation and pain management. Judicious use of fluids should be considered to prevent increase in intraparenchymal hemorrhage, atelectasis, or consolidation by infusing fluids into the injured region of the lung.[12]

Blunt Cardiac Injury

BCI includes myocardial contusion and, less commonly, injury to the ventricular septum, coronary arteries, or cardiac valves. This type of injury usually occurs from a direct impact or compression of the thoracic cavity. The majority of BCIs are caused by MVCs, with motorcycle collisions, falls, and blast injuries being other common mechanisms. Maintain a high index of suspicion for BCI in a patient with an abnormally poor cardiovascular response to his or her injuries.[3,15]

Assessment Findings

Assessment findings include the following:

- Electrocardiogram (ECG) abnormalities, including persistent sinus tachycardia, premature ventricular contractions, atrial fibrillation, ST-segment changes, ischemia, or atrioventricular block[16]
- Hematomas/ecchymosis (chest wall contusion)
- Chest pain

Interventions

Interventions include the following:

- Monitor the heart rate and rhythm.
- Treat dysrhythmias.
- Monitor the patient continuously because the signs and symptoms may not be immediately evident.
- Administer analgesics.
- Perform an echocardiogram.
- Monitor cardiac biomarkers (CK-MB [creatine kinase–muscle/brain], troponin).

- Elevated cardiac troponin levels in a patient with suspected BCI can be a result of skeletal muscle injury and may not necessarily stem from cardiac ischemia.[27]
- BCI can be ruled out if 12-lead ECG and troponin levels are normal within 8 hours of presentation.[22,28]

Cardiac Tamponade

Cardiac tamponade is a collection of blood in the pericardial sac. Typically, the MOI for cardiac tamponade is penetrating trauma, but it can also occur with blunt trauma. Blood that collects between the heart and nondistensible pericardial sac, even as little as 50 mL, compresses the heart and decreases the ability of the ventricles to fill, subsequently causing decreased stroke volume and cardiac output. The decrease in cardiac output is related to both the amount of blood in the pericardial sac and its rate of accumulation.[3]

Assessment Findings

Assessment findings include the following:

- Beck's triad
  - Hypotension
  - Distended neck veins
  - Muffled heart sounds (may be difficult to assess or may be absent)
- Chest pain
- Tachycardia or pulseless electrical activity
- Dyspnea
- Cyanosis
- Pulsus paradoxus

Interventions

Prepare for pericardial decompression:

- A surgical pericardectomy can be done that removes part of the pericardium to create a "window." This pericardial window will prevent blood from accumulating in the pericardial sac.
- Needle pericardiocentesis may also be used to relieve the symptoms of cardiac tamponade, but it is only a temporary solution (**Figure 7-12**). For any patient experiencing a pericardial tamponade and needing pericardiocentesis, surgical evaluation of the heart is required.[3,15]

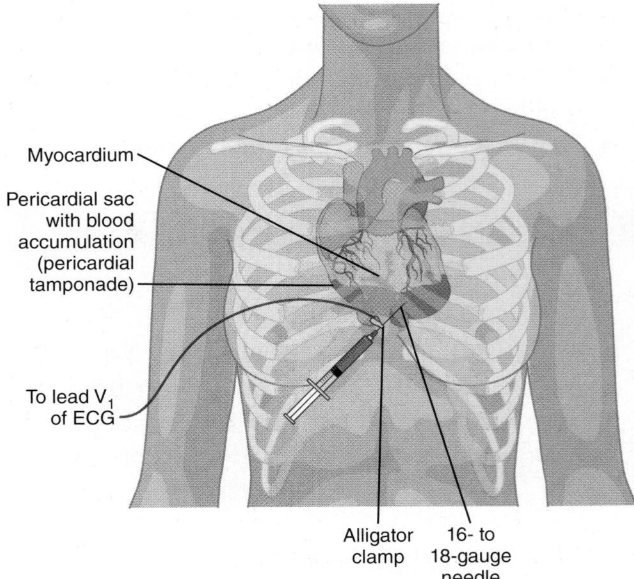

Figure 7-12 *Pericardiocentesis.*

CLINICAL PEARL

Pulsus Paradoxus

Pulsus paradoxus is a decrease of more than 10 mm Hg in the systolic blood pressure that occurs during inhalation (inspiration). It is caused by a fall in cardiac output as a result of increased negative intrathoracic pressure during inhalation. As pressure within the thorax falls, blood pools in the large veins of the lungs and thorax, and stroke volume is decreased.[1]

Aortic Disruption

Injuries to the thoracic aorta are usually caused by blunt trauma but may also be caused by penetrating trauma. The most frequently injured site of the aorta is distal to the left subclavian artery and adjacent to the ligamentum arteriosum. Deaths from aortic injury most commonly occur at the scene; aortic disruption has a mortality rate of approximately 80%.[29] Of those patients who survive to hospitalization, 50% will die within 24 hours of their injury.[29,30]

Assessment Findings

Assessment findings include the following:

- Fractures of the sternum, first or second rib, or scapula
- Cardiac murmurs
- Back or chest pain
- Unequal extremity pulse strength or blood pressure (significantly greater in the upper extremities)
- Hypotension
- Tachycardia

- Skin changes
  - Diaphoresis
  - Pallor
  - Cyanosis
- Paraplegia (due to disruption of spinal perfusion from aortic injury)
- Radiographic findings:
  - Widened mediastinum
  - Right-sided tracheal deviation
  - Left hemothorax

Interventions

Interventions include the following:

- Prepare for angiography or surgery.
- Consider a massive transfusion protocol (see Chapter 5 for more information).
- Consider permissive hypotension.

Ruptured Diaphragm

A ruptured diaphragm is a potentially life-threatening injury. It can be the result of blunt or penetrating trauma, but most commonly occurs from high-speed MVCs. The left hemidiaphragm is more likely to be affected because the right hemidiaphragm is protected by the solid mass of the liver (**Figure 7-13**). When the diaphragm is ruptured, the abdominal contents can herniate into the thoracic cavity, compressing the lung and obstructing the patient's ability to take a breath. If left untreated, this condition may lead to respiratory compromise.[3]

Penetrating trauma below the fourth intercostal space indicates a potential for ruptured diaphragm and concurrent abdominal injury. Without increased awareness and a thorough assessment, this injury may go unrecognized. Penetrating trauma to the lateral chest walls and flanks is also associated with diaphragmatic injuries due to the close proximity, steep slope, and large surface area of the diaphragm.[3,31]

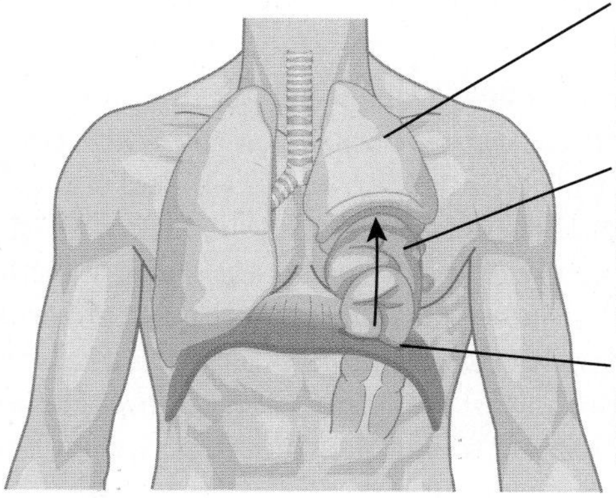

Figure 7-13 *Ruptured diaphragm.*

Assessment Findings

Assessment findings include the following:

- Dyspnea or orthopnea
- Dysphagia
- Abdominal pain
- Pain in the shoulder indicating intraperitoneal bleeding. Left shoulder pain is a classic sign of splenic injury (Kehr's sign)
- Bowel sounds auscultated in the lung fields on the injured side
- Decreased breath sounds on the injured side

Interventions

The intervention is to prepare for surgery.

Reevaluation

Reevaluation begins with imaging studies.

Imaging Studies

Imaging studies include the following:

- A thoracic CT scan can reveal injuries to the thoracic skeletal structure, pulmonary parenchyma, and the aorta.
- Bronchoscopy, laryngoscopy, or esophagoscopy may be indicated in certain neck injuries.
- CT angiography may be used to evaluate suspected vascular injuries in the chest.
- Ultrasound may identify pericardial effusion, hemothorax, pneumothorax and even rib fractures.

Other Studies

Other studies may include the following:

- ECG may identify possible injury to the myocardium.
- An elevated central venous pressure (CVP) may be noted in patients with tension pneumothorax or cardiac tamponade. Patients with hypovolemia may have a low CVP.
- Echocardiography provides an accurate assessment of the cardiac function (wall motion, valvular function, estimated cardiac output) and can identify the presence of pericardial fluid. Transesophageal echocardiography is the most accurate form of this technology.

- Lab studies may also be performed:
  - Arterial blood gases (ABGs)
  - Troponin
  - Amylase
  - Lipase

Chest Drainage Systems

Consider the following points when managing a chest drainage system:

- Be familiar with the facility's equipment and policies and procedures due to variations across products.
- Cover the insertion site securely with tape. Tape all tubing connections between the patient and the chest drainage system to prevent inadvertent disconnection.
- Obtain a chest radiograph to verify improvement in hemothorax or pneumothorax.
- Maintain the chest drainage system below the level of the chest to facilitate the flow of drainage and prevent reflux back into the pleural space. For systems using a water seal, keep the collection chamber upright to prevent loss of the water seal.
- Coil the tubing gently on the bed without any dependent loops or kinks, maintaining the collection chamber below the level of the heart.
- Assess and document the following using the FOCA mnemonic (see **Table 7-3**).
- Troubleshooting for problems should follow the DOPE mnemonic (see Table 7-3).
- Notify the physician of the following and anticipate the need for surgery[3]:
  - If the initial chest drainage is greater than 1,500 mL
  - If there is a continuing blood loss of more than 200 mL per hour for 2 to 4 hours

TABLE 7-3 Assessing and Troubleshooting Chest Drainage Systems

Assessing: FOCA	Troubleshooting: DOPE
Fluctuation in the water seal chamber	**D**isplaced tube
Output	**O**bstruction
Color of the drainage	**P**neumothorax
Air leak present	**E**quipment failure

Note: Fluctuation in the water seal chamber with inspiration and expiration is normal.

- During patient transport, clamping of the chest tube is contraindicated since it may cause the development of a tension pneumothorax.

CLINICAL PEARL

Notify the Physician

Notify the physician of the following and anticipate the need for surgery:

- If the initial chest drainage is greater than 1,500 mL
- If there is a continuing blood loss of more than 200 mL per hour for 2 to 4 hours

CLINICAL PEARL

Do Not Clamp the Chest Tube!

During patient transport, clamping of the chest tube is contraindicated because it may cause the development of a tension pneumothorax.

Autotransfusion

There are risks inherent in receiving a blood transfusion, including infection and anaphylactic reaction. An alternative method for replacing red blood cells with oxygen-carrying capacity is autotransfusion, or the collection of the patient's own blood for reinfusion. There are specific indications and contraindications for autotransfusion, and this modality of treatment remains a controversial intervention.[3] Be familiar with the facility's policies and procedures regarding the use of autotransfusion. See Chapter 5 for more information.

CLINICAL PEARL

Autotransfusion and Chest Tube Drainage

Some commercially available chest drainage systems enable collection of blood and the ability to reinfuse it to the patient to correct blood loss associated with massive hemothorax.[3] Some studies have shown that reintroducing the patient's blood may create a hypercoagulable state[26] and advocate for the use of banked blood to replace what was lost. Massive transfusion protocols can be implemented to replace blood components during the resuscitation phase.[32]

Reevaluation and Post-Resuscitation Care

Reevaluation of the patient with thoracic or neck trauma includes monitoring the following:

- Airway patency, respiratory effort, and ventilation adequacy
- Signs of developing tension pneumothorax following the application of an occlusive dressing
- Neck hematomas for signs of expansion
- Heart sounds
- Vital signs indicating a shock syndrome
- Chest tube drainage systems for the amount of drainage and any change in drainage characteristics
- ABGs for respiratory and/or metabolic acidosis

Definitive Care or Transport

Prepare for surgery, admission, or transport to a trauma center.

Emerging Trends

As the science and evidence of trauma care continue to evolve, tools to improve patient outcomes continue to be trialed and refined. Evidence is tested and replicated, and new standards of care are transitioned into practice. This section on trauma care considerations explores some of the evidence and the potential significance to trauma patient care. In the care of patients with thoracic and neck trauma, stabilization of rib fractures is discussed.

Stabilization of Flail Chest Injuries

Traditional treatment of patients with multiple rib fractures and flail chest injuries has been limited to nonoperative management consisting of pain control, mechanical ventilation with intermittent positive pressure ventilation, and lung and chest physiotherapy. However, even with nonoperative management, patients with severe chest injury remain at high risk for complications such as pneumonia, sepsis, extended hospitalizations and even death.[23] Some research has shown promising results when patients with flail chest injuries have their rib fractures stabilized through various surgical rib stabilization devices; this treatment has been shown to reduce morbidity and mortality by reducing the need for mechanical ventilation, intensive care unit and hospital length of stay, incidence of pneumonia, and the need for tracheostomy.[20,23,24,33]

Summary

Thoracic and neck trauma both have the potential to cause immediate life-threating alterations in airway, breathing, and circulation. Understanding the anatomy, MOI, and pathophysiology related to these injuries can prepare the trauma nurse to accurately and rapidly assess for and proactively and effectively intervene with life-threatening injuries to effect optimal patient outcomes.

References

1. Stacy, K. M. (2018). Pulmonary anatomy and physiology. In L. D. Urden, K. M. Stacy, M. G. Lough (Eds.), *Critical care nursing: Diagnoses and management* (8th ed., pp. 411–430). Maryland Heights, MO: Elsevier.
2. Hartjes, T. M. (Ed.). (2018). *AACN core curriculum for high acuity, progressive, and critical care nursing* (7th ed.). St. Louis, MO: Elsevier.
3. American College of Surgeons. (2018). Thoracic trauma. In *Advanced trauma life support: Student course manual* (10th ed., pp. 62–81). Chicago, IL: Author.
4. Johnson, A. M., Hill, J. L., Zagorski, D. J., McClain, J. M., & Maronian, N. C. (2017). Airway management in a patient with tracheal disruption due to penetrating neck trauma with hollow point ammunition: A case report. *A & A Case Reports*, 1–4. https://doi.org/10.1213/XAA0000000000000675
5. Martin, T. (2015). Neck trauma management. *Surgery, 33*(9), 449–454. https://doi.org/10.1016/j.mpsur.2015.07.002
6. Ibraheem, K., Khan, M., Rhee, P., Azim, A., O'Keefe, T., Tang, A., . . . Joseph, B. (2018). "No zone" approach in penetrating neck trauma reduces unnecessary computed tomography angiography and negative explorations. *Journal of Surgical Research, 221*, 113–120. https://doi.org/10.1016/j.jss.2017.08.033
7. Sell, A., & Patel, A. (2014). Airway trauma. *Anesthesia and Intensive Care Medicine, 15*(5), 242–244. https://doi.org/10.1016/j.mpaic.2014.02.007
8. Morales-Uribe, C., Ramirez, A., Suarez-Poveda, T., Ortiz, M., & Sanabria, A. (2016). Diagnostic performance of CT angiography in neck vessel trauma: Systematic review and meta-analysis. *Emergency Radiology, 23*(5), 421–431. https://doi.org/10.1007/s10140-016-1412-3
9. Bailitz, J., & Hedayati, T. (2013). Thoracic trauma. In J. G. Adams (Ed.), *Emergency medicine: Clinical essentials* (2nd ed., pp. 681–694). Philadelphia, PA: Elsevier Saunders.
10. Denke, N. J. (2010). Thoracic trauma. In P. K. Howard & R. A. Steinmann (Eds.), *Sheehy's emergency nursing: Principles and practice* (6th ed., pp. 285–300). St. Louis, MO: Mosby Elsevier.
11. Frawley, P. M. (2009). Thoracic trauma. In K. A. McQuillan, M. B. Makic, & E. Whalen (Eds.), *Trauma nursing: From resuscitation through rehabilitation* (4th ed., pp. 614–677). St. Louis, MO: Saunders Elsevier.

12. Platz, J. J., Fabricant, L., & Norotsky, M. (2017). Thoracic trauma: Injuries, evaluation, and treatment. *Surgical Clinics of North America, 97*(5), 783–799. https://doi.org/10.1016/j.suc.2017.03.004
13. Sammy, I. A., Chatha, H., Lecky, F., Bouamra, O., Fragoso-Iniguez, M., Sattout, A., Hickey, M., & Edwards, J. E. (2017). Are first rib fractures a marker for other life-threatening injuries in patients with major trauma? *Emergency Medicine Journal, 34*, 205–211. https://doi.org/10.1136%2Femermed-2016-206077
14. Dennis, D. M., Bellister, S. A., & Guillamondegui, O. D. (2017). Thoracic trauma. *Surgical Clinics of North America, 97*, 1047–1064. https://doi.org/10.1016/j.suc.2017.06.009
15. Schellenberg, M., & Inaba, K. (2018). Critical decisions in the management of thoracic trauma. *Emergency Medicine Clinics of North America, 33*(1), 135–147. https://doi.org/10.1016/j.emc.2017.08.008
16. Fallouh, H., Dattani-Patel, R., & Rathinam, S. (2017). Blunt thoracic trauma. *Surgery, 35*(5), 262–268. https://doi.org/10.1016/j.mpsur.2017.02.005
17. Luehrs, P. (2017). Continuous end-tidal carbon dioxide monitoring. In D. L. Wiegand (Ed.), *AACN procedure manual for high acuity, progressive, and critical care* (7th ed., pp. 103–110). St. Louis, MO: Elsevier
18. Brenner, M., Bulger, E. M., Perina, D. G., Henry, S., Kang, C. S., Rotondo, M. F., . . . Stewart, R. M. (2018). Joint statement from the American College of Surgeons Committee on Trauma (ACS COT) and the American College of Emergency Physicians (ACEP) regarding the clinical use of resuscitative endovascular balloon occlusion of the aorta (REBOA). *Trauma Surgery & Acute Care Open, 3*, e000154. https://doi.org/10.1136/tsaco-2017-000154
19. Brasel, K. J., Moore, E. E., Albrecht, R. A., DeMoya, M., Schreiber, M., Karmy-Jones, R., . . . Biffl, W. L. (2016). Western Trauma Association critical decisions in trauma: Management of rib fractures. *Journal of Trauma and Acute Care Surgery, 82*(1), 200–202. https://doi.org/10.1097/TA.0000000000001301
20. Kasotakis, G., Hasenboehler, E. A., Streib, E. W., Patel, N., Patel, M. B., Alarcon, L., . . . Como, J. J. (2017). Operative fixation of rib fractures after blunt trauma: A practice management guideline from the Eastern Association for the Surgery of Trauma. *Journal of Trauma and Acute Care Surgery, 82*(3), 618–626. https://doi.org/10.1097/TA.0000000000001350
21. Majak, P., & Naess, P. A. (2016). Rib fractures in trauma patients: Does operative fixation improve outcome? *Current Opinion in Critical Care, 22*(6), 572–577. https://doi.org/10.1097/MCC.0000000000000364
22. Gross, E. A., Martel, M. L. (2018). Multiple trauma. In R. M. Walls, R. S. Hockberger, M. Gauche-Hill, K. Bakes, J. M. Baren, T. B. Erickson, . . . R. D. Zane (Eds.), *Rosen's emergency medicine: Concepts and clinical practice* (9th ed., pp. 287–300). Philadelphia, PA: Elsevier.
23. Dehghan, N., de Mestral, C., McKee, M. D., Schemitsch, E. H., & Nathens, A. (2014). Flail chest injuries: A review of outcomes and treatment practices from the National Trauma Data Bank. *Journal of Trauma and Acute Care Surgery, 76*, 462–468. https://doi.org/10.1097/TA.0000000000000086
24. Taylor, B. C., Fowler, T. T., French, B. G., & Dominguez, N. (2016, August). Clinical outcomes of surgical stabilization of flail chest injury. *Journal of the American Academy of Orthopaedic Surgeons, 24*, 575–580. https://doi.org/10.5435/JAAOS-D-15-00476
25. Waters, J. (2017). Chest tube placement (assist). In D. L. Wiegand (Ed.), *AACN procedure manual for high acuity, progressive, and critical care* (7th ed., pp. 178–183). St. Louis, MO: Elsevier.
26. Harrison, H. B., Smith, W. Z., Salhanick, M. A., Higgins, R. A., Ortiz, A., Olson, J. D., . . . Dent, D. L. (2014). An experimental model of hemothorax auto transfusion: Impact on coagulation. *American Journal of Surgery, 208*, 1078–1082. https://doi.org/10.1016/j.amjsurg.2014.09.012
27. Leite, L., Goncalves, L., & Vieria, D. N. (2017). Cardiac injuries caused by trauma: Review and case reports. *Journal of Forensic and Legal Medicine, 52*, 30–34. https://doi.org/10.1016/j.jflm.2017.08.013
28. Bellister, S. A., Dennis, B. M., & Guillamondegui, O. D. (2017). Blunt and penetrating cardiac trauma. *Surgical Clinics of North America, 97*, 1065–1076. https://doi.org/10.1016/j.suc.2017.06.012
29. Spencer, S. M., Safcsak, K., Smith, C. P., Cheatham, M. L., & Bhuller, I. S. (2017). Nonoperative management rather than endovascular repair may be safe for Grade II blunt traumatic aortic injuries: An 11-year retrospective analysis. *Journal of Trauma and Acute Care Surgery, 84*, 133–138. https://doi.org/10.1097/TA.0000000000001630
30. Wolf, L., & Zimmermann, P. G. (2013). Abdominal pain and emergencies. In B. B. Hammond & P. G. Zimmerman (Eds.), *Sheehy's manual of emergency care* (7th ed., pp. 291–302). St. Louis, MO: Elsevier Mosby.
31. Ercan, M., Aziret, M., Karaman, K., Bostanci, B., & Akoglu, M. (2016). Dual mesh repair for a large diaphragmatic hernia defect: An unusual case report. *International Journal of Surgery Case Reports, 28*, 266–269. https://doi.org/10.1016%2Fj.ijscr.2016.10.015
32. Malgras, B., Prunet, B., Lesaffre, X., Boddaert, G., Travers, S., Cungi, P. J., . . . Bonnet, S. (2017). Damage control: Concept and implementation. *Journal of Visceral Surgery, 154*, 519–529. https://doi.org/10.1016/j.jviscsurg.2017.08.012
33. Dehghan, N., Mah, J. M., Schemitsch, E. H., Nauth, A., Vicente, M., & McKee, M. D. (2018, January). Operative stabilization of flail chest injuries reduces mortality to that of stable chest wall injuries. *Journal of Orthopedic Trauma, 32*, 15–21. https://doi.org/10.1097/BOT.0000000000000992

CHAPTER 8

Abdominal and Pelvic Trauma

Cynthia M. Bratcher, MSN, APRN, FNP-C, CEN

OBJECTIVES

Upon completion of this chapter, the learner will be able to:

1. Describe the mechanisms of injury associated with abdominal and pelvic trauma.
2. Describe pathophysiologic changes as a basis for the assessment of the trauma patient with abdominal and pelvic injuries.
3. Demonstrate the nursing assessment of the trauma patient with abdominal and pelvic injuries.
4. Plan appropriate interventions for the trauma patient with abdominal and pelvic injuries.
5. Evaluate the effectiveness of nursing interventions for the trauma patient with abdominal and pelvic injuries.

Knowledge of normal anatomy and physiology of the abdominal and pelvic cavity is required to understand the pathophysiologic changes that may occur as the result of trauma; these changes are critical elements in the assessment and care of the trauma patient.[1] The anatomy material is not emphasized in the classroom but may be the basis of skill evaluation assessments and the basis of questions for testing purposes.

Anatomy and Physiology of the Abdominal and Pelvic Cavity

The material in this section begins with a discussion of the abdominal and pelvic cavity itself and then turns to the organs, structures, and vasculature within it.

Abdominal and Pelvic Cavity

The abdominal and pelvic cavity extends from the diaphragm to the groin, and is enclosed by the abdominal wall and the bones and muscles of the pelvis.[2] The abdominal cavity contains the stomach, spleen, liver, gallbladder, small bowel, and some of the large bowel.[2] It is lined with a serous membrane, the peritoneum, that forms a protective cover for many of the abdominal structures. The peritoneum is a single layer in part of the abdomen, double layers over the stomach, and fan shaped over the small bowel to anchor it to the abdominal wall, where the peritoneum is called the mesentery.[2]

The esophagus begins at the hypopharynx and enters the stomach in the upper abdominal cavity, just below the diaphragm. The stomach lies transversely in the upper abdominal cavity, and distally connects to the small bowel. The small bowel is divided into three sections: the duodenum, jejunum, and ileum. It attaches to the pylorus and coils in the abdominal cavity, connecting to the large bowel at the ileocecal valve, which prevents the backward flow of fecal material. The large bowel starts at the ileocecal sphincter and extends to the anus; it includes the cecum, colon, rectum, and anal canal.[2]

The right upper quadrant of the abdominal cavity contains the liver, the gallbladder, the right kidney, and the hepatic flexure of the colon. The pancreas lies behind and beneath the stomach, and the spleen is in the left upper quadrant, above the left kidney and below the diaphragm.[2]

The pelvic cavity is the area surrounded by the pelvic bones, encompassing the lower part of the retroperitoneal and intraperitoneal spaces.[1] It contains portions of the large bowel, the urinary bladder, the internal reproductive organs, and iliac vessels.[1,2]

The flank and back encompass the retroperitoneal space posterior to the peritoneal lining of the abdomen. This area contains the abdominal aorta, inferior vena cava, most of the duodenum, pancreas, kidneys, ureters, and posterior colon.[1] The kidneys, pancreas, adrenal glands, duodenum of the small bowel, ascending and descending colon of the large bowel, inferior vena cava, and portions of the aorta lie in the retroperitoneal space of the abdomen and are only anteriorly covered by the peritoneum.[2]

Abdominal Solid Organs

The abdominal solid organs include the liver, spleen, kidneys, and pancreas. The kidneys and pancreas are discussed later in the section, "Retroperitoneal Organs."

Liver

The liver is the heaviest organ of the body, weighing about 3 pounds in an adult. It is attached to the abdominal wall and diaphragm by the falciform ligament; it is the only digestive organ attached to the anterior abdominal wall.[2] The liver is divided into two main lobes, right and left. The larger right lobe is divided into three sections—the right lobe, the caudate lobe, and quadrate lobe; the smaller left lobe comprises a single section.[2]

The liver has a rich blood supply from both the hepatic artery and the portal vein. The hepatic artery provides oxygenated blood at the rate of 400 to 500 mL/minute, which is approximately 25% of the total cardiac output.[3] The hepatic vein receives deoxygenated blood from the inferior and superior mesenteric veins, the splenic vein, the gastric vein, and esophageal vein; it delivers 1,000 to 1,500 mL/minute of blood to the liver.[2] The liver is highly vascular because of the repeated branching of these vessels.[3] The liver can store a large volume of blood that can be released to maintain systemic volume in the presence of hemorrhage.[3]

Metabolism of carbohydrates, fats, and proteins as well as glucose conversion and release are regulated by the liver. The liver also synthesizes fats from carbohydrates and proteins that have been broken down to amino acids.[3] Bile is excreted from organic waste in the liver; the liver converts fat-soluble waste to water-soluble material that is amenable to renal excretion, approximately 700 to 1,200 mL per day.[3] The liver also synthesizes prothrombin, fibrinogen, and clotting factors. Vitamin K absorption is dependent on the liver producing adequate amounts of bile.[3]

Spleen

The spleen, a fist-sized organ that is the largest of the lymphoid organs, is located in the left upper quadrant of the abdominal cavity. It filters and cleans the blood and serves as a blood reservoir—it can store more than 300 mL of blood.[3] A drop in blood pressure causes the sympathetic nervous system to stimulate constriction of the splenic sinuses, triggering the spleen to expel as much as 200 mL of blood into the venous circulation in an effort to restore blood volume and venous pressure; this process can elevate the hematocrit by 4%.[3] Bloodborne antigens encounter lymphocytes in the spleen, stimulating the body's immune response.

High levels of circulating leukocytes often occur after splenectomy. In addition, iron levels decrease, immune function is diminished, and the blood contains more defective blood cells when the spleen has been removed.[3]

Abdominal Hollow Organs

The abdominal hollow organs include the gallbladder, stomach, small bowel, and large bowel.

Gallbladder

The gallbladder is a pear-shaped sac located in the right upper quadrant of the abdomen, anteriorly on the surface of the inferior liver. The gallbladder stores approximately 90 mL of bile between meals. Within 30 minutes of eating, the gallbladder starts contracting, forcing bile into the duodenum, and prevents duodenal contents from entering the pancreato-biliary system.[3] The gallbladder mucosa absorbs water and electrolytes, leaving behind a high concentration of bile salts, bile pigments, and cholesterol.[3]

Stomach

The stomach is located inferior to the diaphragm in the epigastric, umbilical, and left hypochondriac regions of the abdomen.[2] This J-shaped organ connects the esophagus to the duodenum and the first part of the small bowel. It has four main regions: the cardia, fundus, body, and pylorus. The superior opening of the stomach is surrounded by the cardia, while the fundus is found to the left of the cardia. The largest central portion is called the body. The pylorus connects the stomach to the duodenum.[2] The position and size of the stomach depend on diaphragmatic movement, with the diaphragm moving it inferiorly with inhalation and exhalation pulling it up superiorly.[2] The blood supply to the stomach comes from a branch of the celiac artery; this organ is highly vascular.[3]

Small Bowel

The small bowel is divided into three regions.[2] The shortest region, the duodenum, starts at the pyloric sphincter and extends until it joins the jejunum; it is approximately 25 cm long. The jejunum is approximately 1 m long and extends to the ileum.[2] The ileum is the largest portion, measuring about 2 m long, and joins the large bowel at the ileocecal sphincter. The wall of the small bowel is composed of four layers: mucosa, submucosa, muscularis, and serosa.[2] The superior mesenteric artery supplies blood to the small bowel and proximal colon, with this supply being as much as 800 mL of blood per minute.[3]

Large Bowel

The large bowel begins at the ileocecal sphincter and extends to the anus.[2] The four regions of the large bowel are the cecum, colon, rectum, and anal canal. The cecum is a small, 6-cm pouch the merges with the tube-shaped colon.[2] The colon is divided into the ascending, transverse, descending, and sigmoid sections.[2] The ascending and descending colon lie in the retroperitoneal portion of the abdominopelvic cavity.[2] The ascending colon is found on the right side of the abdomen; it meets the inferior surface of the liver and then turns at the right colic (hepatic) flexure. The colon crosses the abdomen to the left side as the transverse colon, and passes inferior to the iliac crest as the descending colon.[2] The sigmoid colon begins near the left iliac crest and ends at the rectum near the third sacral vertebra.[2] The last 20 cm of the colon constitutes the rectum; it lies anterior to the sacrum and coccyx, with the end of the rectum forming the anal canal.[2] The inferior mesenteric artery supplies the distal colon and rectum with approximately 480 mL of blood per minute.[3]

Pelvic Structures

The pelvic girdle consists of a ring formed by the sacrum, the coccyx, and two innominate bones.[4] Each innominate bone is formed by the fusion of the ilium, ischium, and pubis.[4] The bones are connected posteriorly to the sacrum at the sacroiliac joints and are joined anteriorly at the symphysis pubis.[4] The bony pelvis functions as a stable support for the vertebral column and pelvic organs, serving as a link between the axial skeleton and the lower extremities.[2] The pelvic girdle connects the bones of the lower limbs to the axial skeleton.[2]

Pelvic Organs

The pelvic organs include the bladder, ureters, urethra, and the reproductive organs.

Bladder, Ureters, and Urethra

The ureters are two narrow tubes that lie between the renal pelvis and the urinary bladder in the retroperitoneal cavity and connect to the base of the urinary bladder on the posterior aspect.[2] In males, the urinary bladder is found in the pelvic cavity posterior to the pubic symphysis and anterior to the rectum; in females, it is anterior to the vagina and inferior to the uterus.[2] This distensible organ collapses when it is empty and becomes pear-shaped and rises into the abdominal cavity as urine volume increases.[2] The average urinary bladder capacity is 700 to 800 mL.[2]

The urethra is the terminal portion of the urinary system leading from the floor of the urinary bladder as the outlet of urine from the body.[2] The male urethra passes through the prostate, then through the deep muscles of the perineum, and to the exterior orifice through the penis.[2]

Reproductive Organs

The internal female reproductive organs include the ovaries, fallopian tubes, uterus, and vagina; the external reproductive organs consist of the vulva and the perineum.[2] The floor of the pelvis is formed by the perineal fascia, levator ani, and the coccygeus muscles.[2,5]

The male reproductive organs include the testes, epididymis, ductus deferens, ejaculatory ducts, urethra, seminal vesicles, prostate, scrotum, and penis.[2] The testes are located in the scrotum, and the penis contains the urethra. The penis is attached to the inferior surface of the perineum at the ischial and inferior pubic rami, where this organ is surrounded by muscle. The weight is supported by the fundiform ligament on the inferior part and the suspensory ligament from the pubic symphysis; these ligaments are continuous with the fascia of the penis.[2]

Abdomen and Pelvic Vasculature

Abdominal and pelvic vascular trauma commonly results in hemorrhage in major abdominal vessels, the viscera, and the mesentery, and from the pelvic vasculature.[6] Blood loss within the pelvis can result from fractures or from lacerations or tearing of the vascular structures by bone fragments from fractures.[6,7] Hemorrhage from associated pelvic fractures results in 39% of all trauma

TABLE 8-1 Major Vessels Resulting in Hemorrhage in Abdomen and Pelvic Trauma

Zone 1: Midline Retroperitoneum
Proximal superior mesenteric artery
Proximal renal artery
Superior mesenteric vein
Infrarenal abdominal aorta
Infrahepatic inferior vena cava
Zone 2: Upper Lateral Retroperitoneum
Renal artery
Renal vein
Zone 3: Pelvic Retroperitoneum
Iliac artery
Iliac vein
Zone 4: Portal Hepatic/Retrohepatic Inferior Vena Cava
Portal vein
Hepatic artery
Retrohepatic vena cava

Data from Asensio, J. A., & Feliciano, D. V. (2017). Abdominal vascular injury. In E. E. Moore, D. V. Feliciano, & K. L. Mattox (Eds.), *Trauma* (8th ed., pp. 651–676). Chicago, IL: McGraw-Hill.

deaths.[7] Unstable pelvic fractures have the greatest potential for blood loss and the greatest mortality risk due to increased volume in the pelvis. Pelvic fractures alone may result in significant blood loss that leads to shock and can potentiate shock from other injuries.[1]

Hemorrhage may occur from injury to major vessels such as the external iliac arteries or the hypogastric vascular distribution—a network of small arterial branches that supply blood to the pelvic structures. The midline retroperitoneum, the upper lateral retroperitoneum, the pelvic retroperitoneum, and the portal hepatic/retrohepatic inferior vena cava areas are the four major areas in which bleeding occurs. **Table 8-1** identifies the vessels located in these four zones.[6]

Retroperitoneal Organs

The main retroperitoneal organs are the kidneys and pancreas.

Kidneys

The kidneys are located in the retroperitoneal area between the last thoracic and third lumbar vertebra, where they are partially protected by the eleventh and twelfth ribs. The right kidney is slightly lower than the left kidney because the liver occupies space superior to the right kidney. The average kidney is 10 to 12 cm wide and 5 to 7 cm long.[2] The border of each kidney faces the vertebral column near the renal hilum, where the ureter emerges with blood vessels, lymphatic vessels, and nerves.

The kidneys regulate the concentrations of sodium, potassium, calcium, chloride, and phosphate in the blood. In addition, they regulate blood pH and blood volume by adjusting the conservation or elimination of water in urine.[2] Blood pressure is adjusted through the kidneys' secretion of renin. These organs also produce hormones that stimulate the production of red blood cells. The kidneys can use amino acids to help maintain glucose levels, and they function to excrete waste from the human body.[2]

The kidneys receive 1,000 to 1,200 mL of blood per minute, which accounts for as much as 25% of the cardiac output.[3] Approximately 600 to 700 mL of plasma flows through the kidney each minute (known as the renal plasma flow) in the presence of a normal hematocrit.[3] The plasma moves over the glomerulus capillaries and into the Bowman space, where its filtration results in secretion of wastes and reabsorption of essential electrolytes and organic molecules.[3] The plasma filtration occurs at a rate of approximately 120 mL/minute, called the glomerular filtrate rate (GFR).[3] The GFR affects renal blood flow, and if mean arterial pressure decreases or vascular resistance increases, renal blood flow will decrease.[3] Severe hypoxia and hemorrhage result in sympathetic stimulation and vasoconstriction, such that both GFR and renal blood flow are reduced, which results in decreased organ perfusion.[3]

Pancreas

The pancreas is approximately 12 to 15 cm long and 2.5 cm thick and lies posterior to the stomach. It functions as both an endocrine gland and an exocrine gland.[3] The pancreas consists of a head, a body, and a tail; two ducts connect it to the duodenum.[3] This gland receives its arterial blood supply from branches of the celiac and superior mesenteric arteries. Venous blood leaves the head of the pancreas via the portal vein, and the body and tail are drained by the splenic vein.[3]

The pancreas exocrine cells excrete digestive enzymes called pancreatic juices that enter the small bowel via two ducts. The 1,200 to 1,500 mL of pancreatic juice produced by the pancreas each day contains water, salt, sodium bicarbonate, and ezymes.[3] The enzymes buffer acidic gastric fluids, stop the action of pepsin in the stomach, and create the proper pH of digestive enzymes in the small intestine.[3]

The pancreas endocrine cells, called pancreatic islets, secrete glucagon, insulin, somatostatin, and pancreatic polypetide.[3] Glucagon is released and insulin release is inhibited when blood glucose is too low; conversely, insulin release is stimulated when the glucose level is too high.[3]

Introduction

Abdominal and pelvic trauma can lead to significant blood loss resulting in hypovolemic shock, but often is not clinically apparent on patient arrival.[4] Physical exam findings and knowledge of injury patterns can alert the trauma nurse to patients who are at high risk of hemorrhage and will need aggressive treatment to achieve homeostasis and prevent shock. The absence of abdominal pain or tenderness does not exclude injury because injured intestinal structures may produce minimal hemorrhage.[1] In fact, unexplained hypotension may be the only clinical indicator of pelvic fracture and hemorrhage; its development requires the rapid identification of the cause and prompt intervention.[1] The presence of distracting injuries or intoxication increases the difficulty of the assessment.[1]

Although internal hemorrhage most frequently occurs in the first hour after abdominal and pelvic trauma, it can take several hours before the patient exhibits clinically significant findings.[8] Movement of the patient, particularly log rolling, can cause life-threatening hemorrhage. It is now recommended to avoid log rolling in patients with suspected pelvic fractures prior to imaging to rule out these injuries.[9,10] Log rolling may be indicated if there is suspicion of a penetrating injury causing hemodynamic instability or airway-threatening vomiting that cannot be cleared with suction.[9-11] Preferred methods to move the patient include air-assisted-mattresses, the 6-plus lift-and-slide, and other alternative devices and techniques.[10,11] The trauma nurse must be thorough in the initial assessment, remain vigilant during reassessments, and continuously monitor the vital signs in a patient who has sustained abdominopelvic trauma.

Epidemiology

Abdominal and pelvic trauma is associated with significant morbidity and mortality. An estimated 85% of all abdomen and pelvic injuries are caused by blunt trauma, which most often results in injury to the liver and spleen.[12] Blunt abdomen and pelvic trauma is the seventh leading cause of death in the world and the third most common injury sustained in trauma patients.[12] Injuries to the trunk often cause pelvic fractures, which result in 39% of all trauma deaths and may be associated with injuries to the genitourinary systems.[7] Penetrating abdominopelvic trauma occurs less frequently than blunt trauma but has a higher mortality rate, with gunshot wounds (GSWs) having an eight times higher mortality rate than stab wounds.[13,14]

Mortality from abdominal and pelvic trauma is typically the result of uncontrolled hemorrhage in the early phase of care.[15] Late mortality secondary to abdominal and pelvic trauma occurs when patients experience multisystem failure secondary to sepsis.[16]

Mechanisms of Injury

The mechanism of injury (MOI) for abdominal and pelvic trauma is classified as blunt or penetrating. The injuries sustained during such trauma will be determined by the energy and type of force and the density and strength of the structure receiving the energy. **Table 8-2** summarizes common MOIs and potential resulting injuries.[1,17]

TABLE 8-2 Abdominal and Pelvic Mechanism of Injury History with Implications for Injury

Type of Mechanism	History Questions	Implication for Injury
Motor vehicle collision	What was the type of crash? › Lateral impact (T-bone) › Rear end › Frontal	Provide further clues regarding suspected concurrent injuries.
	› Was the patient restrained? › What type of restraint? • Lap belt • Lap belt and shoulder harness • Air bag deployment › Was it properly positioned?	The locations of restraints can provide further clues regarding suspected injuries. Improper placement may cause compression and rupture of hollow organs and vasculature, as well as laceration of solid organs. This is difficult to determine.

(continues)

TABLE 8-2 Abdominal and Pelvic Mechanism of Injury History with Implications for Injury (*continued*)

Type of Mechanism	History Questions	Implication for Injury
	Was the patient ejected?	Ejection from a compartment may cause penetrating injury in addition to blunt injury. Rapid deceleration can cause vessels to stretch and shear, causing tears, dissection, rupture, or aneurysm formation. Acceleration injuries can result in a hyperextension of the neck, producing "whiplash"-type injuries
	What was the speed of the vehicle?	Speed will influence the severity of injuries.
	› What was the extent of vehicular damage? › How long did extrication take?	The extent of damage and length of the extrication process give an indication of the amount of energy transferred into the passenger compartment and ultimately the patient's body.
	What was the patient's location within the vehicle?	Location, together with extent and type of crash, gives clues for body position and areas possibly injured.
Falls	How far did the patient fall?	Falls from heights from more than 20 feet are associated with increased injury severity (for pediatric patients, height and length of fall are important).
	On what type of surface did the patient land?	Type of surface gives an indication of the severity of energy impact.
	Which body part was the point of impact?	The body part impacted will be the focal point of assessment. If the patient landed on the feet, energy will be transferred from the feet through the body to the head.
Assault/struck by an object	Where on the body was the patient struck?	The location of the point of impact will be the focus of the assessment.
	Has the patient undergone bariatric or other abdominal/pelvic surgery?	Previous surgery to the abdomen may have weakened the musculature and the protection they provide.

Type of Mechanism	History Questions	Implication for Injury
Penetrating trauma	What type of weapon or object was used? › In GSWs, what was the distance from the assailant? What was the caliber and velocity of the weapon? Was special ammunition used, such as exploding bullets, armor-piercing bullets, or buckshot? › What was the estimated blood loss at the scene?	Stab wounds traverse adjacent structures. GSWs may cause additional injuries based on their trajectory, cavitation effect, and bullet fragmentation.

Abbreviation: GSW, gunshot wound.

Data from American College of Surgeons. (2018). Abdominal and pelvic trauma. In *Advanced trauma life support: Student course manual* (10th ed., pp. 83–101). Chicago, IL: Author; Harris, C. (2013). Abdominal trauma. In B. B. Hammond & P. G. Zimmerman (Eds.), *Sheehy's manual of emergency care* (7th ed., 419–426). St. Louis, MO: Elsevier Mosby.

Blunt Trauma

Blunt injuries caused by a direct blow result in compression or crush injuries to the abdominal and pelvic viscera and pelvic bones.[1] Blunt trauma is most often caused by motor vehicle collisions (MVCs), assaults, and falls; less commonly, it occurs in conjunction with blast injuries.[1,13] Blunt trauma can cause injuries to both solid and hollow organs, resulting in hemorrhage or peritonitis.[1] The spleen, liver, and bowel are the organs most commonly injured, but injuries may also occur in the retroperitoneal cavity to the duodenum, kidneys, pancreas, ureters, bladder, and internal reproductive organs in females.[18] The liver, spleen, and kidneys may sustain injury when the anterior abdominal wall is compressed against the thoracic cage or vertebral column, with these organs being lacerated or rupturing.[18] In addition, the following considerations apply in case of blunt trauma:

- Hollow organs are also susceptible to blunt trauma injuries, and restrained occupants of motor vehicles are at higher risk for hollow viscus injuries.[19] The stomach, small bowel, large bowel, uterus, and bladder can rupture when a sudden increase in intra-abdominal pressure occurs.[18] Hollow viscus injuries are more difficult to identify due to their slow leakage of contents, with diagnosis often being delayed until the patient develops fever, unexplained leukocytosis, and increasing abdominal pain.[8,19]
- Deceleration or shearing injuries occur when movable organs sustain trauma between nonfixed anatomy and fixed anatomy. Organs with fixed sites susceptible to sudden deceleration include the small bowel, the large bowel, abdominal vasculature, and pelvic vasculature.[1,7]
- Fractures of the pelvis occur secondary to MVCs, pedestrian injuries, and falls.

Penetrating Trauma

Penetrating trauma occurs as the result of GSWs, stab wounds, or impaled objects.[13] GSWs penetrate the peritoneum 80% of the time, causing vascular or visceral injuries.[14] High-energy GSWs transfer more kinetic energy, and increased damage surrounding the missile track is caused by temporary cavitation; by comparison, low-energy GSWs and stab wounds cause tissue damage by lacerating and tearing structures.[1] Penetrating trauma caused by GSWs most often results in injury to the small bowel, colon, liver, and abdominal vascular structures.[1] The occurrence of visceral injury with GSWs necessitates emergent laparotomy.[14]

Stab wounds most commonly result in injury to the liver, small bowel, diaphragm, and colon.[1] Stab wounds penetrate the peritoneum 66% of the time.[14] Abdominal stab wounds require surgical intervention in the presence of hemodynamic instability, impalement, evisceration, or the development of peritonitis. Penetrating injuries can be more difficult to identify when hidden in the skin folds of obese patients.[1] Patients who are hemodynamically stable can be treated conservatively.[20]

Usual Concurrent Injuries

Trauma to one area of the abdomen or pelvis can result in injuries to more than one body system. The mechanism of injury will raise suspicion for specific injuries. The trauma nurse is alert to concurrent injuries that may include the following:

- Thoracic injuries may include hemothorax, pneumothorax, or lung contusions.[21]
- Lower rib fractures are associated with liver and spleen injuries.[22]
- Lower posterior rib fractures are associated with a higher incidence of renal injuries.[23]
- Complex pelvic fractures are associated with a higher incidence of spleen, liver, bladder, rectal, and urethral injuries.[7,24]
- Lumbar spine fractures are associated with a higher incidence of retroperitoneal hemorrhage.[25]

Pathophysiology as a Basis for Assessment Findings

The two main pathophysiological bases for assessment findings are hemorrhage and pain.

Hemorrhage

Trauma to the abdominal and pelvic cavity can lead to significant hemorrhage from the organs and the bony pelvis.[1] Significant blood loss can be present without changes in the appearance of the abdominal or pelvic cavity.[1] Rapid identification of abdominal and pelvic injury can reduce the risk of death due to hemorrhage.[1] Control of hemorrhage is a priority, with interventions including early administration of blood products and judicious use of isotonic crystalloids.[1] The patient who has profound hemodynamic instability and who has sustained trauma to the torso without other identifiable injuries is assumed to have visceral, vascular, or pelvic injury.[1] See Chapter 5, "Shock," for details on hemorrhage management.

Pain

The trauma nurse's assessment of the abdomen and pelvis includes the subjective complaint of pain. Pain, rigidity, and involuntary guarding can be signs of abdominal and pelvic injury.[1] Palpation of the abdomen can elicit signs of peritoneal irritation. Rebound tenderness is demonstrated when the sudden release of the palpation elicits movement of the peritoneum and internal organs and results in pain.[4,26] Involuntary muscle guarding is a sign of peritoneal irritation; voluntary guarding can result in an unreliable examination.[1] Peritoneal irritation can be caused by the following conditions:

- Hemorrhage
- Leakage of gastric contents
- Leakage of bowel contents

Referred pain can result from abdominal and pelvic trauma, as pain travels along nerve pathways and is referred to a different body part.[27] Examples include the following:

- Left shoulder pain may occur with splenic injury (Kehr's sign).
- Palpation in one quadrant may elicit pain in another quadrant.
- Peritonitis can cause pain to be referred to the genitalia.[27]

Nursing Care of the Patient with Abdominal and Pelvic Trauma

Nursing care of the patient with abdominal and pelvic trauma begins with the primary survey.

Primary Survey

The primary survey may reveal signs of uncontrolled abdominal and pelvic hemorrhage that requires immediate treatment, including application of a pelvic binder, pelvic imaging, or focused assessment with sonography for trauma (FAST) examination.

Chapter 3, "Initial Assessment," describes the systematic approach to the nursing assessment of the trauma patient. The following information is specific to injuries affecting the abdominal and pelvic regions.

Laboratory Monitoring

Laboratory values to monitor include the following:

- Serial laboratory tests are required to evaluate the stability of the patient, and a decrease in hemoglobin (Hgb) and hematocrit (Hct) will be noted in the presence of continued bleeding. Alteration in electrolytes and coagulopathy may occur with the administration of crystalloids and blood products.[28]
- Potassium level may increase with blood transfusions due to the high concentration of potassium in banked blood.
- Calcium levels may drop as calcium citrate in banked blood binds with free calcium in the patient's body.
- Blood urea nitrogen (BUN) and creatinine will rise in patients with poor renal perfusion.[1]

Secondary Survey

The secondary survey begins with a head-to-toe assessment.

CLINICAL PEARL 

Signs and Symptoms

Be aware of these signs during secondary survey:

- *Kehr's sign:* Pain in the shoulder indicating intraperitoneal bleeding. Left shoulder pain is a classic sign of splenic injury.
- *Cullen's sign:* Periumbilical ecchymosis indicating intraperitoneal bleeding.
- *Grey Turner's sign:* Bruising to the flank indicating retroperitoneal bleeding.

H: Head-to-Toe Assessment

Inspect for the following:

- Note any asymmetry, abdominal contour, and abdominal distention.
- Abrasions and contusions from restraint devices can provide clinical indication of injuries. Visible seat belt ecchymosis across the lower abdomen is associated with intestinal perforation in 30% of patients.[29]
- Periumbilical ecchymosis (Cullen's sign) and flank ecchymosis (Grey Turner's sign) may occur several hours after injury.[30]
- Perineal bleeding, rectal bleeding, or the presence of blood at the urinary meatus may indicate urethral injury in males and unstable fractures in females.[7,31]

Auscultate for the presence, hypoactivity, or absence of bowel sounds:

- Bowel sounds may be absent when ileus occurs secondary to trauma.[1]
- Bowel sounds may be decreased or absent when blood or fluid is present in the peritoneum.

Percuss for dullness over solid organs and over hollow organs. Abnormal findings include the following:

- Dullness in the hollow organs, which may indicate fluid or a solid mass
- Hyperresonance, which indicates air over solid organs

Palpate for the following:

- Femoral pulses
- All four quadrants of the abdominal area for tenderness, rebound tenderness, rigidity, voluntary and involuntary guarding
- Pelvic stability (defer for obvious or reported pelvic fractures)
  - Gently apply pressure to both iliac crests downward and medially, assessing for instability.
  - Apply pressure only once to decrease the risk of disrupting early clot formation, which could cause further hemorrhage.[1,32]
- Lightly applying pressure on the iliac crest, which can cause inferior displacement of the leg that indicates vertical instability[1]
- Flanks for tenderness (without turning patient if pelvic fracture is suspected)

General Interventions for All Patients with Abdominal and Pelvic Trauma

Hemodynamic monitoring for patients with suspected abdominal and pelvic trauma begins in the secondary assessment.

- Give 1 L of crystalloids as indicated. If the patient does not show improvement, anticipate rapidly proceeding to blood administration.[1] See Chapter 5 for more information.
- Insertion of a urinary catheter is contraindicated if there is blood at the urethral meatus. Stop catheter insertion if any difficulty is encountered when advancing the catheter, which could indicate a urethral injury.
- The abdominal exam that identifies rebound tenderness with palpation does not proceed with additional assessment if the patient has signs of peritoneal irritation, as it may induce avoidable pain.[1]

Selected Abdominal Injuries

Selected abdominal injuries are described in the following sections. **Table 8-3** summarizes the assessment, diagnosis, and management of abdominal injuries.

Liver Injuries

The liver is the organ most commonly injured as the result of trauma. The posterior superior section of the right lobe is the largest section and most often the site of injury because of its proximity to the ribs and the spine. Suspect liver injury with right-side rib fractures. The liver can have a laceration or hematoma, and even low-grade hepatic trauma can cause hemodynamic instability. The hematoma or laceration is defined by a grading system with grade I as minor and grade VI as most severe (**Table 8-4**).[31,33]

TABLE 8-3 Selected Abdominal Injuries: Assessment, Diagnostics, and Definitive Care

	Liver	Spleen	Pancreas	Small Bowel	Large Bowel and Rectum	Stomach and Esophagus
Assessment						
Inspection	› Nipple line to mid-abdomen, right side › Lacerations › Abrasions › Contusions › Open wounds	› LUQ › Lacerations › Abrasions › Contusions › Open wounds	› Epigastric area radiating to the back, extending to the LUQ › Pain initially minimal, becoming increasingly worse	› Left side of the abdomen › Lacerations › Abrasions › Contusions › Open wounds	› Pelvic and abdominal areas › Lacerations › Abrasions › Contusions › Open wounds	› Neck, chest, and epigastric area › Lacerations › Abrasions › Contusions › Open wounds
Auscultation	Hypoactive or absent	Hypoactive or absent	Hypoactive or absent	Hypoactive or absent	Hypoactive or absent	Hypoactive or absent
Palpation	› RUQ tenderness › Muscle rigidity › Spasm › Involuntary guarding	› LUQ tenderness › Left shoulder pain › Muscle rigidity › Spasm › Involuntary guarding	› Abdominal or LUQ tenderness with deep palpation	› Peritoneal irritation including rebound tenderness and guarding	› Abdominal tenderness or rebound tenderness	› Esophageal: neck, chest, shoulders, or abdomen › Gastric: Pain in epigastric area
Percussion	Dullness	Dullness	Dullness	Dullness	Dullness	Dullness
Reevaluation Adjuncts (Diagnostics)						
Radiographs and Other Diagnostic Tests	› Abdominal radiographs › CT	› Repeat CT imaging to assess for ongoing bleeding	› CT: 80% sensitive; missed diagnosis may occur	› CT › DPL/DPA › FAST (least sensitive)	› CT with oral, IV, and rectal contrast › DPL › Sigmoidoscopy	› Abdominal radiographs › CT › DPL › FAST (least sensitive)
Laboratory Studies	› LFTs › Serial H&H › Coagulation › Profiles	› Serial H&H	› Amylase elevated, but not definitive to diagnose	—	—	—
Definitive Care	› Nonoperative management › Operative management › Angioembolization	› Nonoperative management › Operative management › Angioembolization	› Nonoperative management › Operative management	› Operative management	› Operative management	› Operative management

Abbreviations: CT, computed tomography; DPL/DPA, diagnostic peritoneal lavage/diagnostic peritoneal aspirate; FAST, focused assessment sonography in trauma; H&H, hemoglobin and hematocrit; LFT, liver function tests; LUQ, left upper quadrant; RUQ, right upper quadrant.

TABLE 8-4 Liver Injury Grading

Grade	Injury Description
I	Hematomas: Subcapsular and nonexpanding; affects less than 10% of surface area Lacerations: Less than 1 cm parenchymal depth and nonbleeding
II	Hematomas: 10% to 50% of subcapsular surface; less than 1 cm intraparenchymal hematoma Lacerations: Capsular tear with active bleeding; 1 to 3 cm in length
III	Hematomas: More than 50% surface area or actively bleeding; ruptured subcapsular or parenchymal hematoma; intraparenchymal hematoma more than 10 cm or expanding Lacerations: Less than 3 cm deep into parenchyma
IV	Ruptured parenchymal hematomas with active bleeding or parenchymal disruption involving Affects 25% to 75% of a hepatic lobe
V	Parenchymal disruption involving more than 75% of hepatic lobe Vascular injury involving retrohepatic cava or juxtahepatic venous injury
VI	Hepatic avulsion with avulsion from vascular structures

Data from Bruns, R. B., & Kozar, R. A. (2017). Liver and biliary tract. In E. E. Moore, D. V. Feliciano, & K. L. Mattox (Eds.), *Trauma* (8th ed., pp. 551–574). Chicago, IL: McGraw-Hill.

Assessment Findings

Assessment findings include the following:

- Tenderness, guarding, or rigidity in the right upper quadrant[31]
- Elevated liver function tests without history of liver disease
- Ecchymosis in the right upper quadrant or around the umbilicus (Cullen's sign)

Definitive Care

Definitive care includes the following:

- Nonoperative management is for patients who are hemodynamically stable and have isolated liver injuries, no other intra-abdominal surgical requirements, and no peritoneal signs, and for whom CT scan and intensive care unit beds are available.[31]
- Operative management is considered in hemodynamically unstable patients or those who require other intra-abdominal surgical intervention.
- Angiography—to assess for injury and hemorrhage and embolization, and to control hemorrhage—is used for high-grade liver injuries in patients who are hemodynamically stable.[34]

Spleen Injuries

The spleen is highly vascular, with minimal elasticity and flexibility, and can lacerate under sudden abdominal pressure caused by blunt trauma. Its vascularity makes this organ susceptible to hemorrhage. Splenic injuries occur in patients who have trauma to the left side of the body. Splenic injuries are classified in severity from grade 1 through grade V (**Table 8-5**).[35]

Assessment Findings

Assessment findings include the following[6]:

- Abdominal distention, asymmetry, abnormal contour, or abdominal rigidity
- Abrasions, contusions, ecchymosis, lacerations, or open wounds in the left upper quadrant
- Tenderness or guarding with palpation of the left upper quadrant
- Left shoulder pain when lying supine
- Ecchymosis of the left flank (Grey Turner's sign)
- Contrast extravasation on CT scan

Definitive Care

The goal of spleen injury care is nonoperative management (NOM) to preserve the immunologic function of

TABLE 8-5 Splenic Injury Grading

Grade	Injury	Description
I	Hematoma	Subcapsular, less than 10% surface area
	Laceration	Capsular tear, less than 1 cm parenchymal depth
II	Hematoma	Subcapsular, 10% to 50% surface area Intraparenchymal, less than 5 cm diameter
	Laceration	1–3 cm parenchymal depth not involving a parenchymal vessel
III	Hematoma	Subcapsular, more than 50% surface area or expanding Ruptured subcapsular or parenchymal hematoma Intraparenchymal hematoma of 5 cm or greater
	Laceration	More than 3 cm parenchymal depth or involving trabecular vessels
IV	Laceration	Laceration of segmental or hilar vessels producing major devascularization (more than 25% of spleen)
V	Laceration	Completely shatters spleen
	Vascular	Hilar vascular injury which devascularized spleen

Reproduced from Coccolini, F., Montori, G., Catena, F., Kluger, Y., Biffl, W., Moore, E. E., . . . Ansaloni, L. (2017). Splenic trauma: WSES classification and guidelines for adult and pediatric patients. *World Journal of Emergency Surgery, 12*, 40–66. https://doi.org/10.1186/s13017-017-0151-4.

the spleen. Angiography and embolization may be performed when the patient is hemodynamically stable and has moderate to severe lacerations.[35]

NOM is recommended in patients with the following characteristics:

- Hemodynamically stable
- Age less than 55 years[35]
- Absence of peritoneal signs

Nonoperative management includes the following care:

- Serial abdominal exams
- Serial hemoglobin and hematocrit measurements
- Serial FAST exams
- Admission by a surgeon at a trauma center

Operative management is highly likely when the patient has the following characteristics:

- Age greater than 55 years[35]
- Hemodynamic instability
- Massive transfusion requirements
- Presence of other intra-abdominal injuries requiring laparotomy
- Severe traumatic brain injury limiting the patient's ability to participate in ongoing abdominal exams

Postoperative Considerations

Patients who have undergone splenectomy have permanent immunologic impairment and are at risk for infection in the first 2 years post splenectomy. These patients will need education on the importance of meningococcal, pneumococcal, and influenza vaccines, as recommended by the Centers for Disease Control and Prevention (CDC); the first doses are given within 14 days of splenectomy. The patient is cautioned to seek medical care for minor animal bites, unexplained fever, and prior to traveling to regions with endemic malaria.[35]

Pancreatic Injuries

Pancreatic injuries are less common than other organ injuries, but occur in as many as 12% of cases of abdominal trauma and are frequently accompanied by injury to other upper abdominal viscera.[36] Pancreatic injuries can occur with blunt trauma when the pancreas sustains sudden pressure against the bony spinal column; however, pancreatic trauma occurs more frequently in penetrating trauma.[2,36] Pancreatic injuries are associated with major morbidity and mortality caused by hemorrhage, pancreatic leaks, abscesses, fistula, and pancreatitis.[36]

Assessment Findings

Assessment findings include the following:

- Serial abdominal examinations with serial amylase and lipase are necessary to confirm the suspicion of pancreatic injury. Amylase and lipase may be elevated and help diagnose a pancreatic injury.[37]

- Abdominal tenderness and pain become increasingly worse.
- Epigastric pain radiating to the back.
- The patient has increased rigidity and involuntary guarding.

Definitive Care

Nonoperative management of pancreatic trauma is appropriate for patients who are hemodynamically stable. Damage control laparotomy is indicated for patients with hemodynamic instability.[38]

Small and Large Bowel Injuries

Small bowel injuries occur when blunt trauma compresses the abdominal wall and spine, which can cause perforation, hematoma, or edema that increases the risk of intestinal obstruction. Small bowel injuries occur frequently in the presence of solid-organ and spinal injuries.[39] The difficult diagnosis of small bowel and mesenteric injuries often delays treatment, results in nontherapeutic laparotomies, and results in increased morbidity and mortality.[39]

Traumatic large bowel and mesenteric injuries can be fatal if not identified.[40] Injuries to the large bowel can occur as the result of blunt or penetrating trauma. Blunt trauma can cause a perforation due to increased pressure. Penetrating trauma can result in hemorrhage and intraperitoneal injury.[1]

Assessment Findings

Assessment findings include the following:

- Involuntary guarding and rebound tenderness
- Increasing abdominal pain[19]
- Open abdominal wounds with or without evisceration
- CT scan that shows the presence of free fluid, air, mesenteric hematoma, or intravenous (IV) contrast extravasation in the abdominal cavity[41]
- Hemodynamic instability, persistently elevated white blood cell count, increased amylase, and rising lactic acid[19]

Definitive Care

Nonoperative management includes the following care:

- Serial abdominal examinations
- Serial FAST exams
- Repeat CT scans

Operative management is required when the peritoneum is penetrated, the patient is hemodynamically unstable, or peritonitis develops.[42] Initial surgical management may result in exploratory laparotomy to control hemorrhage and visceral contamination, with delayed fascial closure performed in some instances.[42]

Rectal Injuries

Rectal injuries are uncommon in blunt trauma but do occur with open pelvic fractures. They are more frequently associated with penetrating injury to the pelvis and rectum. Proximal injuries to the rectum are treated as colon or intraperitoneal injuries.[7] The presence of perineal lacerations increases the risk of rectal injuries.[43]

Assessment Findings

Assessment findings include the following:

- External lacerations or hematomas
- Scrotal hematoma
- Foreign objects

Definitive Care

A flexible sigmoidoscope or proctoscope is used to visualize the rectal mucosa so as to determine the presence of injury. Partial-thickness lacerations can extend to full-thickness wounds.[7] Extraperitoneal rectal injuries are managed with repair or diversion via proximal colostomy, with this diversion often being reversed within 2 to 3 months.[7]

Stomach and Esophageal Injuries

Injuries to the stomach and esophagus occur frequently in the presence of other intra-abdominal injuries or with thoracic injury from blunt or penetrating trauma. Injuries to the aorta and thoracic spine raise suspicion for stomach and esophageal injuries, even though these injuries rarely pose an immediate threat to life.[44] Stomach injuries may include hematomas, superficial tears, or full-thickness perforations; such injuries are less common but carry a high mortality rate.[45]

Assessment Findings

Assessment findings include the following:

- Epigastric tenderness or rigidity
- Involuntarily guarding
- Hematemesis or occult blood from a nasogastric (NG) tube[1]

Definitive Care

Operative management is the primary choice for patients with stomach and esophageal injuries. Nonoperative management is also attempted with patients who have minor perforations of the esophagus and who are hemodynamically stable.[46]

Selected Pelvic Cavity Injuries

This section presents selected pelvic cavity injuries.

Reproductive Organs

Injuries to the pelvis and perineum from blunt or penetrating trauma can result in injuries to the reproductive organs. Such injuries are more common in males than in females. Straddle injuries are a common mechanism of injury to the external genitalia.

Male and Female Genitalia

Males sustain genitalia injury most frequently from blunt trauma. The most common injuries are testicular rupture or penile fracture, which often involves injury to the urethra.[24] Injury to the male genitalia may warrant ultrasound to determine the presence of injuries.

Females may sustain injury to reproductive organs from pelvic fractures, straddle injuries, or sexual assaults. Such injuries can result in vaginal and perineal lacerations that extend to the rectum.[7,23] Penetrating trauma may involve the uterus, ovaries, or fallopian tubes. Blood at the vaginal introitus is the most common sign of external genitalia trauma.[7] The trauma nurse assesses for the possibility of sexual assault for any patient who presents with vaginal, perineal, or rectal lacerations in the absence of other trauma.

Assessment Findings

Assessment findings include the following:

- Penile swelling, ecchymosis, and tenderness
- Scrotal and testicular swelling, ecchymosis, and tenderness
- Lacerations or penetrating injuries of the genitalia
- Labial swelling, ecchymosis, and tenderness
- Blood at the vaginal introitus[7]
- Blood at the urinary meatus[23]

Definitive Care

Operative management depends on the location, extent, and the presence of contamination of the wounds. Vaginal wounds may require operative management.[23] Penile fractures will require operative management.[23] Wound care management follows standard wound care guidelines.

Bladder and Urethral Injuries

Bladder and urethral injuries are common with pelvic fractures.[7] The bladder is generally protected by its position in the true pelvis, but rupture may cause extravasation of urine into the peritoneal cavity. Intraperitoneal bladder rupture is caused by a rapid increase in pressure that causes the structure to burst, allowing extravasation of urine into the peritoneum, which can result in a chemical peritonitis.[47] Extraperitoneal bladder rupture occurs more commonly, especially with pelvic fracture, and will result in urine extravasation remaining outside the peritoneum.[48]

The urethral position close to the pubic arc in the pelvis renders the urethra highly susceptible to injury when fractures disrupt the pelvic ring (**Table 8-6**).[22] Pelvic fractures can result in urethral injuries that can cause urinary obstruction, strictures, urinary incontinence, and erectile dysfunction in males.[49] Such injuries are suspected with penile fracture or penetrating trauma to the penis that is accompanied with gross hematuria, inability to urinate, or the presence of blood at the urethral meatus.[24]

Assessment Findings

Assessment findings include the following:

- Blood at the urethral meatus[7]
- Inability to urinate
- Suprapubic hematoma
- Palpable bladder[7]
- Abdominal distention

TABLE 8-6 Simplified Tile Classification of Pelvic Ring Injuries

Type	Stability	Examples
A	Stable	Iliac wing fractures Avulsions or fractures of the iliac spines or ischial tuberosity Nondisplaced pelvic ring fractures
B	Rotationally unstable, vertically stable	Open book fractures Lateral compression fractures Bucket-handle fractures
C	Rotationally unstable, vertically unstable	Vertical shear injuries

Data from Halawi, M. J. (2015). Pelvic ring injuries: Emergency assessment and management. *Journal of Clinical Orthopaedics & Trauma*, 6(4), 252–258. https://doi.org/10.1016/j.jcot.2015.08.002.

- Hematuria
- Rising creatinine/BUN[7]
- Pelvic instability[1,7]

Definitive Care

Extraperitoneal bladder rupture is managed nonoperatively with a urinary catheter and follow-up cystogram. Intraperitoneal bladder rupture requires emergent operative management in the hemodynamically stable patient due to the high risk of peritonitis and inadequate healing without surgical intervention.[7] Suprapubic catheters and delayed reconstruction are frequently required in the presence of hemodynamic instability and with severe urethral injuries, whereas partial urethral tears may be treated with gentle insertion of a urinary catheter during a urethrogram.[7]

Pelvic Fractures

Four patterns of injury may result in pelvic fractures. Three of these patterns are depicted in **Table 8-7**[1,50]; the fourth is a combined mechanism of injury that demonstrates multiple fracture patterns. The most common patterns involve lateral compression and vertical shear fractures.[51]

Pelvic fractures may cause hemorrhage from lacerated veins, arteries, or the fractures themselves.[7,50] Anterior–posterior compression and vertical shear fractures have higher incidence of vascular injury and hemorrhage.[50] Hemorrhage may be severe and cause hemodynamic instability, requiring multiple resources for stabilization.[50]

Assessment Findings

Assessment findings include the following:

- Palpable motion and pain on palpation of the pelvis[1]
- Hypovolemic shock—may or may not be present[1]
- Shortening or abnormal rotation of the leg on the affected side[1]
- Blood at the urinary meatus, hematuria, or intra-abdominal injury[7]
- Rectal bleeding[7]

Definitive Care

Definitive care includes the following measures:

- Early consideration for transfer to a trauma center is essential and is not delayed by obtaining imaging studies.

TABLE 8-7 Classification of Pelvic Fractures

Anterior–Posterior Compression Fracture	Lateral Compression Fracture	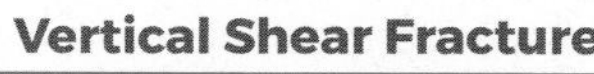 Vertical Shear Fracture
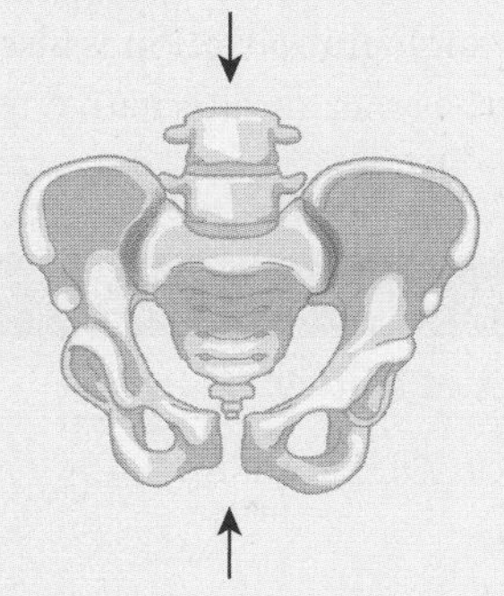	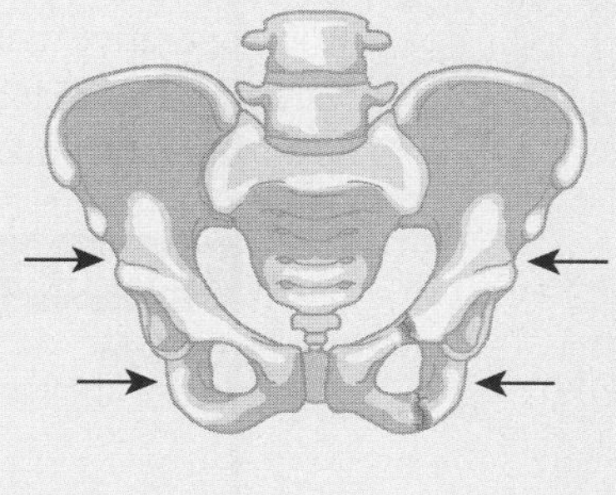	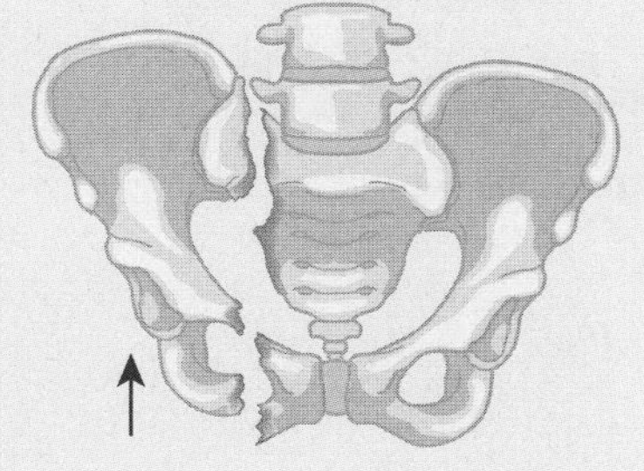
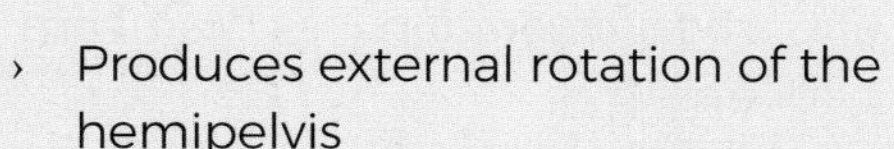 › Produces external rotation of the hemipelvis › Separation of the symphysis pubis that tears the posterior ligaments › Disrupted pelvic ring tears the posterior venous plexus and branches of the iliac arterial system › High incidence of vascular injury and hemorrhage	› Lateral force is directed into the pelvis › Hemipelvis rotates internally, reducing the pelvic volume and injuring the pelvic vascular structure, resulting in hemorrhage › Most common type of fracture	› Occurs secondary to falls when the sacroiliac joint is vertically displaced › Iliac vasculature is disrupted and may result in severe hemorrhage › High incidence of vascular injury and hemorrhage

Data from American College of Surgeons. (2018). Abdominal and pelvic trauma. In *Advanced trauma life support: Student course manual* (10th ed., pp. 83–101). Chicago, IL: Author; Velmahos, G. C. (2017). Pelvis. In E. E. Moore, D. V. Feliciano, & K. L. Mattox (Eds.), *Trauma* (8th ed., pp. 677–692). Chicago, IL: McGraw-Hill.

- Pelvic binder application will help attain stabilization and control hemorrhage by exerting external pressure (**Figure 8-1**). A folded sheet tied around the pelvis at the level of the greater trochanters (**Figure 8-2**) can be utilized if a pelvic binder is unavailable.[52] Internal rotation of the lower extremities after the binder or sheet is applied prevents movement that can potentially worsen the hemorrhage.[1]
- Longitudinal skeletal traction through the skin may be indicated for vertical shear injuries.[1]
- Hemodynamically stable patients may be managed with angioembolization.[1]

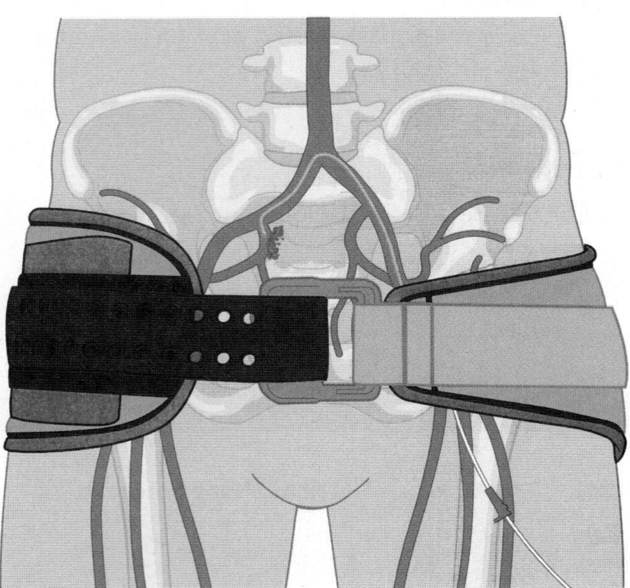

Figure 8-1 *Pelvic binder.*

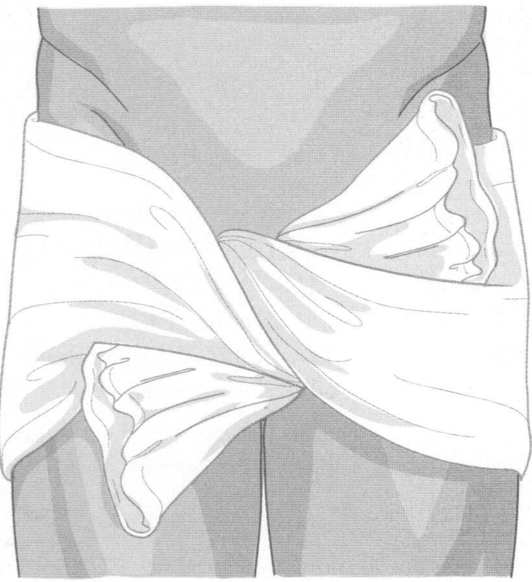

Figure 8-2 *A folded sheet as a pelvic binder.*

- Hemodynamically unstable patients are managed with one or a combination of modalities:
  - Pre-peritoneal packing
  - Pelvic external fixation

Renal Injuries

Renal injuries are classified with a grading system in which grade 1 is the least severe and grade 5 is the most severe (**Table 8-8**).[23] The kidney is the most commonly injured genitourinary organ and is highly susceptible to deceleration injuries because of its fixed position within the renal pelvis and vascular pedicle.[23] Isolated injuries to the renal artery and vein are uncommon except in the multisystem-injured patient.[23]

Assessment Findings

Assessment findings include the following:

- Hematuria—microscopic in minor injuries and gross hematuria in severe injuries[1,49]
- Flank tenderness, abdominal rigidity, costovertebral-angle tenderness, or palpable flank mass
- Ecchymosis over the flank
- Rising BUN and creatinine[53]

Definitive Care

Nonoperative management is recommended in hemodynamically stable patients unless other abdominal organs are injured. Grade V and vascular injuries may require operative management.[23] Renal angioembolization is also used to manage arterial hemorrhage as an alternative to operative management.[54]

TABLE 8-8 Renal Injury Scale

Grade	Description of injury
1	Contusion of subcapsular hematoma
2	Cortical laceration less than 1 cm deep
3	Cortical laceration more than 1 cm without urinary extravasation
4	Laceration into collecting system, segmental vascular injury
5	Shattered kidney, renal pedicle injury or avulsion

Reproduced from Bryk, D. J., & Zhao, L. C. (2016). Guideline of guidelines: A review of urological trauma guidelines. *BJU International, 117*(2), 226–234. https://doi.org/10.1111/bju.13040.

Diagnostics and Interventions for Abdominal and Pelvic Trauma

Reevaluation adjuncts for abdominopelvic trauma include laboratory studies and imaging studies.

Laboratory Studies

Lab studies that aid in diagnosis and management of abdominal and pelvic trauma include the following:

- Type and cross-match
- Complete blood count
- Coagulation studies to assess clotting function and for monitoring for the development of disseminated intravascular coagulopathy
- Baseline BUN and creatinine
- Urine pregnancy test in all females of reproductive age
- Urinalysis for the evaluation of hematuria
- Gastric contents for occult blood
- Serial Hgb and Hct

Imaging Studies

Imaging studies are often done initially and repeated as care is ongoing.

- Plain films can be done at the bedside to evaluate the patient for free air, free fluid, fractures, and foreign bodies.
- Retrograde urethrograms are done prior to insertion of a urinary catheter when a urethral injury is suspected.[7]
- A cystogram is performed to evaluate the bladder and urethra.

FAST Examination

A FAST exam is done at the bedside to identify pathological fluid in the abdominal and pelvic cavities (**Figure 8-3**). The sensitivity and accuracy of this exam depend on the location and quantity of fluid and the provider performing and interpreting the exam. At least 150 to 200 mL of fluid must be present to be identified. Free fluid in the right upper quadrant is identified 66% of the time and fluid originating from injuries to the left upper lobe of the liver is identified more than 93% of the time with a FAST exam.[55] FAST exams reduce the use of more invasive diagnostic peritoneal lavage and can be repeated if clinical changes or hemodynamic changes occur.[56]

- A negative FAST study does not rule out injury and may warrant a follow-up CT scan.[1]

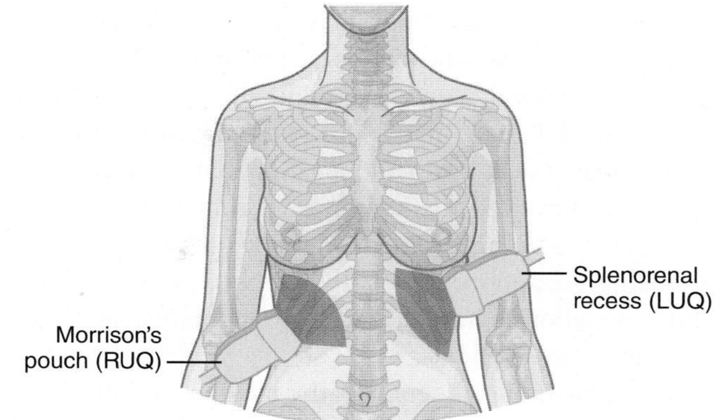

Figure 8-3 *Focused assessment with sonography for trauma.*

- Serial FAST exams can identify increasing abdominal fluid collections from hemorrhage.
- Positive FAST exams in hemodynamically unstable patients indicate the need for emergent operative management.[56]

Computed Tomography

CT scan with IV contrast is the most widely used imaging modality for patients who sustain abdominal and pelvic trauma.[6] Multidetector CT scan has become the standard in trauma centers and is highly reliable in identifying solid organ and intestinal injuries.[57] Only hemodynamically stable patients should undergo CT scanning. A relative contraindication to use of contrast is preexisting renal function abnormality.

CT scan with contrast is used to identify abdominopelvic injuries:

- CT has high reliability in identifying solid-organ injuries and pelvic fractures.[57]
- CT will reveal free air in the abdomen, which is indicative of injury to hollow viscus organs.[1]
- CT will show free fluid, which is a sign of injury that can help identify the extent of organ injury.
- CT may show extravasation of contrast, which is indicative of vascular injury.
- CT can show bowel wall or mesenteric thickening, which can occur with hematoma formation or in the presence of ischemia caused by mesenteric vascular injury.[58]

Angiography

Angiography is provided by interventional radiologists, who deploy a catheter to identify the site of active bleeding of vessels. Embolization places micro-coils, absorbable gelatin (i.e., gel foam), or small occlusion balloons in the vessel to interrupt blood flow and thereby stop hemorrhage.[50] Patients who may benefit from angioembolization are hemodynamically stable and have identified injuries on CT scan. The spleen is the organ most commonly treated with angioembolization, but this technique is also widely used for hemorrhage control in patients with pelvic fractures.[59,60] Angiography and embolization are being used more frequently for hemorrhage control and have allowed for increased nonoperative management of trauma patients.[50]

Contrast-induced nephropathy may occur with angiography and CT scans with contrast, and the risk of this complication increases with advanced age, preexisting renal disease, diabetes, and hypotension. Nephropathy secondary to contrast has been reduced with changes in contrast osmolality.[59]

Diagnostic Peritoneal Lavage/Diagnostic Peritoneal Aspiration

Diagnostic peritoneal lavage (DPL)/diagnostic peritoneal aspiration (DPA) is performed by the surgical team to rapidly identify the presence of hemorrhage in patients who are hemodynamically unstable after experiencing blunt or penetrating trauma.[1] This procedure can also be utilized if FAST and CT are not available and there is suspicion of bleeding in a hemodynamically stable patient. Contraindications to DPL/DPA include previous abdominal surgeries, morbid obesity, known coagulopathy, and advanced cirrhosis. Retroperitoneal injuries will not be identified with DPL/DPA.[1]

Positive DPL/DPA findings will require operative interventions.[1] They include the following results[1]:

- Aspiration of gastrointestinal contents, bile, or vegetable fibers
- Aspiration of greater than 10 mL of blood or greater than 100,000 RBCs/mm^3 on Gram stain
- Aspiration of greater than 500 WBCs/mm^3, food fibers, or bacteria on Gram stain

Procedure

An NG tube and urinary catheter are placed for gastric and urinary decompression prior to the procedure. The DPL is done by either open or closed technique. Sterile technique is maintained by the surgeon performing the procedure. Aspiration of blood is attempted with an 18-gauge needle. If gross blood is aspirated, then operative management is indicated. The absence of gross blood is followed with the instillation of 1 L of warmed isotonic crystalloid solution into the peritoneal cavity through IV blood tubing attached to a catheter. The fluid is spread through the abdomen by gentle agitation. The fluid is drained to a container placed below the level of insertion, and specimens are sent to the lab to evaluate for the presence of RBCs, white blood cells, and bacteria.[1]

Blood tubing is used when infusing isotonic fluid into the abdominal cavity, as traditional IV tubing has a one-way check valve that will prohibit the return of the fluid after the lavage of the abdomen. Blood tubing typically does not include a one-way check valve.

Fluid return from DPL is considered adequate if greater than 20% of the instilled volume is returned. Complications may include hemorrhage, peritonitis from the procedure, laceration of the urinary bladder, injury to other structures requiring operative management, and wound infection at the lavage site.[1]

Selected Nursing Considerations for the Trauma Patient Undergoing Radiologic Evaluation

Remove clothing and metal piercings prior to imaging. Continuous hemodynamic monitoring with the trauma nurse present during imaging is maintained while out of the emergency department or trauma unit.

Specific nursing considerations include the following:

- CT scan
  - IV contrast is widely used, following institutional policy.
  - Ensure the patient is monitored continuously during transport and while in the imaging area.
- FAST examination
  - Transducer gel will be required for the exam.
  - FAST exams have higher reliability when the patient has a full bladder.[1]
- Angiography
  - Ensure the patient is monitored continuously during transport and while in the interventional radiology suite.

Reevaluation and Post-Resuscitation Care

Reassessment is required because patients who sustain abdominal and pelvic trauma can present with subtle clinical indicators of life-threatening injury. The trauma nurse will perform ongoing assessments to identify injuries sustained and provide appropriate interventions. Systematic reassessments are required to identify subtle changes in patient condition. Ongoing reassessments include the following:

- Serial primary survey assessments
- Continuous hemodynamic monitoring

- Serial abdominal examinations
- Frequent reassessment of identified injuries for clinical changes
- Serial lab studies to trend changes

Emerging Trends

As the science and evidence of trauma care continue to evolve, new therapies are being trialed and refined. This section on emerging trends explores some of the resources that may potentially alter care of patients with abdominal and pelvic trauma: resuscitative endovascular balloon occlusion of the aorta (REBOA), nonoperative management of penetrating abdominal wounds, and use of abdominal aortic junctional tourniquets (AAJTs).

Resuscitative Endovascular Balloon Occlusion of the Aorta

REBOA is an emerging trend for hemorrhage control at noncompressible torso sites below the diaphragm.[61,62] REBOA is performed at select trauma centers where surgeons are immediately available when life-threatening hemorrhage is unresponsive to resuscitation.[61]

During REBOA, the femoral artery is cannulated with a balloon catheter and the balloon is inflated to occlude blood flow distally, stopping the life-threatening hemorrhage (see Chapter 5).[61]

Nonoperative Management of Penetrating Abdominal Wounds

Historically, patients with injuries penetrating the abdominal fascia have been treated with surgical exploration and repair as indicated. Today, however, there is a growing trend toward nonoperative management of penetrating abdominal trauma in stab wounds and selective GSWs.[63-65] Patients who would meet the criteria for selective nonoperative management of penetrating abdominal trauma include those who are hemodynamically stable and do not have any peritoneal signs.[63-65] Observation includes 12 hours of nothing by mouth, with abdominal exams by the trauma surgeon occurring every 2 hours for the first 12 hours. If the patient remains stable, the diet is advanced and monitoring continues for 12 to 24 additional hours.[63-65] Following 24 to 48 hours of observation, the patient can be discharged.[63-65]

Abdominal Aortic Junctional Tourniquet: Go for the Green

The AAJT was developed by the U.S. Special Operations Forces and received Federal Drug Administration approval in 2012. The indication for the use of this junctional tourniquet is hemorrhage in the upper extremities, lower extremities, or pelvis, in areas that are otherwise noncompressible.[66,67] This device provides point pressure that can be used to compress the abdominal aorta, axillary vessels, or inguinal vessels. The wider area of compression lowers the risk of the device moving from the required position or tissue injury occurring from compression.[66,67] The junctional tourniquet can be placed by prehospital providers.[66,67]

Summary

Abdominal and pelvic trauma can result in high morbidity and mortality in injured patients. The liver and spleen are the most commonly injured solid organs following blunt trauma, whereas penetrating injuries most frequently affect the large and small bowel. Observation of patients with blunt abdominal trauma includes serial abdominal exams, repeat FAST exams, and repeat lab exams to identify abdominopelvic injury and improve outcomes.

Patients with severe pelvic fractures may sustain hemorrhage that will require rapid intervention by the trauma team, frequent assessments by the trauma nurse, and transfer to a trauma center. Hemorrhagic shock can occur from severe injuries to the abdominal and pelvic region, and these injuries can potentiate shock states from other injuries. Interventions to stabilize the patient with abdominal and pelvic injuries include the administration of blood products, application of the pelvic binder, and preparing the patient for operative management. For some patients with abdominal and pelvic trauma, care has transitioned to nonoperative management. The trauma nurse is essential in providing ongoing assessments to identify changes in patients who have sustained abdominal and pelvic trauma.

References

1. American College of Surgeons. (2018). Abdominal and pelvic trauma. In *Advanced trauma life support: Student course manual* (10th ed., pp. 83–101). Chicago, IL: Author.
2. Tortora, G. J., & Derrickson, B. H. (2017). *Principles of anatomy and physiology* (15th ed.). Hoboken, NJ: Wiley.
3. Huether, S. E. (2017). Structure and function of the digestive system. In S. E. Huether & K. L. McCance (Eds.), *Understanding pathophysiology* (6th ed., pp. 884–902). St. Louis, MO: Elsevier.
4. Ball, J. W., Dains, J. E., Flynn, J. A., Solomon, B. S., & Stewart, R. W. (2015). *Seidel's guide to physical examination* (8th ed.). St. Louis, MO: Elsevier.

5. Venes, D. (Ed.). (2017). *Taber's cyclopedic medical dictionary* (23rd ed.). Philadelphia: F. A. Davis.
6. Asensio, J. A., & Feliciano, D. V. (2017). Abdominal vascular injury. In E. E. Moore, D. V. Feliciano, & K. L. Mattox (Eds.), *Trauma* (8th ed., pp. 651–676). Chicago, IL: McGraw-Hill.
7. Wu, K., Posluszny, J. A., Branch, J., Dray, E., Blackwell, R., Hannick, J., & Luchette, F. A. (2015). Trauma to the pelvis: Injuries to the rectum and genitourinary organs. *Current Trauma Reports, 1*(1), 8–15. https://doi.org/10.1007/s40719-014-0006-3
8. Jones, E. L., Stovall, R. T., Jones, T. S., Bensard, D. D., Burlew, C. C., Johnson, J. L., . . . Moore, E. E. (2014). Intra-abdominal injury following blunt trauma becomes clinically apparent within 9 hours. *Journal of Trauma and Acute Care Surgery, 76*(4), 1020. https://doi.org/10.1097/TA.0000000000000131
9. National Institute for Health and Care Excellence. (2017). Fractures (Complex): Assessment and Management. Retrieved from https://www.nice.org.uk/guidance/ng37/chapter/Recommendations#hospital-settings
10. Rodrigues, I. F. (2017). To log-roll or not to log-roll—that is the question! A review of the use of the log-roll for patients with pelvic fractures. *International Journal of Orthopaedic and Trauma Nursing, 27*, 36–40. https://doi.org/10.1016/j.ijotn.2017.05.001
11. Emergency Nurses Association. (2016). ENA Topic Brief: Avoiding the log roll maneuver: Alternative methods for safe patient handling. Des Plaines, IL: Author. Retrieved from https://www.ena.org/docs/default-source/resource-library/practice-resources/topic-briefs/avoiding-the-log-roll-maneuver.pdf?sfvrsn=78887c44_8
12. Sharma, R. S., Kumar, S., Damole, S., Vivekbhaskar, D., & Gandhi, A. (2017). Clinical study of hollow viscus and solid organ injury in blunt abdominal trauma and its management. *International Journal of Information Research and Review, 4*(4), 3963–3966. Retrieved from http://www.ijirr.com/sites/default/files/issues-files/1940.pdf
13. Bordoni, P. H. C., Santos, D. M. M. D., Teixeria, J. S., & Bordoni, L. S. (2017). Deaths from abdominal trauma: Analysis of 1888 forensic autopsies. *Revista do Colégio Brasileiro de Cirurgiões, 44*(6), 582–595. https://doi.org/10.1590/0100-69912017006006
14. Hamm, A. D., Burlew, C. C., & Moore, E. E. (2018). Penetrating abdominal trauma. In A. H. Harken & E. E. Moore (Eds.), *Abernathy's surgical secrets* (7th ed., pp. 115–120). Philadelphia, PA: Elsevier.
15. Chaudery, M., Clark, J., Wilson, M. H., Bew, D., Yang, G. Z., & Darzi, A. (2015). Traumatic intra-abdominal hemorrhage control: Has current technology tipped the balance toward a role for prehospital intervention? *Journal of Trauma and Acute Care Surgery, 78*(1), 153–163. https://doi.org/10.1097/TA.0000000000000472
16. Giannoudis, P. V., & Pape, H. C. (2017). Principles of damage control for pelvic ring injuries. In H. C. Pape, A. B. Peitzman, P. V. Rotondo, & P. V. Giannoudis (Eds.), *Damage control management in the polytrauma patient* (2nd ed., pp. 219–232). Cham, Switzerland: Springer International Publishing. https://doi.org/10.1007/978-3-319-52429-0_21
17. Harris, C. (2013). Abdominal trauma. In B. B. Hammond & P. G. Zimmerman (Eds.), *Sheehy's manual of emergency care* (7th ed., 419–426). St. Louis, MO: Elsevier Mosby.
18. Diercks, D. B., & Clarke, S. (2018, April 16). Initial evaluation and management of blunt abdominal trauma in adults. *UpToDate*. Retrieved from https://www.uptodate.com/contents/initial-evaluation-and-management-of-blunt-abdominal-trauma-in-adults
19. Matsumoto, S., Sekine, K., Funaoka, H., Funabiki, T., Shimizu, M., Hayashida, K., & Kitano, M. (2017). Early diagnosis of hollow viscus injury using intestinal fatty acid–binding protein in blunt trauma patients. *Medicine, 96*(10), e6187. http://doi.org/10.1097/MD.0000000000006187
20. Biffl, W. L., & Leppaniemi, A. (2015). Management guidelines for penetrating abdominal trauma. *World Journal of Surgery, 39*(6), 1373–1380. https://doi.org/10.1007/s00268-014-2793-7
21. Lee, K., & Lee, J. G. (2016). Management of thoracic aortic injury after blunt trauma: Nine cases at a single medical center. *Journal of Trauma and Injury, 29*(4), 146–150. http://doi.org/10.20408/jti.2016.29.4.146
22. Halawi, M. J. (2015). Pelvic ring injuries: Emergency assessment and management. *Journal of Clinical Orthopaedics & Trauma, 6*(4), 252–258. https://doi.org//10.1016/j.jcot.2015.08.002
23. Bryk, D. J., & Zhao, L. C. (2016). Guideline of guidelines: A review of urological trauma guidelines. *BJU International, 117*(2), 226–234. https://doi.org/10.1111/bju.13040
24. Cheng, M., Cheung, M. T., Lee, K. Y., Lee, K. B., Chan, S. C., Wu, A. C., . . . Yau, K. K. (2015). Improvement in institutional protocols leads to decreased mortality in patients with haemodynamically unstable pelvic fractures. *Emergency Medicine Journal, 32*(3), 214–220. https://doi.org/10.1136/emermed-2012-202009
25. Nakao, S., Ishikawa, K., Ono, H., Kusakabe, K., Fujimura, I., Ueno, M., . . . Matsuoka, T. (2018, January 24). Radiological classification of retroperitoneal hematoma resulting from lumbar vertebral fracture. *European Journal of Trauma and Emergency Surgery*, 1–11. https://doi.org/10.1007/s00068-018-0907-x
26. Perez-Tamayo, A., & Charash, W. E. (2018). Acute abdomen and peritonitis. In P. E. Parsons, J. P. Wiener-Kronish, R. D. Stapleton, & L. Berra (Eds.), *Critical care secrets* (6th ed., pp. 440–445). Philadelphia, PA: Elsevier.
27. Calixte, N., Brahmbhatt, J., & Parekattil, S. (2017). Genital pain: Algorithm for management. *Translational Andrology and Urology, 6*(2), 252. https://doi.org/10.21037/tau.2017.03.03
28. Rossaint, R., Bouillon, B., Cerny, V., Coats, T. J., Duranteau, J., Fernandez-Mondejar, E., . . . Filipescu, D. (2016). The European guideline on management of major bleeding and coagulopathy following trauma: Fourth edition. *Critical Care, 20*(100). https://doi.org/10.1186/s13054-016-1265-x
29. Masudi, T., McMahon, H. C., Scott, J. L., & Lockey, A. S. (2017). Seat belt–related injuries: A surgical perspective. *Journal of Emergencies, Trauma, and Shock, 10*(2), 70–73. https://doi.org/10.4103/0974-2700.201590
30. Revell, M. A., Pugh, M. A., & McGhee, M. (2018). Gastrointestinal traumatic injuries: Gastrointestinal perforation. *Critical Care Nursing Clinics of North America, 30*(1), 157–166. https://doi.org/10.1016/j.cnc.2017.10.014
31. Taha, A. M., Abdallah, A. M., Sayed, M. M., Mohamed, S. I., & Hamad, M. (2017). Nonoperative management of isolated blunt

liver trauma: A task of high skilled surgeons. *Journal of Surgery*, *5*(6), 118–123. https://doi.org/10.11648/j.js.20170506.16

32. Storch, B. (2017, August 22). Pelvic vertical shear fractures. *Core EM*. Retrieved from https://coreem.net/core/pelvic-vertical-shear-fractures/
33. Bruns, R. B., & Kozar, R. A. (2017). Liver and biliary tract. In E. E. Moore, D. V. Feliciano, & K. L. Mattox (Eds.), *Trauma* (8th ed., pp. 551–574). Chicago, IL: McGraw-Hill.
34. Tignanelli, C. J., Joseph, B., Jakubus, J. L., Iskander, G. A., Napolitano, L. M., & Hemmila, M. R. (2018). Variability in management of blunt liver trauma and contribution of level of American College of Surgeons Committee on Trauma verification status on mortality. *Journal of Trauma and Acute Care Surgery*, *84*(2), 273–279. https://doi.org/10.1097/TA.0000000000001743
35. Coccolini, F., Montori, G., Catena, F., Kluger, Y., Biffl, W., Moore, E. E., . . . Ansaloni, L. (2017). Splenic trauma: WSES classification and guidelines for adult and pediatric patients. *World Journal of Emergency Surgery*, *12*, 40–66. https://doi.org/10.1186/s13017-017-0151-4
36. Iacono, C., Zicari, M., Conci, S., Valdegamberi, A., De Angelis, M., Pedrazzani, C., . . . Guglielmi, A. (2016). Management of pancreatic trauma: A pancreatic surgeon's point of view. *Pancreatology*, *16*(3), 302–308. https://doi.org/10.1016/j.pan.2015.12.004
37. Singh, R. P., Garg, N., Nar, A. S., Mahajan, A., Mishra, A., Singh, J., . . . Bawa, A. (2016). Role of amylase and lipase levels in diagnosis of blunt trauma abdomen. *Journal of Clinical and Diagnostic Research*, *10*(2), PC20. https://doi.org/10.7860/JCDR/2016/14346.7308
38. Menahem, B., Lim, C., Lahat, E., Salloum, C., Osseis, M., Lacaze, L., . . . Azoulay, D. (2016). Conservative and surgical management of pancreatic trauma in adult patients. *Hepatobiliary Surgery and Nutrition*, *5*(6), 470. https://doi.org/10.21037/hbsn.2016.07.01
39. Chereau, N., Wagner, M., Tresallet, C., Lucidarme, O., Raux, M., & Menegaux, F. (2016). CT scan and diagnostic peritoneal lavage: Towards a better diagnosis in the area of nonoperative management of blunt abdominal trauma. *Injury, 47*(9), 2006–2011. https://doi.org/10.1016/j.injury.2016.04.034
40. Landry, B. A., Patlas, M. N., Faidi, S., Coates, A., & Nicolaou, S. (2016). Are we missing traumatic bowel and mesenteric injuries? *Canadian Association of Radiologists Journal*, *67*(4), 420–425. https://doi.org/10.1016/j.carj.2015.11.006
41. LeBedis, C. A., Anderson, S. W., Bates, D. D., Khalil, R., Matherly, D., Wing, H., . . . Soto, J. A. (2016). CT imaging signs of surgically proven bowel trauma. *Emergency Radiology*, *23*(3), 213–219. https://doi.org/10.1007/s10140-016-1380-7
42. Demetriades, D., Benjamin, E., & Inaba, K. (2017). Colon and rectal trauma. In E. E. Moore, D. V. Feliciano, & K. L. Mattox (Eds.), *Trauma* (8th ed., pp. 639–650). Chicago, IL: McGraw-Hill.
43. Siada, S. S., Davis, J. W., Kaups, K. L., Dirks, R. C., & Grannis, K. A. (2017). Current outcomes of blunt open pelvic fractures: How modern advances in trauma care may decrease mortality. *Trauma Surgery & Acute Care Open*, *2*(1–4), e000136. Retrieved from http://tsaco.bmj.com/content/tsaco/2/1/e000136.full.pdf
44. Burlew, C. C., & Moore, E. E. (2017). Abdominal esophagus and stomach. In G. C. Velmahos, E. Degiannis, & D. Doll (Eds.), *Penetrating trauma* (pp. 351–356). Berlin, Germany: Springer.
45. Naiem, A. A., Taqi, K. M., Al-Kendi, B. H., & Al-Qadhi, H. (2016). Missed gastric injuries in blunt abdominal trauma: Case report with review of literature. *Sultan Qaboos University Medical Journal*, *16*(4), e508. https://doi.org/10.18295/squmj.2016.16.04.019.
46. Oray, N. C., Sivrikaya, S., Bayram, B., Egeli, T., & Dicle, O. (2014). Blunt trauma patient with esophageal perforation. *Western Journal of Emergency Medicine*, *15*(6), 659. Retrieved from https://westjem.com/case-report/blunt-trauma-patient-with-esophageal-perforation.html
47. Arumugam, P. K. (2017). Isolated intraperitoneal rupture of the urinary bladder following blunt trauma abdomen. *International Surgery Journal*, *4*(5), 1822–1824. https://doi.org/10.18203/2349-2902.isj20171649
48. Shafi, H., Darzi, A., Ahangar, S. K., & Asghari, Y. (2017). Nonoperative management of intraperitoneal bladder rupture due to blunt abdominal trauma. *Trauma Monthly*, *22*(5), e38079. http://doi.org/10.5812/traumamon.3807938079
49. Gómez, R. G., Mundy, T., Dubey, D., El-Kassaby, A. W., Kodama, R., & Santucci, R. (2014). SIU/ICUD consultation on urethral strictures: Pelvic fracture urethral injuries. *Urology*, *83*(3 Suppl.), S48–S58. https://doi.org/10.1016/j.urology.2013.09.023
50. Velmahos, G. C. (2017). Pelvis. In E. E. Moore, D. V. Feliciano, & K. L. Mattox (Eds.), *Trauma* (8th ed., pp. 677–692). Chicago, IL: McGraw-Hill.
51. Khurana, B., Sheehan, S. E., Sodickson, A. D., & Weaver, M. J. (2014). Pelvic ring fractures: What the orthopedic surgeon wants to know. *Radiographics*, *34*(5), 1317–1333. https://doi.org/10.1148/rg.345135113
52. Fitzgerald, M., Esser, M., Russ, M., Mathew, J., Varma, D., Wilkinson, A., . . . Mitra, B. (2017). Pelvic trauma mortality reduced by integrated trauma care. *Emergency Medicine Australia*, *29*(4), 444–449. https://doi.org/10.1111/1742-6723.12820
53. Wells, H., & Somani. B. K. (2015). Current management of renal trauma. *HSOA Journal of Emergency Medicine and Trauma Surgery Care*, *2*(9). https://doi.org/10.24966/ETS-8798/100009
54. Loffroy, R., Chevallier, O., Gehin, S., Midulla, M., Berthod, P. E., Galland, C., . . . Falvo, N. (2017). Endovascular management of arterial injuries after blunt or iatrogenic renal trauma. *Quantitative Imaging in Medicine and Surgery*, *7*(4), 434–442. https://doi.org/10.21037/qims.2017.08.04
55. Bloom, B. A., & Gibbons, R. C. (2017, December 18). Trauma, focused assessment with sonography for trauma (FAST). *StatPearls*. Retrieved from https://www.ncbi.nlm.nih.gov/books/NBK470479/
56. Richards, J. R., & McGahan, J. P. (2017). Focused assessment with sonography in trauma (FAST) in 2017: What radiologists can learn. *Radiology*, *283*(1), 30–48. https://doi.org/10.1148/radiol.2017160107
57. Shah, S., & Pendor, A. (2018). Role of MDCT scanner in evaluation of solid organ injuries in significant blunt abdominal trauma. *International Journal of Scientific Research*, *6*(9). Retrieved from https://wwjournals.com/index.php/ijsr/article/viewFile/388/382

58. Yang, X. Y., Wei, M. T., Jin, C. W., Wang, M., & Wang, Z. Q. (2016). Unenhanced computed tomography to visualize hollow viscera and/or mesenteric injury after blunt abdominal trauma: A single-institution experience. *Medicine (Baltimore), 95*(9). https://doi.org/10.1097/MD.0000000000002884
59. Bhakta, A., Magee, D. S., Peterson, M. S., & O'Mara, M. S. (2017). Angioembolization is necessary with any volume of contrast extravasation in blunt trauma. *International Journal of Critical Illness and Injury Science, 7*(1), 18–22. https://doi.org/10.4103/IJCIIS.IJCIIS_125_16
60. Matsushima, K., Piccinini, A., Schellenberg, M., Cheng, V., Heindel, P., Strumwasser, A., . . . Demetriades, D. (2018). Effect of door-to-angioembolization time on mortality in pelvic fracture: Every hour of delay counts. *Journal of Trauma and Acute Care Surgery, 84*(5), 685–692. https://doi.org/10.1097/TA.0000000000001803
61. Simon, M. A., Russo, R. M., Davidson, A. J., Faulconer, E. R., DeSoucy, E., Loja, M. N., . . . Dawson, D. D. (2017). A case of resuscitative endovascular balloon occlusion of the aorta (REBOA) use in penetrating abdominal aortic injury. *Journal of Endovascular Resuscitation and Trauma Management, 1*(1), 53–57. https://doi.org/10.26676/jevtm,v1i1.12
62. Brenner, M., Bulger, E. M., Perina, D. G., Henry, S., Kang, C. S., Rotondo, M. F., . . . Stewart, R. M. (2018). Joint statement from the American College of Surgeons Committee on Trauma (ACS COT) and the American College of Emergency Physicians (ACEP) regarding the clinical use of resuscitative endovascular balloon occlusion of the aorta (REBOA). *Trauma Surgery & Acute Care Open, 3*(1), e000154. https://doi.org/10.1136/tsaco-2017-000154
63. Goin, G., Massalou, D., Bege, T., Contargyris, C., Avaro, J.-P., Pauleau, G., & Balandraud, P. (2017). Feasibility of selective non-operative management for penetrating abdominal trauma in France. *Journal of Visceral Surgery, 154*, 167–174. https://doi.org/10.1016/j.jviscsurg.2016.08.006
64. Dayananda, K., Kong, V., Bruch, J., Oosthuizen, G., Laing, G., & Clarke, D. (2017). Selective non-operative management of abdominal stab wounds is a safe and cost-effective strategy: A South Africa experience. *Annals of the Royal College of Surgeons of England, 99*, 490–496. https://doi.org/10.1308/rcsann.2017.0075
65. Como, J. J., Bokhari, F., Chiu, W. C., Duane, T. M., Holevar, M. R., Tandoh, M. A., . . . Scalea, T. M. (2010). Practice management guidelines for selective non-operative management of penetrating abdominal trauma. *Journal of Trauma, 68*(3), 721–733. https://doi.org/10.1097/TA.0b013e3181cf7d07
66. Rall, J. M., Redman, T. T., Ross, E. M., Morrison, J. J., & Maddry, J. K. (2018). Comparison of zone 3 resuscitative endovascular balloon occlusion of the aorta and the abdominal aortic and junctional tourniquet in a model of junctional hemorrhage in swine. *Journal of Surgical Research, 26*, 31–39. https://doi.org/10.1016/j.jss.2017.12.039
67. *Trauma System News.* (2018, June 4). Combat-tested abdominal/junctional tourniquet proven equivalent to REBOA. Retrieved from http://trauma-news.com/2018/06/combat-tested-abdominal-junctional-tourniquet-proven-equivalent-to-reboa/

CHAPTER 9

Spinal Trauma

Angela W. Clarkson, BSN, RN-TCRN

OBJECTIVES

Upon completion of this chapter, the learner will be able to:

1. Describe mechanisms of injury associated with spinal cord and/or vertebral column trauma.
2. Describe pathophysiologic changes as a basis for assessment of the trauma patient with spinal cord and/or vertebral column injuries.
3. Demonstrate the nursing assessment of the trauma patient with spinal cord and/or vertebral column injuries.
4. Plan appropriate interventions for the trauma patient with spinal cord and/or vertebral column injuries.
5. Evaluate the effectiveness of nursing interventions for the trauma patient with spinal cord and/or vertebral column injuries.

Knowledge of normal anatomy and physiology serves as a foundation for understanding anatomic derangements and pathophysiologic processes that may result from trauma. The anatomy material is not emphasized in the classroom but may be the basis of skill evaluation assessments and the basis of questions for testing purposes.

Anatomy and Physiology of the Spinal Cord and Vertebral Column

This review begins with the spinal cord and then turns to the vertebral column.

Spinal Cord

The spinal cord is the communication structure between the body and the brain; it is responsible for the two-way communication between the brain and the peripheral nervous system. It occupies the upper two-thirds of the vertebral canal and is wider in the cervical and lumbar areas to accommodate nerve cells supplying the upper and lower limbs. The spinal cord usually ends at the level of the first lumbar vertebra in adults with the sacral nerve roots descending from this point to their appropriate exit points through the intervertebral foramina. Two consecutive rows of nerve roots emerge from each side—the dorsal root and the ventral root. These nerve roots join distally to form 31 pairs of spinal nerves. The end of the

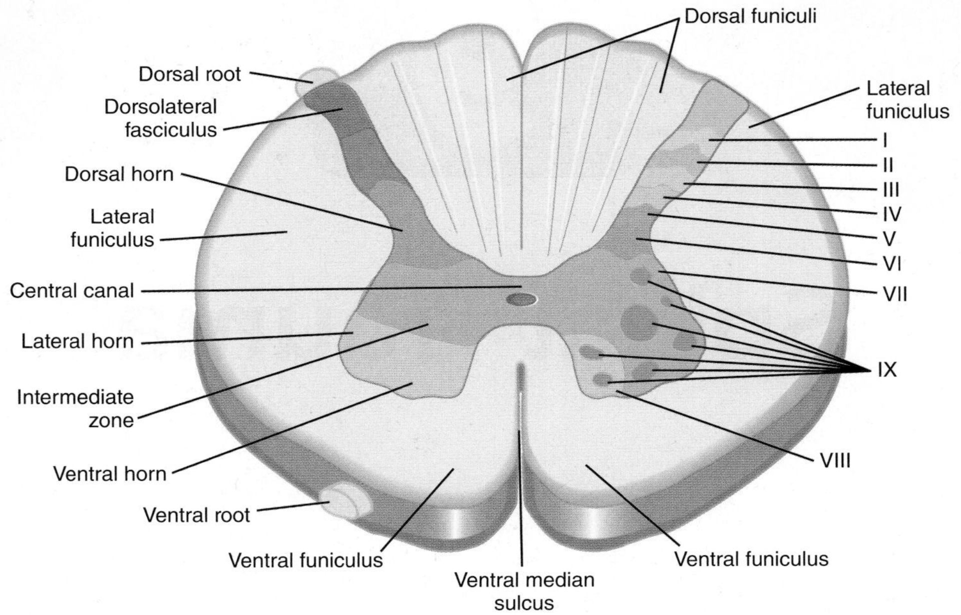

Figure 9-1 *Cross-section of the spinal cord.*

spinal cord, the conus medullaris, is cone shaped. Spinal nerves continue outward from the conus medullaris, forming a nerve bundle known as the cauda equina.[1,2]

The spinal cord is divided into the cervical, thoracic, lumbar, and sacral regions. When viewed in cross-section, the spinal cord has a butterfly- or H-shaped core (**Figure 9-1**). It contains a central mass of gray matter that is divided into three paired horns: ventral (anterior), intermediolateral, and dorsal (posterior). The horns of the spinal cord are responsible for voluntary motor activity. The ventral horn provides the motor components of the spinal nerves. The intermediolateral horn contains the preganglionic sympathetic fibers of the thoracic, lumbar, and sacral spine. The dorsal horn contains peripheral sensory neurons.[1,3,4] Surrounding the gray matter is the white matter, which consists of myelinated nerve fibers and forms three columns: the anterior, the lateral, and the posterior.[1,3-5] Each column contains ascending sensory tracts that carry impulses up the spinal cord to the brain and descending motor tracts that carry motor impulses down the spinal cord.

Motor Function

Impulses are conducted between the brain and the spinal cord through the upper motor neurons.[2] The upper motor neurons form two major systems: the corticospinal tract (**Figure 9-2**), which is responsible for fine motor skills, and the extra-corticospinal tract, which is responsible for gross motor movement (**Table 9-1**).[1,2,4,6] Upper motor neurons cross at the medulla of the brain stem

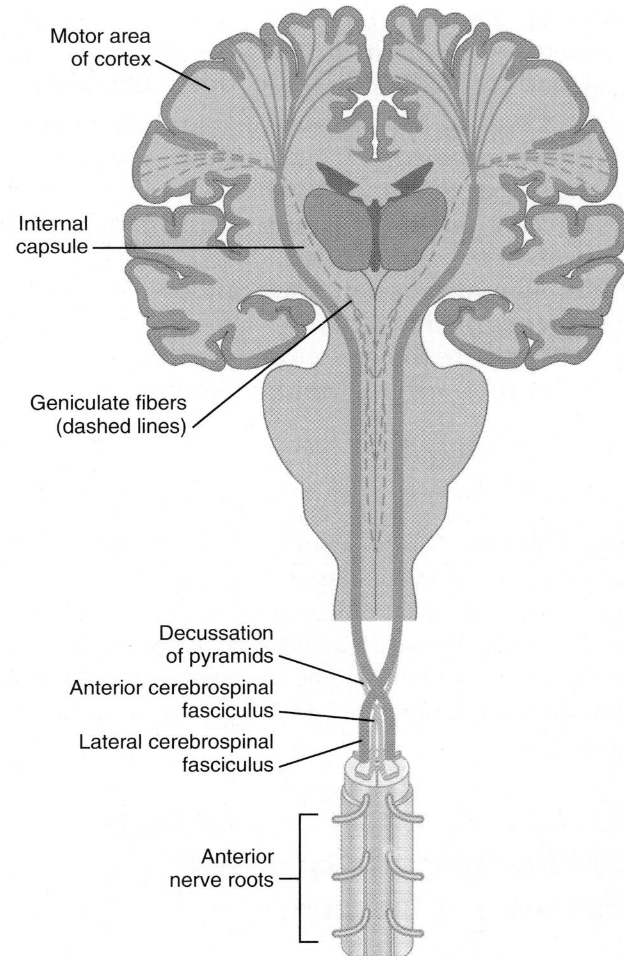

Figure 9-2 *Corticospinal tracts.*

TABLE 9-1 Motor and Sensory Spinal Nerve Tracts

Nerve Tracts	Origin	Function	Location in Spinal Cord
Descending tracts: corticospinal (pyramidal)	Cerebral cortex	Voluntary motor	Anterolateral
Ascending tracts: spinothalamic	Sensory receptors located throughout the body	› Pain › Temperature › Crude touch	Anterolateral
Posterior (dorsal) tracts	Sensory receptors located throughout body	› Proprioception › Fine touch › Two-point discrimination	Posterior (dorsal)

Data from Banasik, J. (2013). Structure and function of the nervous system. In L. Copstead & J. Banasik, *Pathophysiology* (5th ed., pp. 857–897). St. Louis, MO: Saunders/Elsevier.

to the opposite side and descend in the corticospinal tract. This is the basis for loss of movement on the contralateral side from a head injury. Some fibers descend through the white matter on the same side and cross at specific spinal cord segments, resulting in ipsilateral loss of movement when they are damaged.[1,2,5] Impulses that originate in the upper motor neurons are conducted to the lower motor neurons in the spinal cord and innervate the skeletal muscle groups. The cervical nerve fibers from the corticospinal tract, located in the central portion of the ventral horn, innervate the upper extremities. The sacral fibers from the corticospinal tract, located in the peripheral portion of the ventral horn, innervate the lower extremities.[1,3-5]

Sensory Function

Sensory pathways include those impulse routes that can be combined into spinal reflex arcs (sensory) or those transmitted to higher centers in the brain to be interpreted (cortical).

Reflex Arc

The reflex arc is a stimulus-response mechanism that does not require ascending or descending spinal cord pathways to the cerebral cortex to function. Examples of reflex arcs include deep tendon reflexes (e.g., patellar reflex) and the withdrawal reflex to avoid physical injury (e.g., reflexive withdrawal from a hot surface before pain is registered or catching oneself from falling). The reflex arc is the only part of the neural path with withdrawal responses. The stimulus that triggers the withdrawal response continues to travel up the spinothalamic tract to the cortex, registering pain or imbalance.[6]

The essential structures of the reflex arc include the following[7]:

- Receptor (sense organ, cutaneous end organ, or neuromuscular spindle)
- Afferent (sensory) neuron
- Association (interneuron) neuron
- Efferent (motor) neuron
- Effector neuron (muscle, tendon, or gland that produces response)

An anatomically and physiologically intact reflex arc will function even if there is disruption of spinal cord function above the level of the reflex.[4,8]

Cortical Sensation

Cortical sensation includes both simple sensation and deep sensation. Pain, touch, and temperature are known as simple sensations because their detection is carried out by discrete sensory organs, such as the skin. Information from general somatic receptors in the skin is conducted over small-diameter fibers of the spinal nerves into the dorsal horn of the spinal cord's gray matter. Pain and temperature fibers enter the spinal cord and travel within one to two spinal segments, and then cross before ascending in the spinothalamic tract.[9] Light touch sensation fibers cross immediately upon entering the spinal cord and then ascend in the spinothalamic tract.[9]

Deep sensation includes proprioception, vibration sensation, and deep muscle pain.[5] These afferent (ascending) impulses are transmitted by fibers entering the spinal cord via the dorsal roots and ascend in a tract of the spinal cord, depending on the type of sensation. Proprioception and vibration fibers ascend via the posterior column and cross in the medulla. These sensations are referred to as cortical because they require an intact cerebral hemisphere to interpret the impulses.[9]

Spinal Nerves

There are 31 pairs of spinal nerves: 8 cervical pairs, 12 thoracic pairs, 5 lumbar pairs, 5 sacral pairs, and 1 coccygeal pair. Each pair of spinal nerves exits the spinal cord bilaterally, and each has a dorsal and ventral root. The dorsal root transmits sensory impulses, whereas the ventral root transmits motor impulses. The dorsal root of each nerve innervates particular dermatomes in the body (**Figure 9-3**).

The cervical nerves innervate the head, diaphragm, neck, shoulders, and upper arms.[4] The thoracic nerves innervate the thorax, abdomen, and portions of the buttocks and upper arm. The intercostal muscles are innervated by spinal nerves T1 through T12. The lumbar nerves innervate the groin region and lower extremities. The sacral nerves S3 to S5 supply the perianal muscles, which control voluntary contraction of the external bladder sphincter and the external anal sphincter (**Table 9-2**).[4,8,9]

Nerve Plexuses

A plexus is an integral part of the nervous system where nerves converge in small groups. These nerve clusters connect the peripheral and central nervous systems, allowing signals to travel from the brain and spinal cord to

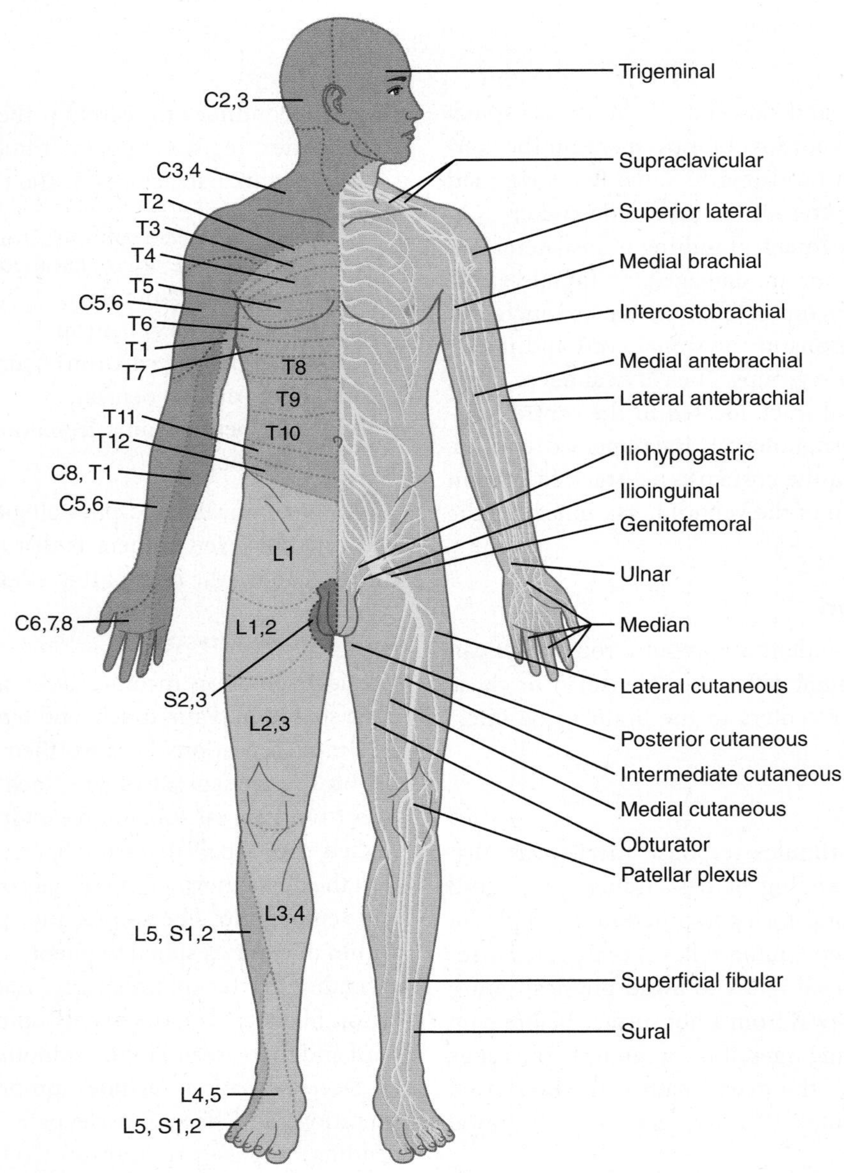

Figure 9-3 *Dermatomes.*

TABLE 9-2 Spinal Nerve Segments and Areas of Innervation

Spinal Nerve Segment	Area Innervated
C5	Area over the deltoid
C6	Thumb
C7	Middle finger
C8	Little finger
T4	Nipple
T8	Xiphisternum
T10	Umbilicus
T12	Symphysis pubis
L4	Medial aspect of the calf
L5	Web space between the first and second toes
S1	Lateral border of the foot
S3	Ischial tuberosity area
S4 and S5	Perianal region

Data from McGee, S. (2012). Examination of the sensory system. In *Evidence-based physical diagnosis* (3rd ed., pp. 567–580). Philadelphia, PA: Elsevier.

the rest of the body. Without these connections, the brain would not be able to communicate with the rest of the body.[6] There are four major nerve plexuses:

- The *cervical* plexus is formed by the first four cervical nerves, which innervate the muscles of the neck and shoulders. In addition, the phrenic nerve arises from C3, C4, and C5; it innervates the diaphragm.[6]
- Spinal nerves C5 to C8, along with T1, form the *brachial* plexus, which supplies motor control and sensation to the arm, wrist, and hand.[3,4] The brachial plexus branches include the ulnar and radial nerves.
- Spinal nerves L1 to L4 form the *lumbar* plexus, which gives rise to the femoral nerve and innervates the anterior portion of the lower body
- Spinal nerves L5 to S4 form the *sacral* plexus, which is the origin of the sciatic nerve. The sacral plexus innervates the posterior portion of the lower body.[4,8]

Autonomic Nervous System

The autonomic nervous system (ANS) fibers innervate smooth muscle, cardiac muscle, and glands, controlling involuntary vital functions such as blood pressure (BP), heart rate, body temperature, appetite, fluid balance, gastrointestinal motility, and sexual function.[2] The ANS has two subdivisions: parasympathetic and sympathetic. The parasympathetic nervous system originates from nerves in the craniosacral regions of the central nervous system, whereas the sympathetic nervous system originates from the thoracolumbar region of the spinal cord. The parasympathetic division regulates bodily functions under normal body conditions. In contrast, sympathetic system activity increases during physiologic and psychological stress. Specific responses from autonomic stimulation depend on the type and number of receptors located within a tissue, organ, or system. The generalized responses resulting from stimulation of both of these systems are listed in **Table 9-3**.[4,6,10]

Vertebral Column

The vertebral column is held together by ligaments and contains 33 vertebrae, including 7 cervical, 12 thoracic, 5 lumbar, 5 sacral, and 4 coccygeal vertebrae (**Figure 9-4**).[6]

The typical vertebra is composed of a weight-bearing body and a vertebral arch. The arch is made of two pedicles (right and left), two laminae, four articular processes (facets), two transverse processes, and one spinous process (**Figure 9-5**). The spinous process can be felt when palpating the back. Together, the arch and the body form an enclosure called the *vertebral foramen* that encircles and protects the spinal cord.[4]

Cervical Vertebrae

The cervical vertebrae are the smallest and most mobile of the vertebrae. The first cervical vertebra, the *atlas*, supports the weight of the head and articulates with the occipital condyles of the skull. The atlas differs from the other vertebrae in that it has no spinous process or vertebral body. In addition, the foramen opening for the spinal cord is larger than in the rest of the vertebrae. The *axis*, C2, has a perpendicular projection called the odontoid process, or *dens*. The atlas articulates with the axis on the odontoid process.

Thoracic Vertebrae

The thoracic vertebrae, T1 through T12, attach to the ribs. This factor limits flexion and extension but permits more rotation than the lumbar region and less than the cervical region. The vertebrae in this region are strong, and additional support is provided by the ribs.

Lumbar, Sacral, and Coccygeal Vertebrae

The five lumbar vertebrae (L1–L5) are the largest and strongest in the vertebral column.[4] This area of the spine has some freedom of movement and rotation, albeit not as much as

TABLE 9-3 Effects of Sympathetic and Parasympathetic Stimulation

Target Tissue, Organ, or System	Result of Sympathetic Stimulation	Result of Parasympathetic Stimulation
Skin	› ↑ Secretions from sweat glands › Piloerection	N/A
Cardiac	› ↑ Heart rate, conduction, and contractility	› ↓ Heart rate, conduction, and contractility
Vascular	› Peripheral vasoconstriction	N/A
Respiratory	› ↑ Respiratory rate › Bronchial dilation › Pulmonary vascular constriction	› Bronchial constriction
Hepatic	› ↑ Glycogen breakdown and synthesis of new glucose	› Promotes glycogen synthesis
Stomach and intestines	› ↓ Motility and tone › Sphincter contraction › ↓ Gastric secretions and mesenteric blood flow	› ↑ Motility and tone › Sphincter relaxation › ↑ Gastric secretions
Renal	› ↑ Renin secretion › Vascular constriction causes ↓ urinary output	N/A
Adrenal medulla	› Catecholamines, norepinephrine, and epinephrine released from adrenal glands	N/A

Data from Banasik, J. (2013). Structure and function of the nervous system. In L. E. Copstead & J. L. Banasik (Eds.), *Pathophysiology* (5th ed., pp. 857–897). St. Louis, MO: Elsevier Saunders; VanPutte, C., Regan, J., Russo, A. Seeley, R. R., Stephens, T., & Tate, P. (2016). *Seeley's anatomy and physiology* (11th ed.). Boston, MA: McGraw-Hill.

the cervical region. The five sacral vertebrae (S1–S5) fuse together to form the sacrum—a solid bone that fits like a wedge between the bones of the hip. The final four coccygeal vertebrae are fused together to form the coccyx.[4,5,11]

Ligaments and Intervertebral Discs

The vertebral bodies are connected by a series of ligaments that provide support and stability for the vertebral column. The anterior and posterior longitudinal ligaments are major ligaments that run the length of the vertebral column and hold the discs and vertebral bodies in position. These ligaments help prevent the vertebral column from experiencing excessive flexion and extension. The spinous and transverse processes act as points of attachment for muscles and other ligaments. Fibrocartilaginous discs are located between the vertebral bodies and act as shock absorbers during weight bearing and as articulating surfaces for the subsequent vertebral bodies. The more flexible cervical and lumbar regions contain thicker intervertebral discs.[5,8]

Vascular Supply

Blood is supplied to the spinal cord from branches of the vertebral arteries and the aorta. Primarily, the cord is perfused from the anterior and posterior spinal arteries, which branch off from the vertebral artery at the cranial base.[1,2,5] Injuries to the spinal cord or surrounding area can lacerate these arteries, resulting in hematoma formation that may compress the cord. Injury to the vessels can be devastating because collateral circulation does not develop in this area.[4]

Introduction

All trauma patients with multiple injuries are at risk for spinal cord injury (SCI), regardless of the presence or absence of neurologic deficit on arrival. Given the

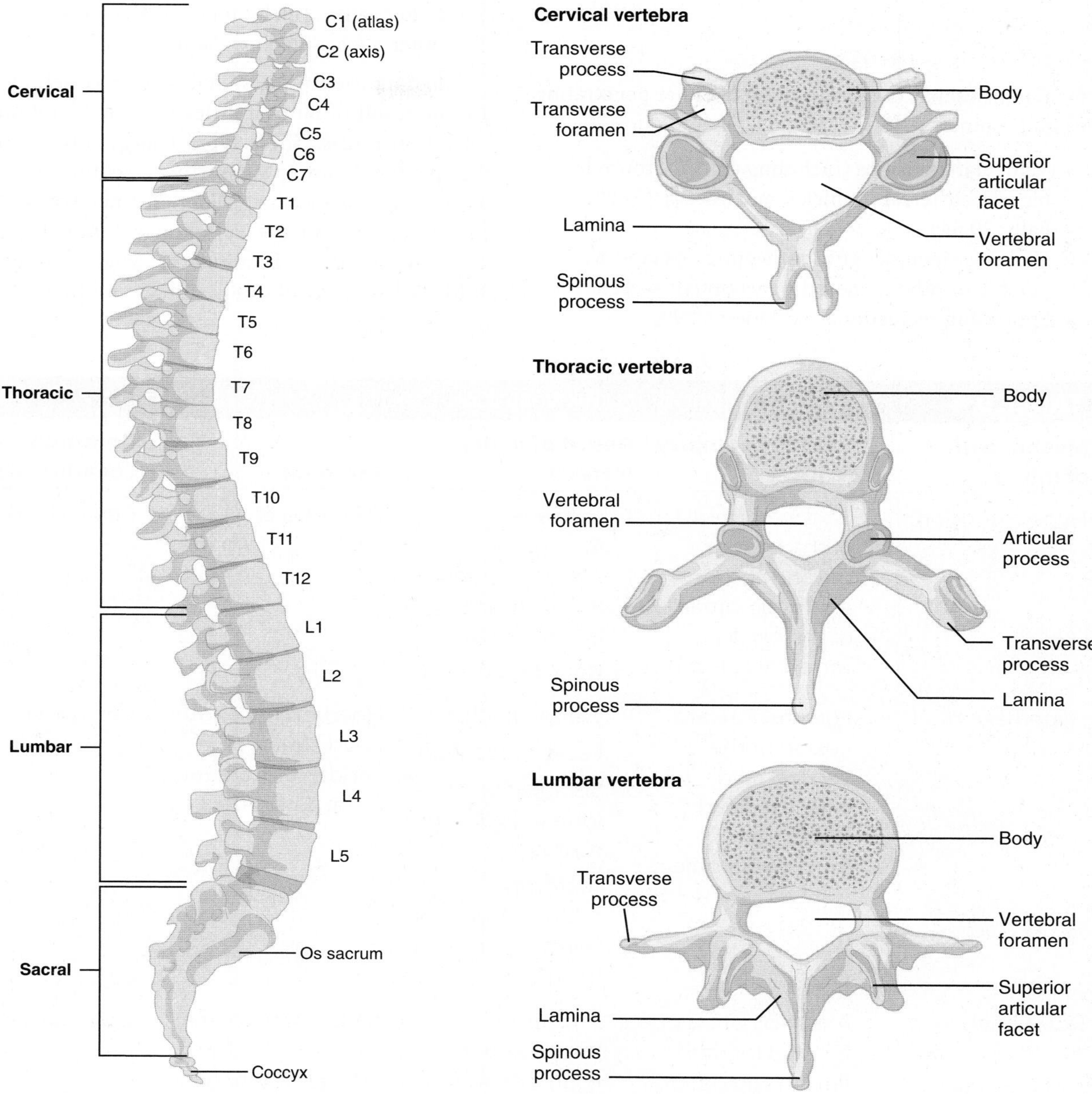

Figure 9-4 *The spine.*

Figure 9-5 *The vertebrae.*

significant impact of a SCI on the patient's health and abilities, it is essential that trauma nurses who care for these patients maintain adequate spinal motion restriction when caring for these patients so as to avoid any excessive manipulation of the spine until injury can be ruled out. In patients with a high index of suspicion for an unstable spine, this includes *not* turning the patient until imaging has ruled out an unstable injury. In patients with an unstable spine, log rolling can cause further injury.[12-19]

Epidemiology

In 2009, the average age of a survivor of a SCI was 40.2 years—an increase over the average age seen in recent years.[9] The percentage of new SCI cases involving individuals older than 65 years increased from 3.1% in the 1970s to 13.2% in 2010 to 2014.[20] Explanations for this trend include improved survival rates for older populations, although most injuries are seen in young adult males.[21]

Mechanisms of Injury and Biomechanics

Spinal injuries may occur as a result of either penetrating or blunt trauma[22]:

- Vehicular collisions (including auto, motorcycle, bicycle, all-terrain vehicles, and boats): 39.08%
- Falls: 29.54%
- Violence (includes gunshot wounds, person-to-person, or other penetrating wounds): 14.41%
- Sports and recreational activities: 8.39%
- Other causes (including pedestrian events and other unclassified mechanisms): 8.57%

Most injuries to the spinal cord or vertebral column are the result of blunt injuries from acceleration or deceleration forces. These rapid energy forces may push the spinal column or supporting structures beyond the usual range of motion.[23] Four distinct types of forces can be applied to the vertebral column: hyperextension, hyperflexion, rotation, or axial loading forces. **Table 9-4** summarizes those forces and their associated injuries.[24-26]

TABLE 9-4 Mechanisms of Injury to the Vertebral Column

Mechanism of Injury	Etiology of Injury (Cause)	Result of Injury (Effect)	Example	Common Location of Injury
Hyperextension	Backward thrust of the head beyond the anatomic capacity of the cervical vertebral column	› Damage to anterior ligaments ranging from stretching to ligament tears › Bony dislocations	Rear-end MVC resulting in whiplash	Cervical spine
Hyperflexion	Forceful forward flexion of the cervical spine with the head striking an immovable object	› Wedge fractures › Facet dislocations › Subluxation (due to ligament rupture) › Teardrop, odontoid, or transverse process fractures	Head-on MVC with head striking the windshield, creating a starburst effect	Cervical spine
Rotational	A combination of forceful forward flexion with lateral displacement of the cervical spine	› Rupture of the posterior ligament and/or anterior fracture › Dislocation of the vertebral body	MVC to front or rear lateral area of the vehicle, resulting in conversion of forward motion to a spinning-type motion	Cervical spine
Axial loading	Direct force transmitted along the length of the vertebral column	› Burst and laminar fractures › Secondary edema of the spinal cord, resulting in neurologic deficits	Diver striking the head on the bottom of the pool or landing on the feet after a long fall	Cervical, thoracic, and lumbar spine

Abbreviation: MVC, motor vehicle collision.

Data from Boss, B. J., & Huether, S. E. (2014). Disorders of the central and peripheral nervous system and the neuromuscular junction. In K. L. McCance & S. E. Huether (Eds.), *Pathophysiology: The biologic basis for disease in adults and children* (7th ed., pp. 581–640). St. Louis, MO: Mosby; Jackson, A. B., Dijker, S. M., Deviv, O. M., & Poczatek, R. B. (2004). A demographic profile of new traumatic spinal cord injuries: Change and stability over 30 years. *Archives of Physical Medicine and Rehabilitation, 85*, 1740–1748; Kaji, A., & Hockberger, R. S. (2018, April 11). Spinal column injuries in adults: Definitions, mechanisms, and radiographs. *UpToDate*. Retrieved from https://www.uptodate.com/contents/spinal-column-injuries-in-adults-definitions-mechanisms-and-radiographs.

Penetrating injuries result from gunshot wounds (GSW) that cause disruption in the integrity of the vertebral column. Stab wounds do not usually cause instability of the vertebral column; however, the wounding object may damage the spinal cord and/or nerve roots.

Types of Injuries

The cervical spine is the most common site for injury because it is the area of spine with the most mobility and exposure.[7,27] An estimated 55% of spinal injuries occur to the cervical vertebrae; 15% of injuries occur to the thoracic vertebral area; and the thoracolumbar junctions and lumbosacral are each involved 15% of the time.[22] Extreme forces are required to produce fractures and dislocations in the thoracic region of the vertebral column; therefore, fractures of the thoracic vertebrae can be frequently accompanied by a SCI.[6]

Usual Concurrent Injuries

Concurrent injuries include closed head injuries, long-bone fractures, thoracic injuries, and abdominal injuries.[28] Approximately 5% of patients with brain injury have an associated spinal injury, and 25% of patients with spinal injury have some mild brain injury.[21] When a patient incurs a cervical spinal fracture, a second non-contiguous vertebral column fracture occurs 10% of the time.[22] Thoracic injuries may be associated with thoracic vertebral injuries,[3] whereas pelvic fractures are frequently associated with injuries to the lumbar spine. A fall from a height, resulting in calcaneus fracture, is an additional pattern of injury associated with compression fractures of the lumbar vertebrae.[27] Patients with SCIs often have decreased or altered sensation and/or proprioception, making it difficult to identify other potentially serious injuries.

Seat belts applied incorrectly may be associated with concurrent injuries. Serious injury to the anterior neck may be associated with the use of diagonal torso belts alone. Lumbar vertebral fractures or dislocations may result from the use of a lap belt only.[27]

Pathophysiology as a Basis for Assessment Findings

To understand a SCI, you must first understand the mechanisms that cause these injuries. When blunt force is applied to spinal tissues or their supporting structures, the effects shown in **Figure 9-6** can be anticipated.

Primary and secondary mechanisms of injury are involved in the pathophysiology of acute SCI. Both may result in neurologic dysfunction.

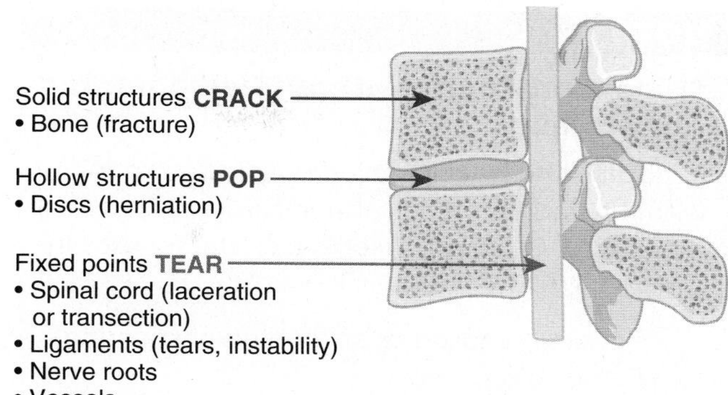

Figure 9-6 *The effects of force on spinal structures.*

Primary Injury

Primary injury refers to the initial mechanical damage to the spinal cord and includes the following conditions:

- Laceration or puncture of the cord from displaced or jagged bone fragments
- Crushed or contused disc material
- Stretching or crushing of the spinal cord
- Torn or strained ligaments
- Bleeding into the vertebral column or edema compressing spinal cord tissue
- Direct injury to the cord including the following:
    - Cord concussion: A transient dysfunction of the spinal cord lasting 24 to 48 hours. This injury may be observed in patients with preexisting degenerative disease and resultant narrowing of the vertebral foramen.[2,29]
    - Cord contusion: Bruising of the neural tissue causing edema, ischemia, and possible infarction of tissue from cord compression. The degree of neurologic deficit depends on the size, location, and local physiologic changes related to the bleeding.[1,2]
    - Cord transection: Complete disruption of the neural elements. With cord transections, all cord-mediated functions below the level of the injury are permanently lost.[1]
    - Incomplete cord transection: An interruption in the vascular perfusion to the spinal cord may result in cord ischemia or necrosis. Ischemia results in temporary deficits; prolonged ischemia results in necrosis of the spinal cord with permanent neurologic deficits.[1]

Healthcare providers' adoption of the "time is spine" concept—an approach intended to ensure rapid identification of patients sustaining acute SCI, early transfer to specialized centers, early decompressive surgery, and early delivery of other supportive treatments (e.g., BP augmentation)—has been shown to improve long-term outcomes for patients with acute SCI.[31]

> **NOTE**
>
> **Spinal Cord Injury without Radiographic Abnormality**
>
> In addition to primary injuries, spinal cord injury without radiographic abnormality (SCIWORA) may occur. Pathophysiological characteristics include the following:
>
> - Generally caused by stretching or shearing of the spinal cord
> - Most frequently seen in young children due to the immature development of their spinal structures[30]

Secondary Injury

Patients with SCI are susceptible to the same secondary injuries found in patients with traumatic brain injury (TBI). These secondary insults are set in motion by biochemical and cellular reactions causing inflammation of tissues and can lead to permanent loss of function if not corrected (**Figure 9-7**). Understanding the pathophysiology related to secondary injury is essential to implementing patient interventions to reduce the amount of cell loss, arrest the secondary injury cascade, and optimize the patient's functional outcome.

Vascular System Response (Neurogenic Shock)

Neurogenic shock occurs when damage to the spinal cord—commonly at T6 or higher—results in disruption of sympathetic innervation and the regulation of vasomotor and vagal tone, producing a loss of vascular resistance and generalized vasodilation (**Table 9-5**).[27,32] Peripheral vasodilation, reduced systemic vascular resistance, decreased venous return, decreased cardiac output, and lowered BP occur due to loss of vascular tone.[1,2,4,28] Although the patient experiences hypotension, it is not the result of a change in blood volume.[6] Instead, neurogenic shock—a form of distributive shock—causes the circulating blood volume to pool in the vasodilated peripheral vasculature with unique assessment findings. See Chapter 5, "Shock," for more information.

Assessment findings include the following:

- Bradycardia
  - Sympathetic innervation to the heart is lost.[3]
  - The body is unable to respond to hypovolemia with a tachycardic response, resulting in an unopposed parasympathetic vagal response.

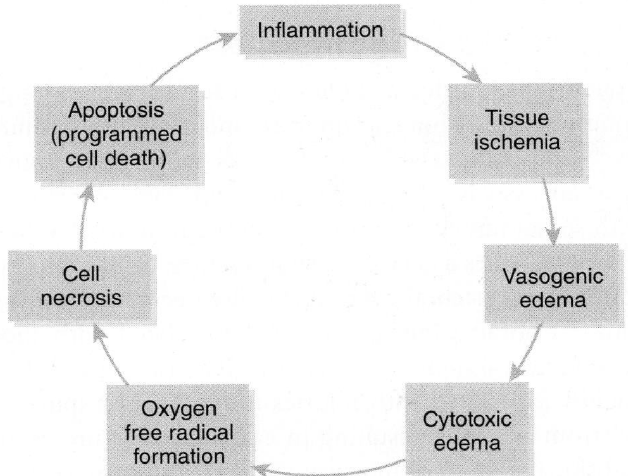

Figure 9-7 *Secondary injury cycle.*

TABLE 9-5 Neurogenic and Spinal Shock

	Neurogenic Shock	Spinal Shock
Precipitating injury	Spinal cord injury at T6 or above	Spinal cord injury at any level
Pathophysiology	Temporary loss of vasomotor tone and sympathetic innervation	Transient loss of reflex (flaccidity) below the level of injury
Duration	Temporary, often lasting less than 72 hours	Variable
Signs/symptoms	› Hypotension › Bradycardia › Loss of ability to sweat below level of injury	› Flaccidity › Loss of reflexes › Bowel and bladder dysfunction

Modified from American College of Surgeons. (2018). Spine and spinal cord trauma. In *Advanced trauma life support: Student course manual* (10th ed., pp. 128–147). Chicago, IL: Author. Data from Fox, A. D. (2014). Spinal shock: Assessment and treatment of spinal cord injuries and neurogenic shock. *Journal of Emergency Medical Services, 39*(11), 64–67.

- Hypotension
  - Loss of sympathetic innervation results in decreased catecholamine (epinephrine) production, which diminishes vasoconstriction.
  - Vasodilation yields a widened pulse pressure with a relative hypovolemia.[30]
  - The decreased cardiac output associated with bradycardia results in a reduction in blood flow and, combined with venous pooling in the periphery, results in decreased BP.
- Warm, normal skin color due to peripheral vasodilation
- Core temperature instability due to the loss of sympathetic response and inability to respond by vasodilation or vasoconstriction

Hypotension from the loss of self-regulation results in a decreased blood supply to the spinal cord, further exacerbating tissue injury. This results in loss of function, which may be either temporary (hours to days) or permanent.[3] Neurogenic shock can occur at the time of injury and, with appropriate supportive measures, usually resolves in weeks to months.[30]

Nervous System Response (Spinal Shock)

Spinal shock occurs when normal activity in the spinal cord at and below the level of the injury ceases because of a disruption or inhibition of impulses in the spinal cord (Table 9-5).[2] When the spinal cord is injured, a cascade of events takes place:

- Blood supply to the cord can be disrupted.
- Axons are severed or damaged.
- Conduction of electrical activity of neurons and axons is compromised.
- All of the above result in loss of function, which can last from several hours to several days. When patients sustain an incomplete SCI, the presence of spinal shock can delay assessment of the full extent of injury until the spinal shock has resolved.[30]

Spinal shock results in a complete loss of reflex function below the level of the injury.[2,22,27] A transient hypotensive period and poor venous circulation may be seen.[2] Disruption in the thermal control centers results in sweating and a lack of ability to regulate body temperature.[2]

Onset of spinal shock is usually immediate or occurring soon after the injury. The timing of resolution of spinal shock is not well established. One model shows spinal shock occurring in four phases, with resolution delayed up to 12 months after injury.[28] The intensity and duration of spinal shock vary with the severity and level of the lesion. The changes are most prominent at the level of the injury and in the two cord segments above and below it.[2]

Additional assessment findings include the following:

- Transient loss of muscle tone (flaccidity) and complete or incomplete paralysis may occur with loss of reflexes and sensation at or below the level of the injury.
- Bowel and bladder dysfunction are noted.
- The return of sacral reflexes, bladder tone, and the presence of hyperreflexia indicates the resolution of spinal shock.[23]
- The presence of rectal tone and intact perineal sensation indicates sacral sparing.

Immune (Inflammatory) Response

Once the spinal cord is damaged, the immune or inflammatory system is activated. The function of immune cells once they enter the damaged spinal cord is not well established.[33] Nevertheless, it is understood that the immune response includes the following effects:

- Within minutes of the injury, the endothelial cells that line the blood vessels in the spinal cord become edematous.[2,5]
- The combination of leaking, swelling, and sluggish blood flow prevents the normal delivery of oxygen and nutrients to neurons.[2,5]
- Edema in the white matter impairs cord circulation and leads to the development of ischemic areas.
- The resulting cellular ischemia may cause a temporary loss of function.

Spinal cord neurons do not regenerate; therefore, severe injury with cellular death may result in the following assessment findings:

- Temporary or permanent loss of function
- Flaccidity
- Loss of reflexes

Other Related Pathophysiologic Changes

Other pathophysiologic changes are respiratory and pain related.

Respiratory System

Respiratory system changes include the following:

- Respiratory arrest: Injury to the cord at the C3–C5 level can cause loss of phrenic nerve function, resulting in a paralyzed diaphragm and inability to breathe.

- Hypoventilation: Injury to the spinal cord between T1 and T11 may result in the loss of intercostal muscles and decreased respiratory effort. Loss of innervation from T7 to T12 may result in loss of the use of abdominal muscles for support of breathing.

Pain

The ability to perceive pain may be disrupted and result in an inadequate physical assessment.

Selected Vertebral Column and Spinal Cord Injuries

This section covers selected vertebral column and SCIs.

Spinal Cord Injuries

SCIs are classified based on the following characteristics[22]:

- Level of injury
- Severity of neurologic deficit
- Spinal cord syndromes

Level of Injury

The vertebral level is the level of vertebrae where the injury occurred. However, the neurologic injury level is determined by clinical assessment and is the lowest level that has positive sensory and motor function.[9] The vertebral level may not be the same as the neurologic level, as the spinal cord tracts are not exactly synonymous with the level of vertebrae. Level of injury usually refers to the neurologic level.

The sensory level is the point of demarcation where there is no or decreased sensation below and normal sensation above.

Severity of Neurologic Deficit

SCI can be characterized as an incomplete or complete lesion.

Incomplete Spinal Cord Lesion

Incomplete lesions are referred to as specific incomplete spinal cord syndromes (**Figure 9-8** and **Table 9-6**).[34] Comparison of motor and sensory function of bilateral upper and lower extremities is important to discern the exact cord syndrome[30]:

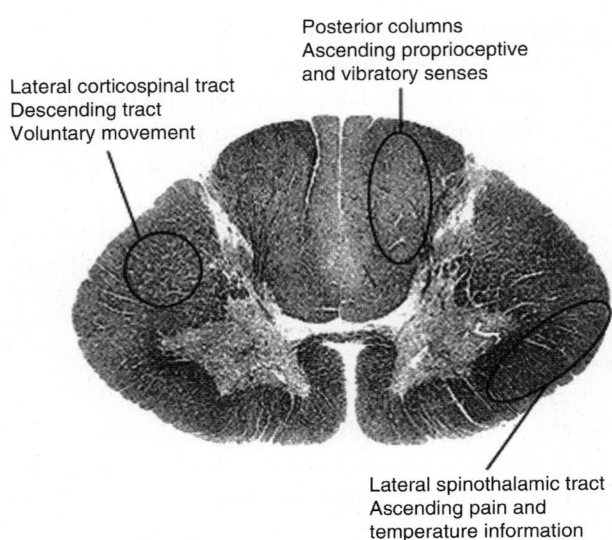

Figure 9-8 *Incomplete spinal cord syndromes.*

Courtesy John Sundsten, Digital Anatomist Project, University of Washington.

- Anterior cord syndrome
  - Also known as anterior spinal artery syndrome.
  - Mechanism of injury often involves extreme hyperflexion.
  - Caused by an injury or disruption of the anterior spinal artery (**Figure 9-9**), which supplies the anterior two-thirds of the spinal cord.
  - Complete motor loss of function below the level of the injury is caused by injury of the spinothalamic tract.
  - Loss of pain and temperature sensation occurs below the level of injury.
  - Urinary retention is present.
  - Outcomes are usually poor, with minimal recovery of function.
  - The dorsal columns remain intact, so the patient retains proprioception and vibratory sensation.
- Posterior cord syndrome (rare injury)
  - Also known as dorsal column syndrome.
  - Mechanism of injury is due to extreme hyperflexion.
  - Caused by an injury or ischemia to the posterior one-third of the spinal cord, which is usually well perfused by the posterior spinal arteries (Figure 9-9).
  - Deficits include loss of deep touch, vibration, and proprioception senses.
  - Motor and most sensory functions are generally spared.
  - Outcomes are variable with many patients experiencing difficulty walking due to the loss of proprioception.[28]
- Central cord syndrome
  - Mechanism of injury can be from hyperextension or hyperflexion. It most frequently occurs due to hyperextension.

TABLE 9-6 Spinal Cord Syndromes

Syndrome	Sensory	Motor	Sphincter Involvement
Central cord syndrome	Variable	Upper-extremity weakness, distal > proximal	Variable
Brown–Sequard syndrome	Ipsilateral position and vibration sense loss Contralateral pain and temperature sensation loss	Motor loss Ipsilateral to cord lesion	Variable
Anterior cord syndrome	Loss of pain and touch sensation Vibration, position sense preserved	Motor loss or weakness below cord level	Variable
Transverse cord syndrome—complete	Loss of sensation below level of cord injury	Loss of voluntary motor function below cord level	Sphincter control lost

Reproduced from Perron, A. D., & Huff, J. S. (2018). Spinal cord disorders. In R. M. Walls, R. S. Hockberger, & M. Gausche-Hill (Eds.), *Rosen's emergency medicine* (9th ed., pp. 1298–1306). Philadelphia, PA: Elsevier.

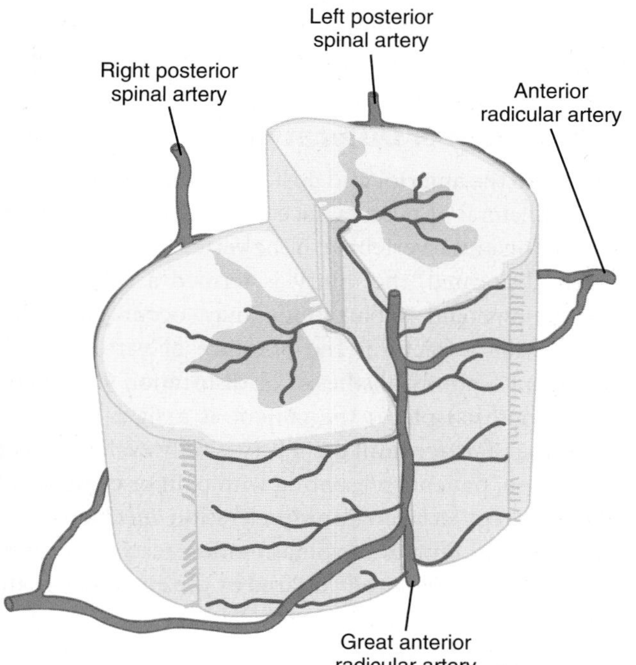

Figure 9-9 *Arterial circulation of the spinal cord.*

- Common in older adults due to chronic cervical spondylosis and often associated with a low-energy fall (e.g., fall from standing).
- Caused by edema or contusion near the center of the spinal cord that essentially squeezes the cord.
- Characterized by loss of motor and sensory function in the upper extremities that is greater than that of the lower extremities. As an example, a patient with a central cord injury might be able to walk but would not be able to use the hands or arms to open the door.
- Fine motor control in the hands is the most common loss of function.
- Outcomes can be positive for return of function as inflammation decreases around the injured cord, but the capacity to regain full function decreases with patient age.

- Brown-Sequard syndrome
  - Also known as hemicord syndrome.
  - Mechanism of injury is from penetrating trauma to the spinal cord but can be from hyperextension or disc herniation.

- Deficits are caused by a partial transection of the spinal cord.
- Classic assessment findings are intact motor function and decreased sensation on one side of the body, while experiencing decreased motor function and intact sensation on the opposite side. An example would be the patient who can pick up a hot pan with his hand but cannot feel his hand burning.
- Outcomes are mixed, but patients can experience some improvement of functioning with time and therapy.

A patient with an incomplete SCI has some sensory and/or motor function below the level of the injury. Sacral sparing is characterized by some structural integrity of the lowest sacral segments of the spinal cord at S4 and S5.[11] Sacral sparing is identified by the following findings[35]:

- Intact perianal sensation
- Voluntary anal sphincter tone
- Voluntary great toe flexor function

Note that a patient with an incomplete lesion may not exhibit sacral sparing in the presence of spinal shock. As spinal shock resolves, sacral sparing may become evident.

Complete Spinal Cord Lesion

Patients with a complete SCI lose all motor and sensory function at and below the level of the lesion. Assessment findings include the following[2,27]:

- Absent motor function below the level of the injury
- Flaccid paralysis and bilateral external rotation of the legs at the hips
- Absent sensory function below the level of the injury, such as loss of pain, touch, temperature, pressure, vibration, and proprioception
- Loss of all reflexes below the level of the injury
- Loss of ANS function
  - Hypotension, resulting in venous pooling in the extremities
  - Bradycardia
  - Poikilothermia, which causes the patient to assume the temperature of the surroundings below the level of the lesion—primarily related to the absence of sympathetic tone and the inability of the patient to shiver or sweat to regulate body temperature
  - Loss of voluntary bowel and bladder function
- Paralytic ileus with abdominal distention
- Priapism
- Respiratory depression

Vertebral Column Injuries

Vertebral column injuries are described as fractures, subluxations/dislocations, or penetrating injuries. They are further classified as stable or unstable.[22]

Atlas and Axis Fractures

The atlas vertebra, C1, and the axis vertebra, C2, provide a wide range of motion. **Table 9-7** describes four fractures and dislocations involving this region.[27,36] Almost one-third of SCIs result from excessive energy transfer to C1 and C2; such an injury can result in death.[22,35] Most fatalities involve cervical spinal injuries at the craniocervical junction, with associated subluxation or dislocation causing loss of central innervation to the phrenic nerve and resulting in apnea.[22,28] The risk of neurologic injury secondary to SCI increases with age-related degenerative changes such as rheumatoid arthritis, ankylosing spondylitis, osteoporosis, and spinal stenosis; specific mechanisms of injury; and specific locations of injury.[33,37]

Vertebral Fracture Stability

Vertebral fractures are frequently classified as stable or unstable. Spinal stability is defined as the ability of the spine to maintain its alignment and protect the neural structures during normal physiologic loads.[33,38]

The integrity of ligamentous and bony structures will dictate the stability of the vertebral column. The loss of ligamentous integrity can result in an unstable spinal injury and subsequent damage to the spinal cord or nerve roots.[33] During resuscitation, treat patients with potential SCI as though they have an unstable injury and maintain spinal motion restriction until SCI can be ruled out (Table 9-7).

Subluxation or Dislocation

Injuries to the anterior and posterior ligaments may produce unilateral or bilateral facet dislocation, resulting in dislocation of the vertebrae. If the vertebrae are not completely dislocated, the injury is termed a subluxation. Dislocations and subluxations may occur simultaneously with a fracture. The presence of vertebral displacement (spondylolisthesis) or dislocation (traumatic spondyloptosis) places the patient at a significant risk for further damage until the injury is fully evaluated. For this reason, patients presenting with pain or evidence of a high-energy acceleration/deceleration mechanism of injury should remain in spinal motion restriction until clinically or radiologically cleared by the emergency care provider.[22,23]

Vertebral Body Fractures

Vertebral fractures most often occur in the vertebral body itself or in combination with an injury to another

TABLE 9-7 C1 and C2 Fractures and Dislocations

Fracture/Dislocation	Mechanism of Injury	Description	Clinical Considerations
(C1) Atlanto-occipital dislocation	Hyperflexion with distracting injury	Dislocation of atlas from the occipital bone	› Commonly fatal › Common cause of death in abusive head trauma
(C1) Atlas fracture, burst fracture, or Jefferson fracture	Axial loading forces transmitted from occiput to spine	› Disrupts anterior and posterior rings of C1 › Lateral displacement of lateral masses › Spinal cord involvement rare	Treat as unstable until definitive evaluation
(C1) Rotary: subluxation	May occur spontaneously or with minor trauma	Persistent rotation of the head (torticollis)	› Most often seen in children › Stabilize in the rotated position
Axis (C2) fractures	Hyperextension	› Occurs in about 18% of axis fractures	› Consider transverse ligament injury
Odontoid fracture:		› Approximately 60% of C2 fractures involve the odontoid process	› Maintain cervical collar until definitive evaluation is complete
› Type I		› Involve tip of the odontoid and are relatively uncommon	
› Type II		› Occur through base of dens and are most common	
› Type III		› Occur at base of dens and extend obliquely into the body of the axis	
Posterior element fracture (hangman's fracture)		› C2 posterior elements are affected	

Data from American College of Surgeons. (2018). Spine and spinal cord trauma. In *Advanced trauma life support: Student course manual* (10th ed., pp. 128–147). Chicago, IL: Author; Davenport, M. (2017, August 18). Cervical spine fracture evaluation workup. *Medscape*. Retrieved from http://emedicine.medscape.com/article/824380-overview.

part of the vertebrae. The mobility of the cervical and lumbar regions results in an increased frequency of these injuries.[2,27]

Fractures of the transverse or spinous processes of the vertebrae are considered minor vertebral fractures, as they do not typically result in associated neurologic compromise and are considered mechanically stable. However, significant forces are required to cause these fractures, so they may be associated with other injuries.[3]

Vertebral fractures of the thoracic and lumbar spine are typically caused by high-energy trauma, and can result in spinal cord damage with neurologic deficits. However, osteoporosis can place the older adult at risk for such fractures even with low-energy trauma.

The unique anatomic and functional features of each vertebral region result in specific injuries. Greater force is required to fracture the thoracic vertebrae due to the support provided by the sternum and the ribs.[39] However, the relative immobility of the thoracic spine as compared to the flexibility of the lumbar spine can result in a fracture at the thoracolumbar junction (T11–L1), most often as a result of acute hyperflexion and rotation.[22] These injuries result in unstable fractures that are vulnerable to rotational movement; thus, great care is required when log rolling these patients.[22] See **Table 9-8** for more information.[27,40]

Nursing Care of the Patient with Spinal Cord or Vertebral Column Injuries

Nursing care of the patient with spinal cord or vertebral column injuries begins with preparation and triage.

Preparation and Triage

Preparation and triage includes safe practice, combined with safe care.

Safe Practice, Safe Care

When considering the nursing care of the trauma patient from the perspective of SCI, a vital aspect of safe care is recognizing when a vague history may indicate a mechanism for spinal injury. An unwitnessed near drowning may be a diving injury; the unconscious patient may have fallen; the unresponsive infant arriving with seizures may have suffered abusive head trauma, which can include a SCI. If the mechanism is unclear, treat these patients as though they have a SCI until they are cleared of this risk.

Triage

The patient with a suspected or confirmed SCI may warrant a high acuity rating for triage for many reasons, including alterations in vital signs from neurogenic shock, diminished respiratory effort from loss of innervation of the muscles of ventilation, and alterations in level of consciousness from concurrent head injury or changes in sensory or motor abilities.

Primary Survey and Resuscitation Adjuncts

Refer to Chapter 3, "Initial Assessment," for a systematic approach to the nursing care of the trauma patient. The following assessment parameters are specific to patients with spinal cord and vertebral column injuries.

TABLE 9-8 Thoracic Vertebral Fractures

Fracture	Mechanism of Injury	Description
Anterior compression (wedge)	› Axial loading › Flexion	› Anterior portion is rarely more than 25% shorter than the posterior body › Most are stable
Burst (comminuted)	Vertical axial compression	› Comminuted fracture of vertebral body › May result in spinal cord injury › Unstable
Chance fracture (seat belt fracture)	Hyperflexion	› Horizontal fracture lines with injury to bone and ligaments › Suspect injuries to organs in the peritoneal cavity › Certain types are unstable
Fracture–dislocation	Extreme flexion	› Disruption of the pedicles, facets and lamina of the thoracic or lumbar vertebrae › Subluxation can result in complete neurologic deficit › Unstable › Relatively uncommon

Data from American College of Surgeons. (2018). Spine and spinal cord trauma. In *Advanced trauma life support: Student course manual* (10th ed., pp. 128–147). Chicago, IL: Author; Ghobrial, G. M. (2016, February 22). Vertebral fracture. *Medscape*. Retrieved from http://emedicine.medscape.com/article/248236-overview#a0104.

A: Alertness and Airway

Cervical spinal motion restriction is always a part of the alertness and airway assessment, but nowhere else is it more important than with the patient with a strong mechanism of injury or indication for spinal injury. Patients with distracting injuries (significant blood loss, open fractures) and those with questionable intoxication or altered mental status are presumed to have sustained a vertebral injury until proven otherwise.[28]

Assessment

Assess cervical spinal motion restriction devices for correct placement and proper fit. Once motion restriction is verified, additional assessment of spinal cord integrity may be deferred until the primary survey is complete.

Intervention

Apply manual stabilization as necessary throughout the primary and secondary surveys, such as when removing the collar to examine the neck.

B: Breathing and Ventilation

Breathing is assessed and ventilation interventions are implemented as indicated.

Assessment

Shallow respirations or evidence of increased work of breathing may indicate a cervical or thoracic SCI. Cervical SCIs can impair the patient's ability to breathe due to loss of phrenic nerve function and use of the diaphragm, whereas thoracic SCIs can result in loss of function of the muscles of respiration (intercostals).

Intervention

Be prepared to support a patient with an inadequate respiratory effort with bag-mask ventilation.

C: Circulation and Control of Hemorrhage

Identify the type of shock.

Assessment

Differentiate signs of hypovolemic shock from signs of neurogenic shock:

- Neurogenic shock presents with assessment findings of impaired cardiac output accompanied by bradycardia, a normal or strong pulse, and warm or flushed skin appearance.
- Hypovolemic shock is characterized by tachycardia, a weak peripheral pulse,[22] and cool or pale skin appearance.

Intervention

Intervention considerations include the following points:

- Use care when administering intravenous fluids to the patient in neurogenic shock to avoid development of pulmonary edema.
- If there is no improvement in hypotension with fluid resuscitation, consider inotropic support.[27]

D: Disability (Neurologic Status)

Assessment

Disability or neurologic status assessment involves the following:

- Be aware that the Glasgow Coma Scale (GCS) motor response score may not be reliable in the patient with SCI. Score patient's GCS as their highest level of motor response. They may be able to shrug shoulders upon command but cannot move arms or legs due to SCI.
- Ineffective breathing from loss of innervation to diaphragm and intercostal muscles may result in anxiety.

E: Exposure and Environmental Control

Identify exposure and environmental control considerations.

- Anticipate temperature instability with neurogenic shock due to peripheral vasodilation.
- External warming measures should be utilized for patients with SCI and can include warm blankets, increased resuscitation room temperature, or external warming devices (e.g., forced-air warming blankets, warming lights). Continue to closely monitor temperature to avoid hypo- or hyperthermia due to potential for poikilothermia (inability to maintain body temperature).

G: Get Monitoring Devices and Give Comfort

Resuscitation adjuncts may include laboratory studies, monitoring, nasogastric or orogastric tubes, and oxygenation and ventilation management.

- **L: Laboratory studies.** Obtain arterial blood gas measurements to determine respiratory status and presence of ineffective gas exchange and cellular perfusion.
- **M: Monitoring.** Monitor cardiac rate/rhythm for bradycardia.
- **N: Nasogastric or orogastric tube.** Consider insertion of an orogastric tube for gastric decompression

to prevent vomiting and potential aspiration of gastric contents in patients who must remain supine in spinal stabilization.

- **O: Oxygenation and ventilation.** Consider weaning oxygen based on oximetry to avoid hyperoxia. Monitor the effectiveness of oxygenation and ventilation with continuous pulse oximetry and capnography. Use capnography for earlier identification of inadequate ventilation that might be masked due to the patient's inability to increase work of breathing.
- **P: Pain assessment and management.** Lack of pain may be a significant finding if SCI is suspected based on mechanism of injury or identified injuries.

Reevaluation

For known SCIs, early evaluation for interfacility transfer is recommended. If transfer is indicated, delegate or begin preparation before continuing to the secondary assessment. The American College of Surgeons (ACS) supports transferring the patient with a known or suspected SCI to a specialized center or trauma center.[27,41] Spinal motion restriction during transport must be ensured.

Secondary Survey

The secondary survey involves the history, head-to-toe assessment, and inspection of posterior surfaces.

H: History

Questions specific to patients with spinal or vertebral injuries include the following:

- Was there a mechanism of injury that is strongly associated with SCI?
- What symptoms were noted in the field—pain in the head or neck, numbness, tingling, loss of motor activity of the extremities, loss of bladder or bowel control? Have the symptoms changed since the patient's arrival at the emergency department (ED)?
- What medications are currently used? Will any affect the assessment parameters in the patient with SCI (changes in heart rate and BP)?
- Is there any past medical history that is significant? Does the patient have diabetic neuropathy, which may affect the central nervous system examination? Is there a history of spinal injury, stenosis, arthritis, or osteoporosis that may increase the suspicion of injury despite a minor mechanism of injury?

Documentation that reflects an accurate and thorough initial assessment and history will facilitate trending of signs and symptoms. The absence of these symptoms with subsequent development later may indicate expansion of a hematoma or edema formation.

H: Head-to-Toe Assessment

Head-to-toe assessment covers the neck and cervical spine, pelvis/perineum, and extremities.

Neck and Cervical Spine

Palpate for the following:

- Use a second person to maintain manual stabilization of the cervical spine while opening the collar for palpation.[22,27] Close the collar after assessment and confirm its proper placement.
- Gently palpate the neck for pain, tenderness, crepitus, subcutaneous emphysema, or step-off deformities between vertebrae.
- Frequently remind the patient to remain still during palpation and examination and to verbalize areas that are painful to examination and not to shake or nod the head.

Cervical Spine Clearance

The prevalence of cervical spinal injury is less than 3% following blunt trauma,[29,42,43] but a timely and accurate diagnosis is imperative in all cases where it is a possibility.[29] There remains some ambiguity around the optimal approach to diagnosing cervical spinal injury.[29,42-44] A more conservative approach to diagnose these injuries is to obtain imaging studies for all trauma patients.[29] Other guidelines recommend using a screening tool to identify those patients with a significant likelihood of clinically important cervical spinal injuries.[29,43] The appropriate screening tool is sensitive, with a low rate of false positives.[29]

Two clinical decision tools are available to assess the patient's need for cervical spine imaging following trauma: the Canadian C-Spine Rule (**Appendix 9-1**) and the National Emergency X-Radiography Utilization Study (NEXUS; **Appendix 9-2**). The aim of both tools is to reduce the unnecessary imaging.[29,33,43] A study published in the *Canadian Medical Association Journal* compared the two screening tools and found the Canadian C-Spine Rule to have better diagnostic accuracy than the NEXUS criteria.[29] The American College of Surgeons Committee on Trauma (ACS-COT) offers guidelines for cervical spinal injury screening (**Table 9-9**).[27] Research is ongoing related to clinical decision rules being utilized by specially trained emergency nurses to allow them to clinically clear cervical spines for low-risk adult patients.[23,45]

TABLE 9-9 American College of Surgeons Guidelines for Screening Patients with Suspected Spine Injury

Cervical Spine Injury

If the patient exhibits paraplegia or tetraplegia, think spinal instability.

In patients who are awake, alert, and not under the influence, and who have no neurologic abnormalities:

- If there is no presence of neck pain, midline tenderness, or distracting injury, an acute cervical spine fracture or instability is unlikely.
  - After removing the collar and performing a manual palpation of the neck, if there is no pain, and the patient is able to move the neck without pain, imaging is not necessary.
- If neck pain and midline tenderness are present, imaging is necessary. Multi-detector axial CT is recommended where available. The alternative is lateral, AP, and open-mouth odontoid radiographs of the cervical spine and axial CT of any suspicious areas or the lower cervical spine if not well visualized on radiographs. Views must include the spine down to T1.
  - If images are normal, the cervical collar can be removed. If suspicion for injury remains, replace the collar and consult a spine specialist.

In patients who have an altered level of consciousness or are nonverbal (e.g., children who cannot describe their symptoms):

- Multi-detector axial CT is recommended where available.
- The alternative is the same as above, with CT optional in children.
- If the cervical spine is normal, the cervical collar can be removed after evaluation by a physician.

When in doubt, leave the collar on.

Consult a physician skilled in evaluating and managing patients with spine injuries when spine injury is suspected or determined.

Evaluate patients with neurologic deficits (paraplegia or tetraplegia) rapidly and remove them from the spine board as soon as possible. This is most safely accomplished using the lift and slide or eight-person lift technique, as log rolling has been shown to cause unacceptable motion in an unstable spine.[13,14,17,46]

In patients who require surgery prior to the completion of a complete spine evaluation:

- Transport the patient carefully and assume an unstable spine injury is present.
- Leave the cervical collar on and use a slide sheet or other lateral transfer device and a team approach to move the patient to and from the operating table.[13]
- Remove the patient from the spine board as early as is safely possible.
- Inform the anesthesiologist and surgical team of the status of the spine evaluation.

Vertebral Column Spine Injury

Paraplegia or sensory loss at the level of the chest or abdomen may indicate spinal instability.

In patients who are awake, alert, and not under the influence, and who have no neurologic abnormalities and midline thoracic or lumbar back pain or tenderness:

- Palpate and inspect the entire spine. If no tenderness is present on palpation and no ecchymosis is noted over the spinous processes, unstable fracture is unlikely and imaging may not be necessary.

(*continues*)

TABLE 9-9 American College of Surgeons Guidelines for Screening Patients with Suspected Spine Injury *(continued)*

In patients with spine pain or tenderness on palpation or with neurologic deficits, an altered level of consciousness, or suspected intoxication: › AP and lateral radiographs are recommended. › Thin-cut axial CT is recommended if suspicious areas are seen on radiographs. › Ensure films are good quality and read by an experienced physician prior to spine clearance.
Consult a physician skilled in evaluating and managing patients with spine injuries when spine injury is suspected or determined.

Abbreviation: AP, anteroposterior; CT, computed tomography.

Data from American College of Surgeons. (2018). Spine and spinal cord trauma. In *Advanced trauma life support: Student course manual* (10th ed., pp. 128–147). Chicago, IL: Author.

Pelvis/Perineum

Assess for the presence of priapism. This may be a sign of loss of sympathetic nervous system control and stimulation of the parasympathetic nervous system.

Extremities

Inspect for the following:

- Ask the patient to wiggle the toes and fingers and to lift the arms and legs to assess extremity movement and control.
  - The inability to perform gross extremity movement indicates the possibility of a SCI at or above the level of the extremity.

Table 9-10 lists normal extremity movement with associated levels of innervation.

Palpate for the following:

- Palpate all extremities for the presence of crepitus, step-off deformity, or early development of edema.
- Palpate for skin temperature.
  - The skin is warm and dry in neurogenic shock, as opposed to cool and moist in hypovolemic shock.
  - If there is concomitant hemorrhage, the skin may become cool.
- Assess all four extremities for muscle strength.
  - Muscle strength is usually graded from 5 (normal) down to 0 (total paralysis).[22]
  - Assess muscle strength bilaterally, in the upper and lower extremities, for comparison.[27]
- Assess sensory function; loss of sensation can affect the patient's ability to identify areas of pain or fractures.
  - *Assess the patient's response to pain.* Use a pinprick to determine levels of sensory function. Begin distally and proceed proximally to aid in localizing the level of injury.[27]
  - *Assess the patient's response to pressure.* Use the head of a pin to determine response to pressure.
  - *Assess proprioception.* This can be tested by moving the great toe up, down, or in a neutral position and asking the patient to describe the position.[27]

TABLE 9-10 Assessment of Innervation Levels

Movement	Innervation
Extend and flex arms	C5 to C7
Extend and flex legs	L2 to L4
Flexion of foot; extension of toes	L4 to L5
Tighten anus	S3 to S5

I: Inspect Posterior Surfaces

If there is a suspected spinal injury, imaging should be obtained prior to inspecting the patient's posterior surfaces. The log roll may be used if needed to protect the patient's airway.[46] If there is a low index of suspicion for an unstable spine, inspect posterior surfaces by log rolling the patient to assess the vertebral column for deformity, tenderness, or open wounds, or impaled objects.

Palpate for the following:

- Palpate the entire vertebral column gently for pain, tenderness, crepitus, or step-off deformities between vertebrae.
- Assess for rectal tone

- An alternative to a digital rectal exam (DRE) is to ask the alert patient to squeeze the buttocks together.
- In the unconscious patient, palpate the anal sphincter.

- Assess for sacral sparing.
  - The presence of perianal sensation and anal sphincter tone when seen in conjunction with focal deficits represents an incomplete SCI.[28] Note, however, that perianal sensation and anal sphincter tone may be absent until the resolution of spinal shock.
- Assess for reflexes.
  - In the presence of spinal shock, the patient may present with diminished or absent reflexes. A Babinski or plantar reflex is a pathologic response in anyone age 1 year or older due to dysfunction of upper motor neurons of the corticospinal tract. See Chapter 12, "Special Populations: The Pediatric Trauma Patient," for more information.
  - Deep tendon reflexes are tested with a reflex hammer by tapping sharply on the tendon and observing for a jerk or contraction of the muscle.

Reevaluation Diagnostic Procedures

Diagnostic procedures include radiographic studies and medications.

Radiographic Studies

Anticipate a CT scan of the cervical, thoracic, and lumbar spine as indicated. If plain radiographic imaging of the cervical spine is used, verify visualization of all cervical vertebrae from the occiput through T1 including lateral, anteroposterior, and open-mouth odontoid views.[27]

Unless contraindicated, magnetic resonance imaging may be used to evaluate ligamentous and cord injuries.[4,27]

Medications

Hypotension should be treated with a cautious combination of fluid resuscitation and vasopressors. Care should be exercised to avoid overhydration in the SCI patient who is already peripherally vasodilated. Complications of excessive fluid resuscitation can include pulmonary congestion, generalized edema, and abdominal compartment syndrome.

The choice of vasopressor for the hypotensive patient with SCI depends on the level of injury. Possibilities generally include dopamine, epinephrine, norepinephrine, and phenylephrine. Dopamine, epinephrine, and norepinephrine are frequent choices for patients with cervical or high thoracic SCI due to their inotropic, chronotropic, and vasoconstrictive properties. Use of phenylephrine in these patients can worsen existing bradycardia due to its sole vasoconstrictive nature. For patients with a low thoracic SCI with hypotension due primarily to peripheral vasodilation, norepinephrine and phenylephrine work well by providing powerful vasoconstrictive effects.[7]

Administer pain management medications as indicated.

Reevaluation and Post-Resuscitation Care

Reevaluation includes trending of neuromuscular status, maintaining homeostasis, and further reevaluation to determine the type and degree of injury. Key points include the following:

- Maintain spinal motion restriction.
- Monitor breathing effectiveness. Patients with disruption of the innervation to the intercostal muscles develop respiratory fatigue and must be monitored closely.
- Monitor changes in sensory and motor function.
- Monitor core temperature to avoid hypothermia.

Definitive Care or Transport

If the decision has not already been made, reassess the patient and prepare for interfacility transfer as needed. Careful attention is given to spinal motion restriction during transport as well as serial assessments for changes in condition.[27]

Emerging Trends

As the science and evidence of trauma care continue to evolve, tools to improve patient outcomes continue to be trialed and refined. Evidence is tested and replicated, and new standards of care are transitioned into practice. This section on trauma care considerations explores some of the evidence and the potential significance to trauma patient care. In the care of patients with spinal cord and vertebral column injuries, evidence related to cervical spinal clearance, stem cell research, and hypothermia for SCIs is discussed.

Stem Cell Research

Stem cells are unspecialized cells capable of regenerating or proliferating through cell division and can be induced to become tissue- or organ-specific cells; they are very proliferative.[21] In contrast, nerve cells do not usually repair, duplicate, or replicate.[21] Demyelination has been documented as a secondary degenerative component of SCIs; however, few studies in humans have explored the exact consequences of this phenomenon for rehabilitation of patients with SCI.[38,47] Chronic demyelination has been observed in the human spinal cord following SCI, suggesting that demyelination contributes to functional disabilities.[48-50] The use of neural stem cells to promote remyelination of nerve cells appears to be promising based on these cells' ability to promote axonal regeneration through development of a foundation for growing axons in the area of ischemia and/or injury.[21,48,49] Stem cell research in patients with SCI is ongoing. Currently, multiple types of cells are used in stem cell research; not all types of cells will have the same effects.[47] Identification of the approach that will have maximal benefit in SCI has yet to occur.[48,49]

Hypothermia

Therapeutic hypothermia remains an experimental clinical approach; however, research and randomized trials are continuing to evaluate therapeutic interventions using this approach. The use of hypothermia in the treatment of SCIs has demonstrated beneficial effects in reducing localized edema and ischemic changes. However, additional research is needed to provide conclusive evidence for the efficacy of its use. Several clinical studies using animal models have shown the use of therapeutic hypothermia to be promising in patients with severe cervical SCI.[29,51-53] Moderate hypothermia (33°C [91.4°F]). introduced systemically by intravascular cooling strategies has been shown to be safe and provides some improvements in long-term recovery of function.[29,51-53]

Spinal Motion Restriction

Prehospital providers have traditionally used longboards when patients have sustained a mechanism of injury forceful enough to have possibly damaged the spinal cord. However, the level of evidence for this practice is considered weak (Level III).[50] Longboard use is associated with clinical complications, with pain being a common complaint. Other potential problems include mild respiratory compromise; pressure ulcers, which can begin forming within 30 minutes of placement on the board; increased intracranial pressure; and, in rare cases, the distracting of an unstable fracture.[49]

A joint position statement from the ACS-COT, the American College of Emergency Physicians, and the National Association of EMS Physicians recommends use of a long backboard, scoop stretcher, vacuum mattress, or ambulance cot for extrication and transfer only. EMS systems and hospitals are advised to remove patients expeditiously from these transfer devices as soon as possible. Spinal motion restriction is maintained with a rigid cervical collar and keeping the head, neck, and torso in alignment on a stretcher. Indications for spinal motion restriction in blunt trauma include an altered level of consciousness, pain or deformity to the spine, focal neurologic deficits, or distracting circumstances. Spinal motion restriction is not indicated in patients with penetrating trauma.[55]

Summary

Blunt and penetrating injuries to the bony vertebral column may result in fractures, subluxations, or dislocations of the vertebral column. Knowledge of the pattern of injury—including the type of forces applied to the vertebral column and the resulting flexion, extension, rotation, or compression/axial loading—is important during the assessment of the trauma patient.

Although many studies are currently examining the ischemic damage to the spinal cord and regeneration of the myelinated nerve fibers, there is no substitution for the initiation and maintenance of spinal motion restriction and good skin care in the ED.

The Canadian C-Spine Rule and the National Emergency X-Radiography Utilization Study created criteria for clearing patients at low risk for unstable fractures or ligamentous injury to reduce unnecessary imaging in this population. Each institution may have its own policies guiding cervical spine clearance, but the examples in Appendices 9-1 and 9-2 are provided for reference. Please refer to your institution's policies.

References

1. Mtui, E., Gruener, G., & Dockery, P. (2016). Midbrain, hindbrain, spinal cord. In E. Mtui, G. Gruener, & P. Dockery, *Clinical neuroanatomy and neuroscience* (7th ed., pp. 26–39). Kidlington, UK: Elsevier.
2. Sugerman, R. A. (2014). Structure and function of the neurologic system. In K. L. McCance, S. E. Huether.,V. L. Brashers, & N. S. Rote (Eds.), *Pathophysiology: The biologic basis for disease* (7th ed., pp. 447–483). St. Louis, MO: Mosby/Elsevier.
3. Russo, T. (2008). Spinal cord injuries. In K. A. McQuillan, M. B. Makic, & E. Whalen, *Trauma nursing: From resuscitation through rehabilitation* (4th ed., pp. 565–613). St Louis, MO: Saunders/Elsevier.
4. VanPutte, C., Regan, J., Russo, A., Seeley, R. R., Stephens, T., & Tate, P. (2016). *Seeley's anatomy and physiology* (11th ed.). Boston, MA: McGraw-Hill.
5. Waxman, S. (2010). *Correlative neuroanatomy.* New York, NY: McGraw-Hill.
6. Banasik, J. (2013). Structure and function of the nervous system. In L. Copstead & J. Banasik, *Pathophysiology* (5th ed., pp. 857–897). St. Louis, MO: Saunders/Elsevier.

7. Schuster, J., & Piazza, M. (2016). How should acute spinal cord injury be managed in the ICU? In C. S. Deutschman & P. J. Neligan, *Evidence-based practice of critical care* (pp. 583–591). St. Louis, MO: Elsevier.
8. Tortora, G., & Derrickson, B. (2017). The spinal cord and spinal nerves. In *Principles of anatomy and physiology* (15th ed., pp. 446–476). New York, NY: Wiley.
9. McGee, S. (2012). Examination of the sensory system. In *Evidence-based physical diagnosis* (3rd ed., pp. 567–580). Philadelphia, PA: Elsevier.
10. Tortora, G., & Derrickson, B. (2017). Nervous tissue. In *Principles of anatomy and physiology* (15th ed., pp. 403–445). New York, NY: Wiley.
11. Tortora, G., & Derrickson, B. (2017). The skeletal system: The axial skeleton. In *Principles of anatomy and physiology* (15th ed., pp. 194–233). New York, NY: Wiley.
12. Prasarn, M., Horodyski, M., Dubose, D., Small, J., Del Rossi, G., Zhou, H., . . . Rechtine, G. (2012). Total motion generated in the unstable cervical spine during management of the typical trauma patient: A comparison of methods in a cadaver model. *Spine, 37*(11), 937–942. https://doi.org/10.1097/BRS.0b013e31823765af
13. Prasarn, M. L., Horodyski, M., DiPaola, M., DiPaola, C., Del Rossi, G., Conrad, B. P., & Rechtine, G. R. (2015). Controlled laboratory comparison study of motion with football equipment in a destabilized cervical spine. *Orthopaedic Journal of Sports Medicine, 3*(9), 1–5.
14. Conrad, B., Del Rossi, G., Horodyski, M., Prasarn, M., Alemi, Y., & Rechtine, G. (2012). Eliminating log rolling as a spine trauma order. *Surgical Neurology International, 3,* S188–S197. https://doi.org/10.4103/2152-7806.98584
15. Conrad, B. P., Marchese, D. L., Rechtine, G. R., & Horodyski, M. (2012). Motion in the unstable thoracolumbar spine when spine boarding a prone patient. *Journal of Spinal Cord Medicine, 35*(1), 53–57. https://doi.org/10.1179/2045772311Y.0000000045
16. Del Rossi, G., Horodyski, M., Conrad, B., DiPaola, C., DiPaola, M., & Rechtine, G. (2008). Transferring patients with thoracolumbar spinal instability: Are there alternatives to the log roll maneuver? *Spine, 33*(14), 1611–1615.
17. Horodyski, M., Conrad, B., Del Rossi, G., DiPaola, C., & Rechtine, G., II. (2011). Removing a patient from the spine board: Is the lift and slide safer than the log roll? *Journal of Trauma: Injury, Infection, and Critical Care, 70*(5), 1282–1285.
18. Leech, C., Porter, K., & Bosanko, C. (2014). Log-rolling a blunt major trauma patient is inappropriate in the primary survey. *Emergency Medicine Journal, 31*(1), 86. https://doi.org/10.1136/emermed-2013-203283
19. Kornhall, D. K., Jørgensen, J. J., Brommeland, T., Hyldmo, P. K., Asbjørnsen, H., Dolven, T., . . . Jeppesen, E. (2017). The Norwegian guidelines for the prehospital management of adult trauma patients with potential spinal injury. *Scandinavian Journal of Trauma, Resuscitation, and Emergency Medicine, 25*(2). https://doi.org/10.1186/s13049-016-0345-x
20. Chen, Y., He, Y., & Devivo, M. J. (2016). Changing demographics and injury profile of new traumatic spinal cord injuries in the United States, 1972–2014. *Archives of Physical Medicine and Rehabilitation, 97,* 1610–1619. https://doi.org/10.1016/j.apmr.2016.03.017
21. National Institutes of Health. (2018, August 27). Stem cell information. Retrieved from https://stemcells.nih.gov/info/basics.htm
22. National Spinal Cord Injury Statistical Center. (2015). Recent trends in causes of spinal cord injury: 2015 SCI data sheet. Retrieved from https://www.nscisc.uab.edu/PublicDocuments/fact_sheets/Recent%20trends%20in%20causes%20of%20SCI.pdf
23. Smith, N., & Curtis, K. (2016). Can emergency nurses safely and accurately remove cervical spine collars in low risk adult trauma patients: An integrative review. *Australian Emergency Care, 19*(2), 63–74. https://doi.org/10.1016/j.aenj.2016.01.003
24. Boss, B. J., & Huether, S. E. (2014). Disorders of the central and peripheral nervous system and the neuromuscular junction. In K. L. McCance & S. E. Huether (Eds.), *Pathophysiology: The biologic basis for disease in adults and children* (7th ed., pp. 581–640). St. Louis, MO: Mosby.
25. Jackson, A. B., Dijker, S. M., Deviv, O. M., & Poczatek, R. B. (2004). A demographic profile of new traumatic spinal cord injuries: Change and stability over 30 years. *Archives of Physical Medicine and Rehabilitation, 85,* 1740–1748.
26. Kaji, A., & Hockberger, R. S. (2018, April 11). Spinal column injuries in adults: Definitions, mechanisms, and radiographs. *UpToDate.* Retrieved from https://www.uptodate.com/contents/spinal-column-injuries-in-adults-definitions-mechanisms-and-radiographs
27. American College of Surgeons. (2018). Spine and spinal cord trauma. In *Advanced trauma life support: Student course manual* (10th ed., pp. 128–147). Chicago, IL: Author.
28. Stahel, P. F., & VanderHeiden, T. (2017). Spinal injuries. In E. E. Moore, D. V. Feliciano, & K. L. Mattox (Eds.), *Trauma* (8th ed., pp. 455–472). New York, NY: McGraw-Hill.
29. Michaleff, Z., Maher, C., Verhagen, A., Rebbeck, T., & Lin, C. (2012). Accuracy of the Canadian C-Spine Rule and NEXXUS to screen for clinically important cervical spine injury in patients following blunt trauma: A systematic review. *Canadian Medical Association Journal, 184*(16), E867–E876. https://doi.org/10.1503/cmaj.120675
30. Criddle, L. M. (2017). Spine and spinal cord injuries. In L. M. Criddle, A. Bellows, J. Fritzeen, T. Goodell, E. Harvey, M. Lanford, . . . C. Wraa (Eds.), *TCAR trauma care after resuscitation* (pp. 147–161). Scappose, OR: TCAR Education Programs.
31. Hachem, L. A. (2017, November). Assessment and management of acute spinal cord injury: From point of injury to rehabilitation. *Journal of Spinal Cord Medicine, 40*(6), 665–675. https://doi.org/10.1080/10790268.2017.1329076
32. Fox, A. D. (2014). Spinal shock: Assessment and treatment of spinal cord injuries and neurogenic shock. *Journal of Emergency Medical Services, 39*(11), 64–67.
33. Kaji, A. H., & Hockberger, R. S. (2018). Spinal injuries. In J. Marx, R. Hockberger, & R. M. Walls (Eds.), *Rosen's emergency medicine: Concepts and clinical practice* (8th ed., Vol. 1, pp. 345–371). Philadelphia, PA: Elsevier/Saunders.

34. Perron, A. D., & Huff, J. S. (2018). Spinal cord disorders. In R. M. Walls, R. S. Hockberger, & M. Gausche-Hill (Eds.), *Rosen's emergency medicine* (9th ed., pp. 1298–1306). Philadelphia, PA: Elsevier.
35. Zhang, S., Wadhwa, R., Haydel, J., Toms, J., Johnson, K., & Guthikonda, B. (2013). Spine and spinal cord trauma: Diagnosis and management. *Neurologic Clinics, 31*(1), 183–206. https://doi.org/10.1016/j.ncl.2012.09.012
36. Davenport, M. (2017, August 18). Cervical spine fracture evaluation workup. *Medscape*. Retrieved from http://emedicine.medscape.com/article/824380-overview
37. Weber, T. (2016). Approach to the patient with metabolic bone disease. In L. Goldman & A. Schafer, *Goldman Cecil medicine* (pp. 1636–1637). New York, NY: Saunders/Elsevier.
38. Khurana, B., Sheehan, S., Sodickson, A., Bono, C., & Harris, M. (2013). Traumatic thoracolumbar spine injuries: What the spine surgeon wants to know. *RadioGraphics, 33*(7), 2031–2046. https://doi.org/10.1148/rg.337135018
39. Wilbeck, J. (2010). Spinal trauma. In P. Howard & R. Steinmann (Eds.), *Sheehy's emergency nursing principles and practice* (6th ed., pp. 272–284). St. Louis, MO: Mosby.
40. Ghobrial, G. M. (2016, February 22). Vertebral fracture. *Medscape*. Retrieved from http://emedicine.medscape.com/article/248236-overview#a0104
41. American College of Surgeons, Committee on Trauma. (2018). *Resources for the optimal care of the injured patient.* Chicago, IL: American College of Surgeons.
42. Barbano, R. (2016). Mechanical and other lesions of the spine, nerve roots, and spinal cord. In L. Goldman & A. Schafer, *Goldman-Cecil medicine* (25th ed., Vol. 2, pp. 2370–2382). Philadelphia, PA: Elsevier Saunders.
43. Como, J. J., Diaz, J. J., Dunham, M., Chiu, W. C., Duane, T. M., Capella, J. M., . . . Winston, E. S. (2009). Practice management guidelines for identification of cervical spine injuries following trauma: Update from the Eastern Association for the Surgery of Trauma Practice Management Guidelines Committee. *Journal of Trauma Injury, Infection, and Critical Care, 67*(3), 651–659. https://doi.org/10.1097/TA.0b013e3181ae583b
44. Rose, M., Rosal, L., Gonzalez, R., Rostas, J., Baker, J., Simmons, J., . . . Brevard, S. (2012). Clinical clearance of the cervical spine in patients with distracting injuries: It is time to dispel the myth. *Journal of Trauma and Acute Care Surgery, 73*(2), 498–502. https://doi.org/10.1097/TA.0b013e3182587634
45. Clement, C., Stiell, I., Davies, B., O'Connor, A., Brehaut, J., Sheehan, P., . . . Beland, C. (2011). Perceived facilitators and barriers to clinical clearance of the cervical spine by emergency department nurses: A major step towards changing practice in the emergency department. *International Emergency Nursing, 19*(1), 44–52. https://doi.org/10.1016/j.ienj.2009.12.002
46. Emergency Nurses Association. (2016). *ENA topic brief: Avoiding the log roll maneuver: Alternative methods for safe patient handling.* Des Plaines, IL: Author. Retrieved from https://www.ena.org/docs/default-source/resource-library/practice-resources/topic-briefs/avoiding-the-log-roll-maneuver.pdf?sfvrsn=78887c44_8
47. Kim, B., Hwang, D., Lee, S., Kim, E., & Kim, S. (2007). Stem cell-based cell therapy for spinal cord injury. *Cell Transplantation, 16*, 355–364.
48. Antonic, A., Sena, E., Lees, J., Wills, T., Skeers, P., Batchelor, P., . . . Howell, D. (2013). Stem cell transplantation in traumatic spinal cord injury: A systematic review and meta-analysis of animal studies. *PLoS Biology*. https://doi.org/10.1371/journal.pbio.1001738
49. Li, J., & Lepski, G. (2013). Cell transplant for spinal cord injury: A systematic review. *BioMed Research International*, 786475. https://doi.org/10.1155/2013/786475
50. Watson, R., & Yeung, T. (2011). What is the potential of oligodendrocyte progenitor cells to successfully treat human spinal cord injury? *BMC Neurology, 11*(113), 1–9. https://doi.org/10.1186/1471-2377-11-113
51. Ahmad, F., Wang, M., & Levi, A. (2014). Hypothermia for acute spinal cord injury: A review. *World Neurosurgery, 82*(1-2), 207–214. https://doi.org/10.1016/j.wneu.2013.01.008
52. Dietrich, W., Levi, A., Wang, M., & Green, B. (2011). Hypothermic treatment for acute spinal cord injury. *Neurotherapeutics, 8*(229). https://doi.org/10.1007/s13311-011-0035-3
53. Maybhate, A., Hu, C., Bazley, F., Qilu, Y., Thakor, N., Kerr, C., & All, A. (2012). Potential long term benefits of acute hypothermia after spinal cord injury: Assessments with somatosensory evoked potentials. *Critical Care Medicine, 40*(2), 573–579. https://doi.org/10.1097/CCM.0b013e318232d97e
54. Morrissey, J. F., Kusel, E. R., & Sporer, K. A. (2014). Spinal motion restriction: An educational and implementation program to redefine prehospital spinal assessment and care. *Prehospital Emergency Care, 18*(3), 429–432. https://doi.org/10.3109/10903127.2013.869643
55. Fischer, P. E., Perina, D. G., Delbridge, T. R., Fallat, M. E, Salomone, J. P., Dodd, J., . . . Gestring, M. L. (2018). Spinal motion restriction in the trauma patient: A joint position statement. *Prehospital Emergency Care*. https://doi.org/10.1080/10903127.2018.1481476

APPENDIX 9-1

Clearing the Cervical Spine

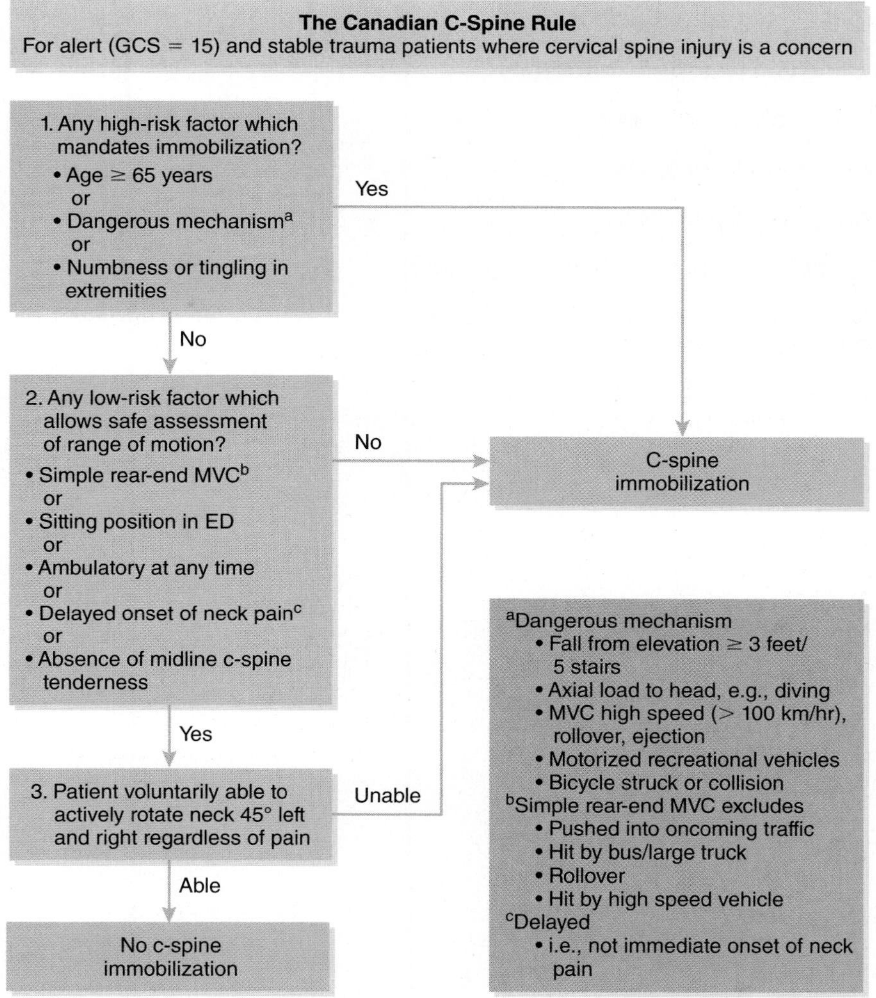

Abbreviations: ED, emergency department; GCS, Glasgow Coma Scale; MVC, motor vehicle collision.

Reproduced from Clement, C. M., Stiell, I. G., Davies, B., O'Connor, A., Brehaut, J. C., Sheehan, P., . . . Beland, C. (2011). Perceived facilitators and barriers to clinical clearance of the cervical spine by emergency department nurses: A major step towards changing practice in the emergency department. *International Emergency Nursing, 19*, 44–52.

APPENDIX 9-2

The NEXUS Criteria for Cervical Spine Clearance

Criteria
› No posterior midline cervical spine tenderness is present
› No evidence of intoxication is present
› The patient has a normal level of alertness
› No focal neurologic deficit is present
› The patient does not have a painful distracting injury

Data from Davenport, M. (2017, August 18). Cervical spine fracture evaluation workup. *Medscape*. Retrieved from http://emedicine.medscape.com/article/824380-workup.

CHAPTER 10

Musculoskeletal Trauma

Kristen M. Cline, BSN, RN, CEN, CPEN, TCRN, CFRN, CTRN, CCRN

OBJECTIVES

Upon completion of this chapter, the learner will be able to:

1. Describe the mechanisms of injury associated with musculoskeletal trauma.
2. Describe pathophysiologic changes as a basis for assessment of the trauma patient with musculoskeletal injuries.
3. Demonstrate the nursing assessment of the trauma patient with musculoskeletal injuries.
4. Plan appropriate interventions for the trauma patient with musculoskeletal injuries.
5. Evaluate the effectiveness of nursing interventions for the trauma patient with musculoskeletal injuries.

Knowledge of normal anatomy and physiology serves as a foundation for understanding anatomic derangements and pathophysiologic processes that may result from trauma. Before reading this chapter, it is strongly suggested that the learner review the following material. This material is not emphasized in the classroom, but rather serves as foundational content. In turn, it may be the basis for some test questions and skill evaluation steps.

Anatomy and Physiology of Musculoskeletal System

The musculoskeletal system provides support, protection, and functional movement to the human body. The system includes bones; joints integrated with tendons, ligaments, cartilage, vessels, and nerves; and muscle. Bones store minerals and lipids and produce blood cells in the red marrow.[1]

Bones and Supporting Structures

Bones are composed of several different types of tissue: cartilage, dense connective tissue, epithelium, adipose tissue, and nervous tissue.[2]

- *Cartilage* is a matrix of cells capable of trapping water, which allows the cartilage to rebound after being compressed, providing strength. Following bones, cartilage is the firmest structure in the body.
- *Dense connective tissue* includes protein fibers that form thick bundles of collagen fibers for structures such as tendons and ligaments. Tendons connect muscles to bones, and ligaments connect bones to bones.

- *Epithelial tissue* covers and protects deeper tissue surfaces.
- *Adipose tissue* contains lipids and functions to insulate, store energy, and protect against injury.
- *Nervous tissue* is characterized by its ability to conduct electrical signals.

The two primary types of bone tissues are compact and spongy (cancellous). *Compact bone* is the strongest form of bone tissue. It is dense and more rigid than cancellous bone and forms the shaft of long bones and the exterior covering of other bones. *Cancellous bone* is located in the interior of the bones, and the macroscopic spaces between its lattice-like columns help make bone lighter. Cancellous tissue is located along stress lines and aids in the bone's resistance to stress without breaking. The cancellous tissue found in the hips, vertebrae, ribs, sternum, and ends of long bones is the storage center for red bone marrow and the location of the bone's blood cell production in adults.[3]

Classification of Bones

The adult human body contains 206 bones; however, infants and children have more bones because some fuse together as the body develops. Most bones can be classified into five categories: long, short, flat, irregular, and sesamoid.[4]

- *Long bones* have greater length than width and have a slight curve for strength. Compact bone tissue composes the shaft of long bones. Long bones include the femur, tibia, fibula, humerus, radius, and ulna.
- *Short bones* are more cube-shaped and consist of cancellous bone except at the surface, which has a thin layer of compact bone. Carpal and tarsal bones are classified as short bones.
- *Flat bones* are usually thin and have a surface of compact bone surrounding a layer of cancellous bone. The cranial bones, the sternum, and the ribs are flat bones.
- *Irregular bones* are complex-shaped bones; the vertebrae, hip bones, and some facial bones are irregular bones.
- *Sesamoid bones* are small bones that develop in tendons for protection from excessive wear. The largest sesamoid bone is the patella.[5]

Structure of Bone

The structural components of long bones (**Figure 10-1**) are as follows:

- Epiphysis: The distal and proximal ends of the bone.
- Epiphyseal plate: A layer of cartilage that allows for bone growth and ossifies when growth stops after puberty and adolescence.[6]

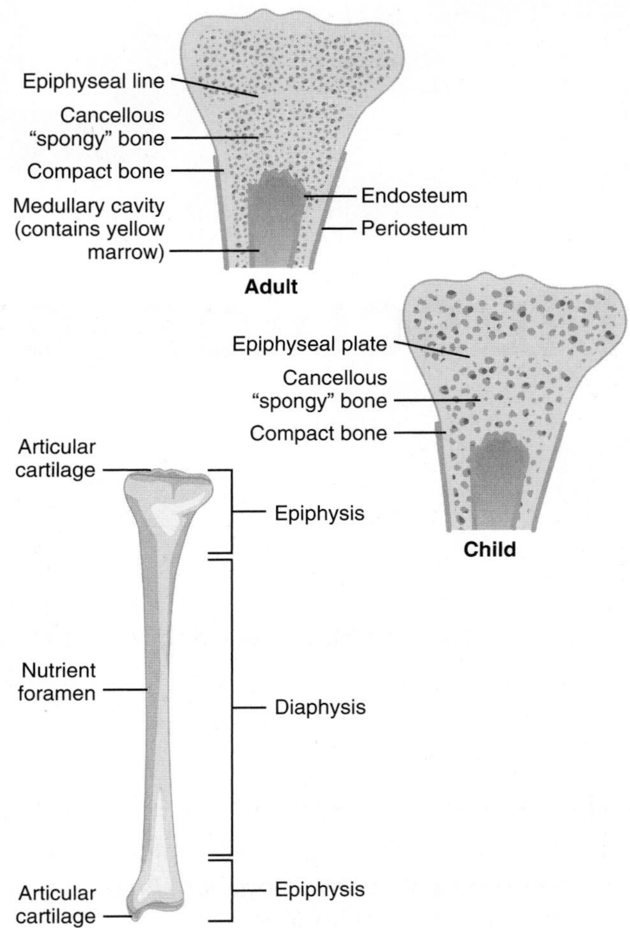

Figure 10-1 *Structural components of long bones.*

- Diaphysis: The main portion of the bone.
- Articular cartilage: A thin layer of cartilage that covers the epiphysis where a bone forms a joint with another bone.
- Periosteum: The connective tissue that covers the bone except at articular surfaces.
- Medullary cavity: The space within the diaphysis that contains yellow bone marrow in adults.[1]

Joints, Tendons, and Ligaments

Joints are classified into three types: synovial, cartilaginous, and fibrous.

- *Synovial joints* have a fluid-filled synovial cavity, and the bones are held together with connective tissue and ligaments. Synovial joints allow free movement and are located at the knee, elbow, and hip.
- *Cartilaginous joints* have no synovial cavity, and cartilage holds the bones together. Cartilaginous joints allow little or no movement and are found at the sternum and vertebra.

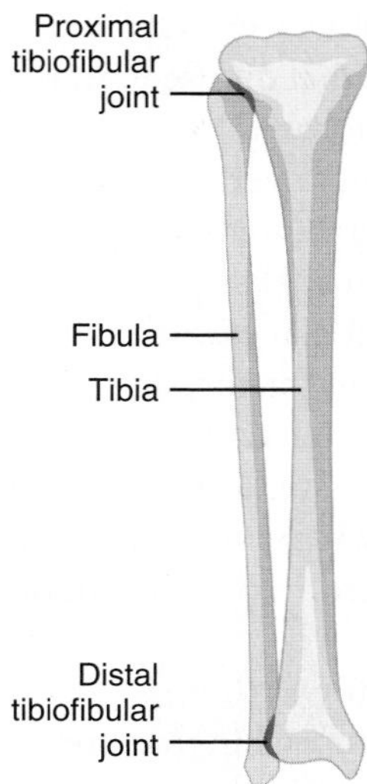

Figure 10-2 *The tibiofibular joint: an example of a fibrous joint.*

- *Fibrous joints* have no synovial cavity, and fibrous connective tissue holds the bones together (**Figure 10-2**). They allow little or no movement and are found in the skull, tibia, and fibula.

Other structures support the musculoskeletal system, including tendons, ligaments, and skeletal muscle.

- *Tendons* are cords of dense tissue that attach muscles to bones and control movement of the extremity by extension or flexion of the muscle groups. The tendon pulls the distal bone in the direction of the muscle group movement.
- *Ligaments* are fibrous capsules that are arranged in parallel bundles of dense connective tissue and are highly resistant to strains. In joints, bones are held together primarily through the strength of ligaments.
- *Skeletal muscle* has striations of dark and light bands containing connective tissues, which surround muscle fibers, blood vessels, and nerves. Skeletal muscle attaches to bone by fibrous connective tissue or tendons.

Blood and Nerve Supply

Bone is highly vascular. Periosteal arteries supply blood to the periosteum and outer part of compact bones, and metaphyseal arteries supply blood to the bone marrow of long bones. Veins are located in the diaphysis, the epiphysis, and the periosteum. The metaphyseal and epiphyseal arteries supply blood to red bone marrow and bone tissue.[3]

Bone is also highly innervated. In particular, the periosteum contains many sensory nerves that carry pain sensations. These nerves are sensitive to tearing or tension that can result in severe pain with fracture.

Introduction

This chapter focuses on musculoskeletal trauma of the extremities. For other selected injuries of the musculoskeletal system, refer to Chapter 8, "Abdominal and Pelvic Trauma," and Chapter 9, "Spinal Trauma." Soft tissue injuries are addressed in Chapter 11, "Surface and Burn Trauma."

Epidemiology

According to the National Hospital Medical Survey 2015, musculoskeletal system diagnoses account for 7.2% of all problems treated in U.S. emergency departments (EDs). Injury and poisoning complaints account for approximately 20% of all ED visits; of these complaints, fractures, sprains, and strains are the most common reason for seeking emergency care.[7]

Mechanisms of Injury

Musculoskeletal trauma can cause single-system or multisystem injuries, which have higher acuity when hemodynamic or neurovascular compromise is present. Injury mechanisms include falls, motor vehicle collisions (MVCs), assaults, sports activities, and home- and work-related activities. Falls are the leading cause of musculoskeletal injury in all age groups except teens and young adults. Falls are the leading cause of injury-related death after age 72 years.[8,9] See Chapter 13, "Special Populations: The Geriatric Trauma Patient," for more information.

Fall Risk

Comorbidities increase the likelihood of poor healing and complications from falls. Specific medications, such as antiplatelet agents and anticoagulants, are associated with a higher incidence of traumatic brain injury in addition to the musculoskeletal injury sustained.[10] Therefore, it is important to evaluate the event that may have precipitated the fall. Consider if the fall was the result of the following:

- A mechanical event (trip or slip)
- A comorbid event (cerebral vascular incident, hypoglycemia, orthostatic hypotension, syncope, myocardial infarction)
- Medication use
- Alcohol use

Drinking two to four alcoholic beverages daily can decrease bone mass and bone mineral density and increase

TABLE 10-1 Classification of Musculoskeletal Injuries

Injury Type	Description
Fracture	Disruption in the continuity of a bone
Dislocation	Ends of two or more bones that make up a joint are forced from their normal position
Amputation	Removal of all or part of a limb
Sprain	Stretch or tear to a ligament
Strain	Stretch or tear to a tendon or muscle
Subluxation	Partial dislocation of two or more bones that make up a joint
Contusion	Area of broken capillaries or venules beneath the skin with extravasation of blood
Avulsion	Tissue is torn away or separated
Crush	Tissue is compressed between two hard surfaces and damaged
Mangled	Injury to three or more systems in a limb (soft tissue, bone, nerve, vascular)

fall risk, including the potential for fractures of the forearm, spine, iliac crest, and greater trochanter.[11]

Types of Injuries

The extremities are the most common site of traumatic injuries.[12] Injuries may involve bone, soft tissue, muscles, nerves, tendons, blood vessels, and joint spaces. Musculoskeletal injuries include fractures, dislocations, amputations, sprains, strains, penetrating injuries, ligament tears, tendon lacerations, and neurovascular compromise. **Table 10-1** provides definitions of these injuries.

Common mechanisms and their associated injuries include the following:

- Falling onto outstretched hands (FOOSH)
  - Colles fracture (distal radius)
  - Scaphoid fracture
  - Monteggia fracture–dislocation (ulnar shaft fracture with radial head dislocation)
  - Galeazzi fracture–dislocation (distal radial fracture with a distal ulnar epiphyseal fracture)
- Jumps/falls with a feet-first landing involve axial loading forces that diffuse upward ("lover's leap" or "Don Juan syndrome")
  - Thoracolumbar vertebral compression fractures
  - Calcaneus fractures (can distract from other injuries due to intense pain)
  - Pelvic/acetabular fractures
  - Tibial plateau fractures
  - Wrist/forearm fractures
- High-impact trauma (passenger-compartment intrusion or when unrestrained occupant is thrown forward into the dashboard of the vehicle)
  - Patella fractures
  - Femur fractures, hip fractures and dislocations, and popliteal artery damage—commonly associated with knee trauma[13]
- Pedestrian-versus-vehicle injuries
  - Bilateral tibia–fibula fractures
  - If the pedestrian is struck by a larger vehicle (sport-utility vehicle, van, or truck), suspect pelvic injuries[14]

Concurrent Injuries

Musculoskeletal injuries can be predictors of concurrent injuries, so knowledge of concurrent injury patterns can help the trauma nurse identify and properly assess for primary and concurrent injuries. In the presence of an open fracture, there is a 70% incidence of associated nonskeletal injury.[15] **Table 10-2** describes injuries associated with musculoskeletal trauma.[15]

Pathophysiology as a Basis for Assessment Findings

The abnormalities seen in patients with musculoskeletal trauma are a result of hemorrhage and disruption of musculoskeletal integrity.

Hypotension

Musculoskeletal trauma can result in large-volume hemorrhage, which is the leading cause of preventable death in trauma.[12,15] Fractures of the femoral shaft resulting from high-energy forces are often associated with other injuries and open wounds. Patients with femur fractures can lose as much as 2 or 3 units of blood as a result of the injury, which can be life threatening.[16]

Alterations in Neurovascular Exam

Musculoskeletal injuries disrupt capillaries and cellular membranes. Hemorrhage in the area surrounding

TABLE 10-2 Injuries Associated with Musculoskeletal Injuries

Injury	Missed or Associated Injury
Clavicular or scapular fracture Fracture and/or dislocation of the shoulder	› Major thoracic injury, especially pulmonary contusion, rib fracture, and great vessel injury
Fracture/dislocation of the elbow	› Brachial artery injury › Median, ulnar, and radial nerve injury
Femur fracture	› Femoral neck fracture › Posterior hip dislocation
Knee dislocation or displaced tibial plateau fracture	› Popliteal artery and nerve injuries
Calcaneal fracture	› Spine injury or fracture › Fracture–dislocation of hindfoot › Tibial plateau fracture
Open fracture	› Associated nonskeletal injury

the injury may be visible or occult. As arterial blood flow becomes obstructed, tissue oxygenation decreases, resulting in tissue ischemia and cellular death. During this progression, pain increases, and pulses may become more difficult to palpate. The extremity becomes pale, cyanotic, and cool, and capillary refill time increases.[17,18]

Bone or joint displacement can compress surrounding nerves, causing pathophysiologic changes distal to the injury. Compressed or lacerated nerves may interrupt conduction pathways, blocking or delaying nerve impulses. The nerve injury can result in alterations in pain sensation and partial or complete loss of motor and sensory function distal to the injured nerve. Increased pain, even when pulses remain present, is a sign of worsening cellular hypoxia, and is often the first sign of increased compartment pressures.[12] However, patients who are unresponsive or intubated will not be able to report this pain. In these patients, it is important to have a high index of suspicion based on the mechanism of injury (MOI). Such patients will need frequent reevaluation to detect subtle changes that are indicative of compartment syndrome.

TABLE 10-3 Classification of Fractures

Fracture	Description
Open	Fracture site is accompanied by compromised skin integrity near or over the fracture.
Closed	Skin is intact over or near fracture site.
Complete	Bony cortex is completely interrupted.
Incomplete	Bony cortex is not completely interrupted.
Comminuted	Bone is splintered into fragments.
Greenstick	Bone bends or is buckled.
Impacted	Bone is wedged into distal and proximal fracture sites.
Displaced	Bone fracture sites are not aligned.

Selected Musculoskeletal Injuries

This section presents selected musculoskeletal injuries.

Selected Fractures

A fracture is a complete or incomplete interruption in the continuity of the bone cortex. **Table 10-3** outlines the classification of fractures. **Figure 10-3** illustrates each type of fracture.

Femur Fractures

Major trauma is often the cause of femoral shaft fractures, which can occur in the proximal, distal, or midshaft femur. Femur fractures can result in significant blood loss due to the rich blood supply they receive. Thus, long bone fractures have the potential to cause shock, especially when these injuries are combined with comorbid factors.[15] Assessment findings with femur fractures may include the following[19]:

- Pain and the inability to bear weight
- Shortening of the affected leg
- Internal or external rotation
- Edema
- Deformity of the thigh
- Evidence of hypovolemic shock
- Evidence of neurovascular compromise in distal extremity

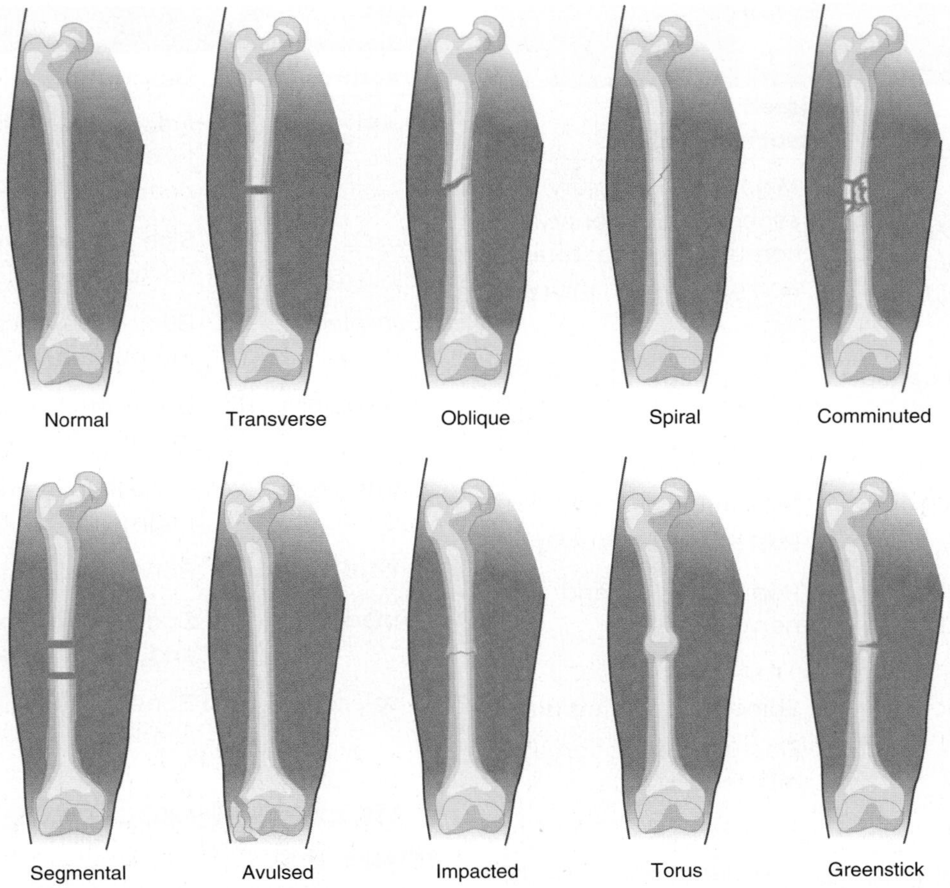

Normal Transverse Oblique Spiral Comminuted

Segmental Avulsed Impacted Torus Greenstick

Figure 10-3 *Types of fractures.*

Fat Embolism Syndrome

Fat from within the medullary cavity is released into the bloodstream when long bones are fractured; fat emboli can be detected in the lungs of as many as 90% of patients with long bone fractures on computed tomography (CT). Nevertheless, most patients do not experience significant symptoms due to the microscopic nature of the majority of fat emboli. Subclinical fat emboli are often found during autopsy of patients with major trauma and other injuries that were incompatible with life.

Of those patients who survive their initial traumatic injuries, 0.5% to 2.2% develop fat embolism syndrome (FES).[20] FES typically occurs between 30 minutes and 48 hours post injury.[20] Its presentation is a result of obstructions caused by fat emboli in the systemic circulation as well as inflammatory mediators released by the presence of lipids in the blood stream.

FES is a clinical diagnosis. Its assessment findings may include the following[21]:

- Presence of a long bone fracture (usually femur)
- Sudden mental status change or focal neurologic findings (when other causes have been ruled out)
- Respiratory distress and hypoxemic respiratory failure
- Tachycardia
- Pyrexia
- Petechial rash (conjunctiva, anterior chest, axilla)
- Visual changes
- Oliguria/anuria
- Thrombocytopenia
- Anemia

Open Fractures

Open fractures are almost always associated with high-energy transfer mechanisms such as MVCs or falls from great heights: One-third of patients with open fractures will have other injuries.[22] All open fractures are considered contaminated due to their exposure to the environment and are at risk for infection. These sites of injury have poor wound healing with a risk of osteomyelitis and sepsis. Table 10-3 describes the classification of open fractures.

Open wounds near a joint may indicate joint space involvement, and some open fractures with neurologic injury, prolonged ischemia, and muscle damage may require amputation.[17] Assessment findings for open fractures include the following[23]:

- Open wound over or near a fracture
- Open wound with protrusion of bone
- Pain
- Neurovascular compromise (in as many as 20% of significant arterial injuries, distal pulses may remain palpable)[22]
- Bleeding (may be controlled or severe)

Amputations

Amputations occur in approximately 1% of all trauma patients, and most victims are males between the ages of 15 and 40. Amputations are associated with substantial morbidity, and their mortality rate approaches 15%.[24,25] Amputations may be partial or complete, and 60% to 80% involve the digits. The lower leg is the next most common amputation, followed by the hand and forearm.[25-27] Amputations often have a dramatic presentation and may be distracting to both the patient and the trauma team. The priority of care is to focus on the overall assessment and resuscitation of the patient so as to establish and maintain hemodynamic stability, including control of hemorrhage.

Assessment findings for an amputation include the following[26]:

- Obvious tissue loss
- Pain
- Bleeding (may be controlled or severe)
  - Complete amputation: Transected vasculature will retract and spasm results in decreased or absent hemorrhage.[26,28]
  - Partial amputation: Vasculature remains connected to the distal body part with blood flow remaining intact, increasing the risk of uncontrolled hemorrhage and exsanguination.[28]
- Hypovolemic shock (may or may not be present)

Crush Injury

A crush injury of a large muscle can be the result of prolonged (greater than 2 hours) compression, entrapment, or a crushing blow.[29] These patients may present after a MVC with prolonged extrication, after a fall, or after being "found down" following a stroke or overdose.[30] Direct muscle injuries may lead to muscle ischemia and ultimately cell death, with subsequent release of myoglobin and other cellular components (potassium and proteolytic enzymes).[31] This injury can result in several complications, including compartment syndrome, hyperkalemia and other acute metabolic derangements (hypocalcemia and hyponatremia), acute prerenal and intrarenal failure, and rhabdomyolysis.

Crush injuries can also cause hemorrhage from the damaged tissue, destruction of muscle and bone tissue, fluid loss due to inflammation, and third spacing resulting in hypovolemic shock and infection. The manifestation of cell death and the release of intracellular contents into systemic circulation following massive crush injuries is known as crush syndrome.[30] Patients who develop crush syndrome may initially appear stable, but can quickly develop life-threatening arrhythmias, shock and hypotension, and eventually renal failure, acute respiratory distress syndrome, disseminated intravascular coagulation, and death.

Mangled Extremity

A rare and severe variant of a crush injury is the mangled extremity (**Figure 10-4**).[31] These injuries typically result from devastating injury mechanisms that are rarely encountered in civilian trauma care, but can occur with high-caliber ballistic injuries, pedestrian-versus-train accidents, or injuries involving machinery or farm equipment. The mangled extremity has extensive injury to bone, soft tissue, nerve, and vasculature, but remains technically attached to the body (a limb may be both mangled and partially amputated).[32] These injuries are often isolated but can also be found in conjunction with multisystem trauma and are, by definition, distracting injuries. Hemorrhage control remains the primary priority for these patients, and wound management is similar to care of an amputated part.

Devastating ischemia can occur in as little as 6 hours, so it is vital to manage these injuries quickly to preserve limb function.[33] The Mangled Extremity Severity Score

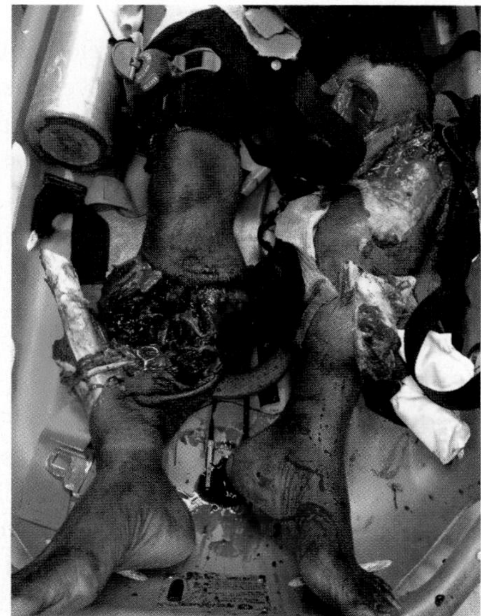

Figure 10-4 *Mangled extremity.*

Reproduced from Bain, K., Parizh, D., Kopatis, A., & Kilaru, R. (2016). Mangled extremity: To salvage or not to salvage? *BMJ Case Reports*. Retrieved from http://casereports.bmj.com/content/2016/bcr-2016-218359.full.

TABLE 10-4 Mangled Extremity Severity Score

	Characteristics	Details	Points
Tissue Injury			
1	Low energy	Stab wound, simple closed fracture, small-caliber bullet	1
2	Medium energy	Open fracture, dislocated, moderate crush	2
3	High energy	Short gun, high velocity	3
4	Massive crush	Logging, railroad	4
Shock			
1	Normotensive	Blood pressure stable	0
2	Transient hypotension	Blood pressure unstable, systolic blood pressure < 90 mm Hg	1
3	Hypotension	In operating room	2
Ischemia			
1	None	No signs of ischemia	0
2	Mild	Diminished pulses	1
3	Moderate	Paresthesias, diminished motor activity	2
4	Advanced	Pulseless, paralysis	3
Age			
1	< 30 years		0
2	> 30 to < 50 years		1
3	> 50 years		2

Data from Loja, M. N., Sammann, A., DuBose, J., Li, C.-S., Liu, Y., Savage, S., . . . Knudson, M. M. (2017). The mangled extremity score and amputation: Time for a revision. *Journal of Trauma and Acute Care Surgery, 82*(3), 518–523. https://doi.org/10.1097/TA.0000000000001339

(MESS) is a decision tool that was developed to assist providers in determining which limbs have a likelihood of successful salvage and which require amputation (**Table 10-4**).[33] Limb salvage often results in prolonged hospitalization, leads to infections, and increases mortality, so it is essential that potentially salvageable limbs are identified immediately, as well as limbs that are beyond saving. This will ensure the patient receives the appropriate interventions that will result in optimal long-term functioning and recovery.[31]

With the advent of aggressive treatment modalities such as fasciotomy, microvascular surgery, tourniquets, vascular shunts, and damage control surgery, mangled limb salvage is increasingly successful.[32] However, the success rate varies and is dependent on available resources and specialties. Hemostasis remains the priority of care and can be difficult to achieve with the widespread tissue damage that occurs with a mangled extremity. Mangled extremities involve ripped tissue and vasculature that can bleed more briskly that a guillotine or clean-cut mechanism.

Compartment Syndrome

Compartment syndrome is a serious complication of musculoskeletal injury that involves increased pressure inside a fascial compartment (**Figure 10-5**).[34] These compartments are nondistensible, so increased pressure is not well tolerated or accommodated. Normal compartment pressures are in the range of 10 to 12 mm Hg. Pain and paresthesia occur at pressures between 20 and 30 mm Hg, which are considered abnormally elevated.[35]

Increased compartment pressures can inhibit blood flow, leading to muscle and nerve damage or destruction. Elevated compartment pressures are commonly caused by hematoma formation secondary to fractures, from increased pressure or decreased space.[18] Increased pressure may occur from internal or external sources. Internal sources of pressure include hemorrhage or edema from fractures or crush injuries; external sources of pressure include casts, dressings, traction splints, air splints, clothing, or jewelry. Patients with a coagulopathy

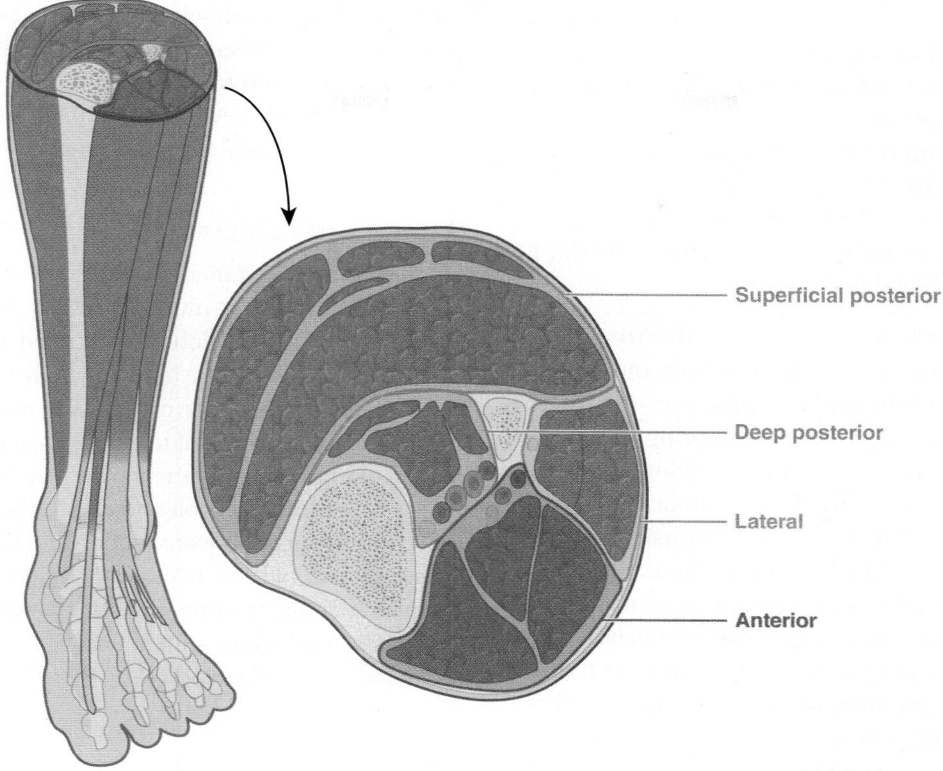

Figure 10-5 *Compartments of the lower leg.*

Data from Mayo Clinic. (n.d.). Chronic exertional compartment syndrome. Retrieved from http://www.mayoclinic.com/health/medical/IM00124.

are at increased risk for developing compartment syndrome. The increased pressure compromises blood flow to nerves, blood vessels, and muscles, resulting in cellular ischemia.

The muscles of the lower leg or forearm are the most frequent sites of compartment syndrome, but this condition can occur in any fascial compartment, including the back, buttocks, thigh, abdomen, and foot.[17,18] The degree of damage depends on the amount of pressure and the length of time for which perfusion is compromised within the compartment. Muscle necrosis can occur within 4 to 6 hours, resulting in permanent loss of function that may require amputation.[17,18] Tissue is less able to tolerate ischemia as compartment pressure increases, so higher pressures result in reduced time to cellular death. Measured compartment pressure elevation confirms compartment syndrome. Basing the diagnosis on the loss of palpable pulse may result in tissue damage, as this is often a late sign.[18] Frequent reassessment and identification of neurovascular compromise can improve patient outcomes.

Assessment Findings

Initial findings in compartment syndrome are a feeling of tightness, pain when the muscle is stretched, and rigidity on palpation. The six P's associated with compartment syndrome or any serious neurovascular compromise to an extremity can be useful in identifying this condition, but other than pain and pressure, the others are late signs and damage may already be irreversible, and any combination of these (or none at all) may be present in the patient with compartment syndrome.[36] The six P's include the following:

- *Pain:* A hallmark sign of compartment syndrome is pain out of proportion to the extent of the injury. Ischemic pain is often described as "burning" and is typically intense and severe. Pain with passive range of motion of the affected compartment can indicate development of or existing compartment syndrome.
- *Pressure:* The compartment or limb will feel tight or tense upon palpation. The skin may appear taut and shiny as the skin stretches.
- *Pulses:* Pulses can remain normal in the presence of compartment syndrome. Once compartment pressures are equal to or exceed the diastolic pressure within the arteries, weak or absent pulses may be noted—they are an ominous finding.[17]
- *Paresthesia:* Numbness, tingling, or loss of sensation may occur as nerves and blood vessels are compressed. With loss of sensation, there may be

a relief of pain. This is indicative of a worsening perfusion, not an improvement.[18]
- *Paralysis:* Motor dysfunction signifies injury to the nervous system.
- *Pallor:* Poor skin color and delayed capillary refill may indicate decreased perfusion.
- *Poikilothermia:* The limb may feel cool or assume the ambient temperature of the environment due to stagnation of blood in the limb.

When a patient is unconscious or otherwise unable to be clinically assessed at regular intervals, the continuous measurement of the intramuscular pressure may be of benefit. Continuous pressure monitoring uses a prescribed perfusion pressure as a threshold for fasciotomy. Perfusion pressure is calculated as diastolic blood pressure minus compartment pressure. Perfusion pressure sustained at less than 30 mm Hg for 2 hours has a 93% positive predictive value for the diagnosis of acute compartment syndrome.[37] Fasciotomy may be safely avoided as long as the perfusion pressure remains greater than 30 mm Hg. Typically, the anterior compartment of the limb is monitored, as the pressures within this compartment tend to be higher. By using this method to assess compartment pressure, emergent fasciotomy can potentially be avoided. **Figure 10-6** illustrates the measurement of compartment pressure in the posterior lower leg.[38]

Hyperkalemia

Potassium exists predominately in the intracellular space, so cellular destruction releases large amounts of potassium into the serum, resulting in hyperkalemia and placing the patient at risk for cardiac dysrhythmias.[39]

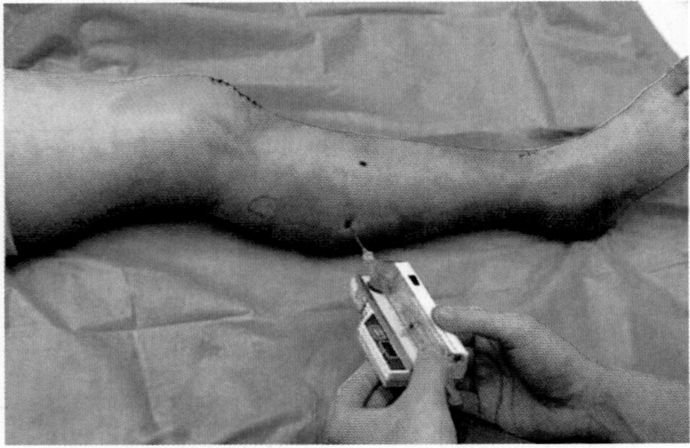

Figure 10-6 *Compartment pressure measurement tool.*

Reproduced from Tepordei, R. T., Stefan, G. T., Cozma, T., Nedelcu, A. H., Ovidiu, A., & Carmen, Z. L. (2014). A comparison of pressure measurement devices used in the acute compartment syndrome of the limbs. *Romanian Journal of Functional and Clinical, Macro- and Microscopical Anatomy and of Anthropology, XIII*(3), 369–372.

Potassium levels peak approximately 12–36 hours after the injury event.[40] This elevation may be seen in the initial resuscitation period following a prolonged extraction or delayed transport. See Chapter 20, "Post-Resuscitation Care Considerations," for more information.

Rhabdomyolysis

Significant muscle damage and cellular destruction also release myoglobin, a muscle protein, into the bloodstream. Because myoglobin is excreted in the kidneys, the risk of acute kidney injury is high in patients with crush injury.[41] The large myoglobin molecules can become trapped in the renal tubules, causing both prerenal and intrarenal failure. Patients with rhabdomyolysis are often profoundly hypovolemic due to the mechanism of muscle injury and vasoconstriction and the third spacing caused by free radicals released during cellular lysis; this intravascular dehydration can exacerbate kidney injuries. The classic triad of assessment findings for rhabdomyolysis includes the following[42]:

- Muscle pain, numbness, or changes in sensation
- Muscle weakness or paralysis
- Dark red, or brown urine (myoglobinuria)

Other assessment findings include the following[42]:

- Extensive soft-tissue edema and bruising
- General weakness or malaise
- Evidence of hypovolemic shock, which may or may not be present
- Elevated creatine kinase levels

Treatment of rhabdomyolysis focuses on early intervention with aggressive fluid resuscitation to flush out myoglobin to prevent renal failure. It is recommended to maintain the patient's urinary output at 100 mL per hour until the myoglobinuria is resolved.[15]

Joint Dislocations

Dislocations occur when the articulating surfaces of the joint become separated. Prolonged separation can cause nerve injury because of the anatomic proximity of nerves to the affected joint.

Assessment findings of joint dislocations include the following:

- Inability to move the affected joint
- Joint deformity
- Pain
- Edema
- Abnormal range of motion
- Neurovascular compromise—diminished or absent pulses; diminished sensory function

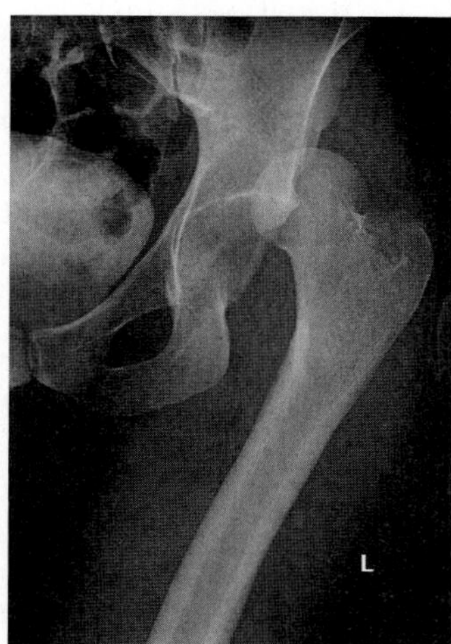

Figure 10-7 *Radiograph of a posterior hip dislocation.*

Courtesy of Dr Hani Salam, Radiopaedia.org, rID: 10397.

Specific joint dislocations can have unique manifestations (**Figure 10-7**)[43]:

- Dislocated hip joints[44]
  - Often associated with significant trauma.
  - Complications of a hip dislocation:
    - Avascular necrosis of the femoral head
    - Sciatic nerve compression
    - Permanent disability
  - Reduction of the dislocated hip is a priority as soon as the patient is stabilized.
- Ankle dislocations may require immediate realignment to restore circulation.[45]
  - May occur in conjunction with open or closed fractures of the tibia/fibula.
- Dislocations of the knee may result in the following[46]:
  - Peroneal nerve injury may occur.
  - Constriction of the popliteal artery and vein is possible if reduction of the dislocation is delayed.
  - Popliteal artery damage may not become apparent for several hours; frequent vascular checks are recommended.

Nursing Care of the Patient with Musculoskeletal Trauma

Nursing care begins with the primary survey.

Primary Survey

See Chapter 3, "Initial Assessment," for the systematic approach to care of the trauma patient. The following assessment parameters are specific to musculoskeletal injuries. Musculoskeletal injuries can have dramatic presentations and, therefore, represent a significant distraction to the trauma team and the patient. It is imperative that the systematic assessment approach proceed as usual for every trauma patient regardless of readily apparent injuries.

Secondary Survey

Secondary survey begins with history.

H: History

The MOI can reveal clues to specific trauma patterns, especially those that occur to certain components of the skeletal structure. It is useful to know where the energy force was applied and where the pain is located. Attempt to reconstruct the event to determine the extent of injury, as well as any potential injuries that may not be apparent. Utilize prehospital personnel to ensure complete understanding of the events surrounding the trauma, position of the patient, length of extrication, and other pertinent factors. See Chapter 2, "Biomechanics, Kinematics, and Mechanisms of Injury," for more information.

Components of the history may include the following:

- MVCs
  - Extent of damage to the vehicle
    - Photographs of the vehicle/scene may be available from prehospital personnel or law enforcement.
  - Point of impact on the vehicle
  - Patient location within the vehicle and location at scene
  - Ejection from vehicle
  - Air bag deployment
  - Use of a seat belt/restraint
  - Speed of the vehicle
- Pedestrian struck by vehicle
  - Speed of the vehicle upon impact
  - Height or size/make of the vehicle
  - Vehicle point of impact
  - Patient point of impact
  - Dragged/thrown by vehicle
  - Presence of "Cinderella sign" (shoes knocked off—a poor prognostic indicator)
- Falls
  - Height of the fall
  - Landing surface: concrete, gravel, sand, grass, and so on
  - Point of impact: feet, head, back, and so on
- Crush injuries
  - Weight of crushing object
  - Length of time compressed/entrapped:
    - Longer periods of compression increase the risk of rhabdomyolysis and hyperkalemia and their speed of onset.
  - Body part or parts affected

- Blast injuries
  - Distance between the patient and the point of blast
  - Flying debris
  - Patient thrown by blast

H: Head-to-Toe Assessment

The secondary survey also involves a head-to-toe assessment.

Head

Sudden vision or mental status changes may indicate a possible fat embolism in the cerebral vasculature.[47]

Chest

Assess for a fat embolism within the pulmonary vasculature, which is a complication of long bone fractures. It may be evidenced by acute respiratory difficulty in a patient with multiple injuries and petechiae on the chest.[47]

Extremities

Inspect and palpate for the following:

- Neurovascular status
- Active, uncontrolled bleeding
- Integrity of the injured area, noting any breaks in the skin and soft-tissue abnormalities that may indicate occult fractures or dislocations
- Deformity or angulation of the extremity
- Color, position, and any obvious differences in the injured extremity as compared to the uninjured extremity, such as shortening, rotation, displacement, or loss of function

The six P's can be helpful to guide the trauma nurse's neurovascular assessment of the extremity[48]:

- Pain
  - Field splints should be removed, at least partially, for assessment.
  - Palpate the entire length of each extremity for pain or tenderness.
  - Assess the quality of pain at identified points.
  - Assess the active and passive range of motion of all extremities. Note pain with movement.
- Pressure
  - The skin may appear shiny as tissue becomes stretched.
  - Palpate the extremity for firmness of compartments and for muscle spasms.
- Pulses
  - Palpate pulses proximal and distal to the injury.
  - Bilateral pulse comparison is necessary to determine the quality of the pulse.
  - The presence of a pulse does not rule out compartment syndrome.
  - Doppler ultrasound may be needed to determine the presence or absence of pulses.
- Paresthesia/paralysis
  - Assess for abnormal sensations such as burning, tingling, and numbness. Ischemic pain is often described as burning.
  - Assess range of motion to determine motor function. Neurologic function is related to mobility.
  - Extremities with obvious injury may require deferment of the range-of-motion assessment due to the risk of increased damage to muscles and nerves.
  - Pain and guarding may limit range of motion assessment.
- Pallor and poikilothermia (assessment is the same for both findings)
  - Assess the color and temperature of the injured extremity.
  - Pallor, delayed capillary refill, and a cool extremity may indicate vascular compromise in a normothermic environment.
  - Assess the ankle brachial index (ABI) or arterial pressure index (API) to detect occult peripheral vascular injuries.[49]

Interventions

Interventions for musculoskeletal injuries include the following:

- Control of hemorrhage by direct pressure, compression dressings, or tourniquets for severe, life-threatening injuries
- Immobilizing the affected extremity to prevent further bleeding, injury, and pain

Splinting

Splinting is usually performed during or after the secondary survey, depending on the risk to the patient. Remove clothing and jewelry prior to splinting and immobilization. Abnormalities that indicate the possible need for splinting include the following:

- Pain
- Deformity
- Bony crepitus
- Edema
- Circulatory compromise

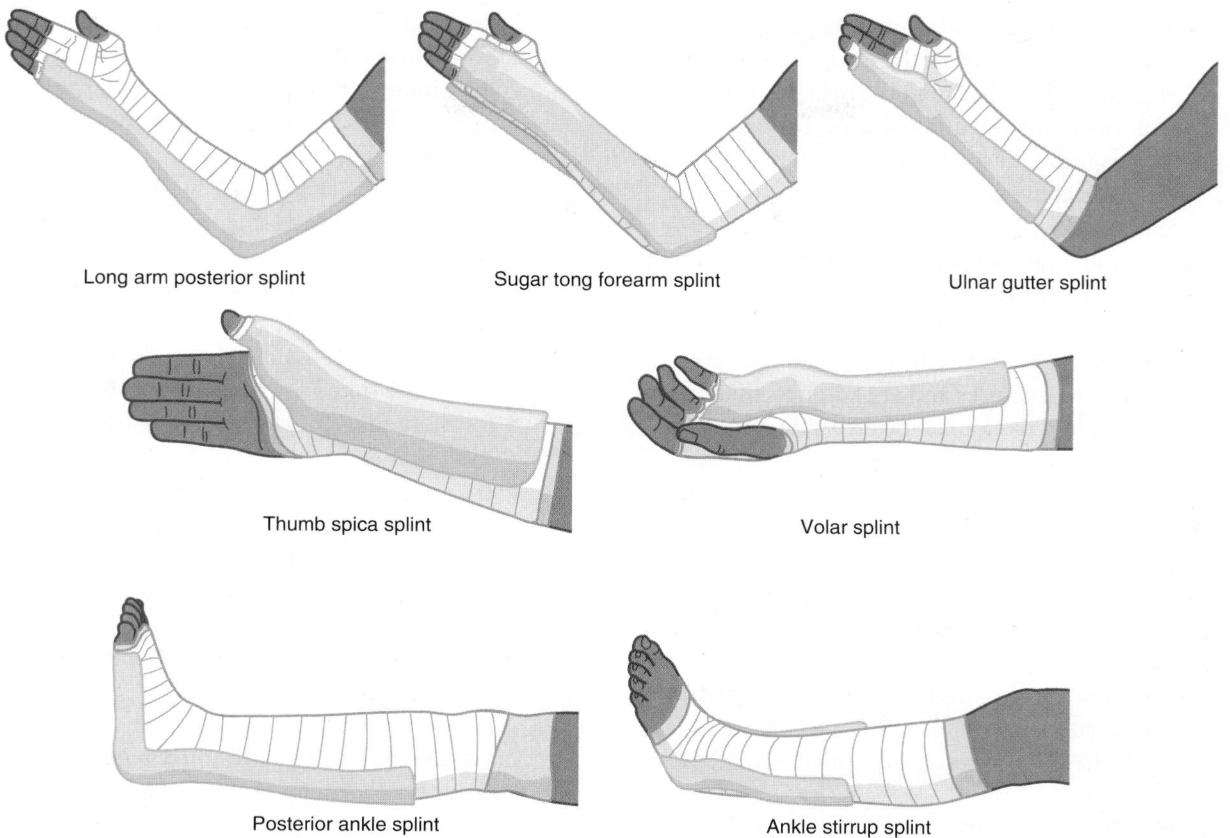

Figure 10-8 *Selected types of splints. The light blue layer is the stockinette, the white layer is the cotton roll, and the beige layer is the splint. A. Long arm posterior splint. B. Sugar tong forearm splint. C. Ulnar gutter splint. D. Thumb spica splint. E. Volar splint. F. Posterior ankle splint. G. Ankle stirrup splint.*

Splinting can also be used to stabilize an impaled object. Types of splints (**Figure 10-8**) include the following:

- Rigid splints, such as cardboard, plastic, or metal splints: Pad to prevent pressure injury to bony prominences.
- Soft splints or air splints.
- Traction splints: Applied for midshaft femur fractures (**Figure 10-9**).
- Custom splints with fiberglass casting materials.

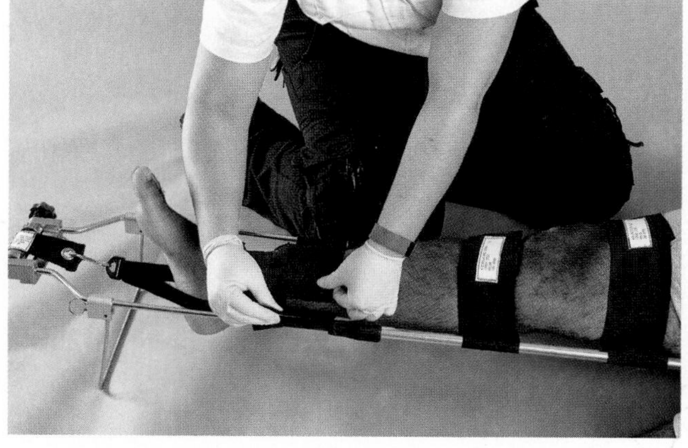

Figure 10-9 *Traction splint for mid-shaft femur fracture.*

Guidelines for splint application include the following[50]:

- If the patient has an obvious deformity or bony protrusion, do not attempt to reposition the limb.
- Assess pulse, temperature, color, and pulse quality before and after each attempt to immobilize the limb or move the patient.
    - Note any losses of a previously palpable pulse; changes in temperature, color, or pulse quality; or increases in pain.
    - If these findings are present, repositioning of the extremity may be indicated. Remove the splints and notify the physician.
- Elevate the extremity.

  - If compartment syndrome is suspected, elevate the limb to the level of the heart.[51] Avoid elevating the limb higher than the heart, as this can reduce circulation and tissue perfusion.[52]
  - If compartment syndrome is not a risk, elevate the limb above the level of the heart to reduce pain and swelling.
- Assess and treat pain, to include administration of pain medications as prescribed.
  - Intravenous (IV) acetaminophen preparations have been shown to effectively manage acute pain from fractures and are adjuncts that can reduce opioid use and associated side effects.[53]
- Prepare for procedural sedation following institutional policy when indicated for reduction of fracture/dislocations.
- Immobilize the joint.
  - When applying a splint or other immobilizing device, include joints above and below the deformity.
  - Avoid movement of the fractured extremity, which can increase bleeding and the risk of fat embolism or can result in an inadvertent open fracture.
- Apply ice to reduce swelling and pain for 20 minutes. Do not place ice directly on the skin. Ice can be reapplied hourly as necessary.[54]
  - If compartment syndrome is suspected, ice is strongly contraindicated, as it can exacerbate already compromised perfusion.

Interventions for Selected Injuries

Interventions for specific injuries follow.

Open Fracture

Interventions for an open fracture include the following:

- Remove gross contaminates.
- Cover open wounds with sterile saline-soaked dressings.[55]
- Administer antibiotics as ordered.
- Administer tetanus prophylaxis according to current Centers for Disease Control and Prevention (CDC) guidelines.

Amputation/Penetrating Injury

Interventions for an amputation/penetrating injury include the following:

- Apply direct pressure over active bleeding or compress the artery above the bleeding site.
- Elevate the extremity.
- Tourniquets are used when pressure and elevation fail to control bleeding.
  - Pneumatic tourniquets (similar to large blood pressure cuffs) may be required for stabilization of complex injuries.[15]
  - Place tourniquets as close to the amputation site as possible to limit ischemia and nerve compression of extremity.
  - Place tourniquets over clothing, with the time of placement clearly marked on the device and documented in the medical record (to track "ischemic time"; tourniquets may be left in place for more than 6 hours with only transient nerve dysfunction).[56]
  - If a single tourniquet fails to control bleeding, a second tourniquet may be placed 2 inches above the first (**Figure 10-10**).[57] This is especially true if clothing is present, the wound is on the thigh, and there is substantial swelling. The first tourniquet may need to be tightened in addition to adding a second one.
  - A tourniquet that is tight enough to control arterial bleeding will be extremely painful to the patient. If a tourniquet is not sufficiently tightened, it may compress veins, but not arteries. This will cause congestion of the limb and paradoxical worsening of bleeding.
  - Do not release the tourniquet unless a physician prepared to manage the bleeding—surgically, if necessary—is present.
  - Tourniquets are valuable as a lifesaving measure for amputations with uncontrolled bleeding and significantly reduce mortality when applied prior to the development of decompensated shock.[58]

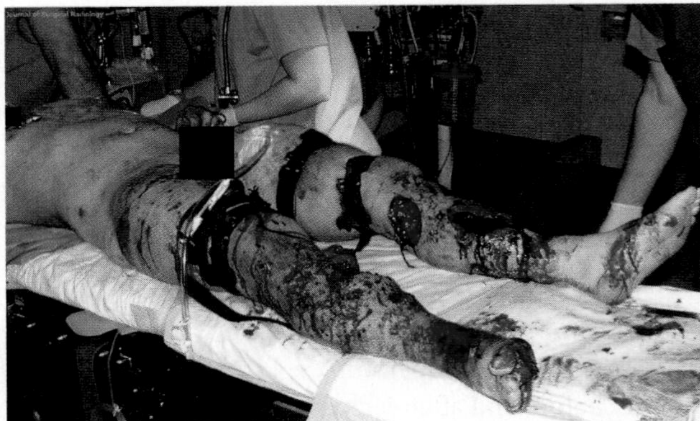

Figure 10-10 *A second tourniquet placed above the first.*

- Remove dirt or debris from the amputated part and the residual limb (**Figure 10-11**).
  - *Residual limb* refers to the part of the body that remains after an amputation. For instance, the part of the thigh that remains following an above-the-knee amputation is the residual limb.[59]
- Keep the amputated part cool by wrapping it in saline-moistened sterile gauze, and then place it in a sealed plastic bag.
  - The bag containing the amputated part is then placed in a second bag containing a mixture of 50% ice and 50% water.
  - Do not allow the amputated part to freeze or be submerged in liquid.
  - Label the bag with appropriate patient identifiers.[58]
- Administer antibiotics as ordered.
- Administer tetanus prophylaxis according to current CDC guidelines.

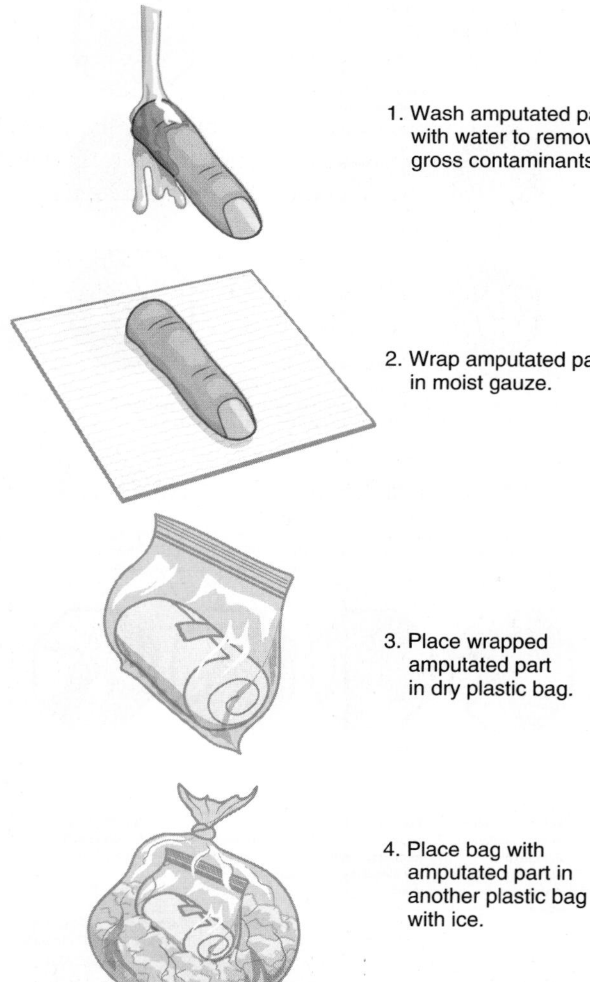

Figure 10-11 *Care of the amputated part.*

Crush Injury and Compartment Syndrome

Interventions for crush injury and compartment syndrome include the following:

- Administer an IV isotonic crystalloid solution to increase urinary output to at least 100 mL per hour to enhance the excretion of myoglobin.[15]
- Remove casts, splints, or dressings.
- Elevate the limb only to the level of the heart to promote circulation.[51]
- Initiate noninvasive hemodynamic and cardiac monitoring to observe for dysrhythmias.
- Prepare for measuring fascial compartment pressure. This is typically performed by a physician inserting a large-caliber needle or catheter into the fascia of the involved muscle and attaching it to a manometer or intracompartmental pressure monitor. A noninvasive method of measuring compartmental pressure is to use near-infrared spectroscopy to measure decreased tissue blood flow.[60] Normal pressure is 0 to 8 mm Hg. Elevated readings of 30 to 40 mm Hg are suggestive of ischemia to muscles and nerves; when pressures exceed 30 mm Hg in any compartment, capillary beds are occluded.
- Anticipate an emergent fasciotomy, if indicated, to decompress the compartment to prevent muscle and/or neurovascular damage and loss of the limb. Surgical debridement or amputation may also be necessary.
- Facilitate emergent transfer either to the operating room or to a center with microvascular surgical capabilities for patients with potentially salvageable mangled extremities.[31]

Diagnostics and Interventions for Musculoskeletal Trauma

Additional diagnostic studies for patients with musculoskeletal trauma include the following:

- Anterior posterior and lateral radiographs of the injured extremity are necessary. Some fractures can be seen only from one angle, which may require an additional oblique view. The images need to include the joints above and below the injury. In children, radiographs of the non-injured extremity may be helpful for comparison.
- CT scan can be used for more definitive evaluation of musculoskeletal trauma and for assessment of damage to surrounding organs. CT scan can also identify organic foreign bodies such as retained splinters.

- Angiography can be performed to identify tears or compressions in the vasculature of the injured extremity.
- Noninvasive near-infrared spectroscopy to measure decreased tissue blood flow can be useful to diagnose compartment syndrome.
- The ABI or API can be obtained to detect occult peripheral vascular injuries.[49]

Reevaluation

Refer to Chapter 3 for a description of reevaluation of the trauma patient. Additional evaluations related to musculoskeletal injuries include the following:

- The six P's
- Urinary output and presence of myoglobinuria
- Control of bleeding (especially after resuscitation with IV fluids or blood products)

Definitive Care or Transport

Prepare the patient for definitive stabilization, operative intervention, hospital admission, or transfer. Definitive stabilization includes the following measures:

- Closed or open reduction
- Traction
- External fixators
- Casting

Emerging Trends

There are several emerging trends related to musculoskeletal trauma.

The Hartford Consensus

With the increase in mass-casualty incidents involving penetrating injuries, a need was identified for increased education and awareness of basic bleeding control techniques. Analysis of events such as the Pulse nightclub shooting in Orlando and the Harvest Music Festival shooting in Las Vegas has led to speculation that the loss of life could have potentially been limited with bystander implementation of these techniques. As a result of this need, the American College of Surgeons released the Hartford Consensus in 2014. This document and the subsequent "Compendium of Strategies to Enhance Victims' Survivability from Mass Casualty Events" report were the results of collaboration between emergency medical services, law enforcement, Homeland Security, and medical professionals. The campaign operates under the goal that "no one should die from uncontrolled bleeding."[61]

The most progressive component of the Hartford Consensus is the "Stop the Bleed" campaign (**Figure 10-12**),

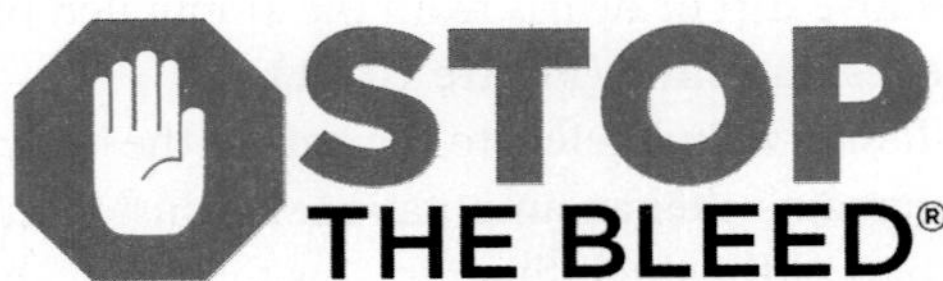

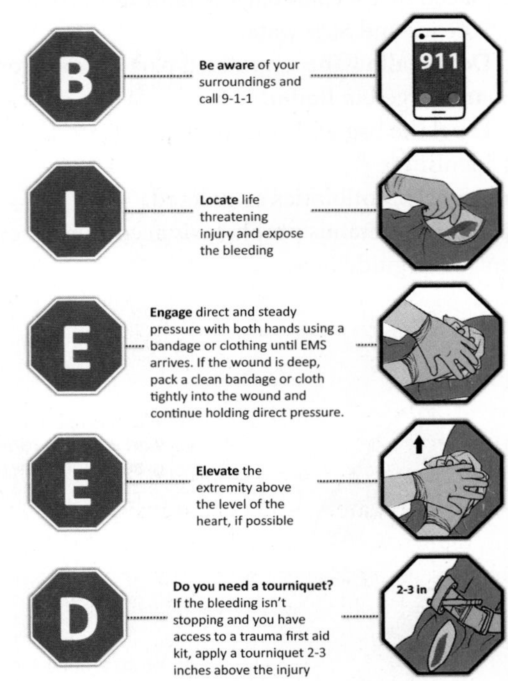

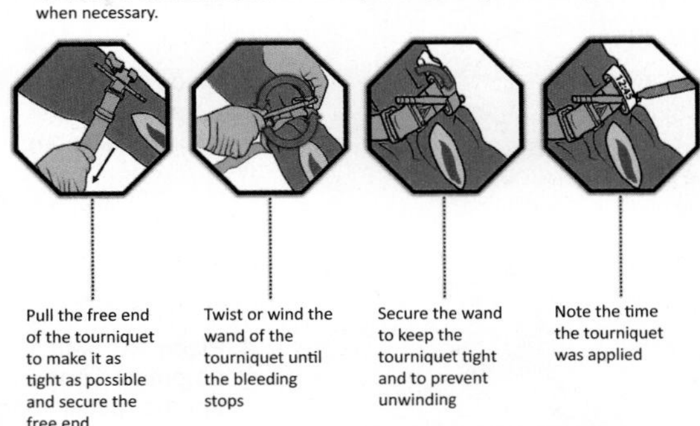

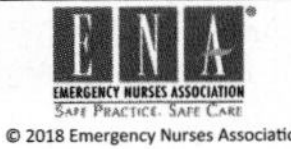

Figure 10-12 *"Stop the Bleed" educational poster.*

a public education initiative aimed at placing bleeding control kits in public spaces, with the goal of decreasing mortality from injuries that would otherwise cause exsanguination prior to the arrival of prehospital providers.[62] The program seeks to replicate the success of publicly accessible automated external defibrillators in improving survival for out-of-hospital cardiac arrest victims. Bystanders are taught to apply direct pressure to bleeding wounds to gain immediate control of active life-threatening hemorrhage. Kits also include gauze impregnated with clotting agents to be packed into bleeding wounds, as well as a tourniquet. As this education campaign and kits become more widely available, more patients may arrive with these measures in place. Emergency nurses are uniquely positioned to actively participate in this campaign by providing community education and increasing the awareness of the importance of bystander involvement as a lifesaving intervention.[63]

Topical Hemostatic Agents

Along with aggressive tourniquet use, topical hemostatic agents have become a mainstay of hemorrhage control in tactical trauma care. Use of these agents on the battlefield has been associated with decreased mortality from extremity injuries and exsanguination.[64] A variety of commercially prepared products are available that can be topically applied to gain control of life-threatening bleeding, including gauze impregnated with concentrated clotting factors and polymers that form mechanical "clots." In addition, clotting factors and polymers are available in bead or granule form that can be poured into the wound bed to achieve the same effect. Currently, fibrin preparations, silver nitrate, and tranexamic acid have all been used topically in the ED to gain control of minor bleeding.[65] More research is needed to determine if these tactical dressings have applications for trauma care in the ED, but they may certainly be useful in resource-poor environments or critical access facilities without immediate access to surgical services.

Summary

Extremity injuries are usually addressed during the secondary survey. However, some injuries may be life threatening and require immediate intervention for uncontrolled hemorrhage during the primary survey. Consideration is also given to injuries that may result in functional disability and loss of limb. The secondary survey is carefully conducted to identify all injuries. Early intervention for suspected fractures, including neurovascular assessment before and after any splint application, can help to prevent further injury. Pain is important to consider in musculoskeletal injuries, and splinting and pain medication can be effective means of pain management.

A systematic approach to the assessment and reassessment of the trauma patient assists in the identification of musculoskeletal injuries and life-threatening sequelae to improve the overall outcome for the patient.

References

1. Fetterman, A., & Horowitz, D. (n.d.). Anatomy of the bone. University of Rochester Medical Center. Retrieved from https://www.urmc.rochester.edu/encyclopedia/content.aspx?ContentTypeID=85&ContentID=P00109
2. Seeley, R., VanPutte, C., Regan, J., & Russo, A. (Eds.). (2016). Skeletal system: Bones and bone tissue. In *Seeley's anatomy and physiology* (11th ed., pp. 165–193). New York, NY: McGraw-Hill.
3. Tortora, G. J., & Derrickson, B. (2017). The skeletal system: Bone tissue. In *Principles of anatomy and physiology* (15th ed., pp. 171–193). Hoboken, NJ: Wiley.
4. Tortora, G. J., & Derrickson, B. (2017). The skeletal system: The axial skeleton. In *Principles of anatomy and physiology* (15th ed., pp. 194–233). Hoboken, NJ: Wiley.
5. O'Toole, M. T. (Ed.). (2016). *Mosby's medical dictionary* (10th ed.). St. Louis, MO: Mosby Elsevier.
6. Gunn, A. (2009). *Essential forensic biology* (2nd ed.). West Sussex, UK: John Wiley and Sons.
7. Centers for Disease Control and Prevention. (2016). National Hospital Ambulatory Medical Care Survey: 2015 Emergency Department Summary Tables. Retrieved from https://www.cdc.gov/nchs/data/nhamcs/web_tables/2015_ed_web_tables.pdf
8. Centers for Disease Control and Prevention. (2017, November). FASTSTATS: Accidental or unintentional injuries. Retrieved from https://www.cdc.gov/nchs/fastats/accidental-injury.htm
9. American College of Surgeons. (2012). Geriatric trauma. In *Advanced trauma life support: Student course manual* (9th ed., pp. 272–285). Chicago, IL: Author.
10. Montali, F., Campaniello, G., Benatti, M., Rastelli, G., Pedrazzoni, M., & Cervellin, G. (2015). Impact of different drug classes on clinical severity of falls in an elderly population: Epidemiological survey in a trauma center. *Journal of Clinical Gerontology and Geriatrics, 6*(2), 63–67. https://doi.org/10.1016/j.jcgg.2015.03.002
11. Cosman, F., Beur, S. J., LeBoff, M. S., Lewiecki, E. M., Tanner, B., Randall, S., & Lindsay, R. (2014). Clinician's guide to prevention and treatment of osteoporosis. *Osteoporosis International, 25*(10), 2359–2381. https://doi.org/10.1007/s00198-014-2794-2
12. Ball, C. G. (2015). Penetrating nontorso trauma: The extremities. *Canadian Journal of Surgery, 58*(4), 286–288. http://doi.org/10.1503/cjs.005815
13. Anwar, R., Tuson, K., & Khan, S. A. (2008). Knee and leg. In *Classification and diagnosis in orthopedic trauma* (pp. 160–174). New York, NY: Cambridge University Press.

14. Desapriya, E., Subzwari, S., Sasges, D., Basic, A., Alidina, A., Turcotte, K., & Pike, I. (2010). Do light truck vehicles (LTV) impose greater risk of pedestrian injury than passenger cars? A meta-analysis and systematic review. *Traffic Injury Prevention, 11*(1), 48–56. https://doi.org/10.1080/15389580903390623
15. American College of Surgeons. (2018). Musculoskeletal trauma. In *Advanced trauma life support: Student course manual* (10th ed., pp. 148–167). Chicago, IL: Author.
16. Zadora, S., Lasik, A., & Bumbasirevic, M. (2016). A case of acute bilateral femur fracture with vascular injury. *Journal of Acute Disease, 5*(1), 86–89. https://doi.org/10.1016/j.joad.2015.07.009
17. Porth, C. (2014). Disorders of the skeletal system: Trauma, infections, neoplasms, and childhood disorders. In *Essentials of pathophysiology: Concepts of altered health states* (4th ed., pp. 1078–1110). Philadelphia, PA: Wolters Kluwer/Lippincott Williams & Wilkins.
18. Percival, T., White, J., & Ricci, M. (2011). Compartment syndrome in the setting of vascular injury. *Perspectives in Vascular Surgery and Endovascular Therapy, 23*(2), 119–124. https://doi.org/10.1177%2F1531003511401422
19. Romeo, N. M. (2018, October 10). Femur injuries and fractures. *Medscape.* Retrieved from https://emedicine.medscape.com/article/90779-overview
20. Kosova, E., Bergmark, B., & Piazza, G. (2015). Fat embolism syndrome. *Circulation, 131*(3), 317–320. https://doi.org/10.1161/circulationaha.114.010835.
21. Tolins, M., & Johnson, N. (2016, January 21). The crashing patient with long bone fractures: A case of fat embolism syndrome. Retrieved from http://www.emdocs.net/the-crashing-patient-with-long-bone-fractures-a-case-of-fat-embolism-syndrome/
22. Ortega, A. (2016, February 10). Open fractures. Retrieved from https://coreem.net/core/open-fractures/
23. Elniel, A. R., & Giannoudis, P. V. (2018). Open fractures of the lower extremity. *EFORT Open Reviews, 3*(5), 316–325. https://doi.org/10.1302/2058-5241.3.170072
24. Delhey, P., Huber, S., Hanschen, M., Häberle, S., Trentzsch, H., Deiler, S., . . . Huber-Wagner, S. (2015). Significance of traumatic macroamputation in severely injured patients. *Shock, 43*(3), 233–237. https://doi.org/10.1097/shk.0000000000000292
25. Barmparas, G., Inaba, K., Teixeira, P., Dubose, J. J., Criscuoli, M., Talving, P., . . . Demetriades, D. (2010). Epidemiology of post-traumatic limb amputation: A National Trauma Databank analysis. *American Surgeon, 76*, 1214–1222.
26. Langdorf, M. I. (2017, September 12). Replantation in emergency medicine. *Medscape.* Retrieved from http://emedicine.medscape.com/article/827648-overview
27. Ziegler-Graham, K., MacKenzie, E. J., Ephraim, P. L., Travison, T. G., & Brookmeyer, R. (2008). Estimating the prevalence of limb loss in the United States: 2005 to 2050. *Archives of Physical Medicine and Rehabilitation, 89*, 422–429. https://doi.org/10.1016/j.apmr.2007.11.005
28. Willis, G., & Reynolds, J. (2011). Traumatic amputations. *Emergency Medicine Reports, 32*, 285–296. Retrieved from https://www.reliasmedia.com/articles/140552-traumatic-amputations
29. Sahjian, M., & Frakes, M. (2007). Crush injuries: Pathophysiology and current treatment. *Nurse Practitioner, 32*, 13–18. https://doi.org/10.1097/01.NPR.0000287464.81259.8b
30. Genthon, A., & Wilcox, S. (2014). Crush syndrome: A case report and review of the literature. *Journal of Emergency Medicine, 46*(2), 313–319. https://doi.org/10.1016/j.jemermed.2013.08.052
31. Bain, K., Parizh, D., Kopatsis, A., & Kilaru, R. (2016). Mangled extremity: To salvage or not to salvage? *BMJ Case Reports.* https://doi.org/10.1136/bcr-2016-218359
32. Weingart, G., & Kumar, S. (2017). Acute compartment syndrome. *Emergency Medicine, 49*(3), 106–115. Retrieved from https://www.mdedge.com/emed-journal/article/132733/pain/acute-compartment-syndrome
33. Loja, M. N., Sammann, A., DuBose, J., Li, C.-S., Liu, Y., Savage, S., . . . Knudson, M. M. (2017). The mangled extremity score and amputation: Time for a revision. *Journal of Trauma and Acute Care Surgery, 82*(3), 518–523. https://doi.org/10.1097/ta.0000000000001339
34. Mayo Clinic. (n.d.). Chronic exertional compartment syndrome. Retrieved from http://www.mayoclinic.com/health/medical/IM00124
35. Ali, P., Santy-Tomlinson, J., & Watson, R. (2014). Assessment and diagnosis of acute limb compartment syndrome: A literature review. *International Journal of Orthopaedic and Trauma Nursing, 18*, 180–190. https://doi.org/10.1016/j.ijotn.2014.01.002
36. Rasul, A. T. Jr. (2018, April 3). Acute compartment syndrome clinical presentation. *Medscape.* Retrieved from http://emedicine.medscape.com/article/307668-clinical#a0256
37. Schmidt, A. (2016). Acute compartment syndrome. *Orthopedic Clinics of North America, 47*, 517–525. https://doi.org/10.1016/l.016.2.001
38. Tepordei, R. T., Stefan, G. T., Cozma, T., Nedelcu, A. H., Ovidiu, A., & Carmen, Z. L. (2014). A comparison of pressure measurement devices used in the acute compartment syndrome of the limbs. *Romanian Journal of Functional and Clinical, Macro- and Microscopical Anatomy and of Anthropology, XIII*(3), 369–372.
39. Copstead, L. E., & Banasik, J. (2018). *Pathophysiology* (6th ed.). St. Louis, MO: Saunders Elsevier.
40. Criddle, L. M. (2003). Rhabdomyolysis: Pathophysiology, recognition, and management. *Critical Care Nurse, 23*, 14–32. Retrieved from http://ccn.aacnjournals.org/content/23/6/14.long
41. Harbrecht, B., Rosengart, M., Zenati, M., Forsythe, R., & Peitzman, A. (2007). Defining the contribution of renal dysfunction to outcome after traumatic injury. *American Surgeon, 73*(8), 836–840.
42. Cervellin, G., Comelli, I., & Lippi, G. (2010). Rhabdomyolysis: Historical background, clinical, diagnostic and therapeutic features. *Clinical Chemistry and Laboratory Medicine, 28*(6), 749–756. https://doi.org/10.1515/CCLM.2010.151
43. Hacking, C., & Gallard, F. (n.d.). Posterior dislocation of the hip. Retrieved from https://radiopaedia.org/articles/posterior-dislocation-of-the-hip?lang=us
44. Anwar, R., Tuson, K., & Khan, S. A. (2008). Hip and thigh. In *Classification and diagnosis in orthopedic trauma* (pp. 134–136). New York, NY: Cambridge University Press.

45. Keany, J. E., & McKeever, D. (2016, April 28). Ankle dislocation in emergency medicine. *Medscape*. Retrieved from http://emedicine.medscape.com/article/823087-overview
46. Kelleher, H. B., & Mandavia, D. (2015, August 24). Knee dislocation. *Medscape*. Retrieved from http://emedicine.medscape.com/article/823589-overview
47. American College of Surgeons. (2012). Ocular trauma. In *Advanced trauma life support: Student course manual* (9th ed., pp. 311–315). Chicago, IL: Author.
48. Johnston-Walker, E., & Hardcastle, J. (2011). Neurovascular assessment in the critically ill patient. *Nursing in Critical Care, 16*(4), 170–177. https://doi.org/10.1111/j.1478-5153.2011.00431.x
49. Feliciano, D. V. (2017). Pitfalls in the management of peripheral vascular injuries. *Trauma Surgery & Acute Care Open, 2*(1), e000110. https://doi.org/10.1136/tsaco-2017-000110
50. Hoyt, K. S. (2009). Plaster and fiberglass splinting. In J. A. Proehl (Ed.), *Emergency nursing procedures* (4th ed., pp. 622–633). St Louis, MO: Saunders Elsevier.
51. Cerepani, M. J. (2010). Orthopedic and neurovascular trauma. In P. K. Howard & R. A. Steinmann (Eds.), *Sheehy's emergency nursing: Principles and practice* (6th ed., pp. 313–339). St. Louis, MO: Mosby Elsevier.
52. Farrow, C., Bodenham, A., & Troxler, M. (2011). Acute limb compartment syndromes. *Continuing Education in Anaesthesia, Critical Care & Pain, 11*(1), 24–28.
53. Bollinger, A. J., Butler, P. D., Nies, M. S., Sietsema, D. L., Jones, C. B., & Endres, T. J. (2015). Is scheduled intravenous acetaminophen effective in the pain management protocol of geriatric hip fractures? *Geriatric Orthopaedic Surgery & Rehabilitation, 6*(3), 202–208. https://doi.org/10.1177/2151458515588560
54. Schmitt, B. D. (2015). *Pediatric telephone protocols* (15th ed.). Itasca, IL: American Academy of Pediatrics Publishing.
55. Mauffrey, C., Bailey, J. R., Bowles, R. J., Price, C., Hasson, D., Hak, D. J., & Stahel, P. F. (2012). Acute management of open fractures: Proposal of a new multidisciplinary algorithm. *Orthopedics, 35*(10), 877–881. https://doi.org/10.3928/01477447-20120919-08
56. Ode, G., Studnek, J., Seymour, R., Bosse, M. J., & Hsu, J. R. (2015). Emergency tourniquets for civilians. *Journal of Trauma and Acute Care Surgery, 79*(4), 586–591. https://doi.org/10.1097/ta.0000000000000815
57. O'Brien P. J., & Cox, M. W. (2011). Stents in tents: Endovascular therapy on the battlefields of the global war on terror. *Journal of Surgical Radiology, 2*(1), 50–56.
58. Mamczak, C. N., Born, C. T., Obremskey, W. T., & Dromsky, D. M. (2012). Evolution of acute orthopaedic care. *Journal of the American Academy of Orthopaedic Surgeons, 20*(suppl 1), S70–S73. https://doi.org/10.5435/JAAOS-20-08-S70
59. Sears, B. (2018, May 29). Residual limb after amputation. *Verywell Health*. Retrieved from https://www.verywell.com/residual-limb-2696169
60. Starks, I., Frost, A., Wall, P., & Lim, J. (2011). Is a fracture of the transverse process of L5 a predictor of pelvic fracture instability? *Journal of Bone & Joint Surgery, 93*(7), 967–969. https://doi.org/10.1302/0301-620X.93B7.26772
61. Jacobs, L. M. (2014). Joint Committee to Create a National Policy to Enhance Survivability from Mass Casualty Shooting Events: Hartford Consensus II. *Journal of the American College of Surgeons, 218*(3). https://doi.org/10.1016/j.jamcollsurg.2013.11.004
62. American College of Surgeons. (n.d.). Stop the Bleed poster. Retrieved from https://www.bleedingcontrol.org/resources/stop-the-bleed-poster
63. U.S. Department of Homeland Security. (n.d.). *Stop the Bleed.* Retrieved from https://www.dhs.gov/stopthebleed/
64. Khoshmohabat, H., Paydar, S., Kazemi, H. M., & Dalfardi, B. (2016). Overview of agents used for emergency hemostasis. *Trauma Monthly, 21*(1). https://doi.org/10.5812/traumamon.26023
65. Georgiev, G. P., Tanchev, P. P., Zheleva, Z., & Kinov, P. (2018). Comparison of topical and intravenous administration of tranexamic acid for blood loss control during total joint replacement: Review of literature. *Journal of Orthopaedic Translation, 13*, 7–12. https://doi.org/10.1016/j.jot.2017.12.006

CHAPTER 11

Surface and Burn Trauma

Courtney Edwards, DNP, MPH, RN, CCRN, CEN, TCRN

OBJECTIVES

Upon completion of this chapter, the learner will be able to:

1. Describe the mechanisms of injury associated with surface and burn trauma.
2. Describe pathophysiologic changes as a basis for assessment of the trauma patient with surface and burn injuries.
3. Demonstrate the nursing assessment of the trauma patient with surface and burn injuries.
4. Plan appropriate interventions for the trauma patient with surface and burn injuries.
5. Evaluate the effectiveness of nursing interventions for the trauma patient with surface and burn injuries.

Knowledge of normal anatomy and physiology serves as a foundation for understanding anatomic derangements and pathophysiologic processes that may result from trauma. Before reading this chapter, it is strongly suggested that the learner review the following material. This material will not be covered in the lectures or tested directly, but it serves as foundational content. Thus, it may be the basis for some test questions and skill evaluation steps.

Anatomy and Physiology of the Integumentary System

The integumentary system, or skin, is the largest organ in the body and is composed of the epidermis, dermis, and hypodermis (**Figure 11-1**). The integumentary system serves many vital functions including the following[1]:

- Protection from environmental hazards, including infection
- Thermoregulation and prevention of excess bodily fluid loss
- Sensory perception
- Vitamin D synthesis

Epidermis

The epidermis is the outermost layer of skin and the body's first line of defense to environmental threat. It is composed of epithelial cells, is avascular, and receives nourishment from the dermis.[1] Melanocytes, which are

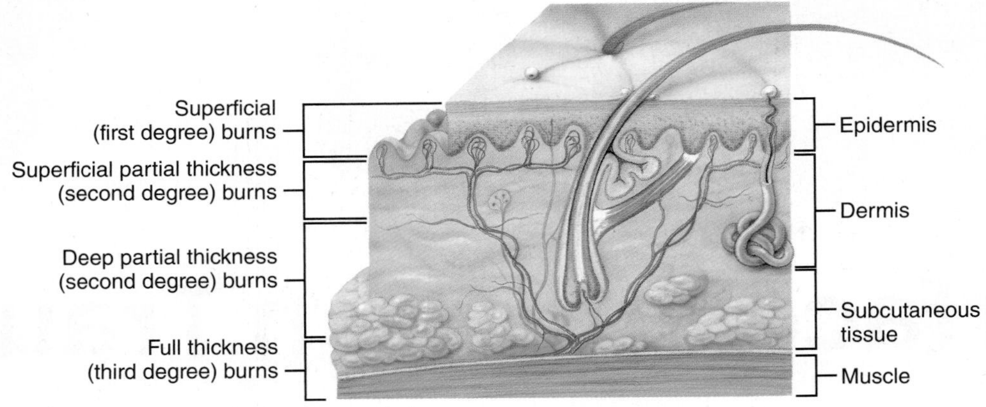

Figure 11-1 *Layers of the skin and depth of burn wound.*
The layers of the skin that are affected differ depending on the depth of a burn injury.

responsible for skin pigmentation, are found within the epidermis. The epidermis is thin in most areas, but is thicker on the soles of feet, hands, and other areas routinely exposed to pressure and friction.[1] The epidermis of the skin is composed of two or more cellular layers; it is constantly shedding cells from the outer layer and developing new cells from the basal cell layer. The epidermal layer of the skin regenerates at a rate of complete replacement every month or faster following an injury. With an intact basal cell layer, regeneration is possible.[1]

Dermis

The dermis is located directly beneath the epidermis, has a strong extracellular matrix and is thicker than the epidermis.[1] The three components of the dermis are *collagen*, a protein that gives skin its mechanical strength; *elastin*, a substance that gives the skin stretch and flexibility; and *ground substance*, which helps to cushion and hydrate the skin.[2,3]

The dermis has two layers. The reticular dermis, the deeper layer, contains nerve endings, hair follicles, sweat and sebaceous glands, finger and toe nails, and blood vessels. The papillary dermis, the superficial layer, aids in healing and provides nourishment to the epidermis.[2,3] This layer of skin is highly vascular and plays a role in fluid, electrolyte, and body temperature regulation.[1-3]

Unlike the epidermis, the dermis does not continuously regenerate new cells. Instead, repair of damaged dermal cells is dependent on the inflammatory and wound healing processes, especially fibroblast infiltration of the area.

Hypodermis

The subcutaneous tissue, sometimes referred to as the hypodermis or superficial fascia, lies beneath the dermis. This layer is rich in fat and connective tissue and attaches the dermis to the underlying structures. It functions as a heat insulator, nutrition supplier, and mechanical shock absorber. Excess fatty tissue, which is not vascular in nature, can delay or complicate wound healing.

Wound Healing

Wound healing is a four-phase process beginning the moment injury occurs[4]:

- Hemostasis
  - Platelet activation and aggregation is triggered.
  - Clotting factors are released, beginning the clotting cascade.
  - Vasoconstriction occurs.
  - A clot is formed.
- Inflammatory phase
  - Vasodilation and capillary permeability increase perfusion to the wound.
  - White blood cells infiltrate the area, removing cellular debris and foreign material, and fighting infection.
- Proliferative phase
  - There is a proliferation and lateral migration of epithelial cells combined with collagen to resurface the wound bed.
  - Activation of keratinocytes assists in closure of the wound and restores the vascular network.
  - Granulation tissue forms; the time needed depends on the depth and severity of the wound.
  - Tensile strength improves.
- Maturation phase
  - This phase can take days to years, depending on when the wound fibroblasts leave the site.

TABLE 11-1 Pressures Involved in Capillary and Fluid Dynamics

Type of Pressure	Effect
Capillary hydrostatic pressure	› Pushes fluid out of the capillary
Tissue (interstitial) hydrostatic pressure	› Pushes fluid into the capillary
Capillary (plasma) oncotic pressure	› Determined by plasma proteins that are relatively impermeable › Prevents movement out of the capillary and pulls fluid into the capillary
Tissue (interstitial) oncotic pressure	› Dependent on the interstitial protein concentration › Prevents movement into the capillary and pulls fluid into the interstitial space

- Tensile strength continues to increase.
- Collagen models scar tissue, reducing the wound's size and visibility.

Capillary and Fluid Dynamics

As noted, the dermis plays a role in fluid and electrolyte balance. Four pressures within the interstitial space and the vasculature play a role in the fluid and electrolyte status of the body, including the skin and its structures (**Table 11-1**).[1] Hydrostatic pressure is the force exerted by a fluid pressing against a wall; it is divided into capillary and tissue pressures. Oncotic pressure is created by the presence of nondiffusible molecules (plasma proteins); like hydrostatic pressure, it is subclassified as either capillary or tissue pressure.

In patients with large burns to the skin, these pressures are disrupted. As a consequence, capillary leak of fluid out of the intravascular space and into the interstitial space occurs and can result in hypovolemia, shock, and death.

Introduction

This chapter addresses both surface trauma and burn injuries, focusing on how the pathophysiology of these injury patterns impacts patient assessment, care, and outcomes. Providing quality care to patients who sustain surface trauma and/or burn injuries is often a labor-intensive process.

A patient who has sustained surface or burn trauma must be managed through the primary and secondary assessments, with any necessary interventions being provided to the patient. Most surface trauma is addressed in the secondary survey; however, some may require immediate intervention to establish an effective airway or control hemorrhage.

Surface Trauma

Surface trauma is defined as a disruption in the normal anatomic structure and function of the integumentary system. It may be the patient's primary traumatic injury, but more often occurs concurrently in a patient with multisystem trauma. Surface trauma includes the following types of injuries:

- Lacerations
- Abrasions
- Avulsions
- Contusions and hematomas
- Puncture wounds
- Missile injuries
- Frostbite

Surface trauma can involve the skin as well as supporting and underlying structures such as muscles, tendons, ligaments, blood vessels, and nerves. It is essential that the seriousness of these seemingly minor injuries is not minimized, as they can result in hemorrhage, loss of limb, and death secondary to infection.

Mechanisms of Injury

The following mechanisms of injury (MOIs) are associated with surface injuries:

- Falls
- Motor vehicle collisions (MVCs)
- Impact with objects
- Overexertion and strenuous movements
- Cutting or piercing objects
- Natural and environmental factors
- Foreign bodies
- Exposure to chemicals or caustic substances

The MOI is essential to predicting injury patterns in the trauma patient. Moreover, assessment findings can provide clues to potential underlying tissue and organ damage. See Chapter 2, "Biomechanics, Kinematics, and Mechanisms of Injury," for more information.

Pathophysiology as a Basis for Assessment Findings

The wound healing process is complex and requires meticulous and ongoing assessment and monitoring to prevent infection, which remains a leading cause of morbidity and mortality.[5]

Certain wound characteristics predispose some injuries to a greater risk of infection:

- Mammalian bites
- Crush injury
- Puncture wounds
- Stellate lacerations
- Wounds with an 8-hour or greater delay in seeking medical treatment

Patients at highest risk for infectious complications include the following groups[5,6]:

- Infants
- Older adults
- Smokers or others with impaired oxygenation and perfusion
- Patients who are immunocompromised or taking immunosuppressants
- Patients with diabetes or renal failure
- Patients with existing vascular disease

Trauma patients with these comorbidities or risk circumstances often benefit from referral to wound clinics that specialize in optimizing the wound healing process with specialized treatments such as leech therapy, hyperbaric oxygen treatments, negative-pressure wound therapy, and specialty dressings (silver-impregnated products, honey, or polyhexamethylene biguanide).[4,5]

Nursing Care of the Patient with Surface Trauma

When caring for trauma patients, keep in mind that surface injuries may be a distraction, especially if they are extensive and obvious, that diverts the provider's attention away from subtle, but potentially more life-threatening injuries such as an ineffective airway.

Primary Survey

The primary survey and all life-threatening injuries are addressed, and the patient is stabilized, before addressing surface trauma. Chapter 3, "Initial Assessment," describes the systematic approach to the nursing care of the trauma patient. Most surface trauma is addressed in the secondary survey; however, some wounds may require immediate intervention to control hemorrhage.

Secondary Survey

The following assessment parameters are specific to patients with surface trauma injuries.

H: History

Questions to ask during history taking include, but are not limited to, the following:

- When and where did this injury occur? How much time has elapsed since injury?
- Was the cause of the injury from a clean or dirty source?
- Was the cause of the wound an animal bite and if so, is the animal known? Is there a risk of rabies exposure?
- Is there a risk of a retained foreign body?
- Is there possible tendon involvement, and does the patient have full or partial range of motion?
- Is there possible nerve involvement, and does the patient have sensation at the site? Is there any numbness or tingling sensations?
- Was the injury intentional or unintentional?
- Is this injury work related?
- Does the patient have a history of medical conditions that may affect wound healing (e.g., diabetes, immunocompromised)?
- Which medications is the patient taking (e.g., anticoagulants, antihypertensives, steroids)?
- Is the patient's tetanus status up to date?
- If the injury involves the hand or arm, what is the patient's hand dominance?

H: Head-to-Toe Assessment

Inspect for the following:

- The location and type of the wound and any associated injuries
- The effectiveness of hemostasis
- The depth, length, and size of the wound
- The color of the tissue and surrounding tissue
- The extent of denuded tissue and underlying structures involved
- Tissue swelling and/or deformity and presence of foreign bodies
- Evidence of any apparent wound contamination or presence of exudate

Palpate for the following:

- Assessment findings suspicious for compartment syndrome, including the following[6]:
  - Pain
    - Is a hallmark of compartment syndrome when it is out of proportion for the injury
    - Often occurs before changes in pulse, color, and temperature of the distal limb
  - Weak or absent distal pulses
  - Delayed capillary refill

- Firmness on palpation of muscle and soft tissue in the surrounding area
- Distal skin that is cool to the touch
- Distal skin that is pale or cyanotic
- Decrease in patient sensation

The six P's mnemonic helps the trauma nurse to remember components of the neurovascular assessment: pain, pallor, pulses, paresthesia, paralysis, and pressure. See Chapter 10, "Musculoskeletal Trauma," for more information.

Interventions

The immediate goal when treating surface trauma is to obtain and maintain hemostasis. This is accomplished by applying direct pressure to the site.[6] For cases that are not resolved by direct pressure, cauterization and suture ligation of isolated vessels may be necessary. In patients who experience limb injuries for which bleeding cannot be controlled with direct pressure, tourniquets have been used successfully.[6] See Chapter 5, "Shock," and Chapter 10 for more information.

Selected Surface Trauma Injuries

The surface trauma injuries discussed in this section include a cross-section of types and causes.

Abrasion

An abrasion is a partial- or full-thickness wound that denudes the skin, exposing the dermis or subcutaneous skin layer.[7] This type of injury commonly occurs with falls and bicycle or motorcycle collisions, where the skin is rubbed off by a hard, rough surface. Abrasions can be mild or severe, and can vary in surface area and depth depending on the mechanism and force involved. Road burn or abrasions, resulting from a low side crash or laying down a motorcycle, is an example of an abrasion involving a large surface area. If the injured area becomes embedded with gravel and dirt despite vigorous wound cleansing and debridement, it can cause a traumatic tattoo effect on the skin, characterized by an irregular black or blue skin discoloration.

Avulsion

Avulsions are full-thickness wounds caused by a tearing or ripping of skin and soft tissue away from underlying tissues.[8] The wound edges are not well approximated.[7] These injuries often involve the fingers, scalp, and nose, and can occur as a result of working with machinery or from MVCs. A degloving injury is an avulsion in which the skin and tissue is removed, exposing underlying structures, including bone, tendons, and ligaments.[8,9] Degloving injuries commonly affect the extremities and scalp.

Avulsions can occur in bone fractures when soft tissue is torn away from the bone. The extent of these injuries can impact other systems. For example, one prognostic indicator for limb salvage after tibia–fibula fracture is the magnitude of avulsed tissue from the bone shaft.[10] When soft tissue is avulsed, the bone may not receive adequate nutrients through the circulation. Exposed bone and mangle injuries are at highest risk for infection.

Treatment for avulsions depends on the body part and the amount of tissue avulsed. Simple wound care may be adequate in a simple skin avulsion, whereas more extensive avulsions, such as degloving injuries, may require surgical intervention for grafting or amputation.[7]

Contusion and Hematoma

A contusion is a closed wound in which a ruptured blood vessel or capillary bed hemorrhages into the surrounding tissue as a result of blunt force trauma.[1] A contusion is synonymous with a bruise. A hematoma occurs when blood leaks under the skin surface and often forms a palpable mass (blood clot) under the skin.[1]

Determining the appropriate treatment requires analysis of the force required to produce the contusion and the potential for trauma to underlying structures such as compression injury to arteries and nerves, causing ischemia.

Laceration

Lacerations are open wounds that result from sharp or blunt forces through the dermis and epidermis with potential involvement of the underlying structures such as muscles, tendons, and ligaments.[9] Common causes of lacerations include injuries from tools or machinery. Exploration of deeper lacerations is required to assess the integrity of underlying structures and to evaluate for foreign bodies. Lacerations differ from cuts or incisions, which have clean, well-approximated edges such as from a knife or broken glass.

Puncture Wound

Puncture wounds occur when a spear-like object creates an open wound deeper than it is wide. Puncture injuries result from various mechanisms including the following:

- Superficial wounds, such as stepping on a tack
- Deeper injuries, such as stab wounds[7]
- Injuries from foreign bodies or implements
- Animal and human bites

Although puncture wounds may appear minor, they carry a potential risk for infection and underlying tissue or organ damage—especially with injuries caused by high pressure (as missile injuries[7]), such as a nail gun injury. See Chapter 2 for more information.

When a patient experiences a missile or impalement injury, the foreign body is often more deeply embedded and impacts underlying tissue. Large foreign bodies are removed after underlying structures have been assessed. Hemorrhage can result after embedded objects are removed because the item may be providing a means of hemostasis. For example, a piece of glass embedded in the hand may be placing pressure on a branch of a capillary, which is serving to control bleeding. Thus, premature removal of the glass will result in bleeding. Large impaled objects are often removed in the operating room by trauma surgeons who can repair damage to deep tissue and vessels.

Puncture wounds carry a high infection rate.[3] Risk factors for infection include the following:

- Large or deep wounds
- Contaminated wounds (bite wounds)
- Wounds with osseous involvement
- High-pressure injuries
- Wounds more than 6 hours old
- Human and animal bites

Rabies, although rare, does occur and is a consideration when managing animal bite wounds. If the animal is known to the patient or family but not current with immunizations or if the animal is unknown or wild, rabies prophylaxis and antibiotic therapy may be indicated.[7]

Missile Injuries

Missile injuries include stab wounds, firearms injuries, and other high-pressure puncture wounds.

Frostbite

Frostbite occurs when exposure to cold causes tissue to freeze and ice crystals to form.[11] Vasoconstriction causes reduced perfusion and injury to the endothelial layer of blood vessels, and a thrombus can form. Frostbite is classified according to the depth and type of tissue involved:

- *Partial thickness:* Skin becomes hyperemic and edematous. Some tingling or burning sensation may be felt.
- *Deep partial thickness:* Clear blisters begin to form. If blood is present in the blister, it may suggest full-thickness damage to the skin. Parathesias and tenderness may be present.
- *Full thickness:* Total skin necrosis reaches into the subcutaneous tissue and involves muscle and bone. The skin turns black, and dry hard eschar forms.

Interventions

Frostbite interventions are summarized **Box 11-1**.

BOX 11-1 Frostbite Interventions

Healthcare professionals in many parts of the United States may never encounter frostbite cases. For others, understanding the interventions required is a necessary part of their practice. Other, less common causes of frostbite, include occupational exposures to very cold liquids or direct contact with extremely cold machinery.

- Start treatment only after it can be confirmed that the affected area will not be at risk for frostbite again after it is rewarmed, as incomplete thawing and refreezing can cause further injury.[11,12]
- Initial treatment consists of quickly rewarming the affected area over a period of 15 to 30 minutes in water that is at a temperature of 37°C to 39°C (98.6°F to 102.2°F). Research has shown that this lower temperature does not substantially increase the time to rewarm but does cause significantly less pain to the individual.[12]
  - Administer pain medication, as the rewarming process can be painful.[11,12]
  - Avoid any friction, rubbing, or massaging of the area to preserve tissue integrity.
  - If possible, immerse the area in warm water at a temperature of 37°C to 39°C (98.6°F to 102.2°F).[3,11,12] Use a method where the temperature of the water can be maintained within the appropriate range, such as a whirlpool with circulating water. The duration of rewarming is approximately 30 minutes; however, clinical findings of sufficient rewarming include return of sensation and presence of flushing in the distal tissues.[12]
  - Large, clear blisters that impede movement may be drained, debrided, and bandaged. Large hemorrhagic blisters that impede movement may be drained, but not debrided. Small blisters are maintained intact.[12,13]
- Guard against further injury to the area. For example, affected extremities can be splinted.

- Prevent or limit the risk of thrombus formation.
  - Administer ibuprofen.
  - The use of tissue plasminogen activator has been effective in maintaining perfusion and decreasing the need for amputation when administered within 24 hours of rewarming.[12]

Diagnostics and Interventions for Surface and Burn Trauma

Reevaluation adjuncts for surface and burn trauma include radiographic studies, laboratory studies, and wound care.

Radiographic Studies

Obtain plain films prior to wound closure to evaluate wounds for foreign bodies and to assess for underlying fractures or joint penetration from any foreign body. Ultrasound may be a more useful tool for determining the presence of plastic or wood than plain radiographs.

Laboratory Studies

Laboratory studies include the following:

- A complete blood count (CBC) with differential may be obtained to assess for anemia and/or thrombocytopenia from blood loss, and for leukocytosis as evidence of possible infection.
- A coagulation profile may be obtained to identify any potential coagulation abnormalities, especially in the setting of deep or large wounds.

Wound culture and sensitivity may be useful in infected wounds to guide appropriate antibiotic therapy.[7] Cultures and sensitivities can be obtained through swab of viable tissues, tissue biopsy, or needle aspiration. This type of study should occur when signs and symptoms of infection are present.

Wound Care

The goals of wound care include the following:

- Promote wound healing
- Prevent complications (infection, limited range of motion)
- Maintain function
- Minimize scar formation

Three basic classifications of closure are used for wound healing: primary, secondary, and tertiary (**Figure 11-2**).[14]

- Primary wound closure is used for wounds with well-approximated borders and minimal tissue destruction. Simple closure techniques, such as suturing, or staples are used.
- Secondary wound closure is used for infection-prone wounds in which the edges are not well approximated. Gauze packing or wound drains may be needed. This method of repair requires formation of granulation tissue from the base of the wound upward.
- Tertiary closure (also known as delayed primary closure) is used for deep wounds that were initially left open and allowed to granulate due to the age of the wound or risk of infection. After this granulation, debridement and sutures are used to bring the wound edges together to promote healing.[4,15]

Nursing considerations include the following:

- All wounds may be cleaned with tap water or normal saline.[16] This is essential and one of the most effective methods to reduce the risk of wound infections.
  - Dirty or deep wounds may require cleansing with alternative antiseptic solutions (e.g., povidone–iodine solution, chlorhexidine, hydrogen peroxide).
  - Use of antiseptics has recently increased because of the emergence of antimicrobial resistance. Follow organizational policy regarding use of cleansing solutions.
- Anesthesia may be required when removing gravel or other foreign materials from the wound or for wound repair.[16]
  - Avoid using lidocaine with epinephrine on the fingers, toes, or any other area where vasoconstriction could cause impaired distal blood circulation.
  - Digital blocks using bupivacaine (Marcaine) or lidocaine may be used for finger or toe injures.
  - Procedural sedation may be needed for repair of extensive wounds or with wound repair in children.
- Hair removal from around the wound is done with scissors or clippers. Shaving is not recommended due to the potential for infection.[17] Eyebrows should never be removed, because their regrowth is not guaranteed. Another option for addressing hair when attempting to create a better field of vision for wound

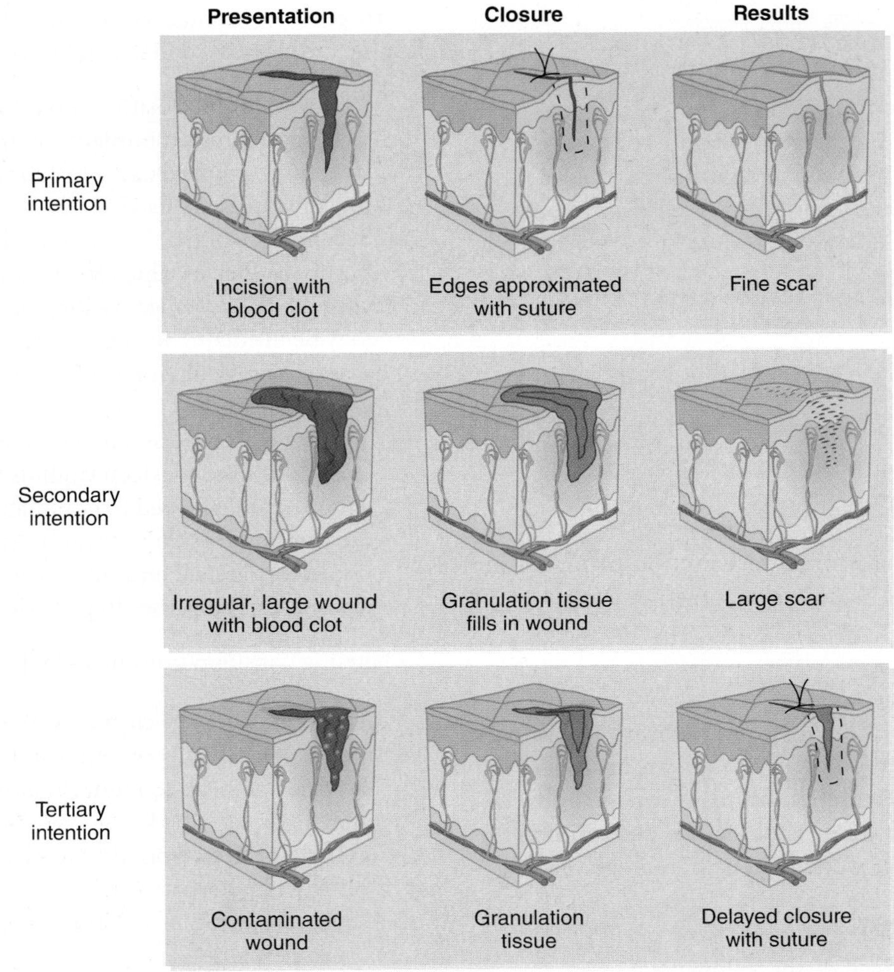

Figure 11-2 *Types of wound healing.*

closure is to lubricate the hair with antibacterial ointment and lay the hair away from the wound edges.

- Wound irrigation can reduce the bacterial contamination of the wound and prevent infection. Use a copious amount of irrigation solution. Low-pressure irrigation, such as with a bulb syringe, will help to remove large contaminants, but high-pressure irrigation works best for smaller contaminants and bacteria. Take care to not destroy viable tissue.[18]
  - Prophylactic systemic antibiotics are not routinely used for acute management surface trauma. Topical antimicrobial agents may be used on the wound to reduce the risk of infection.
- Following organizational policies, consider taking photographs of the injury prior to cleaning or repairing the wounds if the injury was associated with a crime.
- Administer tetanus prophylaxis as indicated (**Table 11-2**)[19]

Reevaluation and Post-Resuscitation Care

Reevaluation and ongoing assessment of new wounds include the following issues:

- The ability of the patient to maintain hemostasis of the wound
- The effectiveness of the wound closure modality

Definitive Care or Transport

Provide the patient and family with education on topics including the following:

- Signs and symptoms of infection including fever, opening of the wound site, drainage from the wound, redness or red streaks progressing up an extremity, excessive pain or swelling at the site, or numbness or tingling at sites distal to the wounds

TABLE 11-2 Guide to Tetanus Prophylaxis with TIG in Routine Wound Management

History of Adsorbed Tetanus Toxoid-Containing Vaccines (Doses)	Clean, Minor Wound		All Other Wounds[a]	
	DTaP, Tdap, or Td[b]	TIG[c]	DTaP, Tdap, or Td[b]	TIG[c]
Unknown or < 3	Yes	No	Yes	Yes
≥ 3	No[d]	No	No[e]	No

Abbreviations: DTaP, diphtheria and tetanus toxoids and acellular pertussis vaccine; HIV, human immunodeficiency virus; Td, tetanus and diphtheria toxoids; Tdap, tetanus toxoid, reduced diphtheria toxoid, and acellular pertussis; TIG, tetanus immune globulin.

[a] Such as, but not limited to, wounds contaminated with dirt, feces, soil, and saliva; puncture wounds; avulsions; and wounds resulting from missiles, crushing, burns, and frostbite.

[b] DTaP is recommended for children < 7 years of age. Tdap is preferred to Td for persons aged 11 years or older who have not previously received Tdap. Persons aged 7 years or older who are not fully immunized against pertussis, tetanus, or diphtheria should receive one dose of Tdap for wound management and as part of the catch-up series.

[c] People with HIV infection or severe immunodeficiency who have contaminated wounds (including minor wounds) should also receive TIG, regardless of their history of tetanus immunizations.

[d] Yes, if ≥ 10 years since the last tetanus toxoid-containing vaccine dose.

[e] Yes, if ≥ 5 years since the last tetanus toxoid-containing vaccine dose.

Data from Centers for Disease Control and Prevention. (May 31, 2018). *Tetanus: For clinicians.* Retrieved from https://www.cdc.gov/tetanus/clinicians.html.

- Bathing information with bandage or dressing supplies
- When to report signs and symptoms to their primary care providers
- Instructions regarding suture removal and follow-up
- Infection prevention

Burn Trauma

Burn injuries can have a lifelong impact on patients due to loss of function, scarring, and psychological trauma. Caring for this patient population can be challenging for the trauma nurse: In addition to life-threatening situations necessitating immediate attention, hypothermia, hypercarbia, and hypoxia may develop. Pain management for these patients can also be difficult. Lengthy recovery, chronic pain, and scarring are common in this patient population.

Epidemiology

Burn injuries continue to be one of the leading causes of unintentional injury in the United States. In the United States, 73% of all burn injuries occur in the home, followed by work (8%) and the street/highway (5%).[20] Fires, flames, and smoke are the fifth leading cause of fatal injury in the home.[21] Cooking is the primary cause of residential fires and home fire injuries, whereas cigarette smoking causes the most fire-related deaths.[21] Alcohol or substance use is implicated as a contributing factor in as many as 14% of home fire-related deaths.[22]

The most vulnerable patient populations at risk for burn trauma include children, elderly, persons with reduced mental capacity (e.g., those with learning disabilities or dementia who may not recognize or react appropriately in a dangerous situation), and individuals with reduced mobility or sensory impairments who might not react quickly to a dangerous situation.[23]

Mechanism of Injury and Biomechanics

Burns are injuries to tissues caused by heat, friction, electricity, radiation, or chemicals. In order of prevalence, the most common mechanisms of burn injury for persons age 5 years and older are the following[24]:

- Fire/flames
- Scald injuries
- Electrical and chemicals

Children younger than 5 years of age are 2.4 times more likely to need emergency medical treatment as a result of a burn injury.[20] Scalds are the most common MOI in young children. Burns from flames are more common for children between the ages of 5 and 16 years.[23]

Burns can be intentional in cases such as assault, abuse, or self-harm. Pattern burns (such as from a cigarette or identifiable object) or immersion burns—such as circumferential and sharply demarcated burns to both feet—should raise suspicion of possible maltreatment. See Chapter 16,

"Special Populations: The Interpersonal-Violence Trauma Patient," for more information.

Burns are classified into four categories based on the source of the burn:

- Thermal
- Chemical
- Electrical
- Radiation

Thermal Burns

Thermal burns result from contact with hot objects (contact burns), hot liquids (scalds), or flames. Flame burns are the predominant cause of burns, particularly in the adult population, for patients who are admitted to burn centers.[23]

Scald burns are thermal burns that result from contact with a hot liquid. Young children are commonly injured by pulling a container of hot liquid onto themselves. Injury severity depends on the temperature of the substance and the length of exposure. For instance, the safety standard for the maximum temperature of U.S. residential water heaters is 48.8°C (120°F).[24] At this temperature, it will take an average of 5 minutes to cause a full-thickness burn on the skin of an adult.[24] By comparison, the temperatures of hot beverages (e.g., coffee, tea) average 71°C to 82°C (160°F to 180°F) and can cause full-thickness burns on contact.[24]

Chemical Burns

Chemical burns result from exposure to acids, alkalis, or organic compounds. Acids are organic or inorganic substances that cause coagulation necrosis. Examples of acids include hydrofluoric acid, carbonic acid, and white phosphorus. Alkalis cause extensive tissue damage by dissolving protein and collagen; thus, they result in deep tissue destruction and necrosis. Examples of alkaline agents include anhydrous ammonia, cement, hydrocarbons, and tar. Organic compounds, such as phenols or petroleum products such as gasoline, tend to dissolve the lipid membrane of the cell wall. Other examples of organic compounds include fertilizers or dyes.

Electrical Burns

Electrical burns are unique in terms of their etiology and severity.

- The cause of electrical burns includes direct exposure to electrical current or a lightning strike. Electrical current can be either direct (DC) or alternating (AC). DC is commonly found in batteries, solar panels, and fuel cells; AC is commonly found in homes and businesses and used in medical devices and electronics. Notably, lightning injuries usually do not traverse the body, but rather flow around it, potentially creating a shock wave capable of causing fractures and other traumatic injuries.
- The severity of injury is determined by many factors, including the voltage, current (amperage), type of current (AC or DC), path of the current flow, duration of contact, resistance at the point of contact, and individual susceptibility.

Radiation Burns

Radiation burn injuries result from exposure to thermal radiation, ultraviolet light, or particulate ionizing radiation.[25] Common causes of radiation burns include the sun, such as a sunburn, and radiation beams used to treat cancer patients. Exposure to radioactive fallout after nuclear explosions or nuclear accidents can also result in beta-radiation burn injuries.

Usual Concurrent Injuries

Patients with selected burn MOIs can be at risk for an inhalation injury, including loss of airway, respiratory failure, and death. Patients who present with thermal burns from fires that occurred in a small or enclosed space are at especially high risk. Other concurrent injuries may be determined by reviewing the MOI and pertinent details from the scene. For example, if the patient jumped from a building during a fire, assess for fractures and organ hemorrhage. If the burn was sustained in an MVC, assess for additional injuries related to the collision. Consider a blunt traumatic injury if the MOI was a blast event. See Chapter 2 for additional information.

Pathophysiology as a Basis for the Assessment Findings of Burn Trauma

The external injury resulting from burn trauma is the destruction of the skin. However, the internal injuries are of equal, if not more, concern in these patients. The pathophysiologic impact of burn injuries primarily depends on the extent of the burn and the depth of the burn.

Airway Patency

Burns to tissue or exposure to heated gases can cause life-threatening airway edema. A hoarse voice, brassy cough, carbonaceous sputum, burns around the mouth or nares, or stridor may indicate burns to the airway. Signs and symptoms of airway obstruction may be subtle, developing over time and not becoming readily apparent until the patient is in extremis.

Hypoxia, Asphyxia, and Carbon Monoxide Poisoning

Hypoxia can result from an inhalation injury or from carbon monoxide (CO) poisoning.[26] Asphyxia occurs from breathing decreased amounts of oxygen in the inspired air, as a result of being in a closed space where oxygen is being consumed by the fire.

CO is a colorless, odorless, and tasteless gas that is released into the air during a fire. CO, which has a higher affinity to the hemoglobin molecule than oxygen, replaces oxygen in the hemoglobin, thereby creating carboxyhemoglobin and reducing the oxygen content of the blood. The patient may complain of headache, confusion, nausea, or vomiting. CO poisoning can also result in coma or death.[27] In assessing the patient with CO poisoning, oxygenation and oxygen saturation are best measured with arterial blood gases (ABGs). The pulse oximeter will not differentiate hemoglobin bound to oxygen from hemoglobin bound to CO, making it unreliable.[26]

Treat the patient with CO poisoning with oxygen until carboxyhemoglobin levels drop to less than 10%. The half-life of CO when a patient is placed on 100% oxygen is decreased to approximately 1 hour; for this reason, patients presumed to have elevated CO levels should be immediately placed on oxygen therapy. Hyperbaric oxygen for CO poisoning has not been definitely shown to improve neurologic outcomes, and its implementation should not delay transfer to a burn center for definitive treatment.[26]

CLINICAL PEARL

The pulse oximeter will not differentiate hemoglobin bound to oxygen from hemoglobin bound to CO, making it unreliable.[26]

Hydrogen cyanide is another product of incomplete combustion of synthetic products such as carpeting, upholstered furniture, plastics, or draperies. When cyanide enters the cells, cells are unable to produce adenosine triphosphate and shift toward anaerobic metabolism. Blood cyanide levels are difficult to measure through routine laboratory studies; therefore, treatment is prophylactically initiated based on the history of being in an enclosed space with symptoms of changes in respiratory rate, shortness of breath, headache, confusion, irritation of the eyes and mucous membranes, or lactic acidosis that persists despite fluid resuscitation.[26] The patient should be treated with a hydroxocobalamin cyanide antidote kit.[26]

Pulmonary Injury

Pulmonary injury doubles the mortality of patients with burns.[27] The process of pulmonary injury includes the following elements[27]:

- Inhalation of the products of combustion, such as particles of carbon and noxious fumes
- Damage to the mucosal cells of the bronchioles
- Increased permeability of cell membranes, allowing leakage from the cells and causing impaired gas exchange
- Sloughing of dead cells, which then obstructs the airways
- Decreased production and/or loss of surfactant, resulting in alveolar collapse
- Spasm of bronchi and bronchioles
- Acute lung injury or acute respiratory distress syndrome (ARDS)
- Secondary complications such as pneumonia

Clinical evidence of a pulmonary injury may not be immediately evident during the resuscitation phase,[27] so it is crucial that the trauma team identify those patients at risk for respiratory compromise and proactively manage and protect the airway.

Capillary Leak Syndrome

Edema formation is one of the more challenging management issues of treating burn injuries. The inflammatory response occurs both locally and, in large burns, systemically, resulting in a shift of fluid from the intravascular fluid into the interstitial space,[28] sometimes referred to as "third spacing." In burned tissue, mediators such as histamine, serotonin, prostaglandins, blood products, complement components, and kinins act to increase the vascular permeability of the capillary membrane.[28] This increased permeability, referred to as *capillary leak*,[29] allows plasma to pass through the damaged membranes, leaving red blood cells in the intravascular space. In areas of undamaged tissue, there can be increased permeability due to the release of the histamines and kinins. Burns greater than 20% total body surface area (TBSA) are most commonly vulnerable to this capillary leak.[28]

During capillary leak, large amounts of the fluid infused during resuscitation can seep from the veins into the tissue.[28] This condition can persist for 6 to 12 hours after the burn injury, until the capillary membranes begin to undergo repair and leakage begins to decrease.[28] However, the edema can last much longer. The rate of fluid lost from intravascular spaces depends on the patient's age, burn size and depth, intravascular pressures, and time elapsed since the burn.[6]

The inflammatory response results in the release of numerous substrates, which then lead to further edema and potential cardiac collapse[6]:

- Release of histamine and prostaglandin leads to vasodilation and increased capillary permeability.
- Thromboxane, a vasoconstrictive substance, causes platelet aggregation and expansion of the zone of coagulation.
- Bradykinin causes increased permeability of the venules, and oxygen-free radicals damage the endothelial cells, which are the basement membrane of new tissue.

Mechanical Obstruction

Circumferential burns to the neck or chest may reduce the ability of the patient to breathe deeply, this is especially prevalent with full thickness burns because the dry, leathery tissue is far less compliant than intact healthy skin.

Loss of Skin Integrity

Loss and destruction of the skin layer results in the loss of vital functions, including thermoregulation and protection against infection. Assessment of the burn surface will reveal a three-dimensional mass of injured tissues (**Figure 11-3**)[30]:

- Zone of coagulation
  - The most severely damaged center of the burn, this area is often necrotic in nature.
  - Debridement of this necrotic tissue is essential for wound healing, as it is not capable of regeneration.
  - Skin grafting is a consideration for burns involving the zone of coagulation.
- Zone of stasis
  - This zone surrounds the zone of coagulation.
  - Tissue in this area has been moderately damaged, resulting in decreased tissue perfusion and edema.
  - If wound treatment is timely and appropriate, this tissue may improve to a zone of hyperemia; if not, it may deteriorate to a zone of coagulation.

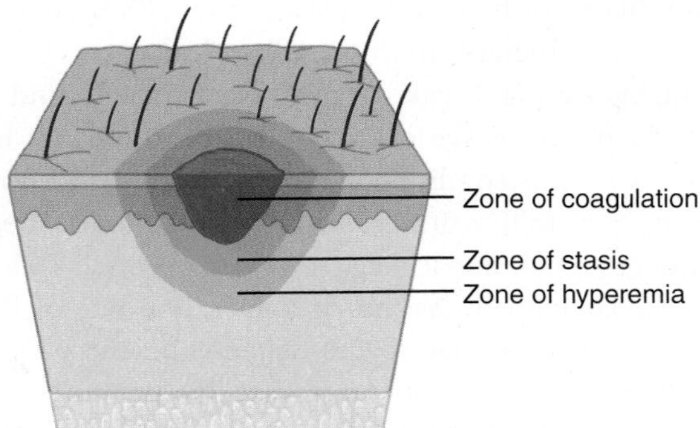

Figure 11-3 *Zones of injury in burns.*

- Zone of hyperemia
  - This is the outermost area of the burn.
  - Due to the inflammatory process, there is increased blood flow to this area, resulting in the best chance for tissue viability, barring infection.

Hypothermia

Patients can become hypothermic owing to disruption of the normal integumentary function of temperature regulation. Hypothermia can help lead to clotting and bleeding disorders such as disseminated intravascular coagulation (DIC).

Nursing Care of the Patient with Burn Trauma

Severe burns can distract from subtler-appearing, yet more life-threatening coexisting injuries such as an ineffective airway. It is imperative that the trauma team maintain focus on treating life threats before treating the burn. Chapter 3 describes the systematic approach to the nursing care of the trauma patient. The following assessment parameters are specific to patients with burn injuries.

Primary Survey and Resuscitation Adjuncts

The primary survey begins with the alertness and airway.

A: Alertness and Airway

Do the following:

- Assess that the patient is alert and can maintain a patent airway.
- If the patient is unable to protect the airway, ensure a patent airway.
- If fire is the mechanism for a thermal burn, inspect for evidence of extensive and deep facial burns, soot, carbonaceous sputum, singed nasal hairs, erythema or swelling of the oropharynx or nasopharynx, brassy cough, or progressive hoarseness—these signs might indicate an inhalation injury. If they are present, consider prophylactic intubation.
- Consider the need for cervical spine protection based on the MOI.

B: Breathing and Ventilation

Do the following:

- Begin administering oxygen at 10–15 L/minute via nonrebreather mask.[31,32]
- After the primary survey is complete, maintain SpO_2 between 94% and 98%.[31,32]
- Ensure effective ventilation. Observe for adequate chest wall expansion.

- Hyperbaric oxygen may be considered for severe CO poisoning after consultation with a medical toxicologist or poison control center outside of the resuscitation phase.[33]

C: Circulation and Control of Hemorrhage

Do the following:

- Avoid obtaining vascular access through burned tissue if possible.
- Follow a fluid resuscitation guideline for calculating the amount of fluid needed to promptly restore intravascular volume and to preserve tissue perfusion to minimize tissue ischemia. More definitive calculation of hourly fluid rates is performed during the secondary survey.
- Prior to calculating the TBSA, the following guidelines are recommended as starting points for fluid resuscitation rates[34]:
  - 14 years and older: 500 mL/hour lactated Ringer's solution
  - 6–13 years of age: 250 mL/hour lactated Ringer's solution
  - 5 years of age and younger: 125 mL/hour lactated Ringer's solution

Adult Fluid Replacement Guidelines

Adult fluid replacement guidelines[15,35] include the following:

- In adults with burn injuries that are more than 20% TBSA, begin fluid resuscitation with lactated Ringer's solution at 2 mL/kg/percentage of TBSA. In adults with electrical burns begin fluid resuscitation, using 4 mL/kg.[36]
- Excessive fluid resuscitation can result in complications such as cerebral edema, pulmonary edema, abdominal compartment syndrome, and ARDS.[28]
- Half of the fluid is given in the first 8 hours from time of the burn injury, and the remainder is given in the remaining 16 hours.
- In an adult, maintain urinary output at 0.5 mL/kg/hour or approximately 30–50 mL/hour (always consider the patient's urinary output, comorbidities, and physiologic response prior to initiating fluid resuscitation). For adults with electrical injuries with evidence of myoglobinuria (dark red or pink-tinged urine), maintain urinary output at 1.0–1.5 mL/kg/hour or approximately 75–100 mL/hour until the urine is clear.
- Fluid resuscitation rate should be adjusted as needed to maintain adequate urine output.

BOX 11-2 Adult Fluid Replacement Recommendations

Formula: Weight in kg × 2 mL × % TBSA = total amount of fluid to be infused in 24 hours from the time of injury

- Give half of the calculated total during the first 8 hours
- Give the remaining half over the next 16 hours

Example: A 100-kg adult patient has sustained a 50% TBSA thermal burn.

- 100 kg × 2 = 200 mL
- 200 mL × 50% TBSA burn = 10,000 mL to be infused over the first 24 hours from the time of the burn
- 5,000 mL (10,000/2 = 5,000) will be given in the first 8 hours
- 5,000 mL will be infused over the remaining 16 hours

Abbreviation: TBSA, total body surface area.

- Ringer's lactated solution is the fluid of choice for fluid resuscitation because it approximates intravascular solute contents.[27,37] Hyperchloremic solutions (e.g., 0.9% sodium chloride) should be avoided.

Box 11-2 provides a sample calculation using this formula.

CLINICAL PEARL

Ringer's Lactated Solution

Ringer's lactated solution is the fluid of choice for fluid resuscitation in burn situations because it approximates the intravascular solute contents. Hyperchloremic solutions (e.g., 0.9% sodium chloride) should be avoided for the burn patient.

Some patients may have greater fluid requirements than the recommended calculations. They include the following groups:

- Infants and children
- Older adults
- Patients with inhalation injury
- Patients with high-voltage electrical injuries
- Intoxicated patients
- Patients who experience a delayed start of fluid resuscitation

Unlike resuscitation for hemorrhage, burn resuscitation is required to replace ongoing losses from capillary leak syndrome. These higher fluid requirements may arise because of an inability to assess the entirety of burn injury such as with inhalational and electrical injuries, or they may result from prior dehydration.

Pediatric Fluid Replacement Guidelines

Pediatric fluid replacement guidelines include the following recommendations[36]:

- For children younger than 14 years or weighing less than 40 kg, give 3 mL/kg per percentage of TBSA, half during the first 8 hours and the remaining half over the next 16 hours.
- For children weighing less than 30 kg, maintain the urinary output at 1 mL/kg/hour. For pediatric patients weighing more than 30 kg, up to age 17, urinary output should be 0.5 mL/kg/hour.
- In addition to resuscitation fluid, infants and young children weighing 30 kg or less should be placed on maintenance fluid containing glucose, specifically D5LR. Maintenance therapy is not titrated to urine output.[27]

D: Disability

Patients with burn injuries are usually alert and oriented. If not, consider associated injuries such as hypoxia, CO poisoning, preexisting medical conditions, or substance use.

E: Exposure and Environmental Control

Maintenance of body temperature is crucial in patients with burns, since they have lost their protective skin barrier. Wet dressings should be avoided.

Exposure

For exposure, do the following[36]:

- Remove all clothing, diapers, and jewelry, especially rings and bracelets that may cause constriction as the extremity swells.
- For superficial burns less than 10% TBSA, cool the burned tissue.
  - Apply cool tap water or saline in any practical manner (e.g., wet cloths, lavage) for a brief period (3–5 minutes).
- Do not apply ice directly to the skin, as it may cause additional tissue damage.
- Do not immerse the burned area in water.

Environmental Control

To maintain environmental control, do the following:

- Use blankets to keep the patient warm.
- Use caution with cooling interventions, as they may contribute to hypothermia.

Reevaluation for Transfer

Consider transfer to a burn center (**Box 11-3**).[38,39] If transferring the patient to a burn center, coordinate with the receiving burn team to determine the recommended wound care prior to transfer.

BOX 11-3 American Burn Association's Burn Injury Referral Criteria

- Partial-thickness burns greater than 10% TBSA
- Burns that involve the face, hands, feet, genitalia, perineum, or major joints
- Third-degree burns in any age group
- Electrical burns, including lightning injury
- Chemical burns
- Inhalation injury
- Burn injury in patients with preexisting medical disorders that could complicate management, prolong recovery, or affect mortality
- Any patient with burns and concomitant trauma (such as fractures) in which the burn injury poses the greatest risk of morbidity or mortality
  - In such cases, if the trauma poses the greater immediate risk, the patient may be initially stabilized in a trauma center before being transferred to a burn unit.
  - Physician judgment will be necessary in such situations and should be developed in concert with the regional medical control plan and triage protocols.
- Burned children in hospitals without qualified personnel or equipment for the care of children
- Burn injury in patients who will require special social, emotional, or rehabilitative intervention

Abbreviation: TBSA, total body surface area.

Data from American Burn Association. (n.d.). Burn center referral criteria. Retrieved from http://ameriburn.org/wp-content/uploads/2017/05/burncenterreferralcriteria.pdf; American College of Surgeons Committee on Trauma. (2014). Guidelines for trauma centers caring for burn patients. In M. F. Rotondo, C. Cribari, & R. S. Smith (Eds.), *Resources for optimal care of the injured patient 2014* (pp. 100–106). Chicago, IL: Author. Retrieved from https://www.facs.org/~/media/files/quality%20programs/trauma/vrc%20resources/resources%20for%20optimal%20care.ashx.

The American Burn Association (ABA) makes the following recommendations in regard to burn care:

- Avoid delays in transport to a burn center.
- Do not debride burns or bullae.
- Do not apply creams, ointments, or topical antibiotics, as they may cause difficulty in assessing the extent of the burn.

F: Full Set of Vital Signs

A reliable blood pressure may be difficult to obtain because of developing edema in the extremities as a result of capillary leak syndrome.

G: Get Monitoring Devices and Give Comfort

Resuscitation adjuncts begin with laboratory studies.

L: Laboratory Studies

Laboratory studies for patients with burns include the following:

- ABGs and oxygenation content of the blood
  - Carboxyhemoglobin levels[35]
    - Normal nonsmoker: 0% to 3%
    - Normal smoker: 0% to 15%
    - Toxic symptoms: 25% to 35%
    - Lethal: more than 60%
- Blood glucose in infants and young children, as hypoglycemia may occur due to their reduced glycogen stores
- CBC, especially white blood cells (WBCs), as an indicator of infection
- Electrolytes, including potassium and magnesium
- Blood urea nitrogen (BUN) and creatinine as indicators of renal function
- Creatinine kinase as an indicator of rhabdomyolysis

M: Monitoring

Monitoring includes the following:

- Continuous cardiac monitoring for dysrhythmias for patients—particularly those with electrical burns, underlying cardiac abnormalities, or electrolyte imbalances—is recommended.
- Insert a urinary catheter to monitor the effectiveness of fluid resuscitation.

N: Nasogastric or Orogastric Tube Insertion

In patients who have burns covering more than 20% TBSA, consider a gastric tube because of the high probability of gastric distention, nausea and vomiting.[36]

O: Oxygenation and Ventilation

Pulse oximetry cannot differentiate oxygen-bound hemoglobin from carboxyhemoglobin, so these readings will not be accurate in the presence of CO saturation. Laboratory analysis of ABGs and carboxyhemoglobin levels is needed to trend changes.

CLINICAL PEARL 

P: Pain Assessment and Management

Pain assessment and management include the following considerations:

- Burns can be very painful, so pain management is a priority.
- Burns cause an increase in metabolism, which can affect medication dosing needs.
- Pain medications should be titrated by administering small, frequent intravascular doses. Do not administer pain medications intramuscularly or subcutaneously.

Reevaluation

Consider transfer to a burn center (Box 11-3).

Secondary Survey

The following subsections discuss the secondary survey and management of the patient with thermal burns. See "Selected Burn Injuries" for a discussion of electrical and chemical burns.

H: History

Example questions specific to patients with thermal burn injuries are as follows:

- If MOI was a fire, where was the fire located (indoors or outdoors)?
- Did the fire occur in a structure? If so, what type (car, house, commercial structure)?
- How long was the patient in the burning structure? Did the patient have to be removed by firefighters or bystanders from the burning structure?
- Was there exposure to chemicals?
- Were other people injured in the fire?
- Was there a fall, or did the patient jump and have associated injuries?
- Was there a blast?
- Are the circumstances of the burn injury consistent with the burn characteristics? Is there a possibility of abuse?

- Obtain an accurate weight of the patient as soon as possible or obtain the patient's pre-burn weight. Fluid resuscitation formulas should be based on the pre-burn weight of the patient.

H: Head-to-Toe Assessment

Determine the depth, extent, and location of the burn wound. All extremities should be examined for pulses, especially in the presence of circumferential burns.

Depth of the Burn

Depth of burn considerations include the following:

- The depth of burn is dependent on four factors:
  - Temperature of the offending agent
  - Duration of contact with the offending agent
  - Thickness of the epidermis and dermis
  - Blood supply to the area
- The depth of the burn is reflective of the layers of skin and tissue affected (**Table 11-3**).[40,41]
- Initial assessment is completed to begin fluid resuscitation. Use only partial-thickness or full-thickness burns to determine the percent of TBSA for the fluid resuscitation formula.
- Definitive assessment of depth may change over the course of the first 24 to 48 hours of the wound.[28]

Extent of the Burn

The Modified Lund and Browder Chart is one method used to determine the TBSA burned in adult and pediatric patients. Thus, assessing the extent of the burn includes the following:

- Determine the extent of partial- and full-thickness burn injury using one of the following:
  - The Modified Lund and Browder Chart is based on age and burned area (**Table 11-4**).
  - The rule of nines (**Figure 11-4**) divides the adult body into areas of 9% or multiples of 9%, except for the perineum, which is 1%.

TABLE 11-3 Differentiating Depth of Wounds

Depth	Appearance	Sensation	Healing Time
Superficial	› Dry, red, pink › Blanches with pressure › Soft › No skin sloughing or blistering	Painful	5–10 days
Superficial partial-thickness	› Blisters › Moist and weeping with serous exudate › Red, pink › Blanches with pressure › Edematous	Painful to temperature and air	7–21 days
Deep partial-thickness	› Blisters › Wet or waxy dry › Red to pale › Does not blanch with pressure	Perceptive of pressure only	› Greater than 21 days › Usually requires grafting
Full-thickness	› Waxy white to leathery gray to charred and black › No blanching with pressure › Dry › Firm › Hair absent	Perceptive of deep pressure only	Requires surgical grafts
Fourth degree (full-thickness)	Extends into fascia and or muscle	Perceptive of deep pressure only or painless	Requires surgical amputation

Data from Black, J. M., & Hawks, J. H. (2009). *Medical–surgical nursing: Clinical management for positive outcomes* (8th ed.). St. Louis, MO: Elsevier; Wolf, S. E. (2016). Burns. In *The Merck manual for health care professionals*. Retrieved from http://www.merckmanuals.com/professional/injuries_poisoning/burns/burns.html.

TABLE 11-4 Modified Lund and Browder Chart

	Age (Years)					
	Birth–1	1–4	5–9	10–14	15	Adult
Burned Area	**Total Body Surface (%)**					
Head	19	17	13	11	9	7
Neck	2	2	2	2	2	2
Anterior trunk	13	13	13	13	13	13
Posterior trunk	13	13	13	13	13	13
Right buttock	2.5	2.5	2.5	2.5	2.5	2.5
Left buttock	2.5	2.5	2.5	2.5	2.5	2.5
Genitalia	1	1	1	1	1	1
Right upper arm	4	4	4	4	4	4
Left upper arm	4	4	4	4	4	4
Right lower arm	3	3	3	3	3	3
Left lower arm	3	3	3	3	3	3
Right hand	2.5	2.5	2.5	2.5	2.5	2.5
Left hand	2.5	2.5	2.5	2.5	2.5	2.5
Right thigh	5.5	6.5	8	8.5	9	9.5
Left thigh	5.5	6.5	8	8.5	9	9.5
Right leg	5	5	5.5	6	6.5	7
Left leg	5	5	5.5	6	6.5	7
Right foot	3.5	3.5	3.5	3.5	3.5	3.5
Left foot	3.5	3.5	3.5	3.5	3.5	3.5

- The rule of palms is used to measure small or scattered burns. A 1% burn is considered to be the size of the patient's hand (including the fingers).[36]
- The percentage of TBSA is essential to calculating fluid resuscitation.

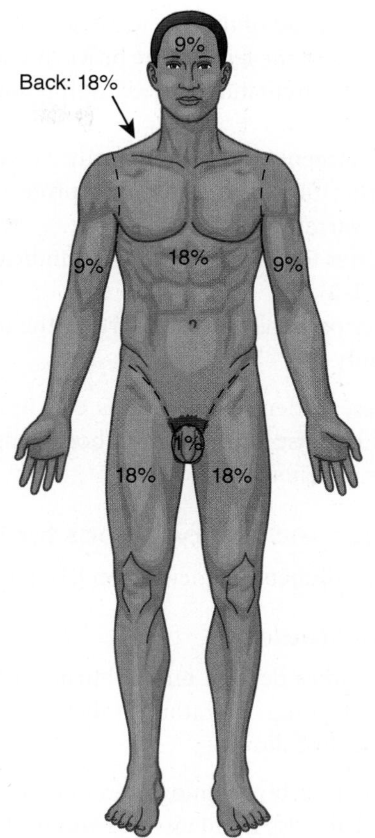

Figure 11-4 *The rule of nines in an adult.*

Location of Burn

Burns identified as high risk include the following[28]:

- Circumferential burns
  - Assess for increasing pressure to the structures located under circumferential burns.
  - Prepare for escharotomy to the chest wall or extremities.
  - Eschar creates restrictive movement and can result in failure to ventilate and/or loss of limb or life.
- Perineal burns
  - These burns are at high risk for contamination or infection.
- Hands or feet burns
  - These burns are at high risk for strictures and require intense rehabilitation.

Interventions

Interventions include the following[28]:

- Assess and manage pain.
- Cover wounds with clean, dry dressings or sheets to minimize exposure to air currents, which can be painful.

- Elevate the head of the bed to 30 degrees and the extremities to the level of the heart (not above) to promote circulation and assist in reduction of edema.
- If maltreatment is suspected, further investigation and notification of social or child protective services is warranted.
- Administer tetanus prophylaxis as indicated (Table 11-2).
- Consider psychological support for the patient and family.

With obese patients, estimations of TBSA are often problematic because of the altered body-mass distribution in these patients.[42]

Diagnostics and Interventions for Burns

Reevaluation adjuncts are focused on laboratory studies.

Laboratory Studies

Laboratory studies depend on the burn type and extent of exposure. Ongoing laboratory studies for patients with burns include the following:

- ABGs with carboxyhemoglobin to follow trends
  - Blood glucose in infants and young children, as hypoglycemia may occur due to their reduced glycogen stores
  - CBC, especially WBC, as an indicator of infection in patients with a delayed presentation of a burn injury or when there is a concern for burn wound infection
  - Serum chemistries/electrolytes
  - Blood urea nitrogen and creatinine to assess renal function
  - Type and screen/cross-match in the setting of associated trauma
  - Urinalysis

Selected Burn Injuries

Selected burn injuries are discussed in this section.

Electrical Burns

History is particularly important to understanding the effects of electrical burns.

H: History

If the patient has experienced an electrical burn, it is important to determine the following:

- The type of current and voltage
  - AC is more dangerous than DC because it causes tetany, which can result in the person tightening his or her grip on the source of current and, therefore, increasing the exposure.[43]
  - The higher the voltage involved, typically 1,000 volts or more, the greater the size of the internal thermal injury. High-voltage injuries tend to spread out to surrounding structures more than do low-voltage injuries.
- The surface area at point of contact, to help identify areas and extent of burn injury
- The points of contact, to anticipate organs damaged along the path of the current
- Duration of contact with the source, to help determine the possible extent of internal injury
- Any loss of consciousness and any concurrent injuries pertinent to the MOI

H: Head-to-Toe Assessment

It is difficult to assess the damage from electrical burns, as much of the injury may be internal. The electrical current enters the body at point of skin contact and travels throughout the body. Thus, it has the potential to damage all types of tissue, including bones, muscles, blood vessels, and nerves—the least resistant to electrical current—before exiting the body.

CLINICAL PEARL

Electrical Burns

Do not label the wounds as "exit" or "entrance," but rather as "contact point."

Assessment findings include the following:

- Wounds or burns to the body (**Figure 11-5**)
  - Document the assessment of the wounds. Do not label the wounds as "exit" or "entrance," but rather as "contact point."

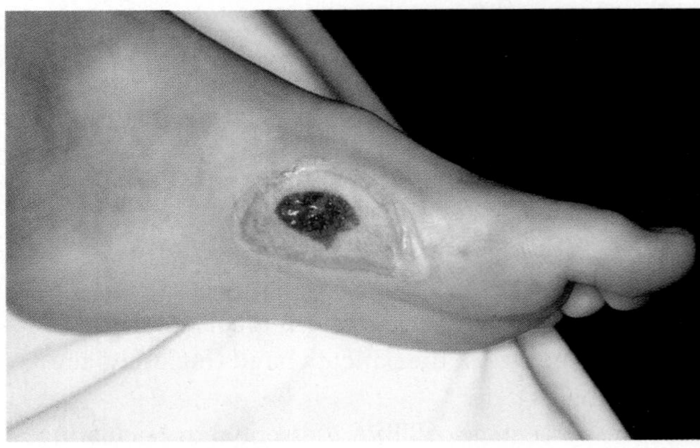

Figure 11-5 *Electrical burn.*

- Cardiac dysrhythmias
  - A frequent cause of death following an electrical injury is cardiac abnormalities.[43] Analyze for abnormal electrocardiogram findings, specifically for ST-segment changes or development of atrial fibrillation, the most common dysrhythmia.
- Rhabdomyolysis with myoglobinuria (see Chapter 20, "Post-Resuscitation Care Considerations," for more information)
  - Urine with myoglobin will appear dark red or brown.
  - Obtain a urinalysis to assess myoglobin levels.
  - Acute kidney injury and renal failure are possible.
  - Obtain BUN and creatinine levels.
  - Determine creatine kinase levels.
  - Consider ABGs with bicarbonate levels for patients with rhabdomyolysis who require alkalization of the urine.
- Fractures
- Seizures

Interventions

Interventions include the following:

- Consider spinal motion restriction based on the MOI.
- Treatment for myoglobinuria includes:
  - Administer an infusion of sodium bicarbonate to alkalize the urine, which promotes the excretion of the myoglobin.[44]
  - Prevent oliguria. Oliguria is frequently the result of insufficient fluid administration.
  - Normalize serum electrolytes.
  - Decompress any areas with compartment syndrome.
- Monitor cardiac rate and rhythm in patients with low- or high-voltage exposure.
- Monitor for signs and symptoms of compartment syndrome and prepare for fasciotomy as indicated.
- Monitor compartment pressures and splint extremities with severe burns.
- Consider tetanus immunization.

Chemical Burns

Care of patients with chemical burns begins with preparation.

Preparation

The first consideration with chemical burns is the safety of the trauma team. Use of personal protective equipment will limit the serious risk of a cross-exposure to the chemical agent, especially during decontamination.

Patient Decontamination

Patient decontamination includes the following:

- Decontamination of dry chemical exposure can generally be accomplished by removal of the patient's clothing. Use caution not to scatter any of the stimulus or causative agent during the removal of clothing and jewelry.
- Lightly brush any remaining dry chemical away.
  - Then dilute by flushing with liberal amounts of water.[36]
- Typically, neutralizing agents are contraindicated because of the exothermic reaction they may create, causing further injury to the patient.[45]

Dry powder and chemical fumes can also cause inhalation injuries.

H: History

When a patient presents with a chemical burn, it is important to determine the following:

- The type of chemical (acid or alkali) and its physical state (liquid, solid, gas)
  - The container with content information can be useful in identifying chemicals.
- The concentration and volume of the chemical
- The route and duration of exposure
- The direct effects of the chemical, such as obvious burning
- Risk for potential systemic effects

Interventions

Interventions include the following:

- Support oxygenation and ventilation and consider the possibility of inhalation injury.
- Remove the chemical by irrigating the skin until the pH is normal. Generally, use of neutralizing agents is contraindicated because of the exothermic reactions that often occur.
  - Normal human skin pH is about 5.3.
  - Tap water may be used. Irrigation should be at low pressures to avoid tissue injury.[45]
  - For extensive acid or alkali burns, it may require several hours of irrigation to achieve neutral pH.[45]
  - Avoid hypothermia by using tepid water.
- Debride any blisters caused by a chemical exposure.[45]
- With tar or asphalt, stop the burning process by using water until the tar or asphalt is cool to the touch, and then use petroleum to assist in removal of the agent.[36,45]

- Phenols are an acidic form of alcohol and are poorly soluble in water. They are found in most household disinfectants and chemical solvents. For patients with phenol burns, provide copious irrigation with water, followed by 50% polyethylene glycol (PEG). PEG increases the solubility of phenols in water. Phenol burns can cause a thick eschar to the affected area, if not removed quickly.[36]
  - Consider liver function tests.
- For hydrofluoric acid (used for glass etching) burns, irrigate for at least 30 minutes.[36]
  - Because hydrofluoric acid can cause depletion of calcium, assess calcium levels. Cardiac dysrhythmias and death from hypocalcemia may occur as the fluoride rapidly binds to free calcium in the blood. Closely monitor for cardiac arrhythmias.
  - Topical calcium gel may be applied to the skin to neutralize the fluoride with hydrofluoric acid burns. This is an instance where a direct neutralizing agent is recommended to treat a chemical exposure.

Reevaluation of the Patient with Burn Injury

Provide frequent and ongoing reevaluation of the following:

- The effectiveness of airway and ventilation, including the ongoing ability of the patient to protect the airway and perform adequate ventilation
- The effectiveness of fluid resuscitation, as evidenced by hemodynamic stability and urine output[36]
  - Monitor urine output every hour.
- All associated injuries and the effectiveness of the interventions
- The patient's temperature, so as to maintain euthermia
- Skin, pulmonary, and systemic signs and symptoms of infections
- The patient's pain level and the pain medication's effectiveness

Post-Resuscitation Care

Post-resuscitation care focuses on wound care but can involve escharotomy.

Wound Care

Wound care includes the following measures:

- Initial wound care varies with the type of wound, but generally includes debridement, topical wound care products, and dressings. This may be done in the emergency department, operating room, or intensive care unit.
- Burn debridement and dressing procedures are very painful, so intravenous pain medication should be administered before and during the process. Monitor patients closely after the procedures for respiratory depression.
- Wounds should be cleansed with soap, baby shampoo, or chlorhexidine, removing dirt and debris.
- Wound care depends on the location, depth, and extent of the burn.
  - Superficial burns may require topical antibiotics but rarely dressings.[30]
  - Early excision and grafting reduce the risk of infection and improves patient outcomes.[42]
  - Skin grafting may be required for deeper wounds.[30]
  - Monitor for hypothermia during wound care. Limit wound care to one extremity or body section at a time.
- Wound healing for larger burns may require weeks or months of inpatient hospital care.
- Reevaluate the effectiveness of interventions.

Escharotomy

An escharotomy is an incision through full-thickness burn eschar down to subcutaneous fat. It relieves external constriction that leads to restriction of the chest wall expansion or loss of peripheral perfusion of an extremity. Generally, escharotomies are not needed until several hours into fluid resuscitation and should be done in consultation with a burn center.

Emerging Trends

As the science and evidence of trauma care continues to evolve, tools to improve patient outcomes continue to be trialed and refined. Evidence is tested and replicated, and new standards of care are transitioned into practice. This section on trauma care considerations explores some of the evidence and the potential significance to trauma patient care. In the care of patients with surface and burn injuries, fluid resuscitation formulas will be discussed.

Pain Management

Uncontrolled pain is a challenge when caring for severely burned patients, particularly during wound care procedures. Side effects and reduced efficacy of narcotic pain medications have led care providers to consider alternative means to manage a patient's pain. This includes development of effective pain medication regimens, but also use of nonpharmacologic techniques. Psychological distraction analgesic options—particularly virtual reality pain distraction—are an emerging trend. Researchers and providers are finding that the use of immersive virtual reality pain distraction used in conjunction with traditional pain medications can significantly reduce pain in those undergoing wound care. Novel techniques for managing patients' experiences of pain will remain a focus of future advances geared toward improving patient outcomes.

Computerized Protocol-Driven Resuscitation

Optimal burn fluid resuscitation ensures that the least amount of sufficient fluid volume is administered to achieve organ perfusion. A computerized decision-support system (CDSS) uses data obtained from a patient's electronic medical record to assist clinicians in making therapeutic or diagnostic decisions. These algorithms typically take into consideration current infusion rates, hourly urine output, burn size, and time since the burn to calculate a recommended infusion rate or adjustment of the current infusion rate. Protocol-driven, CDSS-driven, nurse-driven burn fluid resuscitation allows nurses to make timely and effective changes to the resuscitation rates without a delay while waiting for provider orders. Additionally, these protocols have demonstrated less total volumes delivered while increasing the percentage of time in which the urine output is at goal.

Summary

The integumentary system is the largest organ in the body. The skin serves many vital functions, such as heat regulation, fluid and electrolyte regulation, and sensory relay. It is also the body's first line of defense against environmental hazards. Surface and burn trauma results in alteration of these normal functions. Trauma resuscitation of the patients with skin trauma requires the same resuscitation strategies used for other trauma patients. Once the trauma victim with surface or burn trauma is stabilized, wound care becomes the primary concern. Infection is a leading cause of morbidity and mortality in these patients. The treatment goal is to promote wound healing, maintain function, prevent complications, minimize disfiguring scars, and optimize the patient's return to activities of daily living.

References

1. Lyons, F., & Ousley, L. (2015). Basics of dermatology. In F. Lyons & L. Ousley (Eds.), *Dermatology for the advanced practice nurse* (pp. 15–26). New York, NY: Springer.
2. Wysocki, A. B. (2015). Anatomy of skin and soft tissue. In R. A. Bryant & D. P. Nix (Eds.), *Acute and chronic wounds: Current management concepts* (5th ed., pp. 40–81). St. Louis, MO: Mosby Elsevier.
3. Griffiths, C., Barker, J., Bleiker, T., Chalmers, R., & Creamer, D. (2016). *Rook's textbook of dermatology* (9th ed.). Oxford, UK: Wiley-Blackwell.
4. Doughty, D. B., & Sparks, B. (2015). Wound-healing physiology and factors that affect the Repair Process. In R. A. Bryant & D. P. Nix (Eds.), *Acute and chronic wounds: Current management concepts* (5th ed, pp. 40–62). St. Louis, MO: Mosby Elsevier.
5. Brown, A. (2015). Antibiotic prescribing in wound care. *Nurse Prescribing, 13*(9), 446–450.
6. Moore, E. E., Feliciano, D. V., & Mattox, K. L. (2017). *Trauma* (8th ed.). New York, NY: McGraw-Hill.
7. Ramirez, E.G. (2018). Wounds and wound management. In V. Sweet (Ed.), *Emergency nursing core curriculum* (7th ed., pp. 483–496). St. Louis, MO: Saunders Elsevier.
8. Makic, M. B. F., & McQuillan, K. A. (2009). Wound healing and soft tissue injuries. In K. A. McQuillan, M. B. F. Makic, & E. Whalen (Eds.), *Trauma nursing: From resuscitation through rehabilitation* (4th ed., pp. 306–329). St. Louis, MO: Saunders Elsevier.
9. Herr, R. D. (2013). Wound management. In Emergency Nurses Association, *Sheehy's manual of emergency care* (7th ed., pp. 147–160). St. Louis, MO: Mosby Elsevier.
10. Western Trauma Association. (n.d.). Management of the mangled extremity. Retrieved from http://westerntrauma.org/algorithms/MangledExtremity/Introduction.html
11. Wheeless, C. R. (2016, November 28). Frost bite. In *Wheeless' textbook of orthopaedics*. Retrieved from http://www.wheelessonline.com/ortho/frost_bite
12. Cochran, A., & Morris, S. E. (2018). Cold-induced injury: Frostbite. In D. N. Herndon, *Total burn care* (5th ed., 403–407). St Louis, MO: Elsevier.
13. Zafren, K., & Mechem, C. C. (2018, February 15). Frostbite. *UpToDate*. Retrieved from https://www.uptodate.com/contents/frostbite
14. Denke, N. J. (2010). Wound management. In P. K. Howard & R. A. Steinmann, *Sheehy's emergency nursing: Principles and practice* (6th ed., 111–126). St. Louis, MO: Mosby Elsevier.
15. Brancato, J. C. (2017, December 13). Minor wound preparation and irrigation. *UpToDate*. Retrieved from https://www.uptodate.com/contents/minor-wound-preparation-and-irrigation
16. Fernandez, R., & Griffiths, R. (2012). Water for wound cleansing. *Cochrane Database of Systematic Reviews, 2*, CD003861. https://doi.org/10.1002/14651858.CD003861.pub3

17. Anderson, D. J., Podgorny, K., Berrios-Torres, S. I., Bratzler, D. W., Dellinger, E. P., Greene, L., . . . Kaye, K.S. (2014). Strategies to prevent surgical site infections in acute care hospitals: 2014 update. *Infection Control & Hospital Epidemiology, 35*(6), 605–627. https://dx.doi.org/10.1086%2F676022
18. Gabriel, A. (2017, December 14). Wound irrigation. *Medscape*. Retrieved from http://emedicine.medscape.com/article/1895071-overview
19. Centers for Disease Control and Prevention. (May 31, 2018). Tetanus: For clinicians. Retrieved from https://www.cdc.gov/tetanus/clinicians.html
20. American Burn Association. (2017). Burn incidence and treatment in the United States: 2016. Retrieved from https://ameriburn.org/who-we-are/media/burn-incidence-fact-sheet/
21. National Fire Protection Association. (2018). Fire Loss in the United States During 2017. Retrieved from https://www.nfpa.org/-/media/Files/News-and-Research/Fire-statistics-and-reports/US-Fire-Problem/osFireLoss.pdf
22. National Fire Protection Association. (2011). Possible impairment by alcohol or drugs. Retrieved from https://www.nfpa.org/-/media/Files/News-and-Research/Archived-reports/osalcoholdrugs.ashx?la=en 23.
23. Pruitt, B. A., Wolf, S. E., & Mason, A. D., Jr. (2017). Epidemiological, demographic, and outcome characteristics of burn injury. In D. N. Herndon (Ed.), *Total burn care* (5th ed., pp. 14–27). St. Louis, MO: Elsevier.
24. American Burn Association. (2017). *National Burn Repository 2017 update: Report of data from 2008–2017*. Chicago, IL: Author.
25. American Burn Association. (2016). Appendix 3: Radiation injury. In American Burn Association, *Advanced burn life support provider manual* (pp. 121–124). Chicago, IL: Author.
26. Enkhbaatar, P., Sousse, L. E., Cox, R. A., & Herndon, D. N. (2018). The pathophysiology of inhalation injury. In D. N. Herndon (Ed.), *Total burn care* (5th ed., pp. 174–183). St. Louis, MO: Elsevier.
27. American College of Surgeons. (2018). Thermal injuries. In *Advanced trauma life support: Student course manual* (10th ed., pp. 167–183). Chicago, IL: Author.
28. Cancio, L. C., Bohannon, F. J., & Kramer, G. C. (2018). Burn resuscitation. In D. N. Herndon (Ed.), *Total burn care* (5th ed., pp. 77–86). St. Louis, MO: Elsevier.
29. Stein, D. M., & Scalea, T. M. (2012). Capillary leak syndrome in trauma: What is it and what are the consequences? *Advances in Surgery, 46*(1), 237–253. https://doi.org/10.1016/j.yasu.2012.03.008
30. Makic, M. B. F., & Mann, E. (2009). Burn injuries. In K. A. McQuillan, M. B. F. Makic, & E. Whalen (Eds.), *Trauma nursing: From resuscitation through rehabilitation* (4th ed., pp. 865–888). St. Louis, MO: Saunders Elsevier.
31. Wall, R. M., & Murphy, M. F. (Eds.). (2012). *Manual of emergency airway management* (4th ed.). Philadelphia, PA: Lippincott Williams & Wilkins.
32. American College of Surgeons. (2018). Airway and ventilator management. In *Advanced trauma life support: Student course manual* (10th ed., pp. 23–41). Chicago, IL: Author.
33. Clardy, P. F., Manaker, S., & Perry, H. (2018, June 6). Carbon monoxide poisoning. *UpToDate*. Retrieved from https://www.uptodate.com/contents/carbon-monoxide-poisoning
34. Mlcak, R. P., Buffalo, M. C., & Jimenez, C. J. (2018). Prehospital management, transportation, and emergency care. In D. N. Herndon (Ed.), *Total burn care* (5th ed., pp. 58–65). St. Louis, MO: Elsevier.
35. Thaniyavarn, T., & Eiger, G. (2012, October 25). Carboxyhemoglobin. *Medscape*. Retrieved from http://emedicine.medscape.com/article/2085044-overview
36. American Burn Association. (2016). *Advanced burn life support provider manual*. Chicago, IL: Author.
37. Rice, P. L., Jr., & Orgill, D. P. (2018, March 22). Emergency care of moderate and severe thermal burns in adults. *UpToDate*. Retrieved from https://www.uptodate.com/contents/emergency-care-of-moderate-and-severe-thermal-burns-in-adults
38. American College of Surgeons Committee on Trauma. (2014). Guidelines for trauma centers caring for burn patients. In M. F. Rotondo, C. Cribari, & R. S. Smith (Eds.), *Resources for optimal care of the injured patient 2014* (pp. 100–106). Chicago, IL: Author. Retrieved from https://www.facs.org/~/media/files/quality%20programs/trauma/vrc%20resources/resources%20for%20optimal%20care.ashx.
39. American Burn Association. (n.d.). Burn center referral criteria. Retrieved from http://ameriburn.org/wp-content/uploads/2017/05/burncenterreferralcriteria.pdf
40. Black, J. M., & Hawks, J. H. (2009). *Medical–surgical nursing: Clinical management for positive outcomes* (8th ed.). St. Louis, MO: Elsevier.
41. Wolf, S. E. (2016). Burns. In *The Merck manual for health care professionals*. Retrieved from http://www.merckmanuals.com/professional/injuries_poisoning/burns/burns.html
42. Rowan, M. P., Cancio, L. C., Elster, E. A., Burmeister, D. M., Rose, L. F., Natesan, S., . . . Chung, K. K. (2015). Burn wound healing and treatment: Review and advancements. *Critical Care,* 1–12. https://doi.org/10.1186/s13054-015-0961-2
43. Bernal, E., & Arnoldo, B. D. (2018). Electrical injuries. In D. N. Herndon (Ed.), *Total burn care* (5th ed., pp. 396–402). St. Louis, MO: Elsevier.
44. Cushing, T. A., & Wright, R. (2017, April 2). Electrical injuries in emergency medicine. *Medscape*. Retrieved from http://emedicine.medscape.com/article/770179-overview
45. Williams, F. N., & Lee, J. O. (2018). Chemical burns. In D. N. Herndon (Ed.), *Total burn care* (5th ed., pp. 408–413). St. Louis, MO: Elsevier.

Design credits: Clipboard designed by Vectors Market from Flaticon.

CHAPTER 12

Special Populations: The Pediatric Trauma Patient

Erin Zazzera, MPH, RN, CEN, TCRN

OBJECTIVES

Upon completion of this chapter, the learner will be able to:

1. Describe mechanisms of injury associated with the pediatric trauma patient.
2. Describe anatomic, physiologic, and developmental characteristics as a basis for assessment of the pediatric trauma patient.
3. Demonstrate the nursing assessment of the pediatric trauma patient.
4. Plan appropriate interventions for the pediatric trauma patient.
5. Evaluate the effectiveness of nursing interventions for the pediatric trauma patient.

Introduction

Traumatic injury remains the number one cause of death in children age 1 to 19 years despite significant advances in trauma systems and injury prevention over the past few decades.[1] The American College of Surgeons defines pediatric patients as all children younger than the age of 15 years, although some hospitals use the age of 18 or 21 as a cutoff between pediatrics and adults.

The initial treatment algorithm for pediatric trauma follows the same A–J mnemonic that is used to identify life-threatening injuries in adults. However, growth and development patterns in children make them a unique population to assess and treat. The anatomy and physiology of children, as they move from infancy through adolescence, affect injury patterns after trauma.[2] Growth and development influences the child's behavior and risk of traumatic injury. In addition, assessment and treatment of the injured child requires trauma nurses to adapt to the child's developmental stage. Resuscitation requires smaller equipment for monitoring and weight-based dosages for medication. All emergency departments (EDs) should have pediatric equipment readily available for the initial treatment of an injured child.

Epidemiology

Although the incidence of pediatric mortality from trauma has decreased in the United States, injury remains the primary cause of death in children.[1,3-5] In 2000, pediatric trauma deaths numbered approximately 11,200.[4] In 2013, approximately 6,500 children died from trauma.[4] While deaths may have decreased, inpatient costs for treatment of injured children have increased.[6] Additional considerations related to pediatric trauma are the lifelong need for medical and behavioral health services for survivors, productivity losses, and the costs associated with caregivers' lost earnings.[5] Research has also shown that throughout the United States, the majority of EDs lack pediatric-specific training and equipment to meet the needs of this special population and that most injured children are managed at adult-focused facilities.[7-10] These statistics clearly highlight the need for improved pediatric trauma awareness, education, and preparedness.

Mechanisms of Injury and Biomechanics

Pediatric traumatic events often result in multisystem organ injury. Greater force is distributed throughout the body of pediatric patients as a result of trauma due to the patient's reduced body mass.[2,11-12] This force is transmitted through pliable, incompletely calcified bones, limited connective tissues, weaker abdominal walls, organs that are in closer proximity to other organs and structures, and the pediatric patient's smaller physical stature, frequently resulting in multisystem injury. Knowledge of injury patterns in children allows clinicians to better anticipate and identify injuries and then rapidly intervene in an effort to improve outcomes in the pediatric trauma patient.[11] **Table 12-1** outlines these patterns.[12]

TABLE 12-1 Common Mechanisms of Injury and Associated Patterns of Injury in Pediatric Patients

Mechanism of Injury	Common Patterns of Injury
Pedestrian struck by a vehicle	Low speed: Lower extremity fractures High speed: Multiple trauma, head and neck injuries, lower extremity fractures
Automobile occupant	Unrestrained: Scalp and facial lacerations, head and neck injuries, and multiple trauma Properly restrained: Chest and abdomen injuries, lumbar spinal fractures
Fall from a height	Low: Upper extremity fractures Medium: Head and neck injuries, upper and lower extremity fractures High: Upper and lower extremity fractures, head and neck injuries, multiple trauma
Fall from a bicycle	Without helmet: Head and neck lacerations, scalp and facial lacerations, upper extremity fractures With helmet: Upper extremity fractures Striking handlebar: Internal abdominal injuries

Data from American College of Surgeons. (2018). Pediatric trauma. In *Advanced trauma life support: Student course manual* (10th ed., pp. 188–212). Chicago, IL: Author.

Additional considerations include the following:

- Blunt trauma from motor vehicle collisions (MVCs), suffocation, drowning, and fires and/or burns are the leading causes of injury-related death among children age 14 and younger.[1,3,5]
- Traumatic brain injury (TBI) accounts for more pediatric fatalities than injuries to any other organ systems.[1,13]
- Nonfatal injuries in children age 14 years and younger are most often attributable to unintentional falls.[1]
- Penetrating trauma, most frequently from firearms, most often affects adolescents and carries a high mortality rate.[1,14]
- Youths with assault-related injuries have a high rate of repeat injuries, especially those with a history of drug use.[15]
- Sports- and recreational-related injuries in children demonstrate a significant correlation with TBI and musculoskeletal injuries. These injuries continue to play a significant role in nonfatal, unintentional injuries in pediatric patients.[15,16]
- Injury from child maltreatment reaches across all age groups and both genders, so it is important for the trauma nurse to maintain a high awareness for potential abuse in all pediatric trauma patients. In cases of suspected child maltreatment, the story of injury is often unreliable.[17] Treatment teams should rely on physical exams and imaging studies to identify injuries (see Chapter 16, "Special Populations: The Interpersonal-Violence Trauma Patient," for additional information).

Childhood Growth and Development

Understanding normal childhood growth and development is essential when caring for pediatric trauma patients. Foundational knowledge regarding the pediatric patient's overall body size, larger body surface area, and physiologic and immunologic immaturity inform the care provided to the injured child.[9] Principles such as cephalocaudal and proximodistal define a child's development.[18,19]

- In children, development begins at the head and moves down toward the lower portions of the body in a cephalocaudal progression. This can be seen in the relatively larger size of the head in infants and young children in comparison to their overall body size and in the development of sensory and motor functions, which begin in the upper portions of the body before reaching the lower portions. Thus, children gain control of the use of their hands before the use of their feet.[19]
- Proximodistal development patterns begin from the core of the child's body and move outward as the child grows. An example of this development pattern is a child's control of gross motor movements prior to fine motor control.

Understanding these principles helps the trauma nurse to successfully approach, properly assess, and safely care for the pediatric patient.[18,19] In addition, knowing expected growth and developmental milestones will help the trauma nurse to identify any deviation from established norms. **Appendix 12-1** describes childhood development.

Another reason it is vital that the trauma nurse is familiar with these developmental milestones is to ensure that the story of injury matches the child's developmental level. For example, a 4-month-old presenting with bruising to the lower extremities could not have been injured while attempting to walk or crawl, as these milestones are typically met later in the first year of life.

Children with special healthcare needs often develop at different rates and may have baseline assessment data that differs from accepted norms. In such cases, the nurse can compare assessment findings to the baseline with the caregiver.

Anatomic, Physiologic, and Developmental Differences in Pediatric Trauma Patients

Anatomic and physiologic characteristics unique to the pediatric patient have significant clinical implications. Maintaining an awareness and understanding of these differences can help the trauma nurse optimize care and improve patient outcomes. These unique characteristics are reviewed within each section of the initial assessment.

Selected Developmental Differences

Selected developmental differences include the following[20-22]:

- Children are easily distracted, have a limited grasp of cause and effect, and lack experience with situations that can cause traumatic injury.
- Children have difficulty judging the speed and distance of oncoming vehicles.
- Young children may have trouble localizing sound and recognizing sounds of danger.
- The visual field is primarily at eye level, which is lower in children.
- Toddlers and school-age children are egocentric and believe that if they see the car, the driver sees them.
- Adolescents may be easily distracted by mobile phones while walking near traffic.
- Infants are mobile from birth and can fall off raised surfaces.

Nursing Care of the Pediatric Trauma Patient

Chapter 3, "Initial Assessment," presents the systematic approach to care of the trauma patient. The following assessment parameters are specific to pediatric trauma patients.

Preparation

Preparation begins with safety.

Safe Practice, Safe Care

Because of its complex nature, trauma care creates significant potential for medical errors; the unique anatomic, physiologic, and developmental characteristics of the pediatric patient can further compound this potential.[23,24] Performing a systematic, multisystem assessment in the pediatric patient, despite the specific mechanism of injury (MOI), allows for easier recognition of multi-organ trauma and rapid intervention in life-threatening injuries.

Patient Equipment

Preparation to care for the injured pediatric patient includes ensuring the availability of necessary pediatric-specific equipment (**Appendix 12-2**). Reference materials including normal vital signs ranges by age (**Table 12-2**)[25] and scales configured to read only

TABLE 12-2 Normal Vital Signs Ranges by Age

Respiratory Rate (breaths/min)

Age	Rate
Infant	30–53
Toddler	22–37
Preschooler	20–28
School-age child	18–25
Adolescent	12–20

Heart Rate (beats/min)

Age	Awake Rate	Sleeping Rate
Neonate	100–205	90–160
Infant	100–180	90–160
Toddler	98–140	80–120
Preschooler	80–120	65–100
School-age child	75–118	58–90
Adolescent	60–100	50–90

Data from American Heart Association. (2016). *Pediatric advanced life support: Provider manual.* Dallas TX: Author.

in kilograms can facilitate a thorough assessment. The Emergency Nurses Association (ENA), with the support of other professional healthcare associations, has emphasized the importance of weighing children in kilograms.[26] In addition, length-based resuscitation tapes and guides to appropriately sized equipment and medication dosing promote accurate treatment.

Nursing Preparation

Nursing preparation includes the following:

- Pediatric-specific education and training for trauma nurses, including the Emergency Nursing Pediatric Course (ENPC), can provide them with an understanding of the unique characteristics of the pediatric patient population and the preferred management principles.
- Competency evaluations for all clinical staff to include pediatric skills and skills related to the care of the child with special healthcare needs will increase the trauma team's ability to provide excellent care to the pediatric trauma patient.
- Regular reviews of pediatric trauma cases can assist the trauma team to identify learning, equipment, and policy needs.

Facility Preparation

Facility preparation includes the following:

- Review the care environment, protocols, and guidelines to ensure a proper pediatric focus and safety.
- Ensure policies and agreements are in place for appropriate transfers to definitive care (burn center, pediatric trauma center).

Triage

Triage begins with the Pediatric Assessment Triangle (PAT).[27-29] The PAT is an across-the-room assessment that is completed within 3 to 5 seconds. It evaluates the following aspects of the patient:

- General appearance
  - Muscle tone: Is there normal tone or is the patient limp and floppy?
  - Interactiveness: Does the patient recognize and interact with the caregiver?
  - Consolability: Does the patient respond to soothing attempts by caregiver?
  - Look or gaze: Does the patient maintain visual contact with the caregiver and turn toward the nurse upon entering the room?
  - Speech or cry: Is there a continuous or high-pitched cry or no crying at all?
- Work of breathing
  - Inadequate or excessive
  - Nasal flaring
  - Retractions
  - Accessory muscle use
  - Abnormal upper airway sounds
  - General respiratory rate—too fast or too slow
  - Position of comfort (tripod, sitting up)
- Circulation to the skin
  - Color
  - Mottling or central or peripheral cyanosis
  - Diaphoresis

Primary Survey

While the priorities for the initial assessment of the pediatric trauma patient are the same as they are in the adult patient, anatomic and physiologic differences as well as normal patterns of pediatric growth and development impact the pediatric patient's response to injury. Survival rates in pediatric trauma patients can be directly correlated with rapid airway management, initiation of ventilatory support, and early recognition of and response to intracranial and intra-abdominal hemorrhage.[12] Encourage the caregiver to remain with the child during the initial assessment to help calm the child and gain cooperation during the initial assessment phase.[29]

A: Alertness and Airway

The assessment of alertness and airway begins with anatomic and physiologic characteristics.

Anatomic and Physiologic Characteristics

Anatomic and physiologic characteristics relevant to alertness and airway include the following:

- Infants are obligate nose breathers until 4 to 6 months of age, and may more easily develop respiratory distress as a result of nasal congestion.[30,31]
- Children's relatively smaller airway diameter may cause even minimal amounts of blood, edema, mucus, or foreign objects to partially or completely impede the airway.[2]
- The tongue size is larger in relation to the oral cavity and may require the use of a tongue depressor, positioning, or oral adjuncts to maintain airway patency.[30,31]
- Children's shortened trachea and neck means there is a narrow margin for movement of the endotracheal tube (ETT) before dislodgement, which may lead to increased incidence of right main stem bronchus intubation or inadvertent extubation.[11,12,31]
- The cricoid cartilage is C-shaped in children, allowing for potential increased risk for compression and subsequent airway obstruction with hyperextension or hyperflexion of the neck.[11]
- A large occiput results in passive flexion of the cervical spine while in a supine position that may occlude the airway.[30]
- A large, heavy head, lax neck ligaments, and more flexible joints all contribute to greater energy impact to the neck with angular momentum forces. These characteristics can increase the risk for both head and cervical spinal injuries.[2,11]
- Lax neck ligaments and incompletely calcified vertebrae place the pediatric patient at higher risk for injury to the spinal cord without a fracture, or spinal cord injury without radiographic abnormalities (SCIWORA).[11]
- Vertebral bodies are wedged anteriorly and may tend to slide forward or sublux with flexion due to acceleration/deceleration forces.[12]

Assessment

Use the AVPU mnemonic to assess the mental status of the pediatric patient. See Chapter 3 for more information.

- An alert older infant or toddler will recognize his or her caregiver, be cautious of strangers, and may not respond to commands, which is a normal response.
- It can be difficult to accurately assess the crying child. Look for signs of altered level of consciousness and inconsolability in the young child.[29]
- Assess the child's airway for actual or potential obstructions.
- Loose and missing teeth may be normal findings in school-age children and not the result of oral trauma.
  - Assess for bleeding sockets.
  - Loose teeth can be more easily dislodged and pose a risk for aspiration.
- Assess for cyanosis in the oral mucous membranes.
  - It is a significant finding and indicative of central cyanosis due to either severe respiratory or circulatory issues.

Interventions

Interventions include the following:

- Frequent suctioning or placement of a nasal airway may be required to keep the pharynx clear of secretions and improve ventilation.
- When inserting an oral airway in the unconscious patient by the anatomic insertion method, use a tongue blade and a direct insertion technique, with the oral airway curving downward to avoid damage to the soft palate and to limit the potential for subsequent bleeding.[25,31]
- Previous recommendations suggested the use of uncuffed tubes in children younger than the age of 8 years due to the risk of ischemic damage to the tracheal mucosa from potential compression between a cuff and the cricoid ring. However, ETT cuffs are now designed to be high-volume, low-pressure devices that produce a seal at a lower pressure, and use of cuffed tubes in young children is increasing in EDs and pediatric intensive care units. Be sure to follow manufacturer guidelines regarding air leak and cuff pressure monitoring.[30,32]
- Secure the ETT at the teeth or gums at a depth equal to three times the diameter of the tube until definitive placement can be verified by chest radiograph.[25]
- Gastric tubes decrease gastric distention, facilitate diaphragmatic function and chest expansion, and improve ventilation.[25]

Spinal Motion Restriction

Cervical spinal motion restriction may be an issue in pediatric patients.

Assessment

Assessment includes the following considerations:

- Inspect the position of the infant's or child's occiput in relationship to the body to assure alignment. Pad the upper back to horizontally align the external auditory meatus with the shoulders.[30]
- Assess for appropriate sizing and application of rigid cervical collars to maintain cervical spine stabilization.[33] In the absence of appropriately sized commercial devices, manual stabilization may be required.

Interventions

Interventions include the following:

- Remove the infant from the safety seat while maintaining cervical spinal stabilization.
- One team member stabilizes the infant's head and neck from behind the infant seat, while another lays the infant seat down with the back resting on the stretcher. The infant is removed from the seat and placed onto the stretcher by both team members in a straight motion with support of the body to maintain spinal alignment.

B: Breathing and Ventilation

Breathing and ventilation are surveyed.

Anatomic and Physiologic Characteristics

Anatomic and physiologic characteristics of pediatric patients can create some unique challenges in providing trauma care:

- Children's respiratory rates are faster, as a result of their increased basal metabolic rate (Table 12-2). This contributes to overall insensible fluid losses, resulting in a greater risk for hypovolemia, which is further exacerbated in the presence of hemorrhage.
- An increased metabolic rate inefficiently uses oxygen; limited reserves are quickly depleted in times of physiologic stress such as trauma.
- Children with respiratory distress may increase their respiratory rate and exhibit signs of increased work of breathing to maximize ventilation. This requires a large amount of energy, and the patient will fatigue once physiologic reserves are exhausted, leading to rapid decompensation.
- Due to their horizontally oriented rib cage and weak chest wall and intercostal muscles, young children have smaller tidal volumes with decreased ability to increase their volume during periods of distress.[29]
- Alveoli are fewer and smaller, creating a reduced area for gas exchange in younger children. Existing alveoli have less elastic recoil and lack supportive tissue.[29]
- Younger children have a flat-shaped diaphragm. Since it is the primary muscle for ventilation, gastric distention can greatly limit ventilation.[32]
- Children's thin chest walls contribute to the transmission of breath sounds from one side of the chest to the other, potentially masking the presence of pneumothorax, hemothorax, and tension pneumothorax.[29]
- Younger pediatric patients normally use their abdominal muscles for breathing. Those experiencing abdominal pain may exhibit alterations in respiratory patterns, such as shallow respirations and expiratory grunting.[34]

Assessment

Assessment includes the following:

- Inspect for increased work of breathing:
  - Nasal flaring
  - Retractions
    - Site: Substernal, intercostal, suprasternal, or supraclavicular
    - Severity: Mild, moderate, or severe
  - Head bobbing
  - Expiratory grunting
  - Accessory muscle use—sternocleidomastoid or trapezius
    - Infants normally are diaphragmatic breathers. In these patients, the diaphragm is considered a primary muscle of breathing, not an accessory muscle.
- Auscultate for the following:
  - An appropriately sized stethoscope can assist with the accuracy of auscultating the lung fields and lessen the transmission of lung sounds across the chest.

Interventions

Interventions include the following:

- Blow-by oxygen does not meet oxygen requirements or provide beneficial ventilatory support in the injured child. A tight-fitting, nonrebreather mask with an attached reservoir is recommended for trauma patients.[25]
- If gastric distention develops from either assisted ventilations or air swallowing, a gastric tube can relieve the distention, optimizing lung expansion.

C: Circulation and Control of Hemorrhage

Systemic hypovolemia can produce secondary brain injury and is the single worst risk factor for devastating brain injury.[35]

Anatomic and Physiologic Characteristics

Anatomic and physiologic characteristics to consider include the following:

- Heart rates vary by age (Table 12-2).
- Children have a higher body water composition compared to adults and can easily become dehydrated.
- The myocardium is less compliant in pediatric patients. To maintain cardiac output, heart rate increases to meet systemic demands. A strong compensatory response, as evidenced by tachycardia, may maintain cardiac output in times of increased systemic need for an extended amount of time. When compensatory mechanisms are exhausted, decompensation is sudden and rapid.

Tachycardia and delayed capillary refill of more than 2 seconds are early signs of poor tissue perfusion in the pediatric trauma patient.[12,25] In response to hemorrhagic shock, the initial compensatory mechanism to increase cardiac output is an increase in heart rate. Tachycardia is followed by systemic vasoconstriction to increase systemic vascular resistance, resulting in delayed capillary refill, weak distal pulses, and cool, mottled extremities.

- Systemic vasoconstriction results from stimulation of the sympathetic nervous system, which can maintain adequate systolic blood pressure despite significant blood loss.
- Because children have a larger circulating blood volume to weight ratio, a small volume loss can more quickly result in circulatory compromise than in adult patients.[2]

Hypovolemic shock as a result of hemorrhage is the most common form of shock in the pediatric trauma patient.[2,11] Hypotension (**Table 12-3**) is a late finding, reflecting blood loss of more than 30% of the total blood volume, and indicates severe compromise to organ perfusion.[25]

Signs of late shock are easy to recognize. The challenge for trauma nurses is to watch closely for early signs of shock in children (decreased skin perfusion, altered mental status, and tachycardia) before they decompensate.[2]

TABLE 12-3 Hypotension by Systolic Blood Pressure and Age

Age	Systolic Blood Pressure (mm Hg)
Term neonates (0–28 days)	< 60
Infants (1–12 months)	< 70
Children 1–10 years (5th percentile blood pressure)	< 70 + (age in years × 2)
Children > 10 years	< 90

Data from American Heart Association. (2016). *Pediatric advanced life support: Provider manual*. Dallas TX: Author.

Assessment

Assessment includes the following:

- Palpate central and peripheral pulses. For purposes of determining the need for cardiopulmonary resuscitation, the brachial pulse is palpated in patients younger than the age of 1 year.
- Assess for capillary refill (normal = 2 seconds or less). Blanch the forehead, the sole of the foot, or the palm of the hand and observe time to refill. A nail bed can be used on the older child or adolescent.[36]
- Perform frequent serial assessments and comparison of central and peripheral pulses to determine stability, improvement, or worsening of circulation and perfusion.
- Jugular vein distention can be difficult to assess in young children and infants due to their short necks.[11]

Interventions

Interventions include the following:

- Rapid vascular access with peripheral intravenous (IV) access or intraosseous (IO) access is the priority of care for a patient in shock. It is not necessary to attempt IV access before the use of the IO route. If peripheral perfusion is compromised, IO access may be the best and first choice.[25]
- Immediate, rapid infusion of 20 mL/kg of warmed isotonic crystalloid solution over 5 to 10 minutes with a three-way stopcock and a 20-mL syringe (for a patient weighing 5 kg, fill the 20-mL syringe 5 times to deliver a 20 mL/kg bolus) in the tubing system is an effective way to deliver specific fluid quantities in the injured pediatric patient.[11,37]
  - After administering each bolus of isotonic crystalloid solution, assess bilateral breath sounds for crackles or other signs of fluid excess. Infants

and children with congenital heart defects are susceptible to fluid overload.[37]
- After administering isotonic fluids, consider the use of warmed blood products if the patient continues to show signs of shock. Recent studies in adult trauma patients with hemorrhagic shock have advised minimal use of isotonic fluids in favor of early blood product administration during resuscitation.[12] Although similar studies have not shown a survival benefit in the pediatric population, some pediatric trauma centers have moved toward limiting crystalloids and giving blood early.[12]
- Packed red blood cells are administered as a bolus of 10 mL/kg. Additional products such as plasma and platelets are considered.[12]
- Severely injured children may require large amounts of blood products. Infusing greater than 50% of the child's blood volume in the first 24 hours is commonly referred to as massive transfusion. While research continues to seek the best ratio of fresh frozen plasma to red blood cells to platelets for the benefit of the pediatric trauma patient, most trauma centers currently aim for a 1:1:1 ratio based on studies in the adult population.[2]
- Tranexamic acid (TXA) is an antifibrinolytic infusion that has been associated with decreased mortality in bleeding trauma patients. If used, it must be given within 3 hours of injury.[2,38] Administration of TXA in trauma patients has not been approved by the U.S. Food and Drug Administration (FDA).[39]
- ED thoracotomy is less effective in pediatric trauma patients as compared to adult trauma patients.[2] Children who arrive to the ED in cardiac arrest after injury have a dismal prognosis.[2]
- Resuscitative endovascular balloon occlusion of the aorta (REBOA) is currently being studied in adult and pediatric trauma patients as an alternative to thoracotomy. For patients in uncontrolled hemorrhagic shock, REBOA is a temporary measure to maintain perfusion to the heart and brain while minimizing blood loss.[35]

D: Disability (Neurologic Status)

Disability and neurologic status are considered as well.

Anatomic and Physiologic Characteristics

Anatomic and physiologic characteristic considerations include the following:

- A positive Babinski reflex (**Figure 12-1**) is a normal finding in the young infant.
  - When the sole of the foot is stimulated in a line from the heel to the small toe, the large toe moves upward and the other toes fan out.

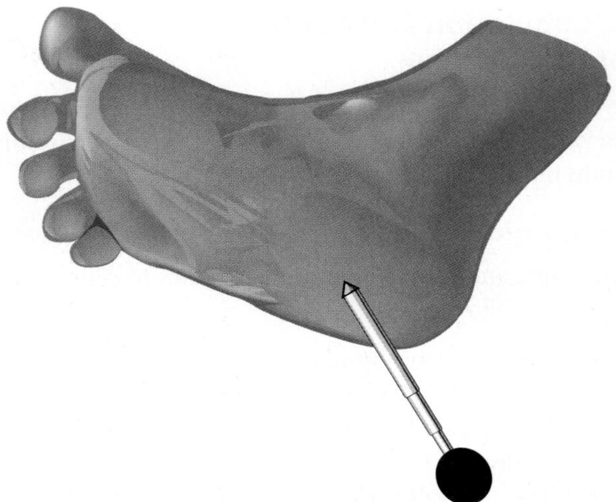

Figure 12-1 *Positive Babinski reflex.*

A positive Babinski reflex is normal in infants. The large toe points upward and the other toes fan out.

- The normal body position in an infant is slightly flexed, with the arms and legs pulled in toward the core.
- The head of the infant and young child is proportionately larger in comparison to overall body size in young children. By age 2 years, the head has achieved 80% of the adult size.[29]
- Children's smaller subarachnoid space and decreased volume of cerebrospinal fluid result in less cushioning for the brain in the event of an injury.
- Infants have unfused cranial sutures and open fontanels that allow for expansion. This means a larger volume of blood can be lost into the cranial vault before assessment findings of increased intracranial pressure (ICP) develop. The posterior fontanel closes at about 8 weeks of age. The anterior fontanel remains open until about 18 months.[40]
- Restlessness, crying, fussiness, agitation, and irritability may be early signs of decreased cerebral perfusion.
- Normal ICPs are as follows[41]:
  - Infants: 2 to 6 mm Hg
  - Young children: 3 to 7 mm Hg
  - Older children: 10 to 15 mm Hg

Assessment

Assessment includes the following:

- Consider any alterations in level of consciousness to be the result of cerebral hypoxia until proven otherwise.
- Restlessness, anxiety, fussiness, crying, irritability, and combativeness can be early signs of hypoxia in the pediatric patient. Be concerned about the older infant and toddler who should express fear or

- anxiety toward a stranger and does not. This may be an altered level of consciousness.[25]
- Calculate the Pediatric Glasgow Coma Scale score (**Table 12-4**).[25]

Interventions

Interventions include the following:

- Consider a bedside glucose measurement to determine if any change in level of consciousness may be related to hypoglycemia.
- Prepare for endotracheal intubation for noted changes in mental status that may indicate decreased cerebral blood flow, hypoxia, or fatigue.
- Hyperventilation ($PaCO_2$ less than 35 mm Hg) causes cerebral vasoconstriction and decreases cerebral blood flow; it is contraindicated in patients with TBI. See Chapter 6 "Head Trauma," for more information.
- Hypotension is associated with poor outcomes in children with TBI.[12,13] Adequate cerebral blood flow must be maintained through the use of IV fluids, blood products, or inotropic drips.

E: Exposure and Environmental Control

Exposure and environmental control for pediatric patients must be considered in terms of their anatomic and physiologic characteristics.

Anatomic and Physiologic Characteristics

Anatomic and physiologic characteristics include the following:

- Children have a large body surface area-to-body mass ratio that increases insensible losses through surface evaporation.
- Young children—specifically infants with a higher percentage of brown adipose tissue, an inability to shiver, and an immature thalamus—have limited ability to regulate temperature.[40]
- Lesser amounts of body fat allow for rapid dissipation of body heat when pediatric patients are exposed to the surrounding environment.
- Hypothermia results in increased oxygen consumption and subsequent hypoxia or acidosis if left uncorrected.[40]

TABLE 12-4 Pediatric Glasgow Coma Scale

Response	Child (1–5 Years)	Infant (<1 Year)	Score
Eye opening	Spontaneous	Spontaneous	4
	To speech	To speech	3
	To pain only	To pain only	2
	No response	No response	1
Best verbal response	Oriented, appropriate	Coos and babbles	5
	Confused	Irritable cries	4
	Inappropriate words	Cries to pain	3
	Incomprehensible sounds	Moans to pain	2
	No response	No response	1
Best motor response[a]	Obeys commands	Moves spontaneously and purposefully	6
	Localizes painful stimulus	Withdraws to touch	5
	Withdraws in response to pain	Withdraws in response to pain	4
	Flexion in response to pain	Abnormal flexion posture to pain	3
	Extension in response to pain	Abnormal extension posture to pain	2
	No response	No response	1

[a] If the patient is intubated, unconscious, or preverbal, the most important part of this scale is motor response. Motor response should be carefully evaluated.

Modified from James, H. E., & Trauner, D. A. (1985). The Glasgow Coma Score and Modified Coma Score for Infants. In James, H. E., Anas, N. G., & Perkin, R. M. (Eds.), Brain insults in infants and children: Pathophysiology and management (pp. 179–182). Orlando, FL: Grune & Stratton, Inc. Copyright Elsevier.

- Hypothermia complicates coagulopathies in the injured pediatric patient and has been correlated with an increased risk of morbidity and mortality in severely injured pediatric patients.[42]
- Children have thinner skin and higher rates of insensible water losses, which render them more susceptible to dehydration, increased severity of burn injuries, and more rapid absorption of dermal toxins.[43]

Assessment

- During clothing removal, take note of any signs or patterns of injuries that might raise an index of suspicion for maltreatment (multiple bruises of varying stages of healing, patterned marks, signs of immersion burns).[44]

Interventions

Interventions include the following:

- Consider continuous temperature monitoring (urinary catheter thermometer, rectal temperature probe) due to the pediatric patient's sensitivity to heat loss.
- A radiant warmer with servo control can provide heat in response to the infant's body temperature while allowing full access for necessary interventions.
- Clothing removal may be upsetting to the pediatric patient. Provide age-appropriate explanations and maintain privacy (Appendix 12-1).

F: Full Set of Vital Signs/Family Presence

Considerations for vital signs and family presence include the following:

- Use appropriately sized equipment to obtain accurate vital signs.
- Respiratory and heart rates can vary with activity, anxiety, and crying. Attempt to measure vital signs when the pediatric patient is calm, and count both for a full minute.
  - Assess the patient while the caregiver holds the child.
  - Count respirations before close interaction or hands-on assessment.
  - Use toys or bright objects to distract the infant during the assessment.
- When using automated blood pressure devices, assure correct sizing of equipment and measure when the patient is calm.
  - Adjust the monitor settings to reflect pediatric or infant parameters.
  - Results may be inaccurate with movement or extreme values.
  - Validate with manual blood pressure.
- Promote family-centered care and recognize that the pediatric patient's family may not just include the caregiver.
- Advocate for and encourage family presence at the bedside throughout the ED stay, especially during invasive procedures and resuscitation. Research supports the development and implementation of structured family-presence programs in the emergency setting.[29] These programs have been shown to have positive effects on patients and caregivers and do not negatively impact clinical care with regard to efficiency and outcomes.[29,45,46]

G: Get Monitoring Devices and Give Comfort

Prepare the resuscitation adjuncts to obtain laboratory analysis.

L: Laboratory Studies

Laboratory studies considerations include the following:

- Use pediatric-specific tubes that can accommodate smaller volumes of blood.
- Perform bedside serum glucose testing and repeat evaluations as needed.
- The metabolic demands of children are higher than those of adults, and glycogen stores in the pediatric liver can be limited. Physiologic stress may rapidly deplete glycogen stores, resulting in hypoglycemia and causing decreased cardiac contractility, alteration in the level of consciousness, seizures, and acidosis.[25]
- Trauma patients in shock may develop coagulopathy, in which the blood fails to clot properly. Traumatic coagulopathy has been linked to increased mortality rates. Thromboelastography (TEG) or rotational thromboelastometry (ROTEM) are used in some trauma centers to evaluate coagulopathy during trauma resuscitation. TEG and ROTEM tests provide a graphical tracing of the components of coagulation and fibrinolysis.[2,47]

M: Monitoring

Monitoring considerations include the following:

- Use appropriately sized pediatric equipment.
- Use noninvasive monitors with caution, knowing that movement and crying, poor perfusion, and extreme values can affect the readings.
- Change monitor alarm settings to reflect normal pediatric parameters for age-based respiratory rate, heart rate, SpO_2, and blood pressure.

N: Nasogastric or Orogastric Tube Consideration

Nasogastric or orogastric tube considerations include the following:

- Crying and bag-mask ventilation can cause children to swallow air and lead to gastric distention. Consider decompression with a nasogastric or orogastric tube. Placement of a gastric tube is considered routine care in the intubated patient to minimize aspiration risk.
- Select appropriate sizes of tubes by using a length-based resuscitation tape.

O: Oxygenation

Oxygenation considerations include the following:

- Apply the pulse oximeter probe to a warm extremity for the most accurate results.
  - A warm pack around the hand or foot may help.
- Other possible locations in the pediatric patient include the side of the hand, the earlobe, or the forehead.

P: Pain Assessment and Management

Pain assessment and management considerations include the following:

- Pain is consistently poorly assessed and managed in pediatric trauma patients.[48,49]
- Children may have difficulty localizing the source(s) of pain and may not be able to effectively communicate that they are experiencing pain.
- Environmental and emotional factors can potentiate the pain experience in pediatric patients.

Assessment and Interventions

Assessment and intervention considerations include the following:

- Use age- and developmentally appropriate pain scales (e.g., **Figure 12-2**) to assess for pain in all injured pediatric patients.
- Nonpharmacologic approaches to pain management for children can be separated into two categories: physical comfort measures and distracting techniques (**Table 12-5**).[48,49]
  - Infants find comfort in oral stimulation (pacifiers, breastfeeding, sucking) and physical contact (swaddling/cuddling, rocking). Cold and heat provide comfort to the older child.
  - Interactive toys, bubbles, art, music, and books all help to distract a young child. Video games and movies are good distraction for the older child.

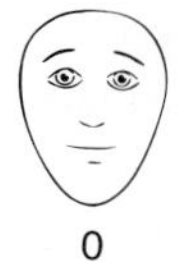

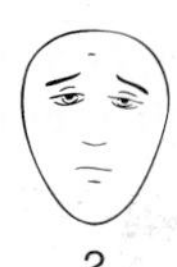

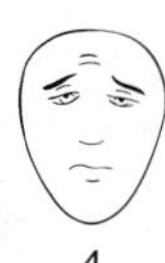

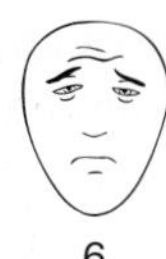

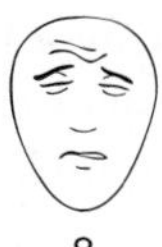

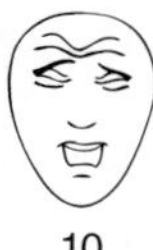

Figure 12-2 *Faces Pain Scale–Revised.*

In the following instructions, say "hurt" or "pain," whichever seems right for a particular child:

"These faces show how much something can hurt. This face [point to left-most face] shows no pain. The faces show more and more pain [point to each from left to right] up to this one. [point to right-most face] It shows very much pain. Point to the face that shows how much you hurt [right now]."

Score the chosen face 0, 2, 4, 6, 8, or 10, counting left to right, so "0" equals "No pain" and "10" equals "Very much pain." Do not use words like "happy" and "sad." This scale is intended to measure how children feel inside, not how their face looks.

Reproduced from Faces Pain Scale-Revised. © 2001. IASP International Association for the Study of Pain. Retrieved from https://www.iasp-pain.org/Education/Content.aspx?ItemNumber=1519&navItemNumber=577. This Faces Pain Scale-Revised has been reproduced with permission of the International Association for the Study of Pain® (IASP). The figure may NOT be reproduced for any other purpose without permission.

TABLE 12-5 Nonpharmacologic Approaches for Pain Management in Children

Physical Comfort (Infants and Young Children)	Distraction Techniques (All Ages)
Rocking	Blowing bubbles
Cuddling/swaddling	Conversation/asking questions
Pacifiers	Sound, music, art
Touch: stroking, rubbing, patting	Books, interactive games, puppets
	Imagery, controlled deep breathing
	Video games

Data from Krauss B., Calligaris L., Green S., & Barbi, E. (2016). Current concepts in management of pain in children in the emergency department. *The Lancet, 387*, 83–92. https://doi.org/10.1016/S0140-6736(14)61686-X.

  - Young children are cognitively immature, so they have difficulty controlling their fears. Distraction techniques are more effective than verbal reasoning in this age group.[48]
- Trauma nurses should continue to advocate for appropriate levels of pain management in all injured pediatric patients.[50] As the use of narcotic prescriptions has decreased, non-opioids and nonpharmacologic methods of pain management will become more prominent.
- Assess for signs and symptoms of traumatic stress (intrusive thoughts or images about the traumatic

event, avoidance of reminders of the event, hyperarousal or exaggerated startle response, emotional or cognitive changes).[51,52]

Reevaluation

Reevaluation considerations include the following:

- Assess for the need of pediatric surgical services, intensive care, or specialists (burn center) at this time and prepare for transport if indicated.
- Determination of the Pediatric Trauma Score (**Table 12-6**) may aid in the determination of the need for transfer to a pediatric trauma center.[12]

Diagnostics and Interventions

The secondary survey starts with history taking.

H: History

History includes the following:

- Obtain additional pertinent history information.
  - Include the caregiver's perception of the child.
  - When asking about last oral intake, also ask about last void/wet diaper.
  - For the child with special healthcare needs, vital signs, work of breathing, color, and mental status may vary from norms. The caregiver should be able to give a description of baseline status for assessment comparison.
- The caregiver may have important insight into the injury.
- Ask EMS personnel if the patient received any prehospital pain management, and document accordingly. Intranasal fentanyl has been shown to be a safe and effective method of delivering analgesia to injured children.[52]

H: Head-to-toe Assessment

Older infants, toddlers, and preschool-age children may respond better to a least invasive to most invasive approach to assessment, rather than a head-to-toe progression.

- Head
  - Palpate the infant for full or bulging fontanels.
- Chest
  - The pediatric patient's ribs are more cartilaginous, so fractures are not common. When present, rib fractures indicate significant force transmitted across the chest, accompanied by the high possibility of damage to underlying structures.
  - A mobile mediastinum allows a greater degree of shift to the right or left in the presence of pneumothorax, hemothorax, and/or tension pneumothorax.
- Abdomen
  - Anatomic and physiologic characteristics
    - The abdominal muscles are thin and less developed, so abdominal organs are not well protected.

TABLE 12-6 The Pediatric Trauma Score

Assessment Component	Pediatric Trauma Score		
	+2	+1	–1
Weight	Weight > 20 kg	10–20 kg	< 10 kg
Airway	Normal	Oral or nasal airway, oxygen	Intubated, cricothyroidotomy, or tracheostomy
Systolic blood pressure	> 90 mm Hg, good peripheral pulses and perfusion	50–90 mm Hg, carotid/femoral pulses palpable	< 50 mm Hg, weak or no pulses
Level of consciousness	Awake	Obtunded or any loss of consciousness	Coma, unresponsive
Fracture	None seen or suspected	Single, closed	Open or multiple
Cutaneous	None visible	Contusion, abrasion, laceration < 7 cm not through fascia	Tissue loss, any gunshot wound or stab wound through fascia

Reproduced from Tepas, J. J., 3rd, Mollitt, D. L., Talbert, J. L., & Bryant, M. (1987). The pediatric trauma score as a predictor of injury severity in the injured child. *Journal of Pediatric Surgery, 22*(1), 14–18. https://doi.org/10.1016/S0022-3468(87)80006-4.

        - The liver is more anterior and less protected by the ribs.
        - The kidneys are more mobile and less protected by fat.
        - The sigmoid colon and ascending colon are more mobile within the peritoneum and at greater risk for deceleration injuries.
        - The duodenum has an increased vascular supply; injury can lead to increased blood loss.[29]
    - Assessment
        - Inspect the abdomen for distention. Determine whether distension may be gastric dilation from swallowing air while crying or with bag-mask assisted ventilations.
        - Crying interferes with the assessment for guarding, tenderness, and rigidity. Provide distraction, involve the caregiver, or take the time for the patient to become calm before assessing.
- Pelvis and genitalia
    - The shallow depth of the pelvis increases risk for bladder rupture, particularly when the bladder is full.[53]
    - Assessing for rectal tone in the pediatric patient can be upsetting and can contribute to a reduction in the patient's cooperation, potentially limiting ongoing systemic assessments.
        - Assess by observing for an anal wink with rectal temperature unless contraindicated.
        - Perform this last and include the caregiver to comfort and hold the patient at the end of the assessment.
- Extremities
    - Pediatric patients have pliable, incompletely calcified bones that may mask significant underlying trauma.
    - Greenstick and buckle/torus fractures of the bones occur frequently in children due to the pliability and cartilaginous nature of young bones.
    - Because of the ossification process in children, comparison views for extremity radiographs will assist in identifying injury.[29]

Diagnostics and Interventions

Diagnostics and interventions revolve around radiographic and sonographic studies.

Radiographic Studies

Trauma centers are limiting the use of unnecessary computed tomography (CT) scans during evaluation of the injured child. Recent research shows that ionizing radiation exposure via CT scanners correlates with an increased lifelong risk of leukemia and solid-tumor cancers.[54-56] Children age 0 to 5 years are most susceptible to ionizing radiation exposure; therefore, it is important to consider the benefit and cumulative radiation dose of each imaging study in this age group. Researchers continue to search for good tools to predict which pediatric trauma patients will benefit from imaging as a diagnostic tool for internal injuries.

Cervical Spinal Trauma

The National Emergency X-Radiography Utilization Study (NEXUS) criteria for cervical spine clearance have demonstrated mixed results in sensitivity in the pediatric population.[57,58] Because young pediatric patients rarely meet the criteria, those younger than 8 years of age may require alternative diagnostic approaches, such as CT. The use of plain cervical radiographs may be useful in limiting exposure to ionizing radiation in children, but CT may still be required if the films are not definitive.[59]

The Pediatric Emergency Care Applied Research Network (PECARN) found that pediatric patients with the following characteristics have a higher risk of cervical-spine injury[60]:

- Altered mental status
- Focal neurologic deficits
- Complaints of neck pain
- Torticollis
- Substantial injury to the torso
- Predisposing condition
- High-risk motor vehicle crash
- Diving

Maintain spinal motion restriction if symptoms exist, even in the face of negative radiographs or CT imaging. SCIWORA can be diagnosed with magnetic resonance imaging (MRI).

Head Trauma

Because the diagnostic value of these images can be crucial when needed, PECARN released guidelines for use of CT in children with head injuries to minimize risk and eliminate unnecessary scans.[61]

Abdominal Trauma

For abdominal trauma in the pediatric patient, diagnostic options continue to evolve. The current recommendations include the following:

- To assess for free air in penetrating abdominal trauma, use CT and upright abdominal radiograph.

- For patients with moderate or severe blunt abdominal trauma[62]:
  - Obtain a CT scan in the stable patient.
  - Use focused assessment with sonography for trauma (FAST) or surgical exploration in the unstable patient.

Focused Assessment with Sonography for Trauma

The FAST exam has limited sensitivity in pediatric patients for identifying peritoneal bleeding but can be useful for the hypotensive patient who is too unstable to undergo CT. Practice in this area is evolving rapidly as studies begin to support FAST use in pediatric trauma management, and as trauma physicians and surgeons develop expertise with the technology.[63]

Diagnostic Peritoneal Lavage

Diagnostic peritoneal lavage (DPL) is no longer considered the preferred diagnostic method to rule out intra-abdominal bleeding in children. Accuracy and expertise with FAST have lessened the popularity of the more invasive DPL.[64]

Selected Injury Findings

This section covers selected injury findings.

Head Injury

Head injury considerations include the following:

- Suspect severe brain injury in a pediatric trauma patient with bulging fontanels. Head ultrasound or CT may be indicated for the infant with bulging fontanel.[65]
- Persistent vomiting post trauma can be an indication of increased ICP.

Traumatic Brain Injury

TBI considerations include the following:

- The assessment goal is to determine if the pediatric patient with TBI requires medical or surgical intervention or if observation and discharge teaching may be indicated.
- The PECARN criteria (**Figure 12-3**) can identify those patients who require observation only, thereby limiting children's exposure to ionizing radiation.[66]

Cervical Spinal Injury

Cervical spinal injury considerations include the following:

- If any signs or symptoms of spinal cord injury are present, despite negative radiographic evidence, assume that an unstable spinal injury exists and maintain spinal motion restriction.
- Appropriate, early removal of cervical collars promotes comfort, decreases anxiety and fear, decreases risk for skin breakdown, and may lower the risk of aspiration in pediatric patients.[67,68]

Abdominal Trauma

Abdominal trauma considerations include the following:

- Because pediatric patients are more susceptible to abdominal injury, bruising, abrasions, or pain to the abdomen may indicate the need for CT or serial assessments.[69]
- The liver, spleen, and kidneys have less protection from the ribs and overlying muscle and fat and, therefore, have the highest risk of injury among the abdominal organs.[29]

Management is based on the patient's hemodynamic stability, the stability of the injured organ, and the need for continued blood replacement therapy. Liver and spleen injuries are managed nonoperatively in the hemodynamically stable pediatric trauma patient.[62] Preservation of the spleen is of utmost importance in this population due to this organ's immunologic functions.[62] Even if surgery is required, the focus is on repair and hemostasis, not removal.

Musculoskeletal Trauma

Injuries involving the growth plates may result in growth abnormalities and have lifelong implications (e.g., length discrepancies in arms or legs, scoliosis, kyphosis, gait disturbances). For the pediatric patient with a growth plate injury, expect referral to an orthopedic specialist for follow-up.

Maltreatment

Care of the pediatric victim of non-accidental trauma or child maltreatment involves several steps: suspicion of abuse, history taking, diagnosis of injuries, treatment, and reporting to child protective services and/or law enforcement.[70] A detailed history should be taken and compared with the physical exam and imaging studies for discrepancies.[17] Also, determine whether MOI is developmentally appropriate for the child's age. See Chapter 16 for more information.

Suspect maltreatment with certain musculoskeletal injury patterns, such as the following[17]:

- Injuries of differing stages of healing and injuries not supported by the reported MOI

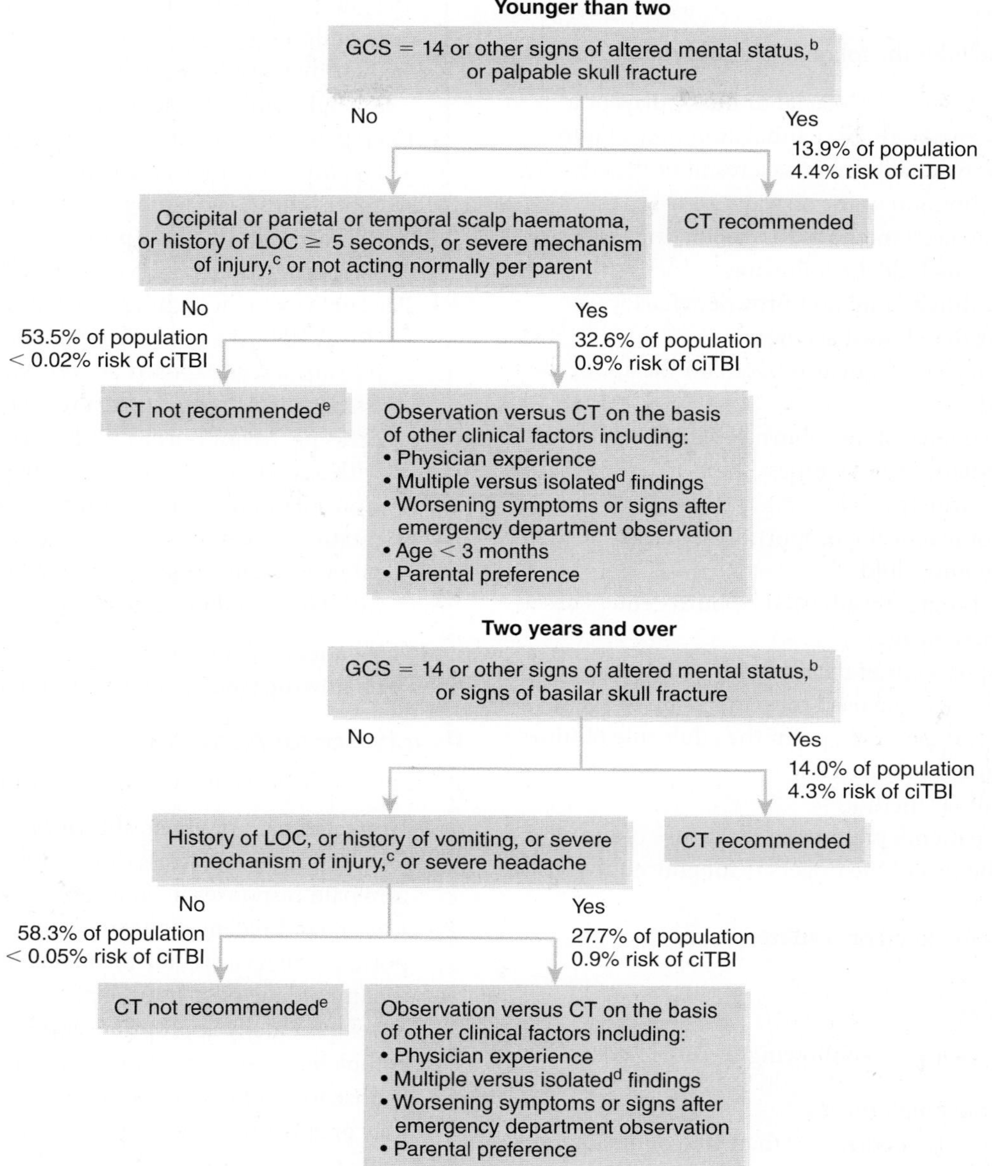

Figure 12-3 *PECARN algorithm.*[a]

Abbreviations: ciTBI, clinically important traumatic brain injury; GCS, Glasgow Coma Scale.

Note: The suggested CT algorithm for children younger than 2 years and for those age 2 years and older with GCS scores of 14 or 15 after head trauma.

[a] Data are from the combined derivation and validation populations.

[b] Other signs of altered mental status: agitation, somnolence, repetitive questioning, or slow response to verbal communication.

[c] Severe mechanism of injury: motor vehicle crash with patient ejection, death of another passenger, or rollover; pedestrian or bicyclist without helmet struck by a motorized vehicle; falls of more than 0.9 m (3 feet) (or more than 1.5 m [5 feet] for panel B); or head struck by a high-impact object.

[d] Patients with certain isolated findings (with no other findings suggestive of traumatic brain injury), such as isolated loss of consciousness, isolated headache, isolated vomiting, and certain types of isolated scalp hematomas in infants older than 3 months, have a risk of ciTBI substantially lower than 1%.

[e] Risk of ciTBI is exceedingly low, generally lower than risk of CT-induced malignancies. Therefore, CT scans are not indicated for most patients in this group.

Reproduced from PECARN.org.

- Rib, scapular, or sternal fractures that require a great deal of force
  - If the MOI does not indicate this level of force, suspect maltreatment.
- Transverse, oblique, and spiral fractures
- Bilateral or symmetrical fractures, bruising, or abrasions

Burn Trauma

The majority of burns in young children are scald burns that occur in the home. Flames are the dominant cause of burn injuries in teenagers, typically from fireworks or flammable substances.[71] (See Chapter 11, "Surface and Burn Trauma," for more information.)

Assessment

Assessment includes the following considerations:

- Pediatric patients with facial or neck burns or a history of enclosed-space inhalation may require rapid airway management as a result of the edema and inflammation in the airway.
- Commonly used methods for calculating burn size in children include the following:
  - The modified Lund and Browder chart[18,29,43]
    - Considered most accurate
    - Estimation of burns is based on the age of the child
    - First choice of most burn centers
  - The pediatric rule of nines[29,43]
    - Most widely used
    - Accounts for the proportionally larger head of the young child
    - May be slightly adjusted by burn centers based on patient age
    - For purposes of determining a higher level of care, can be used for patients up to age 15 years, at which point the adult rule of nines is more accurate
  - The palmar method[29,43]
    - The patient's palm from the crease of the wrist to the tips of the fingers is roughly equivalent to 1%
    - Best for small or scattered burns

Interventions

Interventions include the following:

- Stop the burning process.
  - For superficial burns less than 10% of the total body surface area (TBSA), cool water may be used for 3 to 5 minutes.[72] Never use ice or iced water.[72]
- Provide fluid resuscitation as indicated.
  - The Parkland formula is used to calculate fluid resuscitation in pediatric burn patients and is used when an area of greater than 15% to 20% TBSA exists.[29,43]
  - The Parkland formula for children is 3 mL Ringer's lactate solution multiplied by weight in kilograms multiplied by percent of TBSA including only deep partial-thickness or full-thickness burns (3 mL × weight in kg × %TBSA = 24-hour fluid requirement).[43] Administer the first half of the fluid over the first 8 hours and the remaining half in the next 16 hours.
  - Adequacy of fluid resuscitation is measured by a minimum urine output of 1 to 2 mL/kg/hour.[29]
  - Young children require maintenance IV fluids in addition to burn resuscitation fluids to meet their increased metabolic demands and prevent hypoglycemia and acidosis.[43]
- Keep patients covered to prevent heat loss.
  - Hypothermia increases metabolic demands and contributes to coagulopathy development.
  - Remove wet dressings promptly and implement measures to keep the patient warm.
- Pain management includes the following:
  - Cover all burns to prevent pain from air current passing across exposed nerves. Minor burns (< 10% TBSA) may be covered with a cool moist dressing. Major burns (> 10% TBSA) are covered with a clean dry sheet to avoid hypothermia.[71]
  - Consider opioid treatment at an early stage of treatment. Reassess the patient for pain and relief often, as medication absorption can be unpredictable with fluid shifts.[29]

Refer patients to a burn center per established guidelines for follow-up (see Chapter 11 for more information).

Psychosocial Aspects

Psychosocial aspects include the following:

- Untreated pain has been shown to increase the risk for post-traumatic stress disorder and heighten future pain responses in children.[73]
- Understanding emotional development is important when caring for the pediatric patient in the immediate post-trauma phase. An age- and developmentally appropriate approach facilitates a complete assessment of the pediatric patient's response to traumatic stress. Loss of normal routine may greatly impact younger children, while adolescents may be uneasy because of their sudden loss of independence.[74]
- Play therapy promotes relaxation and helps the young child feel more secure in a strange environment.[74]
- Research indicates that families of pediatric trauma patients experience significant stress. Initiate social support services as early as possible to assist families in their time of crisis.[75]

Disaster Management

Pediatric-relevant information is summarized here, but see Chapter 18, "Disaster Management," for more information.

- Disaster preparedness incorporates addressing pediatric needs, including equipment and resources for staff, by emphasizing weight-based medication principles,

anatomic and physiologic differences in children, normal vital signs ranges, nutritional support, family reunification processes, and mental health resources.[76] Ideally, these resources will be readily available to the trauma team in any mass-casualty incident that includes pediatric patients. Young children and those with limited physical mobility or developmental delays may not be able to remove themselves from unfolding disaster events.
- Children's proximity to the ground and increased respiratory rate may make them more vulnerable to some chemical and biologic agents.
- The thinner skin in pediatric patients leads to increased systemic absorption of biologic and chemical agents.
- JumpSTART is a widely used pediatric mass-casualty triage tool and is discussed more thoroughly in Chapter 18.[77]
- Children may need additional assistance during the decontamination process.
- Use warmed water during decontamination to prevent hypothermia.
- The following measures can promote identification and reunification during a disaster:
  - Document clothing, backpacks, bags, jewelry, and other identifying objects carried or worn by the patient before removing them prior to decontamination.
  - On the child's skin, use a permanent marker to record important identifying characteristics.

Reevaluation and Post-Resuscitation Care

Reevaluation and post-resuscitation care considerations include the following:

- Ongoing assessment and evaluation of interventions include frequent, serial reevaluation of the primary survey, monitoring for changes in vital signs, and continued reevaluation and management of pain and identified injuries. These actions, along with monitoring urine output, will help to guide therapy.
- Continue to monitor and treat serum glucose levels for hypoglycemia, especially in infants and young children, whose glycogen stores may become rapidly depleted.

Patient Safety

Safety of the injured pediatric patient in an adult care setting can consume many resources, but is essential to prevent further injury. Infants and younger children may need constant supervision in the absence of a caregiver and require cribs or isolettes to help prevent falls from a stretcher. Other risks for falls include older children who may attempt to remove themselves from spinal motion restriction devices or may attempt to ambulate unassisted while under the effects of opioids and/or with compromised balance from an injury.

The assistance of social services may be necessary to ensure family reunification if the patient arrives without a primary caregiver. A child life therapist and child life techniques can be helpful to promote normalcy and calmness during difficult procedures.

Definitive Care or Transport

Care and transport considerations include the following:

- Consider the need for transfer to a pediatric trauma center or burn center early in the care and management of the pediatric patient for best outcomes (see Chapter 11 for more information).
- Assessment of the pediatric patient's status, injuries, and needs for definitive care are considered when determining the necessary configuration of the transport team. Pediatric patients have better outcomes and fewer unplanned events when transported by a specialized pediatric team.[78]
- Provide follow-up and clear discharge instructions, including information on gradual and incremental return to play for all patients diagnosed with TBI, including those with concussions. Returning to play while symptoms persist places the patient at risk for secondary brain injury, which is more likely to be fatal in the pediatric patient.[79]
- Have contact information readily available for referral to the closest pediatric trauma center for transfer or consult.

Injury Prevention

Injury prevention education, law enforcement, and product improvement have all played key roles in the reduction of childhood injuries.[80] Successful prevention programs include community involvement to analyze local pediatric-specific trauma statistics, development of initiatives relevant to the local population, and advocacy for child safety legislation within the community. Changing public awareness starts with avoiding terms such as "accident," which makes injuries seem unavoidable or random. The causes of injury are predictable and should be described as preventable events.[81,82]

In the United States, injury prevention is considered a public health priority. Reducing deaths from injury and violence is an objective of the federal government's *Healthy People 2020* initiative.[83] In 2016, the National Academy of Medicine released a report that included a plan and vision to achieve zero preventable deaths after injury.[84] The American College of Surgeons requires that Level I and Level II trauma centers establish injury prevention programs as part of their overall trauma programs.[85] The American Academy of Pediatrics has resources available regarding a wide variety of injury prevention programs. Injury prevention campaigns such as "Head's Up," "Back to Sleep," and programs related to seat belts, safety seats, helmets, water safety, and smoke detector legislation have all worked to increase awareness and decrease unintentional injuries in pediatric patients.

Emerging Trends

Emerging trends in the treatment and prevention of traumatic injuries are occurring on several different fronts.

Reduction of the Use of Unnecessary Radiation During Trauma Evaluations in Children

As outlined in the "Radiographic Studies" section of this chapter, ionizing radiation exposure in children may increase lifetime risk of developing some types of malignancies.[54-56] Treatment teams can use PECARN guidelines, and other evidence-based algorithms, to safely reduce CT scans among hemodynamically stable patients. Some children may undergo MRI, plain films, or ultrasound imaging instead of CT scans.[86] Studies show that nonpediatric trauma centers are more likely to over-radiate pediatric trauma patients.[55,87,88]

Motor Vehicle Design to Reduce Traumatic Injuries in Children

The most common cause of both severe and nonsevere traumatic injuries in children continues to be MVCs involving passengers, drivers, or pedestrians.[6] Any attempts to reduce MVCs through better car design or roadway engineering improvements will decrease the incidence of injured children. In addition, enforcement of better laws addressing child car seats, drunk drivers, and graduated driving laws for teenagers will continue to reduce pediatric injuries.

Progress in Pediatric Concussion Management and Treatment

An estimated 1.1 to 1.9 million children are treated for recreation- and sports-related concussions each year.[89] Most sports-related pediatric TBIs stem from falls or interpersonal contact.[90] Public health programs and state laws have been implemented to help parents and coaches recognize symptoms of concussion on the field and remove affected children from play until they are evaluated by a healthcare professional.[91] Post-concussive symptoms may persist for several weeks after the initial injury. Research continues into better protective gear and more effective treatments of long-term symptoms.

Summary

Pediatric trauma care requires familiarity with the unique responses of the injured pediatric patient. The systematic approach of the primary survey is the same for adults and children, but the clinical manifestations of complications and interventions may vary based on the patient's age, size, and development. Knowledge of normal growth and development assists the trauma nurse in approaching the pediatric patient and providing appropriate care. Family-centered care in the adult population is important; in pediatrics, it is vital. Identification of the primary caregivers and integration of their perspectives and input into care can promote optimal pediatric trauma care. **Table 12-7** identifies Internet resources related to the care of pediatric patients.

TABLE 12-7 Internet Resources

Internet Resource	Web Address
Emergency Nurses Association	www.ena.org
Society of Trauma Nurses	www.traumanurses.org
American Academy of Pediatrics	www.aap.org
American College of Emergency Physicians	www.acep.org
American College of Surgeons	www.facs.org/trauma
Pediatric Trauma Society	www.pediatrictraumasociety.org

Internet Resource	Web Address
Emergency Medical Services for Children National Resource Center	https://emscimprovement.center/
Centers for Disease Control and Prevention	www.cdc.gov/injury
Injury Free Coalition for Kids	www.injuryfree.org
Safe Kids Worldwide	www.safekids.org
Sage Diagram (free TBSA calculator)	www.sagediagram.com
Image Gently Campaign	https://www.imagegently.org/
Pediatric Emergency Care Applied Research Network (PECARN)	www.pecarn.org

References

1. Centers for Disease Control and Prevention, National Center for Injury Prevention and Control. (2016). Web-based Injury Statistics Query and Reporting System (WISQARS). Retrieved from https://www.cdc.gov/injury/wisqars
2. Letton, R. W., & Johnson, J. J. (2017). The ABCs of pediatric trauma. In D. E. Wesson & B. Naik-Mathuria (Eds.), *Pediatric trauma: Pathophysiology, diagnosis, and treatment* (2nd ed., pp. 51–60). Boca Raton, FL: CRC Press.
3. American College of Surgeons. (2016). *National Trauma Data Bank 2016: Pediatric report*. Retrieved from http://www.facs.org/quality-programs/trauma/ntdb/docpub
4. Osterman, M., Kochanek, K., MacDorman, M., Strobino, D., & Guyer, B. (2015). Annual summary of vital statistics: 2012–2013. *Pediatrics, 135,* 1115–1125. https://doi.org/10.1542%2Fpeds.2015-0434
5. Wesson, D. E. (2017). Epidemiology of pediatric trauma. In D. E. Wesson & B. Naik-Mathuria (Eds.), *Pediatric trauma: Pathophysiology, diagnosis, and treatment* (2nd ed., pp. 3–6). Boca Raton, FL: CRC Press.
6. Oliver, J., Avraham, J., Frnagos, S., Tomita, S., & DiMaggio, C. (2018). The epidemiology of inpatient pediatric trauma in United States hospitals. *Journal of Pediatric Surgery,* 53, 758–764. https://doi.org/10.1016/j.jpedsurg.2017.04.014
7. American Academy of Pediatrics. (2015). Ensuring the health of children in disasters (Policy statement). *Pediatrics, 136,* e1407–e1417. https://doi.org/10.1542/peds.2015-3112
8. Ray, K., Olson, L., Edgerton E., Ely, M., Gausche-Hill, M., Schmuhl P., . . . Kahn, J. (2018). Access to high pediatric-readiness emergency care in the United States. *Journal of Pediatrics, 194,* 225–232.e1. https://doi.org/10.1016/j.jpeds.2017.10.074
9. Gausche-Hill, M., Ely, M., Schmuhl, P., Telford, R., Remick, K., Edgerton, E., & Olson, L. (2015). A national assessment of pediatric readiness of emergency departments. *JAMA Pediatrics, 169*(6), 527–534. https://doi.org/10.1001/jamapediatrics.2015.138
10. Peng, J., Wheeler, K., Groner, J., Haley, K., & Xiang, H. (2017). Undertriage of pediatric major trauma patients in the United States. *Clinical Pediatrics, 56,* 845–853. https://doi.org/10.1177/0009922817709553
11. Zonfrillo, M. R. (2015). Evaluation and management of the multiple trauma patient. In R. Shafermeyer & M. Tenenbein (Eds.), *Pediatric emergency medicine* (4th ed., pp. 115–125). New York, NY: McGraw-Hill.
12. American College of Surgeons. (2018). Pediatric trauma. In *Advanced trauma life support: Student course manual* (10th ed., pp. 188–212). Chicago, IL: Author.
13. Quayle, K. S. (2015). Head trauma. In R. Shafermeyer & M. Tenebein (Eds.), *Pediatric emergency medicine* (4th ed., pp. 126–131). New York, NY: McGraw-Hill.
14. Perkins, C., Scannell, B., Brighton, B., Seymour, R., & Vanderhave, K. (2016). Orthopaedic firearm injuries in children and adolescents: An eight-year experience at a major urban trauma center. *Injury, 47,* 173–177. https://doi.org/10.1016/j.injury.2015.07.031
15. Cunningham, R., Carter, P., & Ranney, M. (2015). Violent reinjury and mortality among youth seeking emergency department care for assault-related injury: A 2-year prospective study. *JAMA Pediatrics, 169,* 63–70. https://doi.org/10.1001%2Fjamapediatrics.2014.1900
16. Naranje, S., Eralia, R., Warner, W., Sawyer, J., & Kelly, D. (2016). Epidemiology of pediatric fractures presenting to emergency departments in the United States. *Journal of Pediatric Orthopaedics, 36,* e45–e48. https://doi.org/10.1097/BPO.0000000000000595
17. Cox, C. C., Jackson, M. L., & Aertker, B. M. (2017). Trauma from child abuse. In D. E. Wesson & B. Naik-Mathuria (Eds.) *Pediatric trauma: Pathophysiology, diagnosis, and treatment* (2nd ed., pp. 91–98). Boca Raton, FL: CRC Press.
18. Hogan, M. (2013). *Child health nursing: Pearson reviews and rationales* (3rd ed.). Boston, MA: Pearson.
19. Rodgers, C. C. (2016). Health promotion of the infant and family. In M. Hockenberry, C. Rodgers, & D. Wilson (Eds.), *Wong's essentials of pediatric nursing* (10th ed., pp. 301–309). St. Louis, MO: Elsevier.
20. Rodgers, C. C. (2016). Health promotion of the toddler and family. In M. Hockenberry, C. Rodgers, & D. Wilson (Eds.), *Wong's essentials of pediatric nursing* (10th ed., pp. 370–378). St. Louis, MO: Elsevier.
21. Glass, N., Frangos, S., Simon, R., Bholat, O., Todd, S., Wilson, C., . . . Levine, D. (2014). Risky behaviors associated with pediatric pedestrian and bicyclists struck by motor vehicles.

Pediatric Emergency Care, 30, 409–412. https://doi.org/10.1097/PEC.0000000000000148

22. Stavrinos, D., Pope, C., Shen, J., & Schwebel, D. (2018). Distracted walking, bicycling and driving: Systematic review and meta-analysis of mobile technology and youth crash risk. *Child Development, 89,* 118–128. https://doi.org/10.1111/cdev.12827
23. Parsons, S., Carter, E., Waterhouse, L., Fitzeen, J., Kelleher, D., O'Connell, K., . . . Burd, R. (2014). Improving ATLS performance in simulated pediatric trauma resuscitation using a checklist. *Annals of Surgery, 259,* 807–813. https://doi.org/10.1097/SLA.0000000000000259
24. Wurster, L., Thakkar, R., Haley, K., Wheeler, K., Larson, J., Stoner, M., . . . Groner, J. (2017). Standardizing the initial resuscitation of the trauma patient with the Primary Assessment Completion Tool using video review. *Journal of Trauma and Acute Care Surgery, 82,* 1002–1006. https://doi.org/10.1097/TA.0000000000001417
25. American Heart Association. (2016). *Pediatric advanced life support: Provider manual.* Dallas, TX: Author.
26. Foresman-Capuzzi, J. R. (2020). Triage and prioritization. In D. Brecher (Ed.), *Emergency nursing pediatric course: Provider manual* (5th ed., pp. 109–117). Schaumburg, IL: Emergency Nurses Association.
27. Fernandez, A., Ares, M., Garcia, S., Martinez-Indart, L., Mintegi, S., & Benito, J. (2017). The validity of the Pediatric Assessment Triangle as the first step in the triage process in a pediatric emergency department. *Pediatric Emergency Care, 33,* 234–238.
28. Fuchs, S., Terry, M., Adelgais, K., Bokholdt, M., Brie, J., Brown, K., . . . Marx, W. (2016). Definitions and assessment approaches for emergency medical services for children. *Pediatrics, 138*(6), e20161073. https://doi.org/10.1542/peds.2016-1073
29. Stone, E. (2020). From the start. In D. Brecher (Ed.), *Emergency nursing pediatric course: Provider manual* (5th ed., pp. 13–23). Schaumburg, IL: Emergency Nurses Association.
30. Harless, J., Ramaiah, R., & Bhananker, S. (2014). Pediatric airway management. *International Journal of Critical Illness and Injury Science, 4*(1), 65–70. https://doi.org/10.4103/2229-5151.128015
31. Society of Critical Care Medicine. (2013). *Pediatric fundamental critical care support* (2nd ed.). Mount Prospect, IL: Author.
32. Young, L. L. (2015). Respiratory failure. In R. Shafermeyer & M. Tenenbein (Eds.), *Pediatric emergency medicine* (4th ed., pp. 90–93). New York, NY: McGraw-Hill.
33. National Association of Emergency Medical Technicians & Committee on Trauma of the American College of Surgeons. (2016). *Prehospital trauma life support: Provider manual* (8th ed.). Burlington, MA: Jones & Bartlett Learning.
34. Hockenberry, M. J. (2016). Pain assessment and management in children. In M. Hockenberry, C. Rodgers, & D. Wilson (Eds.), *Wong's essentials of pediatric nursing* (10th ed., pp. 114–149). St. Louis, MO: Elsevier.
35. Norii, T., Miyata, S., Terasaka, Y., Guliani, S., Lu, S., & Crandall, C. (2017). Resuscitative endovascular balloon occlusion of the aorta in trauma patients in youth. *Journal of Trauma and Acute Care Surgery, 82(*5), 915–920. https://doi.org/10.1097/TA.0000000000001347
36. Foote, J. M. (2016). Communication and physical assessment of the child and family. In M. Hockenberry, C. Rodgers, & D. Wilson (Eds.), *Wong's essentials of pediatric nursing* (10th ed., pp. 57–113). St. Louis, MO: Elsevier.
37. Steinman, R. A. (2020). Initial assessment. In D. Brecher (Ed.), *Emergency nursing pediatric course: Provider manual* (5th ed., pp. 45–58). Schaumburg, IL: Emergency Nurses Association.
38. Eckert, M., Wertin, T., Tyner, S., Nelson, D., Izenberg, S., & Martin, M. (2014). Tranexamic acid administration to pediatric trauma patients in a combat setting: The Pediatric Trauma and Tranexamic Acid Study (PED-TRAX). *Journal of Trauma and Acute Care Surgery, 77*(6), 852–858. https://doi.org/10.1097/TA.0000000000000443
39. Napolitano, L. M., Cohen, M. J., Cotton, B. A., Schreiber, M. A., & Moore, E. E. (2013). Tranexamic acid in trauma: How should we use it? *Journal of Trauma and Acute Care Surgery, 74*(6), 1575–1586.
40. Fraser, D. (2016). Health problems of newborns. In M. Hockenberry, C. Rodgers, & D. Wilson (Eds.), *Wong's essentials of nursing* (10th ed., pp. 229–300). St. Louis, MO: Elsevier.
41. Kukreti, V., Mohseni-Bod, H., & Drake, J. (2014). Management of raised intracranial pressure in children with traumatic brain injury. *Journal of Pediatric Neurosurgery, 9*(3), 207–215. https://doi.org/10.4103/1817-1745.147572
42. Perlman, R., Callum, J., Laflamme, C., Tien, H., Nascimento, B., Beckett, A., & Alam, A. (2016). A recommended early goal-directed management guideline for the prevention of hypothermia-related transfusion, morbidity, and mortality in severely injured trauma patients. *Critical Care, 20*(107), 1–11. https:/doi.org/10.1186/s13054-016-1271-z
43. Webman, R. B., Shupp, J. W., & Burd, R. S. (2017). General principles of resuscitation and supportive care: Burns. In D. E. Wesson & B. Naik-Mathuria (Eds.), *Pediatric trauma: Pathophysiology, diagnosis, and treatment* (2nd ed., pp. 75–90). Boca Raton, FL: CRC Press.
44. Cox, C. S., Jackson, M. L., & Aertker, B. M. (2017). Trauma from child abuse. In D. E. Wesson & B. Naik-Mathuria (Eds.), *Pediatric trauma: Pathophysiology, diagnosis, and treatment* (2nd ed., pp. 91–98). Boca Raton, FL: CRC Press.
45. Dudley, N., Ackerman, A., Brown, K. M., Snow, S. K., American Academy of Pediatrics Committee on Pediatric Emergency Medicine, American College of Emergency Physicians Emergency Medicine Committee, & Emergency Nurses Association Pediatric Committee. (2015). Patient and family-centered care of children in the emergency department. *Pediatrics, 135*(1), 1–20. https://doi.org/10.1542/peds.2014-3424
46. Egging, D., Crowley, M., Arruda, T., Proehl, J., Walker-Cillo, G., Papa, A., . . . Bokholdt, M. L. (2011). Emergency nursing resource: Family presence during invasive procedures and resuscitation in the emergency department. *Journal of Emergency Nursing, 37(5),* 469–473. https://doi.org/10.1016/j.jen.2011.04.012

47. Hensch, L., & Teruya, J. (2017). Transfusion therapy in injured children. In D. E. Wesson & B. Naik-Mathuria (Eds.), *Pediatric trauma: Pathophysiology, diagnosis, and treatment* (2nd ed., pp. 109–120). Boca Raton, FL: CRC Press.
48. Krauss, B., Calligaris, L., Green, S., & Barbi, E. (2016). Current concepts in management of pain in children in the emergency department. *The Lancet, 387(10013),* 83–92. https://doi.org/10.1016/S0140-6736(14)61686-X
49. Tepas, J. J., 3rd, Mollitt, D. L., Talbert, J. L., & Bryant, M. (1987). The Pediatric Trauma Score as a predictor of injury severity in the injured child. *Journal of Pediatric Surgery, 22*(1), 14–18. https://doi.org/10.1016/S0022-3468(87)80006-4
50. Young, V. (2017). Effective management of pain and anxiety for the pediatric patient in the emergency department. *Critical Care Nursing Clinics of North America, 29*(2), 205–216. https://doi.org/10.1016/j.cnc.2017.01.007
51. Kassam-Adams, N., Rzucidlo, S., Campbell, M., Good, G., Bonifacio, E., Slouf, K., . . . Grather, D. (2015). Nurses' views and current practice of trauma-informed pediatric nursing care. *Journal of Pediatric Nursing, 30*(3), 478–484. https://doi.org/10.1016/j.pedn.2014.11.008
52. Murphy, A., Hughes, M., McCoy, S., Crispino, G., Wakai, A., & O'Sullivan, R. (2017). Intranasal fentanyl for the prehospital management of acute pain in children. *European Journal of Emergency Medicine, 24*(6), 450–454. https://doi.org/10.1097/MEJ.0000000000000389
53. Hill, J. F., & Robertson, A. K. (2017). Pediatric orthopedic trauma: Spine and pelvis trauma. In D. E. Wesson & B. Naik-Mathuria (Eds.), *Pediatric trauma: Pathophysiology, diagnosis, and treatment* (2nd ed., pp. 263–277). Boca Raton, FL: CRC Press.
54. Puckett, Y., Bonacorsi, L., Caley, M., Farmakis, S., Fitzpatrick, C., Chatoorgoon, K., . . . Vane, D. (2016). Imaging before transfer to designated pediatric trauma centers exposes children to excess radiation. *Journal of Trauma and Acute Care Surgery, 81*(2), 229–235. https://doi.org/10.1097/TA.0000000000001074
55. Pandit, V., Michailidou, M., Rhee, P., Zangbar, B., Kulvatunyou, N., Khalil, M., . . . Joseph, B. (2016). The use of whole body computed tomography scans in pediatric trauma patients: Are there differences among adults and pediatric centers? *Journal of Pediatric Surgery, 51*(4), 649–653. https://doi.org/10.1016/j.jpedsurg.2015.12.002
56. Kharbanda, A., Krause, E., Lu, Y., & Blumberg, K. (2015). Analysis of radiation dose to pediatric patients during computed tomography examinations. *Academic Emergency Medicine, 22*(6), 670–675. https://doi.org/10.1111/acem.12689
57. Vicellio, P., Simon, H., Pressman, B., Shah, M., Mower, W., & Hoffman J. (2001). A prospective multicenter study of cervical spine injury in children. *Pediatrics, 108*(2). https://doi.org/10.1542/peds.108.2.e20
58. Hale, D., Fitzpatrick, C., Doski, J., Stewart, R., & Mueller, D. (2015). Absence of clinical findings reliably excludes unstable cervical spine injuries in children 5 years or younger. *Journal of Trauma and Acute Care Surgery, 78*(5), 943–948. https://doi.org/10.1097/TA.0000000000000603
59. Hannon, M., Mannix, R., Dorney, K., Mooney, D., & Hennelly, K. (2015). Pediatric cervical spine injury evaluation after blunt trauma: A clinical decision analysis. *Annals of Emergency Medicine, 65*(3), 239–247. https://doi.org/10.1016/j.annemergmed.2014.09.002
60. Tat, S., Mejia, M., & Freishtat, R. (2014). Imaging, clearance, and controversies in pediatric cervical spine trauma. *Pediatric Emergency Care, 30*(12), 911–915. https://doi.org/10.1097/PEC.0000000000000298
61. Schonfeld, D., Bressan, S., DaDalt, S., Henien, M., Winnett, J., & Nigrovic, E. (2014). Pediatric Emergency Care Applied Research Network head injury clinical prediction rules are reliable in practice. *Archives of Disease in Childhood, 99*(5), 427–431. https://doi.org/10.1136/archdischild-2013-305004
62. Gillory, L., & Naik-Mathuria, B. (2017). Pediatric abdominal trauma. In D. E. Wesson & B. Naik-Mathuria (Eds.), *Pediatric trauma: Pathophysiology, diagnosis, and treatment* (2nd ed., pp. 215–238). Boca Raton, FL: CRC Press.
63. Mahajan, P., Kuppermann, N., Tunik, M., Yen, K., Atabaki, S., Lee, L., & Holmes, J. (2015). Comparison of clinician suspicion versus a clinical prediction rule in identifying children at risk for intra-abdominal injuries after blunt torso trauma. *Academic Emergency Medicine, 22*(9), 1034–1041. https://doi.org/10.1111/acem.12739
64. Atabaki, S. M. (2015). Abdominal trauma. In R. W. Schafermeyer & M. Tenenbein (Eds.), *Pediatric emergency medicine* (4th ed., pp. 153–165). New York, NY: McGraw-Hill.
65. Fuchs, S. (2015). Altered mental status and coma. In R. W. Schafermeyer & M. Tenenbein (Eds.), *Pediatric emergency medicine* (4th ed., pp. 17–20). New York, NY: McGraw-Hill.
66. Kuppermann, N., Holmes, J., Dayan, P., Hoyle, J. D., Atabaki, S. M., Holubkov, R., & Pediatric Emergency Care Applied Research Network. (2009). Identification of children at very low risk of clinically-important brain injuries after head trauma: A prospective cohort study. *The Lancet, 374*(9696), 1160–1170. https://doi.org/10.1016/S0140-6736(09)61558-0
67. Leonard, J. C., & Leonard, J. R. (2015). Cervical spine injury. In R. W. Schafermeyer & M. Tenenbein (Eds.), *Pediatric emergency medicine* (4th ed., pp. 132–142). New York, NY: McGraw-Hill.
68. Talbot, L. J., & Kenney, B. D. (2017). Clearance of the cervical spine in children. In D. E. Wesson & B. Naik-Mathuria (Eds.), *Pediatric trauma: Pathophysiology, diagnosis, and treatment* (2nd ed., pp. 63–73). Boca Raton, FL: CRC Press.
69. Holmes, J., Kelley, K., Wooton-Gorges, S., Utter, G., Abramson, L., Rose, J., . . . Kuppermann, N. (2017). Effect of abdominal ultrasound on clinical care, outcomes, and resource use among children with blunt torso trauma: A randomized clinical trial. *Journal of the American Medical Association, 317*(22), 2290–2296. https://doi.org/10.1001/jama.2017.6322
70. Nielson, M. H. (2018). Abuse and neglect. In V. Sweet (Ed.), *Emergency nursing core curriculum* (7th ed., pp. 36–46). St. Louis, MO: Elsevier.

71. Lee, C., Mahendraraj, K., Houng, A., Marano, M., Petrone, S., Lee, R., & Chamberlain, R. (2016). Pediatric burns: A single institution retrospective review of incidence, etiology, and outcomes in 2273 burn patients (1995–2013). *Journal of Burn Care and Research, 37*(6), e579–e585. https://doi.org/10.1097/BCR.0000000000000362
72. Rodgers, C. C., Baker, R. U., & Mondozzi, M. A. (2016). Health problems of toddlers and preschoolers. In M. J. Hockenberry, D. Wilson, & C. C. Rodgers (Eds.), *Wong's essentials of pediatric nursing* (10th ed., pp. 393–428). St. Louis, MO: Elsevier.
73. Thrane, S., Wanless, S., Cohen, S., & Danford, C. (2016). The assessment and non-pharmacologic treatment of procedural pain from infancy to school age through a developmental lens: A synthesis of evidence with recommendations. *Journal of Pediatric Nursing, 31*(1), e23–e32. https://doi.org/10.1016/j.pedn.2015.09.002
74. Franklin, Q., & Prows, C. A. (2016). Developmental and genetic influences on child health promotion. In M. J. Hockenberry, D. Wilson, & C. C. Rodgers (Eds.), *Wong's essentials of pediatric nursing* (10th ed., pp. 38–56). St. Louis, MO: Elsevier.
75. Foster, K., Young, A., Mitchell, R., Van, C., & Curtis, K. (2017). Experiences and needs of parents of critically injured children during the acute hospital phase: A qualitative investigation. *Injury, 48*(1), 114–120. https://doi.org/10.1016/j.injury.2016.09.034
76. Chung, S., & Adirim, T. (2015). Disaster preparedness. In R. W. Schafermeyer & M. Tenenbein (Eds.), *Pediatric emergency medicine* (4th ed., pp. 805–809). New York, NY: McGraw-Hill.
77. Nadeau, N., & Cicero, M. (2017). Pediatric disaster triage system utilization across the United States. *Pediatric Emergency Care, 33*(3), 152–155. https://doi.org/10.1097/PEC.0000000000000680.
78. Calhoun, A., Keller, M., Shi, J., Brancato, C., Donovan, K., Kraus, D., & Leonard, J. (2016). Do pediatric teams affect outcomes of injured children requiring inter-hospital transport? *Prehospital Emergency Care, 21*(2), 192–200. https://doi.org/10.1080/10903127.2016.1218983
79. Mahajan, P. (2015). Minor head trauma. In R. W. Schafermeyer & M. Tenenbein (Eds.), *Pediatric emergency medicine* (4th ed., pp. 29–34). New York, NY: McGraw-Hill.
80. Wesson, D. E. (2017). Epidemiology of pediatric trauma. In D. E. Wesson & B. Naik-Mathuria (Eds.), *Pediatric trauma: Pathophysiology, diagnosis, and treatment* (2nd ed., pp. 3–6). Boca Raton, FL: CRC Press.
81. Bonilla-Escobea, F., & Gutierrez, M. I. (2014). Injuries are not accidents: Towards a culture of prevention. *Colombia Medica (Cali), 45*(3), 132–135. Retrieved from http://colombiamedica.univalle.edu.co/index.php/comedica/article/view/1462/2427
82. Moore, K. (2016). Injury prevention and trauma mortality. *Journal of Emergency Nursing, 42(5),* 457–458. https://doi.org/https://doi.org/10.1016/j.jen.2016.06.015
83. *Healthy People 2020.* (2018, February 2). Washington, DC: U.S. Department of Health and Human Services, Office of Disease Prevention and Health Promotion. Retrieved from https://www.healthypeople.gov/
84. National Academies of Sciences, Engineering, and Medicine. (2016). *A national trauma care system: Integrating military and civilian trauma systems to achieve zero preventable deaths after injury.* Washington, DC: National Academies Press.
85. American College of Surgeons. (2014). *Resources for the optimal care of the injured patient.* Chicago, IL: Author.
86. Roguski, M., Morel, B., Sweeney, M., Tatan, J., Rideout, L., Riesenburger, R., . . . Hwang, S., (2015). Magnetic resonance imaging as an alternative to computed tomography in select patients with traumatic brain injury: A retrospective comparison. *Journal of Neurosurgery: Pediatrics, 15*(5), 529–534. https://doi.org/10.3171/2014.10.PEDS14128
87. Nabaweesi, R., Ramakrishnaiah, R., Aitken, M., Rettiganti, M., Luo, C., Maxson, R., . . . Robbins, J. (2018). Injured children receive twice the radiation dose at non-pediatric trauma centers compared with pediatric trauma centers. *Journal of the American College of Radiology, 15*(1), 58–64. https://doi.org/10.1016/j.jacr.2017.06.035
88. Walther, A., Falcone, R., Pritts, T., Hanseman, D., & Robinson, B. (2016) Pediatric and adult trauma centers differ in evaluation, treatment, and outcomes for severely injured adolescents. *Journal of Pediatric Surgery, 51*(8), 1346–1350. https://doi.org/10.1016/j.jpedsurg.2016.03.016
89. Bryan, M., Rowhani-Rahbar, A., Comstock, R., & Rivara, F. (2016). Sports- and recreation-related concussions in US youth. *Pediatrics, 138*(1). https://doi.org/10.1542/peds.2015-4635
90. Yue, J., Winkler, E., Burke, J., Chan, A., Dhall, S., Berger, M., . . . Tarapore P. (2016). Pediatric sports-related traumatic brain injury in United States trauma centers. *Neurosurgical Focus, 40*(4), E3. https://doi.org/10.3171/2016.1.FOCUS15612
91. Silverio, A., Briggs, S., Hasanaj, L., Hurd, J., Jahn, M., Serrano, L., . . . Balcer, L. (2017). Parents take-on concussion: Advances in sideline research and culture in youth sports. *Journal of Sports Medicine and Therapy, 2,* 9–19. https://doi.org/10.29328/journal.jsmt.1001003

APPENDIX 12-1

Childhood Development

Physical and Motor Development	Intellectual or Psychosocial Development	Language Development	Pain	Death
Infant Development (Ages 1 Month–1 Year)				
Growth: Period of most rapid growth; infant weight gain, approximately 28.3 g/day; weight doubles by the age of 6 months and triples by the age of 1 year	Trust versus mistrust (Erikson): When physical needs are consistently met, infants learn to trust self and environment; common fears (after the age of 6 months) include separation and strangers	Sensorimotor period: Infants learn by the use of their senses and activities	Infants do experience pain; the degree of pain perceived is unknown	Infants do not understand the meaning of death; the developing sense of separation serves as a basis for a beginning understanding of the meaning of death
Toddler Development (Ages 1–2 Years)				
Growth: Rate significantly slows down, accompanied by a tremendous decrease in appetite; general appearance is potbellied, exaggerated lumbar curve, wide-based gait, increased mobility, and a hallmark of physical development in the toddler	Autonomy versus shame and doubt (Erikson): Increasing independence and self-care activities; expanding the world with which the toddler interacts; need to experience the joy of exploring and exerting some control over body functions and activity while maintaining support of an "anchor" (primary caregiver); common fears include separation, loss of control, altered rituals, and pain	Sensorimotor period: Cognition and language not yet sophisticated enough for children to learn through thought processes and communication	No formal concept of pain related to immature thought process and poorly developed body image; react as intensely to painless procedures as to those that hurt, especially when restrained; intrusive procedures, such as taking a temperature, are distressing; react to pain with physical resistance, aggression, negativism, and regression; rare for toddlers to fake pain; verbal responses concerning pain are unreliable	Understanding of death still limited; belief that loss of significant others is temporary; reinforced by developing sense of object permanence (objects continue to exist even if they cannot be seen); repeated experiences of separations and reunions; magical thinking; belief in TV shows (cartoon characters)

Physical and Motor Development	Intellectual or Psychosocial Development	Language Development	Pain	Death
Preschool Development (Ages 3–5 Years)				
Growth: Weight gain of 2 kg/year; height gain of 6–8 cm per year; usually are half of adult height by the age of 2 years; general appearance of "baby fat" and protuberant abdomen disappear	Initiative versus guilt (Erikson): Greater autonomy and independence; still intense need for caregivers when under stress; initiate activities, rather than just imitating others; age of discovery, curiosity, and development of social behavior; sense of self as individual; common fears include mutilation, loss of control, death, dark, and ghosts	Preoperational (Piaget): Time of trial-and-error learning; egocentric (experiences from own perspective); understand explanations only in terms of real events or what their senses tell them; no logical or abstract thought; coincidence confused with causation; magical thinking continues; difficulty distinguishing between reality and fantasy; may see illness or injury as punishment for "bad" thoughts or behavior; imaginary friends; fascination with superheroes and monsters	Pain perceived as punishment for bad thoughts or behavior; difficulty understanding that painful procedures help them get well; cannot differentiate between "good" pain (resulting from treatment) and "bad" pain (resulting from injury or illness); react to painful procedures with aggression and verbal reprimands ("I hate you" and "You're mean")	Incomplete understanding of death fosters anxiety because of fear of death; death is seen as an altered state of consciousness in which a person cannot perform normal activities, such as eating or walking; perceive immobility, sleep, and other alterations in consciousness as deathlike states; associate words and phrases ("put to sleep") with death; death is seen as reversible (reinforced by TV and cartoons); unable to perceive inevitability of death as the result of their limited time concept; view death as punishment
School-Age Children (Ages 6–10 Years)				
Growth: Relatively latent period	Industry versus inferiority (Erikson): Age of accomplishment, increasing competence, and mastery of new skills; successes contribute to positive self-esteem and a sense of control; need parental support in times of stress (may be unwilling or unable to ask); common fears include separation from friends, loss of control, and physical disability	Concrete operations (Piaget): Beginning of logical thought; deductive reasoning develops; improved concept of time; awareness of possible long-term consequences of illness; more sophisticated understanding of causality; still interpret phrases and idioms at face value	Reaction to pain affected by past experiences, parental response, and the meaning attached to it; better able to localize and describe pain accurately; pain can be exaggerated because of heightened fears of bodily injury, pain, and death	Concept of death more logically based; understand death as the irreversible cessation of life; view death as a tragedy that happens to others, not themselves; when death is an actual threat, may feel responsible for death and experience guilt

Physical and Motor Development	Intellectual or Psychosocial Development	Language Development	Pain	Death
Adolescent Development (Ages 11–18 Years)				
Growth: For females, growth spurt begins at the age of 9.5 years; for males, growth spurt begins at the age of 10.5 years; at puberty, secondary sex characteristics begin to develop between the ages of 8 and 13 years for females and between the ages of 10 and 14 years for males	Identity versus role confusion (Erikson): Transition from childhood to adulthood; quest for independence often leads to family dissension; major concerns: establishing identity and developing mature sexual orientation; risk-taking behaviors include feeling that nothing bad can happen to them; common fears include changes in appearance or functioning, dependency, and loss of control	Concrete to formal operations (Piaget): Memory fully developed; concept of time well understood; adolescents can project to the future and imagine potential consequences of actions and illnesses; some adolescents do not achieve formal operations	Can locate and quantify pain accurately and thoroughly; often hyperresponsive to pain; react to fear of changes in appearance or function; in general, highly controlled in responding to pain and painful procedures	Understanding of death similar to that of adults; intellectually believe that death can happen to them but avoid realistic thoughts of death; many adolescents defy the possibility of death through reckless behavior, substance abuse, or daring sports activities

Reproduced from Conway, A. (2012). From the start. In *Emergency nursing pediatric course provider manual* (4th ed., pp. 25–49). Des Plaines, IL: Emergency Nurses Association.

APPENDIX 12-2

Guidelines for Care of Children in the Emergency Department

Guidelines for Care of Children in the Emergency Department

This checklist is based on the American Academy of Pediatrics (AAP), American College of Emergency Physicians (ACEP), and Emergency Nurses Association (ENA) 2009 joint policy statement "Guidelines for Care of Children in the Emergency Department," which can be found online at http://aappolicy.aappublications.org/cgi/reprint/pediatrics;124/4/1233.pdf. Use the checklist to determine if your emergency department (ED) is prepared to care for children.

Administration and Coordination of the ED for the Care of Children

- ❍ *Physician Coordinator for Pediatric Emergency Care.* The pediatric physician coordinator is a specialist in emergency medicine or pediatric emergency medicine; or if these specialties are not available then pediatrics or family medicine, appointed by the ED medical director, who through training, clinical experience, or focused continuing medical education demonstrates competence in the care of children in emergency settings, including resuscitation.
- ❍ *Nursing Coordinator for Pediatric Emergency Care.* The pediatric nurse coordinator is a registered nurse (RN), appointed by the ED nursing director, who possesses special interest, knowledge, and skill in the emergency care of children.

Physicians, Nurses and Other Healthcare Providers Who Staff the ED

- ❍ Physicians who staff the ED have the necessary skill, knowledge, and training in the emergency evaluation and treatment of children of all ages who may be brought to the ED, consistent with the services provided by the hospital.
- ❍ Nurses and other ED health care providers have the necessary skill, knowledge, and training in providing emergency care to children of all ages who may be brought to the ED, consistent with the services offered by the hospital.
- ❍ Baseline and periodic competency evaluations completed for all ED clinical staff, including physicians, are age specific and include evaluation of skills related to neonates, infants, children, adolescents, and children with special health care needs. (Competencies are determined by each institution's medical and nursing staff privileges policy.)

Guidelines for QI/PI in the ED

- ❍ The QI/PI plan shall include pediatric specific indicators.
- ❍ The pediatric patient care-review process is integrated into the ED QI/PI plan. Components of the process interface with out-of-hospital, ED, trauma, inpatient pediatric, pediatric critical care, and hospital-wide QI or PI activities.

Guidelines for Improving Pediatric Patient Safety

The delivery of pediatric care should reflect an awareness of unique pediatric patient safety concerns and are included in the following policies or practices:

- ❍ Children are weighed in kilograms.
- ❍ Weights are recorded in a prominent place on the medical record.
- ❍ For children who are not weighed, a standard method for estimating weight in kilograms is used (e.g., a length-based system).
- ❍ Infants and children have a full set of vital signs recorded (temperature, heart rate, respiratory rate) in medical record.
- ❍ Blood pressure and pulse oximetry monitoring are available for children of all ages on the basis of illness and injury severity.
- ❍ A process for identifying age-specific abnormal vital signs and notifying the physician of these is present.
- ❍ Processes in place for safe medication storage, prescribing, and delivery that includes precalculated dosing guidelines for children of all ages.
- ❍ Infection-control practices, including hand hygiene and use of personal protective equipment, are implemented and monitored.
- ❍ Pediatric emergency services are culturally and linguistically appropriate.
- ❍ ED environment is safe for children and supports patient- and family-centered care.
- ❍ Patient identification policies meet Joint Commission standards.
- ❍ Policies for the timely reporting and evaluation of patient safety events, medical errors, and unanticipated outcomes are implemented and monitored.

Guidelines for ED Policies, Procedures, and Protocols

Policies, procedures, and protocols for the emergency care of children should be developed and implemented in the areas listed below. These policies may be integrated into overall ED policies as long as pediatric specific issues are addressed.

- ❍ Illness and injury triage.
- ❍ Pediatric patient assessment and reassessment.

Produced by the AAP, ACEP, ENA, the EMSC National Resource Center, and Children's National Medical Center

Guidelines for ED Policies, Procedures, and Protocols, Cont.

- Documentation of pediatric vital signs and actions to be taken for abnormal vital signs.
- Immunization assessment and management of the under-immunized patient.
- Sedation and analgesia, including medical imaging.
- Consent, including when parent or legal guardian is not immediately available.
- Social and mental health issues.
- Physical or chemical restraint of patients.
- Child maltreatment and domestic violence reporting criteria, requirements, and processes.
- Death of the child in the ED.
- Do not resuscitate (DNR) orders.
- Family-centered care:
  - Family involvement in patient decision-making and medication safety processes;
  - Family presence during all aspects of emergency care;
  - Patient, family, and caregiver education;
  - Discharge planning and instruction; and
  - Bereavement counseling.
- Communication with the patient's medical home or primary care provider.
- Medical imaging, specfically policies that address pediatric age- or weight-based appropriate dosing for studies that impart radiation consistent with ALARA (as low as reasonably achievable) principles.

Polices, Procedures, and Protocols for All-Hazard Disaster Preparedness

Policies, procedures, and protocols should also be developed and implemented for all-hazard disaster-preparedness. The plan should address the following preparedness issues:

- Availability of medications, vaccines, equipment, and trained providers for children.
- Pediatric surge capacity for injured and non-injured children.
- Decontamination, isolation, and quarantine of families and children.
- Minimization of parent-child separation (includes pediatric patient tracking and timely reunification of separated children with their family).
- Access to specific medical and mental health therapies, and social services for children.
- Disaster drills which include a pediatric mass casualty incident at least every two years.
- Care of children with special health care needs.
- Evacuation of pediatric units and pediatric subspecialty units.

Policies, Procedures, and Protocols for Patient Transfers

- Written pediatric inter-facility transfer procedures should be established.

Guidelines for ED Support Services

Radiology capability must meet the needs of the children in the community served. Specifically:

- A process for referring children to appropriate facilities for radiological procedures that exceed the capability of the hospital is established.
- A process for timely review, interpretation, and reporting of medical imaging by a qualified radiologist is established.

Laboratory capability must meet the needs of the children in the community served, including techniques for small sample sizes. Specifically:

- A process for referring children or their specimens to appropriate facilities for laboratory studies that exceed the capability of the hospital is established.

Guidelines for Equipment, Supplies, and Medications for the Care of Pediatric Patients in the ED

- Pediatric equipment, supplies, and medications are appropriate for children of all ages and sizes (see list below), and are easily accessible, clearly labeled, and logically organized.
- ED staff is educated on the location of all items.
- Daily method in place to verify the proper location and function of equipment and supplies.
- Medication chart, length-based tape, medical software, or other systems is readily available to ensure proper sizing of resuscitation equipment and proper dosing of medications.

Medications

- atropine
- adenosine
- amiodarone
- antiemetic agents
- calcium chloride
- dextrose (D10W, D50W)
- epinephrine (1:1000; 1:10 000 solutions)
- lidocaine
- magnesium sulfate
- naloxone hydrochloride
- procainamide
- sodium bicarbonate (4.2%, 8.4%)
- topical, oral, and parenteral analgesics
- antimicrobial agents (parenteral and oral)
- anticonvulsant medications
- antidotes (common antidotes should be accessible to the ED)
- antipyretic drugs
- bronchodilators
- corticosteroids
- inotropic agents
- neuromuscular blockers
- sedatives
- vaccines
- vasopressor agents

Produced by the AAP, ACEP, ENA, the EMSC National Resource Center, and Children's National Medical Center

Equipment/Supplies: General Equipment

- ❍ patient warming device
- ❍ intravenous blood/fluid warmer
- ❍ restraint device
- ❍ weight scale in kilograms (not pounds)
- ❍ tool or chart that incorporates weight (in kilograms) and length to determine equipment size and correct drug dosing
- ❍ age appropriate pain scale-assessment tools

Equipment/Supplies: Monitoring Equipment

blood pressure cuffs
- ❍ neonatal
- ❍ infant
- ❍ child
- ❍ adult-arm
- ❍ adult-thigh

- ❍ doppler ultrasonography devices
- ❍ electrocardiography monitor/defibrillator with pediatric and adult capabilities including pads/paddles
- ❍ hypothermia thermometer
- ❍ pulse oximeter with pediatric and adult probes
- ❍ continuous end-tidal CO2 monitoring device

Equipment/Supplies: Vascular Access

arm boards
- ❍ infant
- ❍ child
- ❍ adult

catheter-over-the-needle device
- ❍ 14 gauge
- ❍ 16 gauge
- ❍ 18 gauge
- ❍ 20 gauge
- ❍ 22 gauge
- ❍ 24 gauge

intraosseous needles or device
- ❍ pediatric
- ❍ adult

- ❍ IV administration sets with calibrated chambers and extension tubing and/or infusion devices with ability to regulate rate and volume of infusate

umbilical vein catheters
- ❍ 3.5F
- ❍ 5.0F

central venous catheters (any two sizes)
- ❍ 4.0F
- ❍ 5.0F
- ❍ 6.0F
- ❍ 7.0F

intravenous solutions
- ❍ normal saline
- ❍ dextrose 5% in normal saline
- ❍ dextrose 10% in water

Equipment/Supplies: Fracture-Management Devices

extremity splints
- ❍ femur splints, pediatric sizes
- ❍ femur splints, adult sizes

- ❍ spine-stabilization devices appropriate for children of all ages

Equipment/Supplies: Respiratory

endotracheal tubes
- ❍ uncuffed 2.5 mm
- ❍ uncuffed 3.0 mm
- ❍ cuffed or uncuffed 3.5 mm
- ❍ cuffed or uncuffed 4.0 mm
- ❍ cuffed or uncuffed 4.5 mm
- ❍ cuffed or uncuffed 5.0 mm
- ❍ cuffed or uncuffed 5.5 mm
- ❍ cuffed 6.0 mm
- ❍ cuffed 6.5 mm
- ❍ cuffed 7.0 mm
- ❍ cuffed 7.5 mm
- ❍ cuffed 8.0 mm

feeding tubes
- ❍ 5F
- ❍ 8F

laryngoscope blades
- ❍ straight: 0
- ❍ straight: 1
- ❍ straight: 2
- ❍ straight: 3
- ❍ curved: 2
- ❍ curved: 3

- ❍ laryngoscope handle

magill forceps
- ❍ pediatric
- ❍ adult

nasopharyngeal airways
- ❍ infant
- ❍ child
- ❍ adult

oropharyngeal airways
- ❍ size 0
- ❍ size 1
- ❍ size 2
- ❍ size 3
- ❍ size 4
- ❍ size 5

stylets for endotracheal tubes
- ❍ pediatric
- ❍ adult

suction catheters
- ❍ infant
- ❍ child
- ❍ adult

tracheostomy tubes
- ❍ 2.5 mm
- ❍ 3.0 mm
- ❍ 3.5 mm
- ❍ 4.0 mm
- ❍ 4.5 mm
- ❍ 5.0 mm
- ❍ 5.5 mm

- ❍ yankauer suction tip

bag-mask device, self inflating
- ❍ infant: 450 ml
- ❍ adult: 1000 ml

masks to fit bag-mask device adaptor
- ❍ neonatal
- ❍ infant
- ❍ child
- ❍ adult

Produced by the AAP, ACEP, ENA, the EMSC National Resource Center, and Children's National Medical Center

Equipment/Supplies: Respiratory, Continued	Equipment/Supplies: Specialized Pediatric Trays or Kits
clear oxygen masks ❍ standard infant ❍ standard child ❍ standard adult ❍ partial nonrebreather infant ❍ nonrebreather child ❍ nonrebreather adult nasal cannulas ❍ infant ❍ child ❍ adult nasogastric tubes ❍ infant: 8F ❍ child: 10F ❍ adult: 14-18F laryngeal mask airway ❍ size: 1 ❍ size: 1.5 ❍ size: 2 ❍ size: 2.5 ❍ size: 3 ❍ size: 4 ❍ size: 5	❍ lumbar puncture tray (including infant/pediatric 22 gauge and adult 18-21 gauge needles) ❍ supplies/kit for patients with difficult airway (supraglottic airways of all sizes, laryngeal mask airway, needle cricothyrotomy supplies, surgical cricothyrotomy kit) ❍ tube thoracostomy tray chest tubes: ❍ infant: 10-12F ❍ child: 16-24 F ❍ adult: 28-40 F ❍ newborn delivery kit, including equipment for resuscitation of an infant (umbilical clamp, scissors, bulb syringe, and towel) ❍ urinary catheterization kits and urinary (indwelling) catheters (6F–22F)

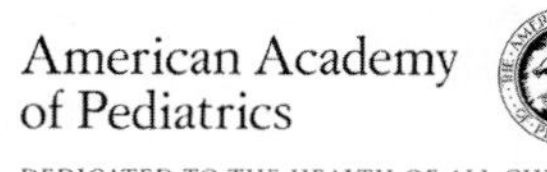

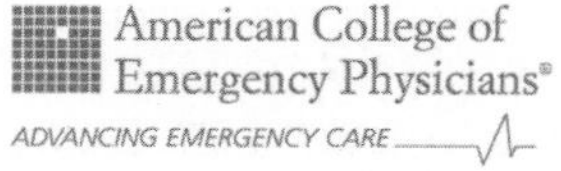

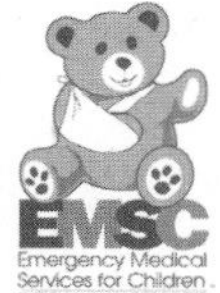

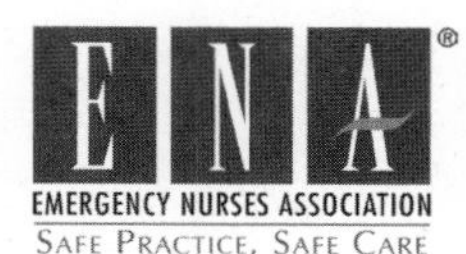

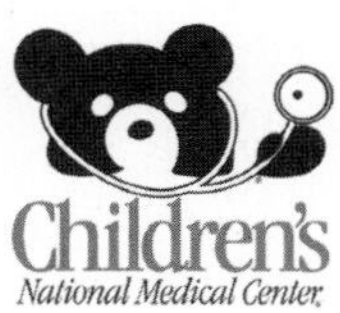

Courtesy of AACP, ACEP, ENA, EMSC National Resource Center, Children's National Medical Center (2009). Guidelines for Care of Children in the Emergency Department. Retrieved from https://www.aap.org/en-us/Documents/Checklist-Guidelines_for_Care_of_Children.pdf.

CHAPTER 13

Special Populations: The Geriatric Trauma Patient

Nancy J. Denke, DNP, RN, ACNP-BC, FNP-BC, CEN, CCRN, FAEN

OBJECTIVES

Upon completion of this chapter, the learner will be able to:

1. Describe mechanisms of injury associated with the older adult trauma patient.
2. Describe age-related anatomic and physiologic changes as a basis for assessment of the older adult trauma patient.
3. Demonstrate the nursing assessment of the older adult trauma patient.
4. Plan appropriate interventions for the older adult trauma patient.
5. Evaluate the effectiveness of nursing interventions for the older adult trauma patient.

Introduction

As the age of the population increases annually, so does the need for an increased knowledge of the unique vulnerabilities seen in the geriatric population, especially as they relate to trauma. Caring for this special population requires nurses to recognize the progressive decline seen at the cellular level with aging. This decline minimizes the reserves and resources that this population has to respond to injury. Appropriate triage and early aggressive management of all trauma (minor and major) can improve outcomes and minimize morbidity and mortality. This chapter focuses on the age-specific considerations of the geriatric patient, considered to be an individual older than the age of 65 years; common mechanisms of injury found in the geriatric population; and the challenges of minimizing morbidity and mortality while mobilizing strategies to improve outcomes.

Epidemiology

The population older than the age of 65 increases annually and is projected to more than double from 46 million today to more than 98 million by 2060. In the United States, 24% of the population will fall into this category.[1] Trauma in older adults due to unintentional injuries accounted for 85% of all injury deaths among adults age 65 and older in the United States between 2012 and 2013, with 55% of these deaths due to falls (**Figure 13-1**).[2] Data for 2015 show that trauma was among the top 10

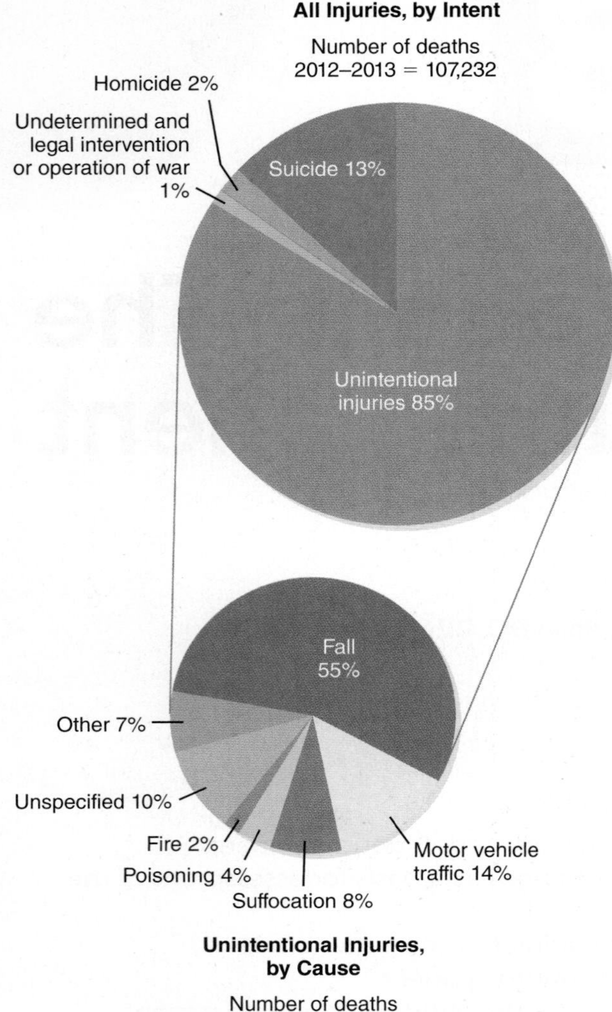

Figure 13-1 *Percent distribution of injury deaths, by intent and cause among adults age 65 and older, United States, 2012–2013.*

Reproduced from Kramarow E., Chen L., Hedegaard H., & Warner, M. (2015). *Deaths from unintentional injury among adults aged 65 and over: United States, 2000–2013. NCHS Data Brief, 199.* Hyattsville, MD: National Center for Health Statistics. Retrieved from https://www.cdc.gov/nchs/data/databriefs/db199.pdf.

causes of death in the geriatric population.[3] Physiological changes and comorbidities may increase the severity of injuries, incidence of complications, and mortality rate in this population. Underestimation of injury severity by healthcare personnel has also been found to increase morbidity and mortality in this age group.[4]

Due in part to an emphasis on preventive medicine and improved healthcare, today's older adults not only live longer than earlier generations, but also live independently and remain more active. Despite their advancing age, a number of older adults still participate in sports and continue to drive their own automobiles. Sometimes we overlook the positive role that exercise plays in helping to keep older drivers safe behind the wheel as they progress through the normal aging process. Exercise can improve flexibility, coordination, strength, balance, and range of motion in these individuals.[5]

The approach and priorities remain the same when caring for the older adult trauma patient; however, special consideration is given to factors that might complicate both the resuscitation and the recovery of these individuals. Since an injury in an older adult, regardless of its severity, may result in a poor outcome, it becomes important to implement the 2012 Eastern Association for the Surgery of Trauma (EAST) Guidelines, which emphasize "a lower threshold for trauma activation should be used for injured patients with advanced age (aged ≥ 65 years) who are evaluated at trauma centers."[6(pS346)] The following factors should be considered and addressed[4]:

- Normal pathophysiologic changes as a result of aging
- Comorbidities
- Medications
- Lower physiologic reserve

In addition to these factors, it is important to understand common mechanisms of injury in this population.

Mechanisms of Injury in the Older Adult

Falls and injuries due to motor vehicle collisions (MVCs) and traffic, including pedestrian-related collisions, are the most common causes of trauma and injury death in adults 65 years and older (Figure 13-1 and **Table 13-1**).[2,7,8]

Falls

In the older adult population, falls are the leading cause of injury-related death and the leading cause of hospital admissions for trauma in the United States and globally.[9] Falls in this patient population are primarily low-energy trauma (LET) events and occur from a standing height or lower, often as a result of conditions such as wet surfaces, poor lighting, inadequate footwear, and cluttered pathways, along with weakness, gait and balance impairments, and use of psychoactive medications.[10] An older adult is often under-triaged after experiencing a LET fall from a standing height. Most falls occur at home (60%), with an additional 30% occurring in the community and 10% in nursing homes or other institutions,[11] often while the older adult patient is engaged in everyday activities such as walking on stairs, going to the bathroom, or working in the kitchen.

TABLE 13-1 Incidents by Mechanism of Injury

Mechanism	Number	Percent	Deaths	Case Fatality Rate
Fall	380,800	44.18	16,623	4.37
Motor vehicle traffic	223,866	25.97	10,343	4.62
Struck by, against	55,662	6.46	755	1.36
Transport, other	39,269	4.56	903	2.30
Cut/pierce	35,565	4.13	776	2.18
Firearm	36,325	4.21	5,557	15.30
Pedal cyclist, other	14,730	1.71	207	1.41
Other specified and classifiable	13,682	1.59	522	3.82
Hot object/substance	8,401	0.97	36	0.43
Fire/flame	7,877	0.91	467	5.93
Unspecified	7,834	0.91	433	5.53
Machinery	8,101	0.94	99	1.22
Natural/environmental, bites and stings	5,868	0.68	62	1.06
Other specified, not elsewhere classifiable	4,059	0.47	74	1.82
Overexertion	2,613	0.30	12	0.46
Pedestrian, other	2,845	0.33	177	6.22
Natural/environmental, other	2,387	0.28	38	1.59
Suffocation	885	0.10	240	27.12
Poisoning	413	0.05	8	1.94
Drowning/submersion	375	0.04	72	19.20
Adverse effects, medical care	224	0.03	11	4.91
Adverse effects, drugs	102	0.01	7	6.86
Not known/not recorded	10,005	1.16	403	4.03
Total	**861,888**	**100**	**37,825**	**4.39**

Reproduced from Committee on Trauma, American College of Surgeons. (2016). *The National Trauma Data Bank 2016 annual report*. Chicago, IL: Author. Retrieved from https://www.facs.org/~/media/files/quality%20programs/trauma/ntdb/ntdb%20annual%20report%202016.ashx. The content reproduced from the NTDB remains the full and exclusive copyrighted property of the American College of Surgeons. The American College of Surgeons is not responsible for any claims arising from works based on the original data, text, tables, or figures.

Falls can also occur as a result of the following factors[10]:

- Syncope due to dysrhythmias, venous pooling, orthostatic hypotension, hypoxia, anemia, or hypoglycemia
- Alcohol and medications (antihypertensives, antidepressants, diuretics, and hypoglycemia agents)
- Changes in postural stability, balance, motor strength, and coordination
- Slower reaction times
- Poor visual acuity and visual attention

Mortality from falls among older men and women has increased sharply over the past decade, and can result in death, serious injury, and loss of independence. Falls account for 25% of all hospital admissions and 40% of all nursing home admissions.[10,11] Of those admitted, 40% do not return to independent living and 25% die within a year.[10,11] In a study done in 2016, females older than 65 years of age had the highest rate of fall-related injuries.[12]

Mortality and disability can be affected by the under-triage of older patients. Falls, or LET, and high-energy trauma, such as MVCs, are categorized and often triaged differently, but the mortality and morbidity rates are similar for both types. Patients with LET should be triaged at a higher level of urgency until they are assessed and all the predisposing factors (medications, medical history) are considered.[6]

The most common injuries resulting from falls in the older adult include the following[7,13]:

- Lacerations and contusions
- Traumatic brain injury
- Fractures, especially of the hip

After a fall, many older adults cannot get up without assistance, which can result in further complications. When a person falls and lies motionless for many hours, the weight of the body results in compression of muscle tissue, placing the patient at risk for rhabdomyolysis (see Chapter 10, "Musculoskeletal Trauma," for more information). Rhabdomyolysis can lead to many serious complications, including the following[14]:

- Acute kidney injury
- Hyperkalemia and other electrolyte imbalances
- Fluid shifting, hypovolemic shock
- Fat embolism and acute respiratory distress syndrome
- Coagulopathies (disseminated intravascular coagulopathy and fibrinolysis)
- Sepsis and multiple organ dysfunction syndrome

Motor Vehicle Collisions

Driving patterns change as people age. Older adults tend to self-regulate their driving behaviors by driving fewer miles, limiting their driving during bad weather and at night, and preferring local roads to expressways and highways. Remaining independent and mobile allows older adults to remain social, thus maintaining their cognitive and mental health. With that in mind, EAST has made recommendations that include encouraging automobile manufacturers to improve safety, civil engineers to improve the visibility of crosswalks, and the consideration of medical screening to obtain continued licensure.[15] The Centers for Disease Control and Prevention (CDC) lists MVCs as the second most common mechanism of trauma in the older adult.[2]

Although the older adult may have more driving experience, normal age-related physiologic changes can affect the ability to drive. These include changes in vision, hearing, perception, muscle flexibility, and reflexes.[5]

MVCs involving older adult drivers are less likely to be related to speed. Instead, the physiologic changes just noted affect the older adult's ability to drive safely in the following situations[5,15]:

- At intersections (due to limited peripheral vision).
- Merging into traffic when another vehicle is traveling faster (due to reduced reaction time).
- When another car is in the older driver's blind spot (due to limited peripheral vision and kyphosis).
- When it is dark (due to loss of visual acuity).
- A single drink can affect the driving ability of older drivers; they may become "intoxicated" below the federal legal blood alcohol concentration level of 0.08%.[16]

Geriatric patients have injury patterns that differ markedly from those seen in younger adults and are susceptible to serious injury from minor trauma. The most commonly injured body regions in the older adults involved in MVCs are the head, chest, and cervical spine.[17] **Table 13-2** describes physiologic changes in older adults that may increase their risk of injury. Additional considerations include the following[18-21]:

- Rib fractures are common due to bone demineralization, with geriatric patients having double the morbidity and mortality of younger adults.
- Complications from these injuries may lead to acute respiratory problems due to hypoventilation such as respiratory failure/hypoxia, pneumonia, and pleural effusion. There is a relationship between the number of ribs fractured and mortality.
- Lower cervical injuries are common due to degenerative changes and relative immobility of the lower cervical spine. There is also an increased incidence of injuries at the craniocervical junction, particularly at C2 and the odontoid.
- Minor head injury can result in a significant intracranial injury, with older adults having three times the incidence of long-term functional disability as younger adults.
- Older patients presenting with lateral pelvic fractures are more likely to hemorrhage.

TABLE 13-2 Anatomic and Physiologic Changes in the Older Adult

System	Changes with Aging
Airway	› Atrophy of oral mucosa may lead to loose or poorly fitting dentures (full or partial) that may obstruct the airway › Relaxed musculature of the oropharynx may result in aspiration › Decreased gag and cough reflexes predispose the older adult to aspiration, infection, and bronchospasm › Temporomandibular and cervical arthritis make intubation more difficult
Cervical spine	Older adults are predisposed to cervical injury and/or discomfort from the rigid spine board due to the following: › Osteoporosis › Changes in bone density › Ankylosing spondylitis › Osteopenia › Development of spinal stenosis › Frequent injury of the odontoid process › Increasing rigidity of the C4 to C6 levels; lever action causes fractures above and below these points › Rigidity from neurologic disorders (Parkinson disease) or from spinal surgery › Kyphosis, which limits cervical range of motion, inhibiting the ability to see oncoming traffic or crossing signals
Breathing	› Older adults experience a loss of strength in the muscles of respiration and diminished endurance, leading to easier fatigue › Costal cartilage calcification decreases inspiratory and expiratory force, and chest expansion/elasticity; increases the respiratory rate; and reduces tidal volume › Respiratory fatigue occurs more easily, resulting in hypoxia › Older adults have a decreased ability to compensate for hypoxia › Older adults have a higher rate of complications, even following minor thoracic injuries, including pulmonary edema, atelectasis, and pneumonia › Decreased cough strength due to anatomic changes of the thorax (anterior curvature or kyphosis; decrease in thoracic cavity size; rib space narrowing, which decreases the length of the intercostal muscles) › Small airways lose recoil, resulting in potential airway collapse, air trapping, and uneven distribution of ventilation › Pain, injury, and extended supine positioning can reduce arterial oxygen saturation and cardiac output
Circulation	› There is a limited ability to increase heart rate and cardiac output in response to physiologic stress › Variations in adrenergic responses due to changes to the parasympathetic and sympathetic systems: • Heart rate > 90 beats/min may indicate significant physiologic stress • Orthostatic hypotension may result from loss of sensitivity of baroreceptors

(continues)

TABLE 13-2 Anatomic and Physiologic Changes in the Older Adult *(continued)*

System	Changes with Aging
	› Hypoperfusion is poorly tolerated due to declining cardiac reserve › Left ventricular thickening and decrease in pacemaker cells in the sinoatrial and atrioventricular nodes decrease filling capacity and delays filling time › Muscle mass reduction and atrial stiffening result in decreased contractility › Reduction in total body water increases risk for dehydration › Anemia is caused by nutritional deficiencies, chronic inflammatory disease, and chronic renal disease
Neurologic	› Brain tissue atrophy results in the following conditions: · Stretching of the parasagittal bridging veins, predisposing them to tearing with injury · Additional space in the cranial vault, resulting in substantial bleeding before the onset of symptoms · Higher incidence of chronic subdural hematomas › Other potential factors include the following: · Anticoagulant therapy (warfarin, novel oral anticoagulants [NOAC] and direct oral anticoagulants [DOAC]) · Antiplatelet therapy (aspirin or adenosine diphosphate receptor [ADP]/P2Y inhibitors. [i.e., clopidogrel, ticagrelor]) · Alcohol abuse, which adds to brain atrophy and causes liver damage that can increase bleeding tendencies · Antipsychotic and dopamine antagonist drugs and medications for glaucoma, which may affect neurologic examination › Nerve cells transmit signals more slowly, reducing reflexes and sensation, leading to problems with movement, safety, and pain perception and control › Accumulation of the protein beta-amyloid, which may signal developing cognitive impairment over time › Increased risk of sleep disorders, delirium, and pain perception
Skin and tissue	› Diminished autonomic response and thinner skin limit thermoregulation (impaired heat conservation, production, and dissipation) › Increased risk of skin breakdown results from: · Skin aging from lifestyle, diet, heredity, sun exposure, and other habits (smoking) · Breakdown of elastin · Obesity · Loss and loosening of subcutaneous fat, thinning of the skin · Decrease in vascular supply to the skin · Decreased ability to sweat › Immobility

System	Changes with Aging
Renal	› Some renal changes may be due to cardiovascular changes › A decreased number of nephrons, loss of renal mass, and loss of functional glomeruli limit the ability to concentrate urine › Decrease in the glomeruli filtration rate impairs electrolytes and water balance › Diminished sense of thirst, leading to dehydration
Musculoskeletal	Fat and fibrous tissue replaces lean body mass, so only 15% of the total body mass is muscle by age 75, producing the following effects: › Diminished force of contractile muscle › Increased weakness and fatigue › Poor exercise tolerance › Slower, limited movement › Slower and shorter gait, unsteadiness
Endocrine	› Thyroid function (T_3 and T_4) decreases, slowing metabolism › Parathyroid levels rise, increasing the risk of osteoporosis › Metabolic syndrome (decreased sensitivity to insulin) increases, blunting the effects of insulin › Aldosterone production drops, predisposing older adults to orthostatic hypotension and dehydration

Data from Jubert, P., Lonjon, G., Garreau de Loubresse, C., & Bone and Joint Trauma Study Group. (2013). Complications of upper cervical spine trauma in elderly subjects. A systematic review of the literature. *Orthopaedics & Traumatology: Surgery & Research, 99*, S301–S312. https://doi.org/10.1016/j.otsr.2013.07.007; Lee, S. Y., Shih, S. C., Leu, Y. S., Chang, Y. H., Lin, H. C., & Ku, H. C. (2017). Implications of age-related changes in anatomy for geriatric-focused difficult airways. *International Journal of Gerontology, 11*, 130–133. https://doi.org/10.1016/j.ijge.2016.11.003; Sadro, C. T., Sandstrom, C. K., Verma, N., & Gunn, M. L. (2015). Geriatric trauma: A radiologist's guide to imaging trauma patients aged 65 years and older. *RadioGraphics, 35*(4), 1263–1285. https://doi.org/10.1148/rg.2015140130; Smith, C. M., & Cotter, V. T. (2016). Age-related changes in health. In M. Boltz, E. Capezuti, T. Fulmer, & D. Zwicker (Eds.), *Evidence-based geriatric nursing protocols for best practice* (5th ed., pp. 23–42). New York, NY: Springer.

Older adults can experience the same injury patterns as their younger counterparts, but require a lengthier recovery time, which may result in increased deaths among the geriatric population.[18]

Pedestrian-Related Collisions

Most pedestrians struck by vehicles receive injuries from contact with the vehicle as well as from the subsequent ground contact. While the probability of a vehicle colliding with a pedestrian has decreased in recent years, the probability of a pedestrian fatality has increased, especially in the geriatric population.[22] The CDC notes the that the overall pedestrian death rate could increase with the aging of the U.S. population.[23] Greater severity of injury and poorer outcomes for adults age 50 years and older are also associated with low-velocity pedestrian collisions.[22] Older adults are at high risk for pedestrian-related collisions and have higher rates of morbidity and mortality.[22] Strategies to prevent pedestrian deaths should include consideration of the needs of the older population.[23] See Chapter 2, "Biomechanics, Kinematics, and Mechanisms of Injury," for more information.

The geriatric population has also been found to sustain more tibial, pelvic, chest, spinal, and brain trauma after pedestrian MVCs compared to the pediatric population, with similar hollow viscus and solid organ injuries.[19,23] Age-related (physical and mental) changes also can contribute to these pedestrian-related collisions,[19] including the following factors:

- Kyphosis, which can decrease cervical range of motion, limiting the older adult's ability to see oncoming traffic or crossing signals
- Inability to walk quickly—due to potential decreases in agility, gait, balance, and coordination
- Reduced reaction time. with slowing of processing powers
- Decreased hearing
- Loss of visual acuity and peripheral vision due to vestibular apparatus changes

Age-Related Anatomic and Physiologic Changes

Two categories of factors impact the older patient's response to illness and injury. Nonmodifiable changes occur as a result of the natural aging process (Table 13-2), while other changes are due to modifiable factors, such as lifestyle.

Nonmodifiable factors that occur through aging can affect how the older adult responds to stress, illness, temperature, medications, trauma, and blood loss. Each patient is unique in their response to aging, illness, and injury.

Modifiable factors that influence the older adult's ability to respond to illness and injury include the following:

- Lifestyle
  - Use/misuse of alcohol or tobacco
  - Use of illicit drugs
  - Misuse of prescription medication and/or polypharmacy
  - Weight (obesity)
- Socioeconomic characteristics
  - Live alone
- Diet
  - Healthy diet
  - Unhealthy diet
  - Failure to eat due to illness or depression, loss of appetite, or financial restrictions
- Physical activity
  - Active
  - Inactive

Nursing Care of the Geriatric Trauma Patient

Refer to Chapter 3, "Initial Assessment," for the systematic approach to the nursing care of the trauma patient. The following assessment parameters are specific to the older adult trauma patient. An important concept to remember is that older adults may display atypical presentations of disease, infection and trauma.

Preparation and Triage

Prehospital and ED triage of the older adult can be challenging. The mechanism of injury and vital signs can be misleading triage tools in older adult trauma patients due to their susceptibility to significant injuries from even relatively minor mechanisms or trauma.[18] This leads to a lower threshold for field triage of older trauma patients directly to a designated/verified trauma center.[6]

Primary Survey and Resuscitation Adjuncts

Primary survey and resuscitation adjuncts begin with the patient's alertness and airway.

A: Alertness and Airway with Cervical Spine Stabilization

Aging changes body structure, so the older adult may be prone to structural and functional changes surrounding the airway. In opening and clearing the airway of the older adult patient, also assess for the following[20]:

- Decreased gag reflex and diminished cough reflex
- Presence of full or partial dentures or the attrition of teeth
- Thin, smooth, and dry oral mucosa with a loss of elasticity
- Musculoskeletal degenerative changes such as osteoarthritis
- Increased body mass index—"double chin"
- Possible neurologic sequelae due to strokes, such as a loss of or decrease in the function of the glossopharyngeal or hypoglossal nerves, resulting in diminished control in swallowing and tongue movement

Interventions

Interventions include the following:

- Since loss of muscle mass, osteoporosis, osteoarthritis, and kyphosis can contribute to discomfort and skin breakdown in the older patient, consider padding bony areas and facilitate removal from the spine board as quickly as possible.
- The routine use of the "neutral position" adopted for cervical spine stabilization may not be appropriate in the older patient. This may inappropriately hyperextend the cervical spine. Using the "chin–brow horizontal" angle may be more appropriate.[24] The chin–brow horizontal angle is the angle of a line running from the brow to the chin when the patient is horizontal on a flat surface.
- Keep in mind that the mucosa is thinner in older adults and that the older patient may be on anticoagulant therapy; use caution when inserting an oral or nasal airway and when suctioning. Either of these procedures can result in swelling, bleeding, or hemorrhage.[20]

B: Breathing and Ventilation

Breathing and ventilation considerations include the following:

- Assess and monitor the work of breathing, as older adults may have a lack of physiologic reserves.

- Consider early ventilatory support, especially with multiple rib fractures.
- Consider leaving dentures in place if they fit well and the patient requires bag-mask ventilation, as intact dentures may help ensure a tighter-fitting mask.

Interventions

Interventions include the following:

- If spontaneous breathing is present, deliver supplemental oxygen delivery using the most appropriate method the patient will tolerate.
- All seriously injured individuals should have oxygen delivered at the highest concentration in a manner that is appropriate for their medical condition and history.
- Consider using a non-rebreather at a flow rate sufficient to keep the reservoir inflated during inspiration, usually 12–15 liters.
- Use care during intubation, since arthritis and osteoporosis have the following effects:
  - Limited visualization of the vocal cords from decreased mobility with the jaw thrust
  - Increased possibility of cervical spine injury during instrumentation[20]

C: Circulation and Control of Hemorrhage

Maintenance of homeostasis in an older adult trauma patient can be difficult. Owing to their limited cardiac reserves, older adults may deteriorate quickly without exhibiting the usual expected changes in vital signs, urinary output, and physiologic responses.[19]

The normal older adult's heart and baroreceptors have a limited response to the body's normal release of catecholamines (adrenaline and norepinephrine), which are needed to increase heart rate and cardiac output.[19] The administration of medications such as beta blockers and cardiac glycosides can further limit this response. Regardless of the history of the older adult patient, a heart rate of greater than 90 beats per minute may indicate significant physiologic stress and increases the risk of mortality.[25]

Interventions

Interventions include the following:

- Consider smaller fluid boluses, with reassessment for signs of fluid overload (increased work of breathing or crackles on auscultation of lung sounds) after every bolus.
- Consider early administration of packed red blood cells to maintain adequate tissue perfusion and oxygenation while correcting any coagulopathy.[26,27]
- If indicated, initiate hemorrhage control measures such as pressure dressings, a tourniquet, and vitamin K for control of internal and external bleeding if the patient takes any anticoagulant medications.[26]
- Trend endpoints of resuscitation as well as lactate and/or base deficit levels.
- Consider the use of thromboelastography, rotational thromboelastometry (TEG, ROTEM) in monitoring coagulation in patients with trauma-induced coagulopathy.[6,26,27]

Cardiac dysfunction may be the cause or the result of trauma in the older adult. Any complaint of chest pain warrants further investigation for either a pathophysiologic or traumatic cause. When assessing the older adult patient, ask questions including the following:

- Did the pain begin before the injury, possibly precipitating the injury?
- Did the pain begin directly after the trauma, possibly indicating tissue damage?
- Was there shortness of breath or any other symptoms prior to the chest pain?

D: Disability (Neurologic Status)

Head trauma can result in both acute and chronic subdural hematoma. Cerebral atrophy causes tension on the parasagittal bridging veins, making them more susceptible to rupture and increasing the risk for subdural hematoma even with minor trauma to the head. There is also an increased incidence of intracerebral hematomas, which may be caused by anticoagulant use.

Severe head injury with hypotension is associated with high mortality (an 18.8% increase in odds of dying).[28] Cerebral atrophy causes increased space within the skull and allows bleeding to accumulate before the patient exhibits signs and symptoms of increased intracranial pressure (ICP). Consider the following factors:

- Maintain a high index of suspicion for bleeding to the brain.
- Consider the need for computed tomography (CT) of the brain early in the resuscitation.
- Continuously monitor the patient for signs of increased ICP.

Altered mental status in the older adult patient may have several possible causes aside from the traumatic injury. Changes in neurologic status require a full investigation to rule out the following conditions:

- Hypoglycemia
- Hypoxia
- Hyperthermia or hypothermia
- Anxiety, disorientation, agitation, and confusion
- Dementia or mental health issue

Interventions

Interventions include the following:

- If a head injury is suspected in the older adult, the trauma management is the same, and early CT is recommended.
- Close monitoring and frequent reorientation are needed for the confused patient.

E: Exposure and Environmental Control

Older adults are at increased risk for hypothermia and resulting complications. As the adult ages, normal body temperature becomes more difficult to regulate (Table 13-2). Factors contributing to the risk of compromised thermoregulation include the following:

- Loss of subcutaneous fat and thinning of the skin
- Decreased ability to sweat
- Neurologic changes
- Chronic cardiac or thyroid conditions
- Poor nutrition
- Psychotropic medications

The risk is increased when the older adult is exposed to temperature extremes at the site of the trauma or in the ED. Such a patient may present with either hypothermia or hyperthermia. When obtaining a history from the patient, family, or EMS providers, identifying the location where the trauma occurred is important. For instance, determine if there was prolonged extraction from a vehicle with exposure to high or low temperatures.

Hyperthermia should be considered, especially following a fall where exposure and environmental temperature is a factor. Signs and symptoms of hyperthermia include the following[29]:

- Headache
- Vertigo
- Syncope
- Dehydration
- Rapid respirations
- Confusion
- Agitation
- Delirium
- Hallucinations
- Convulsions

Interventions

Because maintenance of normothermia is so important in the older adult trauma patient, regulate the ambient temperature in the trauma room as needed, apply warm blankets, and administer warmed intravenous fluid. When using mechanical warming devices, such as forced-air blankets or fluid warmers, monitor the temperature closely to avoid thermal burns to fragile skin.

Resuscitation Adjuncts

Resuscitation adjuncts include vital signs, laboratory studies, monitoring, and pain assessment and management.

F: Full Set of Vital Signs

In addition to comorbidities and medication history, baseline changes in respiration and pulse may be present in the older adult's vital signs.

G: Get Monitoring Devices and Give Comfort

Get the following resuscitation adjuncts.

L: Laboratory Studies

It is important to perform glucose (point-of-care testing), arterial blood gas (base excess), lactate, prothrombin time, partial thromboplastin time, and coagulation studies, along with the use of thromboelastography.[6,26,30] Note that the use of anticoagulants and antiplatelet medications is common among older adults. Use of alcohol and changes in the liver can also affect clotting. An increased international normalized ratio has been associated with increased mortality in the older adult trauma patient.[6,31] Both an elevated lactate level (greater than 2) and an abnormal base deficit (less than –6) have been associated with major injury and mortality in trauma patients.[28,30]

M: Monitoring

An electrocardiogram may be indicated, particularly if there is a history of cardiac disease or if the patient has since developed signs and symptoms of myocardial ischemia surrounding the traumatic event.

N: Nasogastric or Orogastric Tube

Consider the need for placement of a nasogastric or orogastric tube to evacuate stomach contents and relieve gastric distention. If the patient has been intubated, place a gastric tube to decrease gastric distention and increase diaphragmatic excursion. Consider additional interventions listed in Chapter 3.

O: Oxygenation and Ventilation

Pulse oximetry measures oxygenation, not ventilation. Consider weaning oxygen based on oximetry to avoid hyperoxia. Use end-tidal carbon dioxide monitoring for intubated or sedated patients to measure ventilation. Consider additional interventions listed in Chapter 3.

P: Pain Assessment and Management

The older adult trauma patient who is anxious, is confused, or has dementia may not be able to accurately report pain, so it is important for trauma nurses to assess behavioral cues, subtle signs of discomfort, and common pain responses to injuries. Older adults are frequently undermedicated due to the failure to appropriately assess them for pain and the fear of overmedicating them.[31]

When using opioids for pain relief, consider the following:

- Obtain an accurate body weight prior to starting opioid administration and calculate doses accordingly
- Use of smaller doses is indicated. Remember to "start low, go slow."
- Monitor the patient closely for decreased respirations and blood pressure.
- Monitor any alteration in level of consciousness and any reports of dizziness.

Since some age-related compromise to the respiratory system is likely to exist in older adults, failure to aggressively manage pain from rib contusions and fractures results in increased respiratory complications and disability.[20]

Controlling pain in patients with fractured ribs is essential for preventing secondary complications (i.e., atelectasis, pneumonia, and even progression to chronic pain). Alternatives to opioid use in pain management include continuous intercostal nerve blocks for rib fractures using long-acting anesthetics. These nerve blocks can be placed safely in a patient who is anticoagulated.

Reevaluation

Reevaluation includes the following:

- Consider early transfer to a trauma center.
- If signs of internal hemorrhage are present, consider a focused assessment with sonography for trauma ultrasound and/or chest, and/or pelvis radiograph.

Secondary Survey and Reevaluation

The secondary survey and additional diagnostics and interventions start with the history.

H: History

For the older adult patient, a pertinent medical history is crucial. In addition to the findings in the primary survey, it is important that the trauma nurse ask about a patient's comorbidities and all current and recently discontinued medications. Include questions about multiple prescribers, compliance, or obstacles to taking prescribed medications.

Comorbidities

As a result of advances in medicine, more adults are living longer with chronic diseases and comorbidities, necessitating the use of multiple medications. These comorbidities, as well as medication effects, affect the number and severity of complications and the mortality and morbidity experienced by older patients.

Older adult patients may present with preexisting conditions, so it is important for the trauma nurse to consider their impact on patient assessment and interventions. Comorbidities may result in a cascade of effects, where one system impacts another, resulting in increased morbidity and mortality.[6] Other factors may also contribute to the morbidity and mortality of older adult trauma patients. Cirrhosis, coagulopathy, ischemic heart disease, chronic obstructive pulmonary disease, diabetes, renal disease, and malignancy all increase mortality risk in older adults.[6,18]

Comorbid factors to be assessed in the older trauma patient who has experienced a fall include the following[10]:

- Acute problems
  - Cardiac disease, such as myocardial infarction or arrhythmia
  - Stroke
  - Postural hypotension
  - Hypovolemia
- Chronic problems
  - Neurologic disease, such as dementia or parkinsonism
  - Neuropathy
  - Balance problems that can occur post stroke or brain injury
  - Medication such as analgesics, antihistamines, anticoagulants, sleeping aids, or antidepressants

In addition to the aging process, comorbidities can decrease the physiologic reserves in the older adult trauma patient.[6,19] In other words, the body loses its ability to function above its basic level in times of stress. This may be the result of the sympathetic response being circumvented by cardiac disease, pacemakers, or medications. The inability to increase heart rate so as to compensate for decreased volume can conceal the fact that a patient is hemorrhaging, so it is essential for the trauma nurse to consider the complete presentation and history to obtain a true representation of the patient's condition.

Loss of physiologic reserve is a primary factor resulting in the following outcomes[6,19]:

- Increased complications
- Decreased independence
- Increased morbidity or mortality following a traumatic event

Medications

It is important to obtain a current list of medications, herbal supplements, illicit drugs, and over-the-counter (OTC) medications that the patient is using and to consider their potential contributing and complicating effects[32]:

- Antihypertensives
  - Beta blockers are used to treat hypertension and cardiac arrhythmias. They can prevent the increase in heart rate that is an expected response in patients with hypovolemia, shock states, pain, or stress.
- Antiplatelet medications: aspirin, adenosine diphosphate receptor (ADP)/P2Y inhibitors (i.e., clopidogrel, ticagrelor), or anticoagulants (warfarin [Coumadin], heparin, enoxaparin [Lovenox], NOAC, and/or DOAC)
  - These medications are the most frequently prescribed in the older adult[27,28,30] and increase the possibility of intracranial, internal, or retroperitoneal bleeding.
- Diabetes medications: biguanides, dipeptidyl peptidase-4 (DPP-4) inhibitors insulin, or glucagon-like peptides
  - If a patient is taking any diabetes medications, a change in the level of consciousness or mentation may be due to abnormal blood sugar levels.
- Medications that depress the central nervous system, such as opioids, benzodiazepines, anticholinergic, alcohol and illicit drug use
  - These medications can be the cause of a traumatic injury by impairing balance and judgment.
  - Check the patient for any extra pain patches that they may have forgotten to remove.
  - Ask if the patient has received any pain medications in the past or currently on any pain medications.
    - If so, what was prescribed, how much, and how did the patient respond or react?
    - Did the medication cause excessive sedation?
    - What, if any, adverse effects did the patient experience?
  - Inquire and observe for behaviors of misuse of a prescription and OTC medication. Be sure to obtain an alcohol level and drug(s) of abuse screen.
- Nitroglycerin
  - Use can increase the chance of injury secondary to a drop in blood pressure.

H: Head-to-Toe Assessment

Head-to-toe assessment considerations for the older adult trauma patient may include consideration of urinary catheterization.

Urinary Catheter Considerations

Insertion of a urinary catheter to assess output related to circulation and renal function may increase the risk of a catheter-acquired urinary tract infection. This type of infection is more common and can result in more severe complications (i.e., sepsis; prostatitis, and epididymitis in males; pyelonephritis; endocarditis; and increased length of stay) in the older adult population. Consider alternative methods of output measurement before inserting a urinary catheter.[33]

I: Inspect Posterior Surfaces

To help prevent pressure sores and decrease the discomfort associated with being immobilized on a spine board, expedite removing the board. If not done earlier, this can be done when inspecting the posterior if there are no contraindications to log rolling. If unable to log roll the patient due to potential unstable spine, pelvis, or other injuries, alternate techniques such as the lift and slide are advised to remove the spine board. In the older adult, even 30 to 45 minutes of lying on a spine board can cause skin breakdown.[34,35] Physiologic changes due to osteoporosis, osteoarthritis, and kyphosis increase the discomfort of the rigid spine board in older adults, and the loss of subcutaneous fat and thinning of the skin with aging means that they have less padding. The skin's blood vessels are more fragile, resulting in easier bruising, bleeding under the skin, and skin tears in the older adult. Once off the board, frequent turning may help to prevent the formation of pressure sores.

Reevaluation and Post-Resuscitation Care

The older adult has limited physiologic reserves, so frequent reevaluations are important to determine any changes in vital signs, pain, injuries, and the effectiveness of any interventions implemented. Reassessment of the primary survey is also necessary in this population.

Definitive Care or Transport

Two important topics related to definitive care or transport of the older adult trauma patient are the relationship between length of stay and adverse events and the risk of rib fractures.

Length of Stay and Adverse Events

Increased length of stay in the ED has been associated with poorer outcomes and increased mortality across all trauma patient populations, but in the older adult trauma patient, ED boarding is more likely to result in an adverse event.[6,36] The older adult tends to take more medications and have more comorbidities, and these factors increase the risk of an adverse event. This is why older adults should be prioritized for admission while waiting for an inpatient bed.[36]

Rib Fractures

Blunt chest trauma from falls, MVCs, and physical assault are common sources of rib fractures in older adults, whose morbidity and mortality increase with each additional rib fractured.[37] The National Trauma Data Bank revealed an all-cause mortality rate of 5.8% for those persons who sustain a single traumatic rib fracture, increasing to 34% for those persons with seven or more rib fractures.[37]

Many times, older adults with rib fractures are discharged from the ED with mild oral analgesia and possibly an incentive spirometer. Many of these individuals develop pulmonary complications due to tenderness around the injured area and pain during movement, coughing, and/or breathing. These complications can be seen within 48 to 72 hours post injury due to inadequate respiratory effort, and lead to increased work of breathing, atelectasis, and an inability to clear secretions.[37] Given this risk, it is imperative that analgesia for rib fracture be started early, not just for pain management and patient comfort, but also as an attempt to prevent the complications that may follow over the subsequent days. Pain management may consist of the following:

- Simple analgesia: nonsteroidal anti-inflammatory drug (NSAID), either oral or transdermal
- Lidocaine transdermal patches (also can be purchased as OTC products)
- An opioid alone or in conjunction with the NSAID
- Regional anesthetic (thoracic epidural)
- Continuous intercostal nerve block with the use of an On-Q pump, which has been found to decrease hospital length of stay[38] (**Figure 13-2**)
- Operative fixation for multiple rib fractures

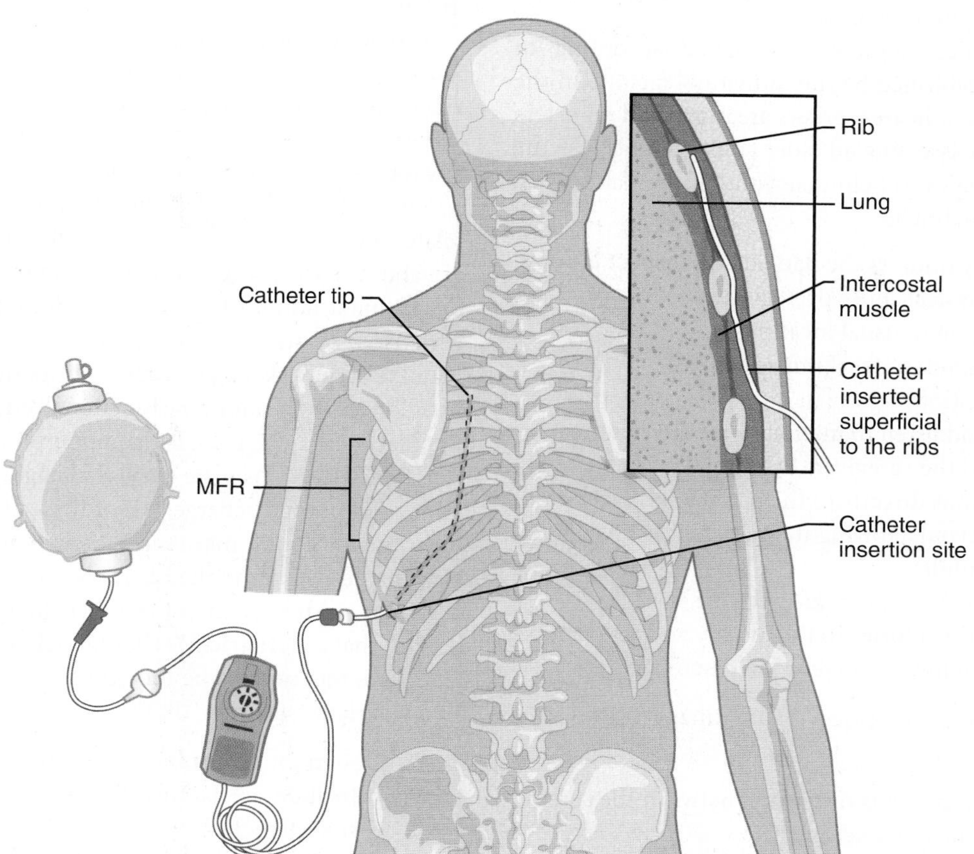

Figure 13-2 *Continuous intercostal nerve block with use of On-Q.*

Elder Maltreatment

According to the American Psychological Association (APA), approximately 2.1 million older adults in the United States are victims of physical abuse, emotional abuse, neglect, or other forms of maltreatment.[39] For this reason, when an older adult who was injured at home or in a nursing facility presents to the ED, the patient should be assessed for signs of elder maltreatment and appropriately referred.

It is estimated that 1 out of 10 older adults experiences abuse or neglect by a caregiver each year.[40] As older adults acquire more physical limitations, they become more vulnerable to maltreatment. Limitations in mobility, vision, and hearing can make them a target. Mental or physical ailments may add to stress for caregivers.[39]

Visits related to healthcare may be the only human contact the older adult has other than with the abuser.[39] Fear of retribution, losing their home, or isolation often keeps older adults from self-reporting instances of elder maltreatment. For every case of elder maltreatment that is reported to authorities, an estimated five cases have not been reported.[39] Recent research suggests that older adults who have been abused tend to die earlier than those who are not, even in the absence of chronic conditions or life-threatening disease.[40]

Suspected maltreatment is reported according to the protocol established by the individual facility. In the United States, healthcare workers are mandated reporters of abuse. When assessing all older adult patients, use the following strategies to help determine if the patient is a victim of maltreatment:

- Completely undress the patient and inspect for any signs of physical abuse or neglect:
  - Bruising in unusual locations
  - Dehydration or fecal impaction
  - Malnutrition
- Observe and listen to interactions between the patient and the caregiver.
- Ask questions directly to the patient and listen to answers. Avoid allowing the caregiver to answer for the older adult.
- Ask if the patient feels safe at home.
- Compare the injuries to the history and reported mechanism for concurrence or discrepancy.

Signs of potential elder maltreatment include the following[39,40]:

- Frequent arguments or tension between the caregiver and the older adult
- Reported changes in personality or behavior in the older adult when the abuser is present
- Caregiver's refusal to allow the older adult to be seen alone
- Caregiver's dismissive attitude or statements about injuries
- History of visiting different EDs for repeated injuries
- Threatening, belittling, or controlling behavior by the caregiver
- Behavior from the older adult that mimics dementia, such as rocking, sucking, or mumbling to oneself

See Chapter 16, "Special Populations: The Interpersonal-Violence Trauma Patient," for more information regarding signs and symptoms of maltreatment.

Emerging Trends

Increases in the older population have posed significant challenges to available healthcare resources. A report from the Institute of Medicine, "Retooling for an Aging America: Building the Health Care Workforce,"[41] details the impending shortage of qualified care providers for the nation's Baby Boomers and recommends solutions that, if adopted now, can help forestall a major deficiency in care for older adults. Here are just a few of the trends that are surfacing.

Promotion of geriatric-focused emergency medicine services and EDs is the number one challenge for ED providers. Not only do we want to improve the care of the geriatric patient, but we must also have the resources to allow for safe care within the department and on discharge. A few of the challenges facing dedicated Geriatric EDs relate to ED staffing, training, and education; availability of validated screening tools; and sustained support from the hospital administration.[42] We must remember that geriatric patients do not come in just with a chief complaint, but may also have comorbidities that may need to be addressed. In addition, functional limitations in this population may be a challenge upon presentation to the ED. Social issues can be very challenging, but must be addressed upon discharge. All of these challenges, if not taken into account, may "send the patient" into a trajectory that leads back to the ED in the form of readmission.

As we address some of these challenges, we will describe what a Geriatric ED should look like. Here are five essentials that need to be thought through when designing a "geriatric-friendly" ED[43]:

1. Design the right physical setting.
   - Include special furniture, equipment, and visual elements:
     - Nonskid and non-glare floors
     - Pressure-reducing mattresses

- Quieter areas
- Low beds
- Extra glasses to be able to read forms

2. Build an interdisciplinary team to address some of the complex issues with which these patients present.
3. Hone the screening and triage processes.
   - Screen for dementia, delirium, and geriatric syndromes. Recognizing delirium among older adult ED patients is challenging, however.
   - Screening instruments include the following:
     - Use of the modified Confusion Assessment Method for the Emergency Department (mCAM-ED) tool to assess delirium in the ED. It can be used to assess patients with and without dementia, and applies a minimal screening and assessment burden on the patient.[44]
     - Patient vulnerability assessment tool.
     - Stop and watch tool (used in assisted living but can easily be used at triage).[45]
     - SPICES (Skin integrity, Problems eating, Incontinence, Confusion, Evidence of falls, Sleep distrubrance)—a screening tool for frailty risks.[46]
4. Provide a robust geriatric training/educational program for all providers.
5. Be vigilant about metrics. Monitor hospital admission rates, readmission rates, transfers, patient outcomes, and patient experience.

Other Trends

Use of telehealth to improve transitions of care to home. Telehealth can offer immediate virtual rounding that takes place while a home health nurse or therapist is visiting with a patient. These collaborative "virtual visits" can improve teamwork between agencies and primary care physicians while improving the patient experience and decreasing readmission rates.

Domestic violence advocates throughout the United States are attempting to bring visibility to interpersonal violence experienced by older adults. June 15, 2017, was designated as the international World Elder Abuse Day. This day brought awareness to some of the obstacles and challenges that elder abuse patients face. The National Clearinghouse on Abuse in Later Life (NCALL) has a course dealing with some of the challenges that elder abused individuals face when seeking shelter[47]:

- Misalignment between the older survivors' needs and traditional safety planning
- True peer advocacy for older adults who find they are the only survivors of their age group in the program
- Accessibility and restrictive policies

Summary

Normal age-related changes can complicate the assessment of the older adult trauma patient. Any presence of comorbidity and the individual response to illness and injury make each patient unique. Failure to recognize the impact of those age-related changes, acknowledge the patient's medications and history, and understand the older adult's response to physical and emotional stress can result in poorer outcomes. For an older adult with multiple injuries, early consideration of transfer to a trauma center may reduce mortality and morbidity.

References

1. Mather, M. (2016). Fact sheet: Aging in the United States. Retrieved from https://www.prb.org/aging-unitedstates-fact-sheet/
2. Kramarow, E., Chen, L., Hedegaard, H., & Warner, M. (2015). *Deaths from unintentional injury among adults aged 65 and over: United States, 2000–2013. NCHS Data Brief, 199.* Hyattsville, MD: National Center for Health Statistics. Retrieved from https://www.cdc.gov/nchs/data/databriefs/db199.pdf
3. Centers for Disease Control and Prevention. (2017). 10 leading causes of injury deaths by age group highlighting unintentional injury deaths, United States—2015. Retrieved from https://www.cdc.gov/injury/images/lc-charts/leading_causes_of_death_age_group_2015_1050w740h.gif
4. Braun, B. J., Holstein, J., Fritz, T., Veith, N. T., Herath, S., Mörsdorf, P., & Pohlemann, T. (2016). Polytrauma in the elderly: A review. *EFORT Open Reviews, 1*(5), 146–151. https://doi.org/10.1302/2058-5241.1.160002
5. Gurwell, M. (2017). The role of exercise in older driver safety. Retrieved from http://www.legalexaminer.com/automobile-accidents/the-role-of-exercise-in-older-driver-safety-2/
6. Calland, J. F., Ingraham, A. M., Martin, N., Marshall, G. T., Schulman, C. L., Stapleton, T., & Barraco, R. D. (2012). Evaluation and management of geriatric trauma: An Eastern Association for the Surgery of Trauma practice management guideline. *Journal of Trauma Acute and Care Surgery, 73*, S345–S350. https://doi.org/10.1097/TA.0b013e318270191f
7. American College of Surgeons. (2016). National Trauma Data Bank 2016: Annual Report. Retrieved from https://www.facs.org/~/media/files/quality%20programs/trauma/ntdb/ntdb%20annual%20report%202016.ashx
8. Committee on Trauma, American College of Surgeons. (2016). *The National Trauma Data Bank 2016 annual report.* Chicago, IL: Author. Retrieved from https://www.facs.org/~/media/files/quality%20programs/trauma/ntdb/ntdb%20annual%20report%202016.ashx

9. Centers for Disease Control and Prevention. (2017). Important facts about falls. Retrieved from https://www.cdc.gov/homeandrecreationalsafety/falls/adultfalls.html
10. Lukaszyk, C., Harvey, L., Sherrington, C., Keay, L., Tiedemann, A., Coombes, J., . . . Iver, R. (2016). Risk factors, incidence, consequences and prevention strategies for falls and fall-injury within older indigenous populations: A systematic review. *Australian and New Zealand Journal of Public Health, 40*(6), 564–568. https://doi.org/10.1111/1753-6405.12585
11. Lee, A., Lee, K. W., & Khang, P. (2013). Preventing falls in the geriatric population. *Permanente Journal, 17*(4), 37–39. https://doi.org/10.7812%2FTPP%2F12-119
12. Verma, S. K., Willetts, J. L., Corns, H. L., Marucci-Wellman, H. R., Lombardi, D. A., & Courtney, T. K. (2016). Falls and fall-related injuries among community-dwelling adults in the United States. *PLoS One 11*(3), e0150939. https://doi.org/10.1371/journal.pone.0150939
13. Deprey, S. M., Biedrzycki, L., & Klenz, K. (2017). Identifying characteristics and outcomes that are associated with fall-related fatalities: Multi-year retrospective summary of fall deaths in older adults from 2005–2012. *Injury Epidemiology, 4*(21). https://doi.org/10.1186%2Fs40621-017-0117-8
14. Wongrakpanich, S., Kallis, C., Prasad, P., Rangaswami, J., & Rosenzweig, A. (2018). The study of rhabdomyolysis in the elderly: An epidemiological study and single center experience. *Aging and Disease, 9*(1), 1–7. https://doi.org/10.14336%2FAD.2017.0304
15. Crandall, M., Streams, J., Duncan, T., Mallet, A., Greene, W., Violano, P., . . . Barraco, R. (2015). Motor vehicle collision–related injuries in the elderly: An Eastern Association for the Surgery of Trauma evidence-based review of risk factors and prevention. *Journal of Trauma and Acute Care Surgery,* 79, 152–158. https://doi.org/10.1097/TA.0000000000000677
16. Sklar, A. L., Boissoneault, J., Fillmore, M. T., & Nixon, S. J. (2014). Interaction between age and moderate alcohol effects on simulated driving performance. *Psychopharmacology (Berlin), 231*(3), 557–566. https://doi.org/10.1007/s00213-013-3269-4
17. Labib, N., Nouh, T., Winocour, S., Deckelbaum, D., Banici, L., Fata, P., . . . Khwaja, K. (2011). Severely injured geriatric population: Morbidity, mortality, and risk factors. *Journal of Trauma, 71*(6), 1908–1914. https://doi.org/10.1097/TA.0b013e31820989ed
18. Sadro, C. T., Sandstrom, C. K., Verma, N., & Gunn, M. L. (2015). Geriatric trauma: A radiologist's guide to imaging trauma patients aged 65 years and older. *RadioGraphics, 35*(4), 1263–1285. https://doi.org/10.1148/rg.2015140130
19. Smith, C. M., & Cotter, V. T. (2016). Age-related changes in health. In M. Boltz, E. Capezuti, T. Fulmer, & D. Zwicker (Eds.), *Evidence-based geriatric nursing protocols for best practice* (5th ed., pp. 23–42). New York, NY: Springer.
20. Lee, S. Y., Shih, S. C., Leu, Y. S., Chang, Y. H., Lin, H. C., & Ku, H. C. (2017). Implications of age-related changes in anatomy for geriatric-focused difficult airways. *International Journal of Gerontology, 11*, 130–133. https://doi.org/10.1016/j.ijge.2016.11.003
21. Jubert, P., Lonjon, G., Garreau de Loubresse, C., & Bone and Joint Trauma Study Group. (2013). Complications of upper cervical spine trauma in elderly subjects: A systematic review of the literature. *Orthopaedics & Traumatology: Surgery & Research, 99*, S301–S312. https://doi.org/10.1016/j.otsr.2013.07.007
22. Baltazar, G. A., Bassett, P., Pate, A. J., & Chendrasekhar, A. (2017). Older patients have increased risk of poor outcomes after low-velocity pedestrian–motor vehicle collisions. *Pragmatic and Observational Research,* 8, 43–47. https://doi.org/10.2147%2FPOR.S127710
23. Centers for Disease Control and Prevention. (2013). Motor vehicle traffic-related pedestrian deaths—United States, 2001–2010. *Mortality and Morbidity Weekly Report, 62*(15), 277–282. Retrieved from https://www.cdc.gov/mmwr/preview/mmwrhtml/mm6215a1.htm
24. Rao, P. J., Pha, K., Mobbs, R. J., Wilson, D., & Ball, J. (2016). Cervical spine immobilization in the elderly population. *Journal of Spine Surgery, 2*(1), 41–46. Retreived from https://www.ncbi.nlm.nih.gov/pmc/articles/PMC5039838/pdf/jss-02-01-041.pdf
25. Navaratnarajah, A., & Jackson, S. H. D. (2017). The physiology of ageing. *Medicine, 45*(1), 6–9. https://doi.org/10.1016/j.mpmed.2016.10.008
26. Wise, R., Faurie, M., Malbrain, M., & Hodgson, E. (2017). Strategies for intravenous fluid resuscitation in trauma patients. *World Journal of Surgery, 41*, 1170–1183. https://doi.org/10.1007/s00268-016-3865-7
27. Mador, B., Nascimento, B., Hollands, S., & Rizoli S. (2017). Blood transfusion and coagulopathy in geriatric trauma patients. *Scandinavian Journal of Trauma Resuscitation and Emergency Medicine, 25,* 33. https://doi.org/10.1186/s13049-017-0374-0
28. Levine, M. (2016). Geriatric trauma and medical illness: Pearls and pitfalls. *emDocs*. Retrieved from http://www.emdocs.net/geriatric-trauma-medical-illness-pearls-pitfalls/
29. Centers for Disease Control and Prevention. (2017, November 3). Warning signs and symptoms of heat-related illness. Retrieved from https://www.cdc.gov/disasters/extremeheat/warning.html#text
30. Bar-Or, D., Salottolo, K. M., Orlando, A., Mains, C. W., Bourg P., & Offner, P. J. (2013). Association between a geriatric trauma resuscitation protocol using venous lactate measurements and early trauma surgeon involvement and mortality risk. *Journal of the American Geriatrics Society, 61*, 1358–1364. https://doi.org/10.1111/jgs.12365
31. Hogas, A. L., Grall, M., & Hoon, S. L (2016). Pain management. In M. Boltz, E. Capezuti, T. Fulmer, & D. Zwicker (Eds.), *Evidence-based geriatric nursing protocols for best practice* (5th ed., pp. 263–282). New York, NY: Springer.
32. Dalton, T., Rushing, M. R., Escott, M. E. A., & Monroe, B. J. (2015, November 2). Complexities of geriatric patients. *Journal of Emergency Medical Services*. Retrieved from https://www.jems.com/articles/print/volume-40/issue-11/features/complexities-of-geriatric-trauma-patients.html
33. Galen, B. T. (2015). Underpad weight to estimate urine output in adult patients with urinary incontinence. *Journal of*

Geriatric Cardiology, 12, 189–190. https://doi.org/10.11909%2Fj.issn.1671-5411.2015.02.016

34. Ham, W., Schoonhoven, L., Schuurmans, M. J., & Leenen, L. (2014). Pressure ulcers from spinal immobilization in trauma patients: A systematic review. *Journal of Trauma and Acute Care Surgery, 76*(4), 1131–1141. https://doi.org/10.1097/TA.0000000000000153
35. Ham, W., Schoonhoven, L., Schuurmans, M. J., & Leenen, L. (2017). Pressure ulcers in trauma patients with suspected spine injury: A prospective cohort study with emphasis on device-related pressure ulcers. *International Wound Journal, 14*(1), 104–111. https://doi.org/10.1111/iwj.12568
36. Kinney, E. P., Gursahani, K., Armbrecht, E., & Dalawari, P. (2015). Does emergency medicine length of stay predict trauma outcomes at a Level 1 trauma center? *Journal of Hospital Administration, 4*(5), 1–7. https://doi.org/10.5430/jha.v4n5p1
37. Britt, T., Sturm, R., Ricardi, R., & Labond, V. (2015). Comparative evaluation of continuous intercostal nerve block or epidural analgesia on the rate of respiratory complications, intensive care unit, and hospital stay following traumatic rib fractures: A retrospective review. *Local and Regional Anesthesia, 8*, 79–84. https://doi.org/10.2147/LRA.S80498
38. Halyard Health. (2015). On-Q* pain relief system. Retrieved from https://www.halyardhealth.co.uk/media/17525923/mk-00781-emea_on-q_ribfracturetrauma_2015.pdf
39. American Psychological Association. (n.d.). *Elder abuse and neglect: In search of solutions.* Retrieved from http://www.apa.org/pi/aging/resources/guides/elder-abuse.aspx
40. Hoover, R. M., & Pollson, M. (2014). Detecting elder abuse and neglect: Assessment and intervention. *American Family Physician, 89*(6), 453–460. Retrieved from https://www.aafp.org/afp/2014/0315/p453.html
41. Institute of Medicine. (2008). Retooling for an aging America: Building the health care workforce. Retrieved from http://nationalacademies.org/hmd/~/media/Files/Report%20Files/2008/Retooling-for-an-Aging-America-Building-the-Health-Care-Workforce/ReportBriefRetoolingforanAgingAmericaBuildingtheHealthCareWorkforce.pdf
42. Schumacher, J. G., Hirshon, J., Hogan, T., Magidson, P., & Chrisman, M. (2017). Trends in geriatric emergency medicine for older adult patients. *Innovation in Aging, 1*(Suppl. 1), 111. https://doi.org/10.1093/geroni/igx004.461
43. Ponte, M. (2016). 5 essentials of a geriatric emergency department. Retrieved from https://www.healthleadersmedia.com/clinical-care/5-essentials-geriatric-emergency-department?page=0%2C5
44. Hasemann, W., Grossmann, F. F., Stadler, R., Bingisser, R., Breil, D., Hafner, M., Kressig, R. W., & Nickel, C. H. (2017). Screening and detection of delirium in older ED patients: Performance of the modified Confusion Assessment Method for the Emergency Department (mCAM-ED): A two-step tool. *Internal and Emergency Medicine.* https://doi.org/10.1007/s11739-017-1781-y
45. National Center for Assisted Living. (2014). Stop and watch tool. Retrieved from http://www.pathway-interact.com/wp-content/uploads/2017/04/Assisted-Living-Stop-and-Watch.pdf
46. Aronow, H. U., Borenstein, J., Haus, F., Braunstein, G. D., & Bolton, L. B. (2014). Validating SPICES as a screening tool for frailty risks among hospitalized older adults. *Nursing Research and Practice*, 846759. http://doi.org/10.1155/2014/846759
47. Slye, S., & Brandl, B. (2017). Recognizing the emergency housing & shelter needs of older survivors on world elder abuse awareness day. Retrieved from https://nnedv.org/latest_update/housing-shelter-world-elder-abuse/

CHAPTER

14

Special Populations: The Bariatric Trauma Patient

Nycole D. Oliver, DNP, APRN, CEN, ACNPC-AG, FNP-C

OBJECTIVES

Upon completion of this chapter, the learner will be able to:

1. Describe mechanisms of injury associated with the bariatric trauma patient.
2. Describe pathophysiologic changes as a basis for assessment of the bariatric trauma patient.
3. Demonstrate the nursing assessment of the bariatric trauma patient.
4. Plan appropriate interventions for the bariatric trauma patient.
5. Evaluate the effectiveness of nursing interventions for the bariatric trauma patient.

Introduction

The word *bariatric* comes from the Greek word *baro*, meaning "heavy or large,"[1] and describes patients who are overweight. However, more specific definitions are necessary to identify and classify bariatric patients and discuss trauma care for this unique patient population.

The World Health Organization (WHO) uses body mass index (BMI) to define the degree to which a person is considered overweight.[2] BMI is calculated by dividing a person's weight in kilograms by the individual's height in meters squared. The WHO has developed the following classifications for obesity[2]:

- Underweight: BMI less than 18.5 kg/m^2
- Normal weight: BMI between 18.5 kg/m^2 and 24.9 kg/m^2
- Overweight (pre-obese): BMI between 25 kg/m^2 and 29.9 kg/m^2
- Obese: BMI of 30 kg/m^2 or greater

When a patient reaches a BMI of 40 kg/m^2 or greater, the individual is considered morbidly obese. Such a patient's health is often significantly impacted by diseases such as hypertension, hyperlipidemia, obstructive sleep apnea (OSA), diabetes, and others.[3] Many of these disorders may also be present at lower BMI levels, although a higher BMI increases the risk of these diseases and others. In children and teens, age- and gender-specific tables are used that take into account developmental changes to determine BMI and degree of obesity.[4]

For the purposes of this chapter, the *bariatric patient* is typically a patient with a BMI of 30 kg/m^2 or greater, unless otherwise specified.

Epidemiology

The rates of obesity are increasing in the United States and around the world. In 2015, 38.2% of adults and 31% of children in the United States were identified as obese.[5] Worldwide, obesity has increased in developed countries, with rates of obesity in Mexico now surpassing those in the United States, and lower, yet still significant rates of obesity being seen in Korea, Japan, and China. **Figure 14-1** shows the increase in levels of obesity in countries in North America, Europe, and Asia.[5] Australia shows similar growth in obesity rates; in 2014–2015, 28% of Australian adults were considered obese.[6]

In keeping with this trend, increasing numbers of bariatric trauma patients are presenting to the emergency department for care. Both physicians and nurses report challenges in the assessment and care of this group, including difficulties with vital signs measurement, venipuncture, intravenous (IV) cannulation, patient positioning and mobilization, and other general procedures.[7] Difficulty finding appropriately sized equipment is common.[1] Education regarding this population can assist the trauma nurse to be better prepared to care for these patients.

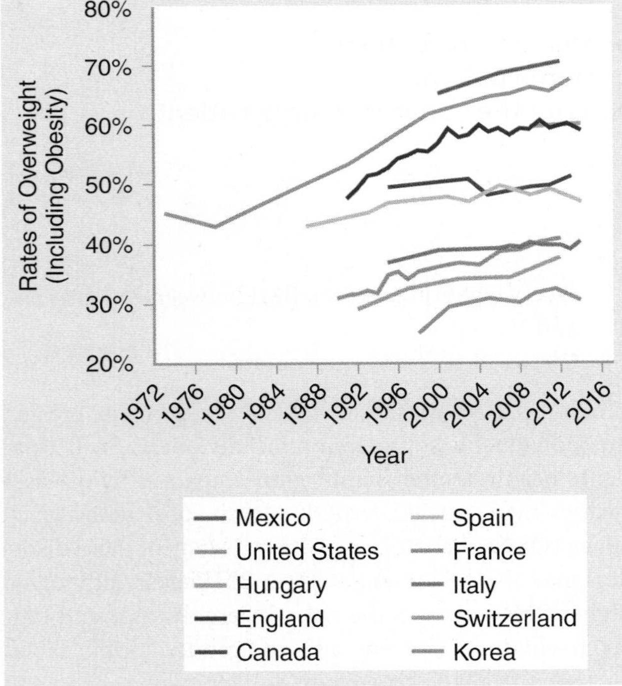

Figure 14-1 *World obesity.*

Reproduced from Organisation for Economic and Co-operative Development. (2017). *Obesity update 2017*. Paris, France: Author. Retrieved from https://www.oecd.org/els/health-systems/Obesity-Update-2017.pdf.

Mechanisms of Injury and Biomechanics

Research related to patterns and severity of injury in bariatric patients show mixed data over the past few decades. BMI has been identified as an independent risk factor for mortality and other adverse outcomes following blunt trauma, such as infectious complications, acute respiratory distress syndrome (ARDS), hematologic complications, and decubitus ulcers.[8] Once injured, bariatric patients have an increased incidence of complications. When they experience orthopedic trauma, bariatric patients have higher rates of complications and hospitalization than patients of more normal weight.[9] In addition, evidence shows that bariatric patients have an increased risk of abdominal compartment syndrome, ARDS, and cardiac arrest with increased mortality attributed not to obesity alone, but also to comorbid diseases, such as diabetes.[10] Other studies show no correlation between obesity and mortality, length of hospital stay, comorbid disease, or complications.[11]

Several factors are associated with the higher mortality rates for bariatric patients, including higher incidence of specific injuries, the inability to use or improper fit of safety equipment and practices, and comorbidities in patients with increased BMI.[12] Notably, studies have found increased mortality for bariatric patients involved in frontal motor vehicle collisions (MVCs).[13] Specific injuries more common in bariatric patients include head, thoracic, pelvic, and lower extremity fractures.[13-15] While bariatric patients may initially sustain fewer injuries, their injuries tend to be more severe. These patients have longer hospital and intensive care unit lengths of stay, with worse survival rates compared to those of patients who are of a normal weight.[9,13,14,16,17]

Morbidly obese drivers in severe MVCs have an increased mortality rate, with one study demonstrating a 52% greater risk of mortality compared to drivers of a normal weight, and an 84% increase in mortality in motorists with morbid obesity who did not use protective equipment.[12,18] These outcomes may result from a decrease in seat belt usage in morbidly obese drivers and passengers. In one of the largest studies to date, researchers found normal-weight drivers were 67% more likely to wear seat belts than morbidly obese drivers.[19] Inappropriate or inadequate restraint points for body habitus and different energy distribution have been offered as theories to explain these injury patterns.[20] In the past, little research has been conducted regarding MVC mechanics, including data related to increased BMI.[11] Currently, statistics and data from research regarding obese patients are based on standard height and weight projections of a BMI of 30 or higher.[16,18,20] Patients who wear seat belts experience fewer injuries than patients who do not, among individuals of all weights.[21]

Comorbid conditions and factors often associated with bariatric patients, such as sleep apnea, obesity hypoventilation syndrome (OHS), decreased endurance and reserve, diabetes, and gastroesophageal reflux disease (GERD), affect the risk for and response to injury. Drivers with untreated sleep apnea have a 243% higher risk for vehicular collisions than drivers without sleep apnea due to drowsiness while driving.[22,23] Bariatric patients with limited endurance and reserves are at greater risk for falls and delayed recovery from decreased mobility.[14,16] Diabetes affects sensation of injury, healing, and metabolism. Patients with GERD have a higher risk of aspiration and pneumonia, which can delay recovery from injury.[24]

Pathophysiologic Differences in the Bariatric Trauma Patient

Bariatric patients with BMI greater than 30 kg/m^2 can have both functional and physiologic differences relative to normal-weight patients, which may contribute to poorer outcomes and delay functional recovery following traumatic injury.[24] An increased BMI has also been associated with dyslipidemia, diabetes, and cardiovascular disease.[11]

Airway changes in obese patients can include a larger neck circumference, increased chin and neck tissue, and extra parapharyngeal tissue, which can increase resistance of the upper airway.[25] Increased abdominal mass can also limit diaphragm expansion.[24] The airway of a patient of normal weight is often maintained best in a supine position; for the bariatric patient, the opposite may be true. In the supine position, the chest and diaphragm of the latter patient can become obstructed due to excess abdominal mass, hindering effective ventilation.[25] **Figure 14-2** shows the difference between the airway of a bariatric patient and a normal-weight counterpart.[26] These differences can lead to intubation difficulties; such challenges have also been attributed to increased neck circumference, shorter thyromental and sternomental distances, and increased accumulation of fat in the oral cavity and cheeks of bariatric patients.[25,27]

Obesity can have a significant effect on the respiratory system.[28] In a patient with excessive weight, expiratory reserve volume is reduced, which in turn reduces the functional residual capacity. Closure of the smaller airways leads to collapsed alveoli and a chronic state of micro-atelectasis in the bases of the lungs.[28] Dyspnea at rest, a higher respiratory rate, lower tidal volumes, and increased minute ventilation have also been identified in obese individuals.[28] In addition, obesity has been identified as a major risk factor in OSA and GERD.[23,28]

Bariatric patients who are morbidly obese have increased abdominal and visceral adipose tissue. This is

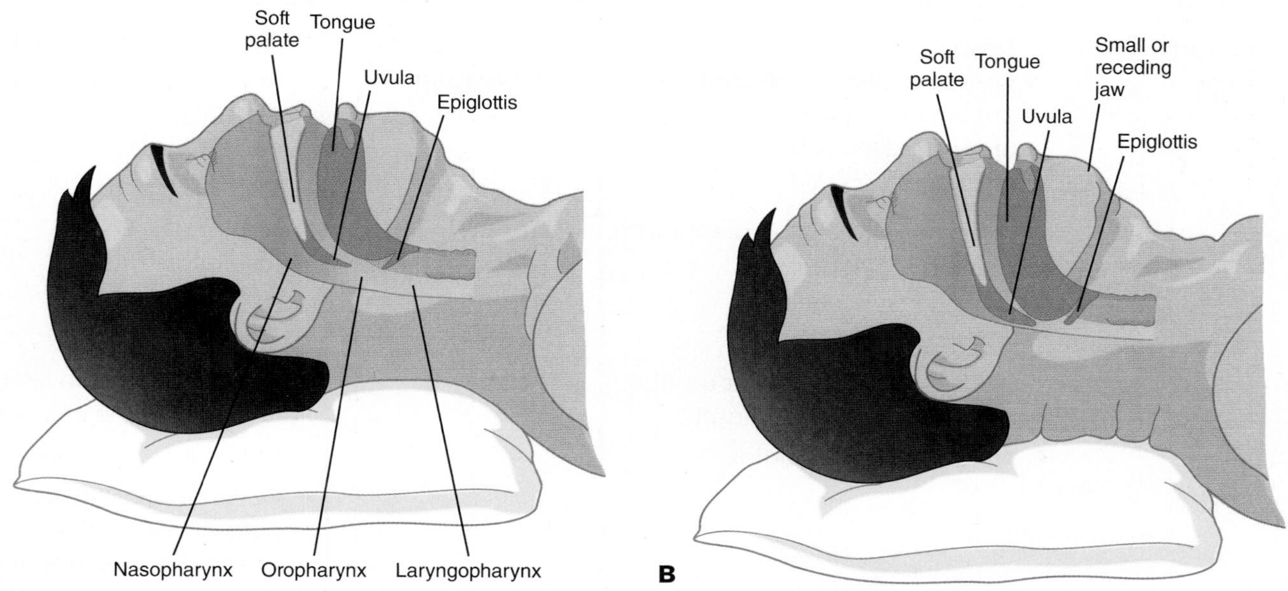

Figure 14-2 *Airways of a normal body weight patient and an obese patient.* ***A.*** *Airway of a normal-body-weight patient.* ***B.*** *Airway of an obese patient.*

associated with a multitude of comorbid conditions, including the following[28,29]:

- Respiratory compromise and OHS
- Hypertension and cardiovascular disease
- GERD
- Depression
- Idiopathic intracranial hypertension (formerly called pseudotumor cerebri)
- Deep vein thrombosis (DVT) and pulmonary embolism
  - Delayed venous return resulting from increased intra-abdominal pressure creates a high risk for DVT and pulmonary embolus in the bariatric patient.
  - Compromise from injury and/or decreased mobility due to lower extremity injury further increases the risk.
  - Decreased blood circulation in the legs creates a prothrombotic milieu, which increases the risk of DVT.[30]

Pharmacokinetic factors associated with obesity may affect medication metabolism and pharmacodynamics. Bariatric patients have both increased lean body mass and increased fat mass. Muscle tissue holds more water than fat tissue does, so medications that are hydrophilic are distributed more to lean tissue and less to adipose tissue. In general, hydrophilic medications (such as morphine) are dosed based on ideal body weight (IBW) and not on actual weight.[31] Lipophilic medications (such as fentanyl) are better absorbed by adipose tissue and may be dosed based on actual body weight.[31] These agents have a longer half-life, which means their elimination is relatively slow, prolonging their effects. Renal function is also a factor in medication clearance, especially in patients with comorbidities of diabetes or hypertension.[31] Consider consultation with a clinical pharmacist to review appropriate drug dosing in bariatric patients.[2]

In many patients, obesity causes alterations in joint cartilage and bone metabolism. A BMI greater than 30 kg/m^2 is linked to an increase in musculoskeletal injuries, leading to early development of osteoarthritic disorders.[32] Complications postoperatively following orthopedic surgery have been associated with obesity, perhaps due to preoperative comorbidities in obese patients.[32] **Table 14-1** outlines both physiologic changes seen in obesity and signs and symptoms related to the changes.

TABLE 14-1 Pathophysiologic Changes Related to Obesity and Morbid Obesity

System	Alterations	Related Disorder	Signs and Symptoms Affecting Trauma Patients
Pulmonary/airway	› Respiratory insufficiency due to chest-wall weight, decreased chest-wall compliance, and increased airway resistance[10,23,25,31,33]	› Increased work of breathing	› Dyspnea with very mild exertion, positional dyspnea
	› IAP leads to elevated diaphragm, chronic atelectasis	› Obesity hypoventilation syndrome, also known as OSA	› Higher baseline respiratory rate
	› Narrowed airway, larger tongue, relaxed pharyngeal muscle › Nocturnal gastric reflux	› Asthma	› Oxygen saturation likely lower in supine position › Hypoxia, hypercapnia › Daytime drowsiness common in undiagnosed sleep apnea; may contribute to MVCs

System	Alterations	Related Disorder	Signs and Symptoms Affecting Trauma Patients
Cardiovascular	Ventricular remodeling[9,10,17,18,25,30,34]: › Left ventricle hypertrophy and decreased compliance › Increased cardiac output › Diastolic dysfunction	Hypertension	Muffled heart sounds
	Accelerated rate of coronary atherosclerosis › Increased IAP thought to contribute to development of hypertension as well as lower extremity circulatory disorder › Venous insufficiency	Right- and left-sided heart failure › Pulmonary hypertension › Varicose veins	Compensatory tachycardia ECG changes: › PR, QRS, and QT intervals prolonged › ST depression, or flattening of T waves › Low QRS voltage
	Elevated blood viscosity due to increased leptin	› Venous stasis › Pulmonary embolism	Arrhythmias › Higher incidence of atrial fibrillation › Premature ventricular contractions common › Edema in the lower extremities
Endocrine	Elevated insulin levels and resistance to endogenous insulin, cholesterol production[30,34]	› Metabolic syndrome › Type 2 diabetes › Dyslipidemia › Polycystic ovarian syndrome	Elevated blood glucose levels
Musculoskeletal	Weight-bearing joint deterioration due to excess weight [9,14,35]	Osteoarthritis	Degenerative symptoms: › Joint pain, particularly in the lower hips, knees, and ankles › Limited range of motion of extremities › Limited flexibility
	Compression of spinal vertebrae due to weight load	Low back pain	Back pain, neurologic symptoms
	› Increase in uric acid › Gait and balance changes related to weight distribution with increased BMI	Gout	› Pain, swelling, and redness of affected area › Decreased mobility

(continues)

TABLE 14-1 Pathophysiologic Changes Related to Obesity and Morbid Obesity (*continued*)

System	Alterations	Related Disorder	Signs and Symptoms Affecting Trauma Patients
Gastrointestinal	Increased IAP, inability to lower esophageal sphincter to withstand this pressure[25]	Gastroesophageal reflux	Reports of reflux from awake patient or potential aspiration symptoms in altered consciousness
	Increased liver size due to fatty deposits	Nonalcoholic fatty liver disease	Elevated liver function studies, often asymptomatic
	Abdominal muscle-wall weakness, increased IAP	Hernias	Pain, bulging on palpation of abdomen
Genitourinary	Insulin resistance and IAP causation[25,31,36]	Renal dysfunction	Elevated BUN and creatinine levels
	Increased urinary bladder pressure related to IAP	Urinary stress incontinence	Urinary urgency, leakage
Neurologic	Increased intracranial pressure due to IAH[37]	Idiopathic intracranial hypertension (pseudotumor cerebri)	Headaches, visual disturbances
Skin	Venous stasis in lower extremities	Cellulitis	Early breakdown of skin in moist area, and areas of pressure points, including occiput
	Excess skin accumulation	Intertrigo under skin folds	
Psychological		› Depression › Low self-esteem › Social isolation	

Abbreviations: BMI, body mass index; BUN, blood urea nitrogen; ECG, electrocardiogram; IAH, intra-abdominal hypertension; IAP, intra-abdominal pressure; MVCs, motor vehicle collisions; OSA, obstructive sleep apnea.

Nursing Care of the Bariatric Trauma Patient

Nursing care of the bariatric trauma patient begins with proper preparation and is followed by primary survey.

Preparation

It is important to be prepared before the trauma patient's arrival with equipment in a variety of appropriate sizes, such as stretchers, blood pressure cuffs, and cervical spine collars. Education regarding the special considerations of caring for bariatric patients can also serve as a foundation for the trauma team to provide competent, safe, and sensitive trauma care.

Primary Survey and Resuscitative Measures

Bariatric patients with lower BMI levels may be able to adequately compensate with little noticeable difference in their assessment parameters. As the BMI level increases, expect physiologic and functional changes to become increasingly severe. The initial assessment focuses on establishing a baseline to determine which findings can be attributed to a known, suspected pre-injury cause and which may be related to potential traumatic injury.

A: Alertness and Airway

Assess and consider interventions needed.

Assessment

Bariatric patients are at high risk for gastric reflux or aspiration, especially those patients with altered levels of consciousness.

Interventions

Interventions may include the following:

- Cervical spinal stabilization
  - Blanket rolls, wedges, and tape can be used to assist stabilization.[25] Commercially available stabilization devices may not fit the bariatric patient who has a shorter, thicker neck.
  - Anticipate the need for additional personnel when log rolling or repositioning the patient.
- Airway
  - Use a two-handed bilateral jaw-thrust maneuver with airway adjuncts for optimal airway control.[35]
  - Anticipate the need for early intubation if airway compromise is a risk.
  - The reverse Trendelenburg position will benefit the patient in terms of both airway maintenance and work of breathing.[25]
- Place the patient in a position with the head elevated during intubation, with the external auditory canal parallel with the sternal notch to allow for better visualization of pharyngeal landmarks.[25] This position is known as the *ramped* position (**Figure 14-3**).[26,38] Blankets can be used to elevate the head and torso into this position.
- Awake intubation using fiberoptic technology may be preferable in bariatric patients, as it preserves pharyngeal and laryngeal muscle tone.[25] Fiberoptic visualization also provides a superior view of the glottis in many patients.[25]
- Selection of the provider with the most experience in difficult airway management is recommended.[25,33]

Rapid-Sequence Intubation

Rapid-sequence intubation dosage for bariatric patients remains controversial.

- Evidence at this time supports using lean body weight (LBW) when determining the dose for induction agents, IBW for rocuronium and other nondepolarizing agents, and total body weight (TBW) for succinylcholine.[39] **Table 14-2** provides information that can be used to rapidly estimate medication dosages in emergent situations.[25,26,38]
- Monitor the patient closely for desaturation. Increased oxygen consumption leads to rapid desaturation in the obese patient; a patient with

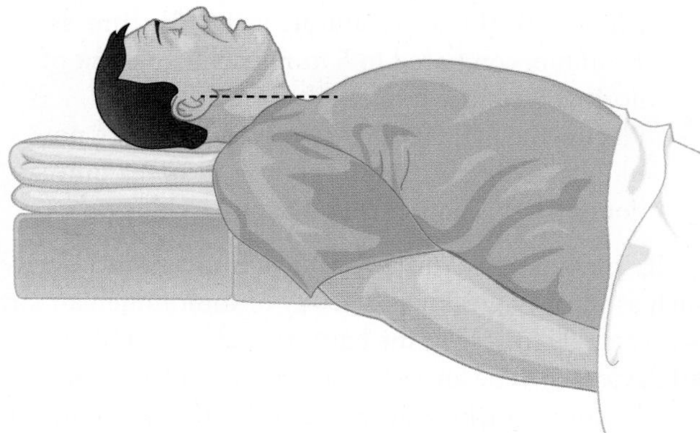

Figure 14-3 *Patient in ramped position for better visualization with intubation.*

TABLE 14-2 Information for Rapidly Estimating Medication Dosage to Facilitate Intubation

Height (in.)	Height (cm)	IBW[a] (kg)	Approximate LBW in Class III Obesity[b] (kg)
Female			
60	152	46	52
65	165	57	60
70	178	68	70
75	191	80	80
Male			
60	152	50	63
65	165	62	73
70	178	76	85
75	191	89	97
80	203	103	112

Abbreviations: BMI, body mass index; IBW, ideal body weight; LBW, lean body weight; TBW, total body weight.

[a] IBW male = 50 + (2.3 × height in inches over 5 feet); IBW female = 45.5 + (2.3 × height in inches over 5 feet).

[b] Approximate LBW in class III obesity (BMI 40–45 kg/m^2) for dosing emergency medications; LBW estimate (kg) = (9270 × TBW)/(A + B × BMI), where A and B are 6,680 and 216, respectively, for males and 8,780 and 244, respectively, for females.

Data from Arbelaez, C., Bartels, S., & Brown, C. A. (2018). Emergency airway management in the morbidly obese patient. *UpToDate*. Retrieved from https://www.uptodate.com/contents/emergency-airway-management-in-the-morbidly-obese-patient.

a higher BMI may desaturate in as little time as 1 minute, compared to 6 minutes in a patient of normal weight.[25,33]

- Placing the patient in reverse Trendelenburg position to 25 degrees prolongs the safe apnea time, as does preoxygenation with a bag-mask device.[25,33]

If intubation is unsuccessful, a supraglottic device such as the laryngeal mask airway or multilumen airway is acceptable for use in the bariatric patient.[33] Other useful devices include an endotracheal tube introducer.

Obtaining tracheal access may be necessary in patients when intubation fails. In such a case, surgical cricothyrotomy is the technique of choice.[40] Use of an endotracheal tube is recommended, as the standard cricothyrotomy tube may be too short.[40] Tracheostomy is less desirable in this patient population due to increased complications and procedure difficulty.[40]

B: Breathing and Ventilation

Assess the patient and consider interventions needed.

Assessment

Assess as follows:

- Inspect for the following:
  - Increased work of breathing, especially when in a supine position. Weakened respiratory muscles may quickly lead to fatigue and respiratory failure.
  - Monitor level of consciousness; lethargy, mental status changes, and restlessness that may indicate hypoxia.
- Auscultate for the following:
  - Breath sounds can be muffled through additional soft tissue.[33]
  - Displace skin folds over the lung area to auscultate lung sounds.

Interventions

Interventions include the following:

- As soon as the cervical spine is cleared, place the patient in an upright position to improve access and chest excursion.
  - Placing the patient in a lateral left position or elevating the head of the bed in reverse Trendelenburg position at 45 degrees may help the patient with adequate ventilation.[25,33]
- Anticipate potential use of bilevel positive airway pressure (BiPAP).
  - This can be a useful intervention prior to intubation to provide adequate ventilation, especially in patients with a history of sleep apnea.[41]
  - BiPAP can be useful in patients with flail chest injury or any other blunt chest trauma.[41]
  - Prior to application, assure that the patient has an intact swallow function, gag reflex, and cough mechanism.[41]
- Use two-person bag-mask ventilation with oropharyngeal or nasopharyngeal airways in place, unless contraindicated, if manual ventilation is required.[25,33]

C: Circulation and Control of Hemorrhage

Assess and consider interventions needed.

Assessment

Subcutaneous emphysema over chest wall is significant, as auscultation of breath sounds and percussion may not be as useful in detecting chest injuries due to the effects of subcutaneous tissue in muffling accurate sound transmission from the lungs.[42]

Interventions

Interventions include the following:

- Monitor the volume of fluid resuscitation closely to avoid overload—some bariatric patients with cardiac comorbidities may not tolerate aggressive fluid administration.[34]
- Use guided ultrasound for catheter placement if there is difficulty obtaining IV access.[43]
- Consider use of intraosseous access devices. External jugular cannulation attempts may be impaired due to increased adipose tissue in the neck area; however, if landmarks can be visualized, these sites can be used after the cervical spine has been cleared.
- Burn management may require higher levels of fluid replacement, and patients with burn injuries will be at high risk of infection.[44]

Resuscitative Measures

Accuracy of vital signs can be a problematic issue with the bariatric patient.

F: Full Set of Vital Signs

Obtaining an accurate blood pressure in the bariatric patient can be a challenge. The following recommendations include those resulting from research using automated blood pressure devices:

- Use an appropriately sized cuff.
- A cuff that is too small can produce a false high pressure reading.[45]

- The forearm can be used for blood pressure measurement; however, results may be higher than pressures taken in the upper arm.[45]
- Obtaining the correct cuff size for the forearm is essential, and the circumference of the forearm should be measured midway between the elbow and wrist.
- Center the cuff between the elbow and the wrist, with the arm supported at the level of the heart.[45]

Conduct palpation of anatomic landmarks before performing an electrocardiogram (ECG). Placement of ECG leads in bariatric patients may be difficult,[46] but these leads should be placed under the breast-area tissue when possible. If the patient goes to the operating room, the anesthesia provider may remove all chest leads for surgical preparation and instead place them on the shoulders and left leg. Greater chest circumference will cause lead placement that is wider than on a standard-sized person; however, the landmarks of the midclavicular and midaxillary lines are the same for all patients.

G: Get Monitoring Devices and Give Comfort

Address the L, N, O, and P elements:

- L: Laboratory studies
  - Additional laboratory studies related to comorbid conditions as indicated
  - Arterial blood gases to evaluate ventilation status
  - Liver function studies and renal studies to compare to baseline values and rule out significant pathology
- N: Nasogastric or orogastric tube consideration
  - If a patient's history includes recent bariatric surgery, blind placement of a nasogastric or orogastric tube is contraindicated, as it may disrupt the suture lines of the new stomach or perforate the smaller stomach.
  - Tubes may be safely placed using fluoroscopy if indicated.[47]
- O: Oxygenation and ventilation
  - Continuously monitor oxygenation status and capnography.
  - Higher concentrations of supplemental oxygen may be necessary to achieve adequate oxygenation.
  - Conversely, obese patients have higher rates of chronic obstructive pulmonary disorder, so the risk of hyperoxia includes loss of ventilatory drive as well as hyperoxia. Monitor and maintain SpO_2 between 92% and 96%.[48]
- P: Pain assessment and management
  - Pain medication dosing is based on IBW or normal weight parameters and not on actual weight.[32]
  - Lipophilic medications are taken up by adipose tissue and released slowly back into the bloodstream. Medications that are lipophilic—including benzodiazepines, propofol, and fentanyl—should be titrated according to effects and the patient's response monitored closely.[32]

Emergency Resuscitation

While obesity can make resuscitation efforts more challenging, no modifications to basic or advanced life support procedures are recommended by the American Heart Association's Advanced Cardiac Life Support Guidelines.[49] Defibrillation is best accomplished using a biphasic defibrillator, which delivers energy from one contact point or pad to the other and then reverses direction back to the source. There is no current evidence that supports the need for higher energy levels, larger pads, or any change in the algorithm for defibrillation with bariatric patients.[49]

Secondary Survey

The secondary survey includes the history and head-to-toe assessment.

H: History

The trauma nurse should consider several questions when obtaining the history of a bariatric patient.

- What is the patient's current weight and height?
  - Weight may be used for adequate medication dosing. Studies have shown that physicians and nurses are able to estimate a patient's weight within 10% of the actual weight less than 60% of the time, and that patient estimates are most accurate.[50]
  - Use of a bed or stretcher with weight measurement capability is ideal for the bariatric patient who may lack mobility. Check this equipment for upper weight limits before use.
- What medical problems does the patient have?
  - Known medical history and potential undiagnosed conditions are both important factors.
  - Be alert for signs of comorbidities that have yet to be identified.
    - Ask about increased thirst, urination, dry mouth, headaches, or fatigue, as they may indicate the presence of metabolic syndrome or elevated glucose levels.

  - Symptoms such as snoring, daytime drowsiness and fatigue, frequent night awakening, observed apnea, or a choking sensation during sleep can indicate undetected sleep apnea.[23]
- Does the patient have a history of bariatric surgery?
  - A patient who has undergone surgery may be in one of several stages of weight loss, have achieved limited success, or have rebounded with weight gain occurring at some point after the original surgery.
  - Determine the type of procedure, any complications, and when it was performed.
  - Patients who have not been compliant with dietary and vitamin recommendations may have deficiencies in their protein or vitamin levels. Patients who have undergone gastric bypass, for example, are more likely to have iron and vitamin B_{12} deficiencies and may have a baseline anemia that affects laboratory studies.
- Which medications is the patient taking?
  - Bariatric patients may be currently treated for several comorbid conditions. It is important to determine the patient's use of the following medications:
    - Antidiabetic medications, including last dose
    - Diuretics
    - Antihypertensives
    - Antilipidemics
    - Anticoagulants and salicylates
    - Antianginals, including calcium-channel blockers, beta-adrenergic blockers, and nitrates
    - Antacids and histamine antagonists
    - Antidepressants
    - Bronchodilators and corticosteroids
    - Appetite suppressants: May cause tachycardia, increased blood pressure, paresthesia, dyspepsia, and abdominal pain, which can be confused with trauma-related injury symptoms[51]
    - Chronic pain medications, including nonsteroidal anti-inflammatory medications
  - Because of altered absorption following bariatric surgery, many patients may be taking vitamin supplements.
  - Ask about over-the-counter medications, alternative and herbal remedies, and the use of energy supplements or drinks.

H: Head-to-Toe Assessment

Peripheral pulses may need to be assessed using Doppler ultrasound.

Reevaluation Measures

Of particular concern is thromboembolism prevention.

Thromboembolism Prevention

The bariatric patient is at higher risk for thrombus formation and for serious complications from thromboembolism. Standard prevention measures include sequential compression devices, prophylactic anticoagulant therapy, and early mobilization.

Patients who are discharged with reduced mobility after fractures may need anticoagulation as well as discharge instructions related to signs and symptoms of thromboembolism. Fracture stabilization choices may be altered due to the need for custom-fit splints, which allow for the anticipated swelling.[52] Bariatric patients with a BMI greater than 40 kg/m^2 will need specialty beds to help prevent complications of immobility.

Computed Tomography

Be aware of weight limits and size restrictions of the computed tomography (CT) scanning equipment. Prepare alternative options in advance.

Staff and Patient Safety

Staff safety during procedures is a consideration when caring for bariatric patients. The weight of an extremity in a bariatric patient with a BMI greater than 40 kg/m^2 may exceed the safe lifting load for a single caregiver, and lifting devices should be used to help prevent staff and patient injury in all aspects of care. Consideration should be given to preplanning and training in the use of techniques and devices to assist in transfer, positioning, and nursing care procedures.

Lateral transfer devices should be used to help prevent skin shearing and staff injury. Such devices include slider boards and friction-reduction devices, as well as air-assisted lateral transfer aids. Friction-reduction sheets and air transfer cushions need to be placed on the stretcher prior to patient use. With the lateral air transfer device, air flows through the inflated mattress to provide a thin cushion of air to move the patient laterally, reducing the work of transfer.[53]

Providing a safe environment for the bariatric patient involves the following key components:

- Knowing the weight capacity of conventional equipment (stretchers, wheelchairs, toilets) and the capacity and size of openings of CT and magnetic resonance imaging tables and openings
- Being familiar with safe use of the bariatric equipment available in the department

- Demonstrating confidence in the ability to safely care for the bariatric patient and ensure the safety of other caregivers

Patient Dignity

Bariatric patients often experience discrimination and bias in healthcare settings.[54,55] Physicians, nurses, and other staff members may have negative beliefs and opinions about causes of obesity and characteristics of obese patients, which can translate into care that lacks sensitivity or even displays open prejudice. The challenges of providing care to bariatric patients can also lead to frustration for the trauma nurse. This behavior may be perceived by patients as a negative reaction directed at them.

To provide sensitive care for the bariatric patient, follow these guidelines:

- *Protect patient privacy.* Provide adequately sized gowns and draping, and obtain the patient's weight in a discreet manner.
- *Demonstrate tact regarding weight issues.* References to "large size," "big boy," "obesity," or "excess fat" are often offensive to bariatric patients. Terms such as "weight problem" or "excess weight" are often less emotionally charged.[54,55]
- *Be sensitive to the bariatric patient's past encounters with healthcare providers.* Many bariatric patients have suffered embarrassment from use of improperly sized equipment, insensitive comments, and even openly discriminatory behavior. Be aware of nonverbal communication.

A heightened sensitivity to these issues is needed in the care of the bariatric patient to overcome self-protective barriers and develop a trusting relationship that will facilitate care.[54,55]

Reevaluation and Post-Resuscitation Care

Continued assessment of the airway and oxygenation are the highest priority in bariatric trauma patients, to include monitoring for the following conditions:

- Signs of impending airway or respiratory compromise
- Signs of gastric reflux, which can lead to pulmonary aspiration, particularly in a supine patient
- Signs and symptoms of pulmonary embolism, since both obesity and trauma are independent risk factors for this complication[9,31,55]

Due to the numerous challenges in evaluation and treatment of bariatric patients, prolonged immobilization can occur.[55] Ongoing reevaluation includes monitoring for the following complications:

- Pressure-induced rhabdomyolysis from muscle breakdown (see Chapter 10, "Musculoskeletal Trauma")
- Acute compartment syndrome in compromised extremities (see Chapter 10)
- Skin breakdown, particularly on the occiput area of the head and between skin folds in bariatric patients, along with areas of bony prominence[55]
- If using BiPAP, monitor for the following[41]:
    - Skin breakdown across the bridge of the nose due to mask pressure
    - Gastric insufflation and potential regurgitation and aspiration

Disposition or Transport

Bariatric centers of excellence are located throughout the United States. Consider if the patient needs to be cared for at a trauma center and/or bariatric center of excellence.

Emerging Trends

Bariatric trauma patients can require special handling to prevent injuries to both the patient and staff. Assistive devices such as bariatric hospital beds, overhead/ceiling lifts, stand-up lifts, and sliding boards can greatly increase safety when caring for these patients.[56] Consulting with a bariatric nurse coordinator (if available) when planning care/protocols specifically for bariatric trauma patients will significantly improve safe patient handling for both obese patients and healthcare workers.

Summary

Trauma nurses are encountering increasing numbers of trauma patients who are overweight or obese. This bariatric patient population is a vulnerable group due to the presence of functional and physiologic changes, and is at high risk of airway and breathing complications. Standard assessments and interventions may need to be modified, and equipment needs to be available for use in a variety of sizes. Trauma care goals are aimed at diagnosis and management of injury, despite challenges presented by body habitus and limited diagnostic capabilities, while preserving the dignity of the patient.

References

1. Mills, C., & Dee, S. (2016). Challenging perceptions of body image using a bariatric weight suit with female university dancers. *Journal of Obesity and Bariatrics, 3*(1). https://doi.org/10.13188/2377-9284.1000019
2. World Health Organization. (20188). *Obesity and overweight (Fact sheet)*. Geneva, Switzerland: Author. Retrieved from http://www.who.int/mediacentre/factsheets/fs311/en/
3. Copstead, L. E., & Banasik, J. (Eds.). (2014). *Pathophysiology* (5th ed.). St. Louis, MO: Elsevier Saunders.
4. Hales, C. M., Carroll, M. D., Fryar, C. D., & Ogden, C. L. (2017). Prevalence of obesity among adults and youth: United States, 2015–2016. *NCHS Data Brief*, No. 288. Hyattsville, MD: National Center for Health Statistics. Retrieved from https://www.cdc.gov/nchs/data/databriefs/db288.pdf
5. Organisation for Economic and Co-operative Development. (2017). *Obesity update 2017*. Paris, France: Author. Retrieved from https://www.oecd.org/els/health-systems/Obesity-Update-2017.pdf
6. Australian Institute of Health and Welfare. (2016). *Australia's health 2016*. Australia's Health Series No. 15. Cat. No. AUS 199. Canberra, Australia: Author. Retrieved from https://www.aihw.gov.au/getmedia/9844cefb-7745-4dd8-9ee2-f4d1c3d6a727/19787-AH16.pdf.aspx
7. Sabol, V. K., & Molloy, M. A. (2015). GAPNA Section. Aging and obesity: General assessment and management considerations. *Geriatric Nursing, 36*(5), 407–409. https://doi.org/10.1016/j.gerinurse.2015.08.008
8. Ditillo, M., Pandit, V., Rhee, P., Aziz, H., Hadeed, S., Bhattacharya, B., . . . Joseph, B. (2014). Morbid obesity predisposes trauma patients to worse outcomes: A National Trauma Data Bank analysis. *Journal of Trauma and Acute Care Surgery, 76*(1), 176–179. https://doi.org/10.1097/TA.0b013e3182ab0d7c
9. Childs, B. R., Nahm, N. J., Dolenc, A. J., & Vallier, H. A. (2015). Obesity is associated with more complications and longer hospital stays after orthopaedic trauma. *Journal of Orthopaedic Trauma, 29*(11), 504–509. https://doi.org/10.1097/BOT.0000000000000324
10. Hwabejire, J. O., Nembhard, C. E., Obirieze, A. C., Oyetunji, T. A., Tran, D. D., Fullum, T. M., . . . Greene, W. R. (2015). Body mass index in blunt trauma patients with hemorrhagic shock: Opposite ends of the body mass index spectrum portend poor outcome. *American Journal of Surgery, 209*(4), 659–665. https://doi.org/10.1016/j.amjsurg.2014.12.016
11. Lee, F. A., Hervey, A. M., Berg, G. M., Acuna, D. L., & Harrison, P. B. (2016). Association of injury factors, not body mass index, with hospital resource usage in trauma patients. *American Journal of Critical Care, 25*(4), 327–334. https://doi.org/10.4037/ajcc2016665
12. Joseph, B., Hadeed, S., Haider, A. A., Ditillo, M., Joseph, A., Pandit, V., . . . Rhee, P. (2017). Obesity and trauma mortality: Sizing up the risks in motor vehicle crashes. *Obesity Research and Clinical Practice, 11*(1), 72–78. https://doi.org/10.1016/j.orcp.2016.03.003
13. Chuang, J., Rau, C., Kuo, P., Chen, Y., Hsu, S., Hsieh, H., & Hsieh, C. (2016). Traumatic injuries among adult obese patients in southern Taiwan: A cross-sectional study based on a trauma registry system. *BMC Public Health, 16*(275), 1–9. https://doi.org/10.1186/s12889-016-2950-z
14. Chuang, J., Rau, C., Liu, H., Wu, S., Chen, Y., Hsu, S., . . . Hsieh, C. (2016). Obese patients who fall have less injury severity but a longer hospital stay than normal-weight patients. *World Journal of Emergency Surgery, 11*(3), 1–6. https://doi.org/10.1186%2Fs13017-015-0059-9
15. Ebinger, T., Koehler, D. M., Dolan, L. A., McDonald, K., & Shah, A. S. (2016). Obesity increases complexity of distal radius fracture in fall from standing height. *Journal of Orthopaedic Trauma, 30*(8), 450–455. https://doi.org/10.1097/BOT.0000000000000546
16. Osborne, Z., Rowitz, B., Moore, H., Oliphant, U., Butler, J., Olson, M., & Aucar, J. (2014). Obesity in trauma: Outcomes and disposition trends. *American Journal of Surgery, 207*(3), 387–392. https://doi.org/10.1016/j.amjsurg.2013.10.013
17. Peitz, G., Peitz, G. W., Troyer, J., Jones, A. E., Shapiro, N. I., Nelson, R. D., . . . Kline, J. A. (2014). Association of body mass index with increased cost of care and length of stay for emergency department patients with chest pain and dyspnea. *Circulation: Cardiovascular Quality and Outcomes, 7*(2), 292–298. https://doi.org/10.1161/CIRCOUTCOMES.113.000702
18. Desapriya, E., Giulia, S., Subzwari, S., Peiris, D. C., Turcotte, K., Pike, I., . . . Hewapathirane, D. S. (2014). Does obesity increase the risk of injury or mortality in motor vehicle crashes? A systematic review and meta-analysis. *Asia-Pacific Journal of Public Health, 26*(5), 447–460. https://doi.org/10.1177/1010539511430720101053951 1430720
19. Jehle, D., Doshi, C., Karagianis, J., Consiglio, J., & Jehle, G. (2014). Obesity and seatbelt use: A fatal relationship. *American Journal of Emergency Medicine, 32*(7), 756–760. https://doi.org/10.1016/j.ajem.2014.01.010
20. Rupp, J. D., Flannagan, C. A., Leslie, A. J., Hoff, C. N., Reed, M. P., & Cunningham, R. M. (2013). Effects of BMI on the risk and frequency of AIS 3+ injuries in motor-vehicle crashes. *Obesity, 21*(1), E88–E97. https://doi.org/10.1002/oby.20079
21. Han, G., Newmyer, A., & Qu, M. (2017). Seatbelt use to save money: Impact of hospital costs of occupants who are involved in motor vehicle crashes. *International Emergency Nursing, 31*, 2–8. https://doi.org/10.1016/j.ienj.2016.04.004004
22. Pucher, P. H., Tanno, L., Hewage, K., & Bagnall, N. M. (2017). Demand for specialized training for the obese trauma patient: National ATLS expert group survey results. *Injury, 48*(5), 1058–1062. https://doi.org/10.1016/j.injury.2017.02.027
23. Gurubhagavatula, I., Sullivan, S., Meoli, A., Patil, S., Olson, R., Berneking, M., & Watson, N. F. (2017). Management of obstructive sleep apnea in commercial motor vehicle operators: Recommendations of the AASM sleep and transportation safety awareness task force. *Journal of Clinical Sleep Medicine, 13*(5), 745–758. https://doi.org/10.5664/jcsm.6598
24. Dhungel, V., Liao, J., Raut, H., Lilienthal, M. A., Garcia, L. J., Born, J., & Choi, K. C. (2015). Obesity delays functional

recovery in trauma patients. *Journal of Surgical Research, 193*(1), 415–420. https://doi.org/10.1016/j.jss.2014.07.027

25. Hanlon, P. (2016). Intubation and airway management for the bariatric patient. *RT: The Journal for Respiratory Care Practitioners, 29*(5), 10–13.
26. Hostetler, M. A. (2008). Use of noninvasive positive-pressure ventilation in the emergency department. *Emergency Medical Clinics of North America, 26,* 929–939. https://doi.org/10.1016/j.emc.2008.07.008
27. Welliver, M., & Bednarzyk, M. (2009). Sedation considerations for the nonintubated obese patient in critical care. *Critical Care Nursing Clinics of North America, 21*(3), 341–352. https://doi.org/10.1016/j.ccell.2009.07.001
28. Ciernak, M., Sobczak, R., Timler, D., Wieczorek, A., Borkowski, B., & Gaszynski, T. (2016). The degree of intubation difficulties and the frequency of complications in obese patients at the hospital emergency department and the intensive care unit. *Medicine, 95*(52), e5777. https://doi.org/10.1097%2FMD.0000000000005777
29. Brazzale, D. J., Pretto, J. J., & Schachter, L. M. (2015). Optimizing respiratory function assessments to elucidate the impact of obesity on respiratory health. *Respirology, 20*(5), 715–721. https://doi.org/10.1111/resp.12563
30. Skolnik, N. S., & Ryan, D. H. (2014). Pathophysiology, epidemiology, and assessment of obesity in adults. *Supplement to the Journal of Family Practice, 63*(7), S1–S10.
31. Klovaite, J., Benn, M., & Nordestgaard, B. G. (2015). Obesity as a casual risk factor for deep vein thrombosis: A Mendelian randomization study. *Journal of Internal Medicine, 277*(5), 573–584. https://doi.org/10.1111/joim.12299
32. Velissaris, D., Karamouzos, V., Marangos, M., Pierrakos, C., & Karanikolas, M. (2014). Pharmacokinetic changes and dosing modification of aminoglycosides in critically ill obese patients: A literature review. *Journal of Clinical Medicine Research, 6*(4), 227–233. https://doi.org/10.14740%2Fjocmr1858w
33. Hodgson, E. (2016). Airway management of the morbidly obese patient. *Journal of Perioperative Practice, 26*(9), 196–200. https://doi.org/10.1177/175045891602600902
34. Bhupathiraju, S. N., & Hu, F. B. (2016). Epidemiology of obesity and diabetes and their cardiovascular complications. *Circulation Research, 118*(1), 1723–1735. https://doi.org/10.1161/CIRCRESAHA.115.306825
35. Werner, B. C., Burrus, M. T., Looney, A. M., Park, J. S., Perumal, V., & Cooper, M. T. (2015). Obesity is associated with increased complications after operative management of end-stage ankle arthritis. *Foot and Ankle International, 36*(8), 863–870. https://doi.org/10.1177/1071100715576569
36. Saccomani, S., Lui-Filho, J. F., Juliato, C. R., Gabiatti, J. R., Pedro, A. O., & Costa-Paiva, L. (2017). Does obesity increase the risk of hot flashes among midlife women? A population-based study. *Menopause, 24*(9), 1065–1070. https://doi.org/10.1097/GME.0000000000000884
37. Stevens, S. M., Rizk, H. G., Golnik, K., Andaluz, N., Samy, R. N., Meyer, T. A., & Lambert, P. R. (2018). Idiopathic intracranial hypertension: Contemporary review and implications for the otolaryngologist. *Laryngoscope, 128*(1), 248–256. https://doi.org/10.1002/lary.2658126581
38. Arbelaez, C., Bartels, S., & Brown, C. A. (2018). Emergency airway management in the morbidly obese patient. *UpToDate.* Retrieved from https://www.uptodate.com/contents/emergency-airway-management-in-the-morbidly-obese-patient
39. Baerdemaeker, L. D., & Margarson, M. (2016). Best anaesthetic drug strategy for morbidly obese patients. *Current Opinion in Anesthesiology, 29*(1), 119–128. https://doi.org/10.1097/ACO.0000000000000286
40. Takashi, A., & Asai, T. (2016). Surgical cricothyrotomy, rather than percutaneous cricothyrotomy, in "cannot intubation, cannot oxygenate" situation. *Anesthesiology, 125*(2), 269–271. https://doi.org/10.1097/ALN.0000000000001197
41. Shebl, R. E., Samra, S. R., Abderaboh, M. M., & Mousa, M. S. (2015). Continuous positive airway pressure ventilation versus bilevel positive airway pressure ventilation in patients with blunt chest trauma. *Egyptian Journal of Chest Diseases and Tuberculosis, 64*(1), 203–208. https://doi.org/10.1016/j.ejcdt.2014.11.016
42. Young, A. M., Joseph, A. P., & Jackson, A. (2015). Crush injury by an elephant: Life-saving prehospital care resulting in a good recovery. *Medical Journal of Australia, 203*(6), 264–265. https://doi.org/10.5694/mja15.00519
43. Bahl, A., Pandurangadu, A. V., Tucker, J., & Bagan, M. (2016). A randomized controlled trial assessing the use of ultrasound for nurse-performed IV placement in difficult access ED patients. *American Journal of Emergency Medicine, 34*(10), 1950–1954. https://doi.org/10.1016/j.ajem.2016.06.098
44. Peeeters, Y., Vandervelden, S., Wise, R., & Malbrain, M. L. (2015). An overview on fluid resuscitation and resuscitation endpoints in burns: Past, present, and future. Part 1: Historical background, resuscitation fluid and adjunctive treatment. *Anaesthesiology Intensive Therapy, 47*(1), s6–s14. https://doi.org/10.5603/AIT.a2015.00630063
45. Arnold, A., & McNaughton, A. (2018). Accuracy of non-invasive blood pressure measurements in obese patients. *British Journal of Nursing, 27*(1), 35–40. https://doi.org/10.12968/bjon.2018.27.1.35
46. Day, K., Olivia, I., Krupinski, E., & Marcus, F. (2015). Identification of 4th intercostal space using sternal notch to xiphoid length for accurate electrocardiogram lead placement. *Journal of Electrocardiology, 48*(6), 1058–1061. https://doi.org/10.1016/j.jelectrocard.2015.08.019
47. Thorell, A., MacCormick, A. D., Awad, S., Reynolds, N., Roulin, D., Demartines, N., . . . Lobo, D. N. (2016). Guidelines for perioperative care in bariatric surgery: Enhanced Recovery After Surgery (ERAS) Society recommendations. *World Journal of Surgery, 40*(1), 2065–2083. https://doi.org/10.1007/s00268-016-3492-3
48. Beasley, R., Chien, J., Douglas, J., Eastlake, L., Farah, C., King, G., . . . Walters, H. (2017). Target oxygen saturation range: 92–96% versus 94–98%. *Respirology, 22*(1), 200–202. https://doi.org/10.1111/resp.12879

49. Kleinman, M. E., Goldberger, Z. D., Rea, T., Swor, R. A., Bobrow, B. J., Brennan, E. E., . . . Travers, A. H. (2018). 2017 American Heart Association focused update on adult basic life support and cardiopulmonary resuscitation quality: An update to the American Heart Association guidelines for cardiopulmonary resuscitation and emergency cardiovascular care. *Circulation, 137*(1), e7–e13. https://doi.org/10.1161/CIR.0000000000000539
50. Young, K. D., & Korotzer, N. C. (2016). Weight estimation methods in children: A systematic review. *Annals of Emergency Medicine, 68*(4), 441–451. https://doi.org/10.1016/j.annemergmed.2016.02.043
51. Hocking, S., Dear, A., & Cowley, M. A. (2017). Current and emerging pharmacotherapies for obesity in Australia. *Obesity Research & Clinical Practice, 11*(5), 501–521. https://doi.org/10.1016/j.orcp.2017.07.002
52. Padegamas, E. M., & Ilayas, A. M. (2015). Distal radius fractures: Emergency department evaluation and management. *Orthopedic Clinics of North America, 46*(2), 259–270. https://doi.org/10.1016/j.ocl.2014.11.010
53. Barlow, R. D. (2018). No time to rest. *Healthcare Purchasing News, 42*(2), 40–42. Retrieved from https://www.hpnonline.com/no-time-rest/
54. Smigelski-Theiss, R., Gampong, M., & Kuraski, J. (2017). Weight bias and psychosocial implications for acute care of patients with obesity. *AACN Advanced Critical Care, 28*(3), 254–262. https://doi.org/10.4037/aacnacc2017446
55. Berrios, L. A. (2016). The ABCDs of managing morbidly obese patients in intensive care units. *Critical Care Nurse, 36*(5), 17–26. https://doi.org/10.4037/ccn2016671
56. Choi, S. D., & Brings, K. (2016). Work-related musculoskeletal risks associated with nurses and nursing assistants handling overweight and obese patients: A literature review. *Work, 53*(2), 439–448. https://doi.org/10.3233/WOR-152222

CHAPTER 15

Special Populations: The Pregnant Trauma Patient

Kristine K. Powell, MSN, RN, CEN, NEA-BC, FAEN

OBJECTIVES

Upon completion of this chapter, the learner will be able to:

1. Describe mechanisms of injury associated with the pregnant trauma patient and fetus.
2. Describe physiologic and developmental changes as a basis for assessment of the pregnant trauma patient and fetus.
3. Demonstrate the nursing assessment of the pregnant trauma patient and fetus.
4. Plan appropriate interventions for the pregnant trauma patient and fetus.
5. Evaluate the effectiveness of nursing interventions for the pregnant trauma patient and fetus.

Introduction

Resuscitation priorities for the injured pregnant patient are identical to those for the nonpregnant patient.[1] Assessment of the pregnant trauma patient, however, is complicated by maternal anatomic and physiologic adaptations designed to nourish the second patient, the fetus. During the resuscitative phase of treatment, pregnancy should not limit or restrict any diagnostic or pharmacologic treatment.[2,3] Indeed, optimal resuscitation of the mother affords the best fetal outcome.[4] It is important to access obstetric consultation in the resuscitation process[4] as the trauma team simultaneously manages two patients—the mother and the fetus. The Emergency Nurses Association recommends routine needs assessments, specialized education, training, and competencies, and policies and procedures to support emergency nurses in providing the expected standards of care.[5]

Epidemiology

Trauma is not only the leading cause of death among women of childbearing age, it is the leading non-obstetric cause of maternal death and disability during pregnancy.[1,2] It is estimated that 7% of all pregnancies are complicated by trauma, with death occurring in 6% to 7% of the population of injured mothers.[4] The hormonal and physiologic differences during the gestational period appear to provide a survival advantage to the injured mother over her nonpregnant injured peers.[2] Pregnancy alters the pattern of injury, and the gravid patient is more prone to abdominal trauma as gestation progresses.

Head injury and hemorrhagic shock remain the leading causes of maternal death. The most common cause of fetal death is maternal death. Fetal mortality rates are as high as 61%; in the presence of maternal shock, this rate may increase to 80%.[4] Evidence suggests that premature delivery, low birth weight, and fetal demise are post-traumatic issues, even when the mother experiences no or minor injuries.[2] Minor trauma accounts for as many as 50% of fetal deaths.[1]

Mechanisms of Injury and Biomechanics

Blunt trauma is responsible for the vast majority of maternal injuries, and occurs 10 times more often in this population than penetrating trauma.[2] The most common mechanisms of injury (MOIs) include motor vehicle collisions (MVCs), falls, and violence.[1] MVCs and penetrating trauma are responsible for the highest proportion of maternal deaths.[2] Falls, which become increasingly common as pregnancy progresses, account for the majority of minor injuries. The incidence of intentional injury from interpersonal violence rises during pregnancy, ultimately occurring in as many as 20% of all pregnancies.[1] Penetrating trauma from gunshot wounds (GSWs) or stab wounds may occur during interpersonal violence and suicide attempts.[1] As the pregnancy progresses, the growing uterus is often targeted with direct impact or penetrating trauma.[1] MOIs such as falls or MVC might also be caused by pregnancy-related pathology (e.g., seizure from pregnancy-induced hypertension).[3]

The potential for direct injury to the fetus increases with each trimester. With blunt maternal abdominal trauma or pelvic fractures, it is important to assess for fetal injuries, including skull fractures and intracranial hemorrhage. Clavicle and long-bone injuries may also occur in utero. GSWs to the maternal abdomen and uterus are frequently associated with fetal injury and death.

Anatomic and Physiologic Changes During Pregnancy as a Basis for Assessment Findings

Anatomic and physiologic changes in pregnancy can confound the typical assessment findings associated with trauma. Understanding these changes is critical to the accurate assessment and evaluation of the pregnant trauma patient.

Cardiovascular Changes

Cardiovascular changes include the following:

- Pregnancy results in a hypervolemic, hyperdynamic state. Total blood volume increases, improving maternal tolerance to hemorrhage. The pregnant patient can lose as much as 30% to 40% of her circulating volume before a significant drop in blood pressure occurs.[2]
- Resting heart rate increases 10 to 20 beats per minute to help meet the increased metabolic demands of mother and fetus and results in increased cardiac output.[6] Patients with heart rates greater than 100 beats per minutes are assessed for shock or other causes of tachycardia.[3]
- Increased hormonal levels (estrogen, progesterone) cause vasodilation, resulting in a decrease in systemic vascular resistance and pulmonary vascular resistance.[6] Peripheral resistance decreases, causing a small decrease in systolic blood pressure and a more marked decrease in diastolic blood pressure. The pregnant patient in shock may appear warm and dry due to this vasodilation.
- Supine hypotension syndrome (aortocaval compression) may occur after 20 weeks' gestation as the aorta and inferior vena cava are compressed by the uterus and its contents when the patient is supine. Venous return decreases, and cardiac output falls.[1-3] The patient may report acute nausea and dizziness, appearing pale and diaphoretic.
- Increased blood flow to the uterus and placenta and engorged pelvic vessels increase the risk of retroperitoneal hemorrhage with maternal pelvic fractures.[1]
- Catecholamine-mediated vasoconstriction of uterine vessels in response to hemorrhage shunts blood to the mother and away from the fetus. Fetal hypoperfusion, evidenced by fetal tachycardia or bradycardia and changes in fetal movement, can occur before signs of maternal shock become apparent.

Respiratory Changes

Respiratory changes include the following:

- Capillary engorgement of the upper respiratory passages increases the risk of nasopharyngeal bleeding and upper airway obstruction.
- Minute ventilation—the amount of air inhaled and exhaled in 1 minute—increases as respiratory rate and tidal volume—the amount of air moved in and out with each breath—increase.
- Oxygen consumption increases, placing the mother and fetus at increased risk for hypoxia.
- As the gravid uterus presses on the diaphragm, functional residual capacity decreases. In turn, the pregnant patient breathes at a faster rate, decreasing the partial pressure of carbon dioxide (PCO_2) levels and resulting in a state of respiratory alkalosis.[3,6]

- The diaphragm is pushed upward by the expanding uterus, and chest tube placement is one to two intercostal spaces higher.[7,8]

Hematologic Changes

Hematologic changes include the following:

- By week 30 of a pregnancy, the amount of circulating plasma has increased to 30% to 50% above its original volume, resulting in a dilutional or physiologic anemia and a proportional decrease in hematocrit.[3,6]
- An increase in fibrinogen levels and clotting factors results in a hypercoagulable state that increases the risk for thromboembolism and DIC.[1,2]

Gastrointestinal Changes

Gastrointestinal changes include the following:

- The abdominal organs are displaced laterally and cephalad by the enlarging uterus.
- The abdominal wall muscles are stretched and lax and may mask typical findings of guarding and rigidity.[4] Abdominal palpation is less reliable.
- Bowel sounds are less audible.
- The prolonged emptying time of the gastrointestinal tract increases the risk of aspiration.[2,3]
- An increase in gastric secretions makes the gravid patient more prone to gastric reflux, passive regurgitation, and aspiration.

Renal Changes

Renal changes include the following:

- Urinary stasis increases the risk for urinary tract infection.
- Urinary frequency increases due to the increase of renal blood flow and resulting increased glomerular filtration rate.[6] The mother feels additional pressure as the uterus compresses the bladder.

Musculoskeletal Changes

Musculoskeletal changes include the following:

- Softening and relaxation of the sacral ligaments and pubic symphysis make the pelvis more flexible.
- The widening pelvis and heavy abdomen results in an unsteady gait, predisposing the gravid patient to falls.

Selected Injuries and Emergencies

The selected injuries and emergencies to the pregnant patient and fetus discussed here include preterm labor, abruptio placentae, uterine rupture, and maternal cardiopulmonary arrest/fetal delivery.

Preterm Labor

Preterm labor is the most common obstetric complication in the pregnant trauma patient, occurring in as many as 25% of patients. Contractions are usually noted in alert patients but may go undetected in unconscious or intubated patients. Common causes of premature labor include placental abruption, hypoxia, and hypovolemia.[8] Assessment findings for preterm labor include the following:

- More than six uterine contractions per hour
- Abdominal or low back pain, pressure, or cramping
- Vaginal bloody show or bleeding
- Rupture of amniotic membranes
- Cervical dilation and/or effacement

Interventions for preterm labor include ongoing monitoring of fetal heart rate and uterine contractions, admission or transfer to a tertiary care unit, and neonatology consultation.[7] Tocolytic agents such as magnesium sulfate or terbutaline may be effective in halting preterm labor in the hemodynamically stable patient. With preterm labor or high risk of preterm labor at 24 or more weeks' gestation, the administration of betamethasone for fetal lung maturation is considered even with minor trauma.[1]

Abruptio Placentae

Abruptio placentae, or placental abruption, is the premature separation of a portion of the placenta from the uterine wall, which disrupts maternal–fetal circulation. Acceleration/deceleration forces can shear the relatively inelastic placenta from the elastic uterus, resulting in abruption. The effects on the fetus depend on the amount of functional placenta that remains attached to the uterine wall. Any blunt abdominal trauma places the pregnant patient at risk. Maternal mortality is low; however, fetal mortality rates are higher with placental abruption than any other cause pregnancy-related injury.[8] Placental abruption may also cause premature labor.[7]

Assessment findings for abruptio placentae include the following[9]:

- Dark red vaginal bleeding (amount is variable and may be absent due to concealed hemorrhage)
- Abdominal or back pain (sudden onset, sharp, constant)
- Fetal distress (alteration in fetal heart rate and rhythm)
- Uterine irritability and rigidity with tetanic contractions (board-like uterus)

- Preterm labor
- Maternal shock presentation disproportionate to the amount of visible vaginal bleeding
- Rising fundal height
- DIC developing as late as 48 hours after the initial trauma

Interventions for placental abruption include close monitoring of maternal vital signs for a progressing shock condition, aggressive management of hypovolemic shock, ongoing monitoring of the fetal heart rate and uterine contractions, and admission or transfer to a tertiary care unit with appropriate consultations to obstetrics and neonatology providers. Sonography may be a possibility, but is not considered a reliable test for placental abruption and should not delay treatment.[7] Serial coagulation studies will assist with recognizing DIC.[7] In extreme cases, an emergent transfer to the operating room for cesarean section may improve maternal survival with a nonviable fetus or may improve maternal and fetal survival even if premature delivery becomes necessary.[7]

Uterine Rupture

Actual tearing or laceration of the uterus is rare,[8] but may occur in patients with extreme compression injury or with a history of prior cesarean sections. Uterine rupture is associated with high maternal and fetal mortality.[1,8]

Assessment findings for uterine rupture include the following[8]:

- Sudden onset of sharp abdominal or suprapubic pain
- Asymmetry of the uterus (possible to palpate fetal parts outside the uterus)
- Maternal shock
- Slowing or absent fetal heart tones
- Vaginal bleeding (may or may not be present)

With uterine rupture, fetal survival is rare. Aggressive shock management and emergent laparotomy with bleeding control are needed to improve the chance of maternal survival.[7]

Maternal Cardiopulmonary Arrest/Fetal Delivery

If any moribund patient is at 24 weeks' gestation (the accepted standard age of fetal viability) or later, it is important to consider a perimortem cesarean section.[2] Delivery of the fetus may improve the effectiveness of resuscitative efforts when the uterus is no longer gravid and potentially causing aortocaval compression.[7,10] Estimation of gestational age and assessment of fetal heart activity can be rapidly obtained while cardiopulmonary resuscitation (CPR) is being performed.

To optimize the fetal outcome, the American Heart Association recommends that cesarean section be initiated within 4 minutes of maternal arrest[1] and that the fetus be delivered within 5 minutes of any unsuccessful maternal resuscitative attempts.[10] It is essential that a team capable of neonatal resuscitation be present.[1] Begin basic life support and advanced life support protocols and continue them throughout the procedure.[10] Remember the following points when performing CPR on a pregnant patient:

- Perform chest compressions higher on the sternum, slightly above the center of the sternum.
- Displace the uterus laterally during chest compressions to minimize aortocaval compression for any pregnant patient with gestational age greater than 20 weeks or if the fundal height is above the level of the umbilicus.[10]

Nursing Care of the Pregnant Trauma Patient

Nursing care of the pregnant trauma patient begins with triage and prioritization.

Triage and Prioritization

A valid and reliable triage method is used to prioritize patients in the emergency care setting. The Maternal Fetal Triage Index (MFTI), which was developed by the Association of Women's Health, Obstetric and Neonatal Nurses (AWHONN), is a valid and reliable five-level triage tool that may assist in the triage of obstetric trauma patients.[5,11]

Primary Survey

See Chapter 3, "Initial Assessment," for the systematic approach to care of the trauma patient. The following assessment parameters are specific to pregnant trauma patients.

C: Circulation

Position the patient on the side to prevent supine hypotension from aortocaval compression if she is greater than 20 weeks' gestation. A 15-degree tilt of the long board or lateral displacement of the uterus can release pressure on the inferior vena cava.[1,3,4,7] The left lateral position is preferred, but tilting to either side may be beneficial if the patient has injuries that interfere with left lateral positioning. Displacing the uterus off the vena cava may increase cardiac output by as much as 30%.[1]

Secondary Survey

The secondary survey begins with the history.

H: History

Ask these questions when taking the patient's history:

- What was the MOI?
  - For events related to MVCs:
    - Was the patient wearing a safety restraint device?
    - How was the restraint positioned?
  - For falls:
    - What was the height of the fall?
    - What was the surface on which the patient landed?
    - Which body part impacted the surface?
- When was the last normal menstrual period? Consider the possibility of pregnancy in any female of childbearing age.[2,7]
- When is the expected date of confinement (EDC)? To estimate the EDC, count back 3 months from the first day of the last known menstrual period and add 7 days.
- Which problems or complications have occurred during this or other pregnancies?
- Is there a possibility of more than one fetus?
- Is there vaginal bleeding?
- Are uterine contractions or abdominal pain present?
- Is there fetal activity?
  - If available, begin monitoring as soon as possible to trend the fetal heart rate.
- Is there a suspicion that injuries have been caused by interpersonal violence?

H: Head-to-Toe Assessment

Inspect for the following:

- The shape and contour of the abdomen: A change in shape may indicate concealed hemorrhage or uterine rupture.
- Signs of fetal movement.
- Vaginal bleeding or the presence of amniotic fluid around the perineum.
  - The patient may describe having had a sudden gush of fluid. This may be an indication of a spontaneous bladder void or premature rupture of the amniotic membranes.
- Crowning or any abnormal fetal presentation at the vaginal opening.
  - Prolapse of the cord is rare. If present, relieve cord compression immediately. If positioning the mother to relieve pressure on the cord is contraindicated, manual displacement of the presenting part of the cord may be needed.

Auscultate for the following:

- Fetal heart tones and rate
  - The pregnant patient, owing to her increase in circulating blood volume, can better compensate for blood loss. Fetal distress may be the first indication of maternal shock.
  - Fetal heart rate is an indicator of the well-being of both the mother and the fetus. The normal range for fetal heart rate is between 120 and 160 beats per minute. Fetal heart tones may be heard using a Doppler ultrasound by 10 weeks' gestation.[12(p234)]
  - Continuous fetal monitoring (cardiotocography) is recommended for all pregnant patients of more than 20 weeks' gestation to assess fetal well-being. Abnormal fetal heart rate may also serve as an early warning of maternal decompensation.[2]

Palpate for the following:

- The height of the fundus
  - Fundal height is an indicator of gestational age. The fundus is measured in centimeters from the symphysis pubis to the top of the fundus and approximates the number of weeks' gestation. The fundal height reaches the symphysis at 12 weeks, the umbilicus at 20 weeks, and the costal margin at 36 weeks (**Figure 15-1**).
  - Fundal height may be elevated with a concealed intrauterine bleed from placental abruption.[9]
  - Generally, a fundal height indicating 23 or more weeks' gestation is consistent with a viable fetus.[8]
- Tenderness or contractions of the uterus or abdomen
- Fetal parts outside the uterus

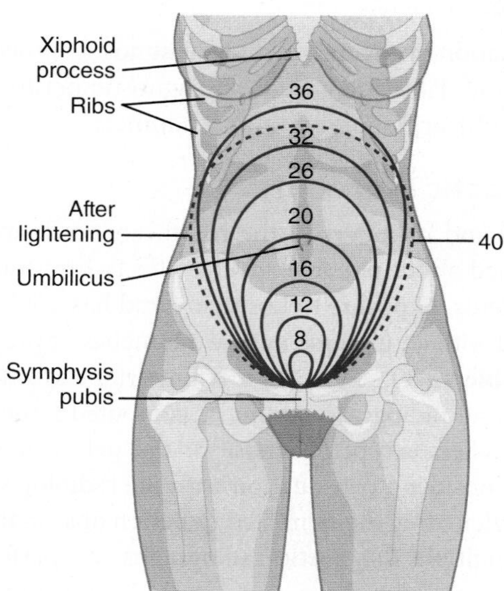

Figure 15-1 *Uterine size and location reflecting gestational age.*

Interventions

Maternal stabilization is the priority with a pregnant trauma patient, so the initial interventions are focused on resuscitation of the mother. Interventions specific to the pregnant trauma patient include the following:

- Administer O-negative blood products to avoid alloimmunization in Rh-negative mothers. When available, type and cross-matched blood may be administered.[12]
- Obtain obstetric consultation in all cases of injury in pregnant patients.[1,4] A multidisciplinary team approach is recommended, in which team members have defined roles and follow established protocols.[1]
- Monitor fetal heart rate and uterine contractions in all pregnancies greater than 20 weeks' gestation.
  - Initiate continuous fetal monitoring (cardiotocography) early in the resuscitation of the mother for pregnancies at 20 weeks' gestation or more.[2]
  - Cardiotocography monitors both the fetal heart rate and uterine contractions.
  - It is essential that a healthcare provider experienced in the interpretation of fetal monitoring be present to assist in the care of the patient.
  - An abnormal fetal heart rate response to uterine contractions may be the result of maternal hypovolemia or fetal hypoxia from underlying pathology such placental separation or uterine rupture.
  - Continue fetal monitoring for a minimum of 6 hours for any viable pregnancy[4] and up to 24 hours if there are abnormal findings.[1,3,7]

Reevaluation

Reevaluation measures include diagnostic procedures, ultrasound, laboratory studies, diagnostic peritoneal lavage (DPL), and some additional adjuncts.

Diagnostic Procedures

Patients and members of the healthcare team are often concerned about possible adverse effects from radiation on the fetus. Exposure to less than 5 rad has not been associated with an increase in fetal anomalies or pregnancy loss (**Table 15-1**).[4] Even so, it is important to shield the fetus for all radiographic films or computed tomography (CT) studies, except for those of the pelvis or lumbar spine. Consider a consultation with the radiologist to assist in calculating the estimated radiation dose to the fetus when multiple diagnostic radiographs are performed.[4] Imaging procedures not associated with ionizing radiation are recommended instead of radiographs whenever possible.[4,8]

TABLE 15-1 Estimated Fetal Exposure for Various Radiographic Studies

Examination Type	Estimated Fetal Dose per Examination (rad)
Plain Radiograph	
Cervical spine	0.002
Chest (two views)	0.00007
Pelvis	0.04
Thoracic spine	0.009
Lumbosacral spine	0.359
CT Scans	
Head	< 0.05
Chest	< 0.1
Abdominopelvic	2.6

Data from Barraco, R. D., Chiu, W. C., Clancy, T. V., Como, J. J., Ebert, J. J., Hess, L., & Weiss, P. M. (2010). Practice management guidelines for the diagnosis and management of injury in the pregnant patient: The EAST practice management guidelines work group. *Journal of Trauma, 69*(1), 211–214. https://doi.org/10.1097/TA.0b013e3181dbe1ea.

Ultrasound

Ultrasound involves the use of sound waves and is not a source of ionizing radiation. Uterine views are being incorporated with the focused assessment with sonography for trauma at some trauma facilities to screen for pregnancy in patients who cannot communicate or do not know if they are pregnant. A more comprehensive ultrasound may be performed during the secondary survey to determine the following:

- Gestational age
- Fetal weight
- Fetal heart rate and variability
- Placental location

Sonography has demonstrated poor sensitivity for diagnosing placental abruption, missing 50% to 80% of these injuries.[7,8]

Laboratory Studies

In addition to routine trauma laboratory studies, other laboratory studies to consider in the pregnant trauma patient include the following[9]:

- Prothrombin time and partial thromboplastin time and serial coagulation studies
- Beta human chorionic gonadotropin (βHCG)

  - It is recommended that all female patients of childbearing age with significant trauma have a pregnancy test and be shielded for radiologic imaging whenever possible.[2] βHCG in blood confirms pregnancy as early as 1 to 2 weeks after conception and in urine 2 to 4 weeks after conception.
- Kleihauer–Betke (KB) test
  - The KB serum test detects fetal red cells in the maternal circulation, indicating hemorrhage of fetal blood through the placenta. A KB analysis is recommended for all pregnant patients of more than 12 weeks' gestation.[4]
  - The KB test is important in determining the need to administer Rh immune globulin when the mother is Rh negative and the fetus is Rh positive, so as to prevent maternal alloimmunization. Studies have shown that the KB test is an important predictor of abuptio placentae and preterm labor[4]; it may also be used to determine the correct dosage of Rh immune globulin.[1,8]

Diagnostic Peritoneal Lavage

Although rarely done, DPL can be safe in pregnant trauma patients when other imaging options are not available.[3] Insert a gastric tube and urinary catheter prior to the procedure.

Additional Reevaluation Measures

Some additional diagnostics and interventions include the following:

- Perform a pelvic examination.
  - The cervix is assessed to determine if the cervical os is closed and the membranes are intact. If not, there is a risk for preterm delivery and the patient may need to be admitted.
  - Test any obvious fluid in the vaginal vault for presence of amniotic fluid. Strongly consider rupture of membranes if pH of any vaginal fluid is greater than 4.5.[12]
- Provide psychosocial support and realistic reassurance related to the well-being of the fetus; allay maternal and family concerns related to fetal safety during diagnostic procedures.[5]
- Screen the patient for intimate partner violence.[2]

Reevaluation and Post-Resuscitation Care

In addition to those assessments described in Chapter 3, reevaluation of the pregnant trauma patient includes the following steps:

- Monitor the amount of uterine and/or vaginal blood loss.
- Measure and record fundal height every 30 minutes.
- Monitor the fetal heart rate and activity and assess uterine activity.
  - Use cardiotocographic monitoring for a minimum of 6 hours in all women of greater than 20 weeks' gestation who experience trauma.[4] This monitoring is commonly initiated in the emergency department and continued in the labor and delivery or inpatient area.

Definitive Care or Transport

Prepare the patient for hospital admission, operative intervention, or transfer, as indicated. Patients who are discharged receive instructions for follow-up with an obstetrician, management of injuries, community resources, and injury prevention teaching (e.g., seat belt use, alcohol and substance abuse, and interpersonal violence risks).[2]

Summary

The consequences of trauma during pregnancy may include the following:

- Maternal or fetal injury
- Preterm labor and delivery
- Maternal or fetal hemorrhage
- Uterine rupture
- Maternal or fetal death

The pregnant trauma patient presents the team with unique challenges and responsibilities related to assessing and managing two patients—the mother and the fetus. The resuscitation priorities for the injured pregnant patient are identical to those of any injured patient. Fetal well-being is dependent on adequate blood flow to the uterus and placenta; therefore, the best chance for fetal survival is optimal resuscitation of the mother.

References

1. Pearce, C., & Martin, S. R. (2016). Trauma and considerations unique to pregnancy. *Obstetrics & Gynecology Clinics of North America, 43*(4), 791–808. https://doi.org/10.1016/j.ogc.2016.07.0083
2. Lucia, A., & Dantoni, S. E. (2016). Trauma management of the pregnant patient. *Critical Care Clinics, 32*(1), 109–117. https://doi.org/10.1016/j.ccc.2015.08.008

3. American College of Emergency Physicians. (n.d.). *Trauma in the obstetric patient: A bedside tool.* Irving, TX: Author. Retrieved from https://www.acep.org/by-medical-focus/trauma/trauma-in-the-obstetric-patient-a-bedside-tool/#sm.00001qaywj7yeld1xy3qntc0x7jmp
4. Barraco, R. D., Chiu, W. C., Clancy, T. V., Como, J. J., Ebert, J. J., Hess, L., & Weiss, P. M. (2010). Practice management guidelines for the diagnosis and management of injury in the pregnant patient: The EAST practice management guidelines work group. *Journal of Trauma, 69*(1), 211–214. https://doi.org/10.1097/TA.0b013e3181dbe1ea
5. Bush, K. (2017). *Obstetrical patients in the emergency care setting (Position statement).* Des Plaines, IL: Emergency Nurses Association. Retrieved from https://www.ena.org/docs/default-source/resource-library/practice-resources/position-statements/obpatientined.pdf?sfvrsn=e02a3d6c_10
6. Sanghavi, M., & Rutherford, J. D. (2014). Cardiovascular physiology of pregnancy. *Circulation, 130*, 1003–1008. https://doi.org/10.1161/CIRCULATIONAHA.114.009029
7. Venu, J., Chari, R., Maslovitz, S., & Farine, D. (2015). Guidelines for management of a pregnant trauma patient. *Journal of Obstetrics and Gynaecology Canada, 37*(6), 553–571. https://doi.org/10.1016/S1701-2163(15)30232-2
8. Krywko, D. M., & Bhimji, S. S. (2017). Pregnancy, trauma. *StatPearls.* Retrieved from https://www.ncbi.nlm.nih.gov/books/NBK430926/
9. Jordan, K. S. (2017). Obstetric and gynecologic emergencies. In V. Sweet (Ed.), *Emergency nursing core curriculum* (7th ed., pp. 366–386). St. Louis, MO: Saunders.
10. Lavonas, E. J., Drennan, I. R., Gabrielli, A., Heffner, A. C., Hoyte, C. O., Orkin, A. M., Sawyer, K. N., & Donnino, M. W. (2015). Part 10: Special circumstances of resuscitation: 2015 American Heart Association guidelines update for cardiopulmonary resuscitation and emergency cardiovascular care. *Circulation, 132*, S501–S518. https://doi.org/10.1161/CIR.0000000000000264
11. American College of Obstetricians and Gynecologists Committee on Obstetric Practice. (2016). Hospital-based triage of obstetric patients (Committee Opinion No. 667). Retrieved from https://www.acog.org/-/media/Committee-Opinions/Committee-on-Obstetric-Practice/co667.pdf?dmc=1&ts=20170606T1551428741
12. American College of Surgeons. (2018). Trauma in pregnancy and intimate partner violence. In *Advanced trauma life support: Student course manual* (10th ed., pp. 226–239). Chicago, IL: Author.

CHAPTER 16

Special Populations: The Interpersonal-Violence Trauma Patient

Patricia A. Normandin, DNP, RN, CEN, CPN, CPEN, FAEN

OBJECTIVES

Upon completion of this chapter, the learner will be able to:

1. Identify the risk factors for and types of interpersonal violence.
2. Discuss assessment priorities in the care of the patient experiencing interpersonal violence.
3. Apply appropriate medical and forensic interventions for the patient who has experienced interpersonal violence.
4. Summarize the role of the nurse in support of prevention programs for interpersonal violence.

Introduction

Interpersonal violence is a global epidemic. More than 1.3 million people worldwide die each year from all forms of violence. Between the year 2000 and the publication of its report on this subject in 2014, the World Health Organization (WHO) estimates 6 million people globally were killed in acts of interpersonal violence. This makes homicide a more frequent cause of death than all wars combined during this period. Nonfatal interpersonal violence is significantly more common than homicide and has serious and lifelong health and social consequences for its survivors.[1] WHO also estimates that tens of thousands of survivors of interpersonal violence seek emergency care for injuries sustained from encounters involving interpersonal violence.

As of 2018, statistics show that in 1 year, more than 10 million men and women are physically abused by their intimate partner. This equates to about 20 people per minute who are survivors of physical intimate-partner violence (IPV). During their lifetime, 1 in 3 women experience IPV and 1 in 4 men experience IPV.[2]

Violence is the intentional use of physical power or force, actual or threatened, against a person (self or other) or community. This chapter focuses on interpersonal violence, which is specifically violence between or against family members, intimate partners, friends, acquaintances, and strangers that carries an extreme probability that death, injury, psychological damage, poor development, or deprivation will occur. Interpersonal violence includes elder abuse, child maltreatment, violence against women (such as sexual violence and IPV), and youth violence (gang association). Cultural considerations may influence the type of interpersonal violence that occurs, although this type of violence occurs across all cultures and environments.[1] People who experience interpersonal violence do not always report the actual mechanism of injury, but are often treated in the emergency department (ED). Trauma nurses and teams have the unique opportunity to assess for and identify these injuries, protect and care for these patients in a safe environment, and advocate for their well-being.

In addition, emergency nurses must remember to wear a forensic lens during care of the interpersonal-violence trauma patient. Caring for this particularly vulnerable population requires a paradigm shift in identification, terminology, treatment, referral, and medico-legal documentation. It begins with education and awareness, recognition of patterns of injuries, preservation and collection of evidence, documentation, and reporting to appropriate jurisdictional law enforcement agencies, as aspects of patient assessment and care may pertain to criminal investigations.[3] It always involves every interdisciplinary trauma team member understanding and applying the trauma-informed framework.[4]

Epidemiology

WHO has identified two distinct categories of interpersonal violence[1]:

- *Family and intimate-partner violence* typically occurs within a family unit or between partners. It includes child maltreatment, IPV, and elder maltreatment.
- *Community violence* occurs between people who may be strangers or acquainted but are not related. It includes youth violence, random violence, rape or sexual violence, and institutional violence in schools, workplaces, prisons, and care facilities.

Some types of violence classified as family/intimate-partner violence or community violence (**Figure 16-1**[5]) have similarities and may fall under both categories. For example, sex trafficking (under community violence) can involve a stranger or an intimate partner or child. These crimes are similar in the use of power and control by the perpetrator as a method of abuse. Psychological coercion, physical assaults, isolation, and other abusive power strategies are utilized by perpetrators of both IPV and trafficking to maintain control over the victims.[6]

Risk Factors

Interpersonal violence is seen across all cultures and environments. However, some characteristics place certain

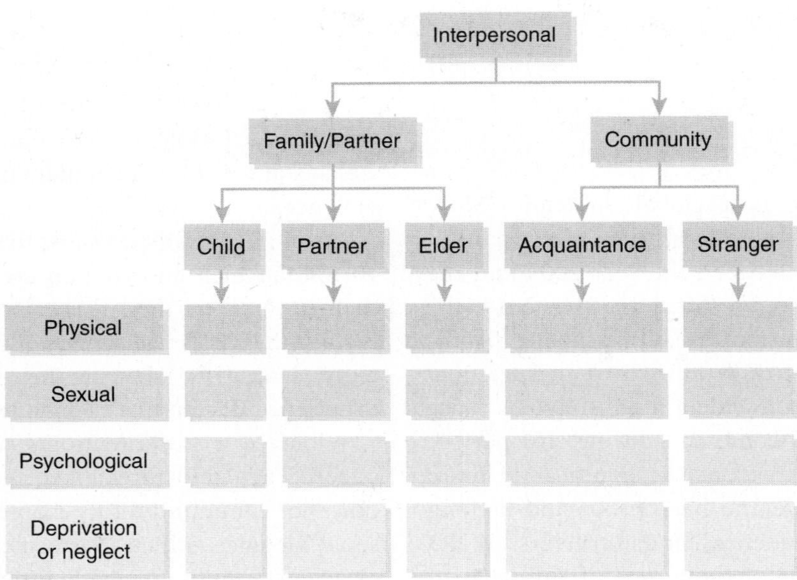

Figure 16-1 *Typology of interpersonal violence.*

Reproduced from Violence Prevention Alliance. (2018). *Definition and typology of vilence.* Geneva: World Health Organization. Retrieved from http://www.who.int/violenceprevention/approach/definition/en/.

people at higher risk for being subjected to this type of violence. **Table 16-1** lists some of the individual, relational, community, and societal risk factors. Trauma team members must maintain a high index of suspicion for identifying interpersonal violence in high risk populations.[1-4,8-13]

Patterns of Abusive Behavior

The Power and Control Wheel (**Figure 16-2**), developed by Domestic Abuse Intervention Programs and produced and distributed by the National Center on Domestic and Sexual Violence, is a powerful tool for understanding the full picture of the types and patterns of abusive behavior.[14] The Power and Control Wheel describes behavior abusers use to gain power and control over another person.[15] Power and control can even result from infrequent assault. The threat of future violence is enough to enable the abuser to exert control.

Types of Interpersonal Violence

To understand interpersonal violence, it is useful to consider the various types.[16]

Child Maltreatment

Child maltreatment is the neglect or abuse of a person younger than 18 years of age. It involves emotional or physical abuse, negligence, commercial exploitation, or other abusive or exploitative behavior.[17,18] Children's exposure to IPV is often included as a form of child maltreatment.[16]

Child abuse and neglect can be defined as any act or patterns of acts that are committed or omitted by parent or a caregiver (teacher, coach, clergy, person of authority over child) that results in harm, threat of harm, or potential harm to a child.[19] Acts of commission, which are intentional or deliberate, are words or actions that can cause harm, threat of harm, or potential harm, even if harm was not the intended consequence. Physical abuse, psychological abuse, and sexual abuse are examples of acts of commission. Acts of omission, or child neglect, are failure to protect from harm or potential for harm, and/or failure to provide for the child's needs. Examples include physical neglect, emotional neglect, educational neglect, inadequate supervision, exposure to violent environments, or medical and dental neglect.[19,20] Current statistics report that 676,000 children are victims of child maltreatment annually—including 1,750 child deaths from maltreatment.[21,22] Of those 676,000 children, 74.8% are victims of neglect, 18.2% are victims of physical abuse,

TABLE 16-1 Interpersonal Violence Risk Factors

Individual	Interpersonal Relationship	Community and Social	Society or Macro-Level Factors
Personal attitude and beliefs that tolerate IPV Age › Youth due to immaturity › Adolescent dating population Pregnancy, child birth, postpartum Gender › Women age 12–25 years Vulnerable persons › Linguistic isolation › Minority ethnic status › Cultural beliefs such as patriarchal gender beliefs, collectivism, power distance › Prior abuse history › Poverty or inadequate resources	Relationship with peers involving dominance and control Family violence Exposure to interpersonal violence as a child Human trafficking › Runaways › Rural area › Inadequate support by family including migration › Labor trafficking	Social vulnerability[8] › Poverty › Lack of access to services or transportation › Crowded housing Schools with economic disadvantage and lack of safety Children in foster care Children involved in human trafficking	Gender inequality › Belief in traditional gender roles and norms

(continues)

TABLE 16-1 Interpersonal Violence Risk Factors *(continued)*

Individual	Interpersonal Relationship	Community and Social	Society or Macro-Level Factors
Antisocial personality traits › Substance use disorders › Heavy alcohol use › Behavioral health disorders Special populations › People covered by the Americans with Disabilities Act, such as the deaf and blind › Lesbian, gay, bisexual, transgender, queer or questioning individuals › Institutionalized individuals: · Nursing homes · Assisted living facilities · Correctional facilities/ juvenile system Isolation › Unemployment › Homeless › Lack of education › Marginalized persons	Relationship with Partners › Marital conflict › Unstable marriages › Divorce › Separation › Financial stress › One partner displaying dominance and control in the relationship	Workplaces › Low economic social situations Neighborhoods › Poverty › Overcrowding › Weak community response to IPV	Religious or cultural beliefs Society norms Economic or social policies

Abbreviation: IPV, intimate-partner violence.

Data from Agency for Persons with Disabilities. (2017). Common signs and symptoms of abuse, neglect, and exploitation. Retrieved from http://apd.myflorida.com/zero-tolerance/common-signs/; Beal, J. A. (2017). Healthcare of the transgender youth still inadequate . . . still at risk. *Journal of Maternal/Child Nursing, 42*(5), 296. https://doi.org/10.1097/NMC.0000000000000362; Campana, D. (2018). Hidden in plain sight: Labor trafficking victims in the ED. *ENA Connection, 42*(1), 16–19; Centers for Disease Control and Prevention. (2018). Social Vulnerability Index (SVI) (Factsheet). Retrieved from https://svi.cdc.gov/Documents/FactSheet/SVIFactSheet.pdf; Chisolm-Straker, M., & Stoklosa, H. (2017). *Human trafficking is a public health issue.* Cham, Switzerland: Springer; Mills, T. J. (2015, February). Elder abuse. *Medscape*. Retrieved from https://emedicine.medscape.com/article/805727-overview; National Coalition Against Domestic Violence. (2018). Domestic violence national statistics. Retrieved from www.ncadv.org/statistcs; Tracy, E. E., & Macias-Konstantopoulos, M. (2018, March 16). Human trafficking: Identification and evaluation in the health care setting. *UpToDate*. Retrieved from https://www.uptodate.com/contents/human-trafficking-identification-and-evaluation-in-the-health-care-setting.

8.5% are victims of sexual abuse, and 6.9% are victims of psychological maltreatment.[21] See Chapter 12, "Special Populations: Pediatric Trauma," for additional physical signs of child maltreatment.

Intimate-Partner Violence

Commonly referred to as domestic violence, IPV is a grave public health problem that affects more than 10 million people annually.[2] Domestic violence is the willful intimidation, physical assault, battery, sexual assault, and/or other abusive behavior as part of a systematic pattern of power and control perpetrated by one intimate partner against another. It includes physical violence, sexual violence, threats, and emotional/psychological abuse. The frequency and severity of domestic violence varies dramatically,[2] as it includes both acts of violence or threats of violence by a current or former intimate partner.[19] In the United States, 1 in 3 women and 1 in 4 men have been victims of some form of physical violence by an intimate partner.[2] On a global scale, the prevalence

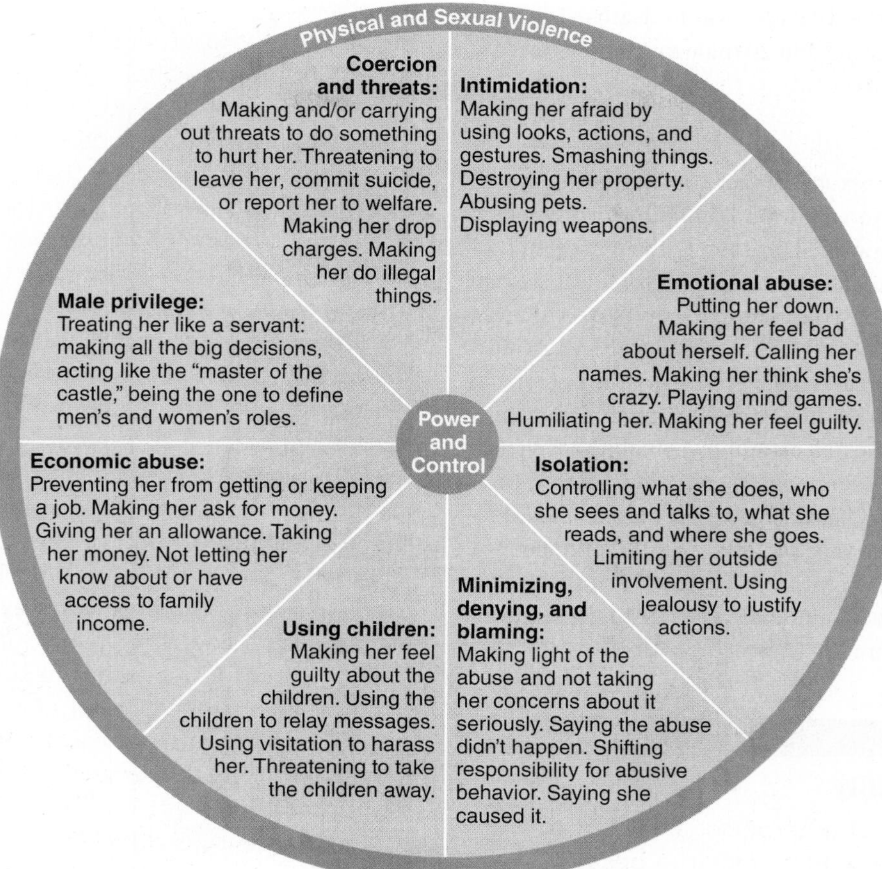

Figure 16-2 *The Power and Control Wheel.*

Reproduced from National Center on Domestic and Sexual Violence. *Power and control wheel.* Austin, TX: Author. Retrieved from http://www.ncdsv.org/images/powercontrolwheelnoshading.pdf.

of IPV averages 30%. The statistics are higher in low- to middle-income regions (up to 37%) around the globe, whereas countries in high-income regions fall just below the average (23%).[23]

Physical Assault

Women between the ages of 18 and 34 years are the most common victims of IPV. A majority of physical abuse is perpetrated by dating partners rather than spouses.[2] Approximately 41% of female IPV survivors and 14% of male IPV survivors experience some form of physical injury related to their experience of relationship violence.[24]

Victims are likely to incur injuries to the head, neck, or face. They are also likely to have injuries in multiple locations, including the torso or limbs.[25] Types of physical violence cover a wide range of actions, such as pushing, slapping, punching, choking, arm twisting, hair pulling, and slamming against a wall.

Strangulation is recognized as the most predictive factor for risk of homicide.[26] This type of severe violence is related to a 7.5-fold increased risk of homicide.[27] The most common form of strangulation in IPV is applied by using the hands, forearms, or other limbs to place pressure over the neck of the victim. This tactic is often repetitive and used by the perpetrator to subdue the victim and demonstrate power/control. Victims who experience strangulation often do not seek medical treatment—because injuries are usually not visible—unless they are referred by law enforcement for forensic evaluation.[28]

Having a partner with an alcohol use disorder issue and having a partner with mental illness are major risk factors for IPV. A victim whose partner misuses alcohol is 3.6 times more likely to be assaulted by the partner.[25] The consumption of alcohol during a dispute is likely to decrease inhibitions and increase impulsivity, thereby creating an opportunity for an argument to escalate into a physical altercation. Drinking may or may not be the cause of the violence, but alcohol-related disorders could introduce more tension into the relationship, which can lead to aggression and violence, as well as presence of a weapon in the home.[29]

In the extreme case, IPV can lead to death—1 in 3 female murder victims and 1 in 20 male murder victims are killed by intimate partners.[2]

Sexual Assault

Sexual assault is any sexual contact—including attempted rape, actual penetration of the body, fondling or any sexual touching—that is unwanted, or forcing the person to perform sexual acts. It can include child sexual abuse, sexual assault of men and boys, intimate-partner sexual violence, incest, and drug-facilitated sexual assault (DFSA). Almost half of female (46.7%) and male (44.9%) victims of rape in the United States are raped by an acquaintance. Acquaintance rape is forced sexual assault by someone the victim knows—for example, someone the victim is related to, is in a relationship with, has dated, or just met. Of these victims, 45.4% of female rape victims and 29% of male rape victims are raped by an intimate partner.[2] The survivor is less likely to report acquaintance rape due to the relationship with the perpetrator.[30]

NOTE

Tonic Immobility

Many survivors of interpersonal violence find themselves feeling guilt or shame because they "froze" or didn't "fight back." This initial "freeze" response is triggered by the amygdala, which is responsible for emotions such as fear. It signals the brain to prepare for a sympathetic response associated with the fight-or-flight response. Freezing can be a short response if the prefrontal cortex, which is responsible for rational thought and planned responses, can inhibit the amygdala's reactivity to fear.

The victim of sexual assault is sometimes able to make attempts to fight back, plan an escape route, or at least scream to alert others. However, the information that is transferred into the victim's brain during an assault can be highly traumatic, threatening, and perceived as entrapment; the cortisol and norepinephrine may be at such high levels that they actually impair cognitive functioning of the prefrontal cortex. The victim is unable to logically plan steps to defend or remove themselves. In such a case, the body "freezes" by eliciting a temporary unresponsiveness to external stimuli. This physiologic state, called tonic immobility, is marked by decreased respirations, eye closure, and muscular paralysis. Similar to freezing, it is characterized by the absence of movement in response to severe threat, but occurs after fight, flight, and freezing are no longer optimal for survival.[31] Tonic immobility is an involuntary motor and vocal inhibition reaction, which features changes in heart rate and body temperature. Memory and learning, however, remain intact. Approximately 50% to 70% of rape victims experience tonic immobility during a sexual assault.[32]

If the state of tonic immobility is not viable, the parasympathetic nervous system remains active and takes over in the stage of collapse. Endogenous opioids are also released in very high levels and block the physical and emotional pain in preparation for a mental state of surrender, impending injury, or death. Collapsed immobility can cause the heart rate and blood pressure to decrease, so that the victim may lose consciousness or feel "sleepy" or faint during the assault. It is common to encounter a survivor whose affect is flat or unemotional after an assault; this response is a protective mechanism to minimize the risk of injury that would otherwise occur with fighting back.

The mere size difference often found between men and women, even without an expressed threat or weapon, can elicit this instantaneous and natural response. It is important for the trauma nurse to avoid placing blame on the survivor, who may feel shame or guilt for "failing to resist." It is also expected that the survivor may not recall the details of the event immediately after the assault. Catecholamines and glucocorticoid levels may remain high in the aftermath of such trauma, and their elevations are correlated to impaired memory retrieval.[33]

Depression and post-traumatic stress disorder (PTSD) are closely associated with the experience of tonic immobility in an assault.[32]

Interpersonal Violence During Pregnancy

Pregnancy can be a particularly vulnerable time for women experiencing interpersonal violence. A number of physical, emotional, social, and economic changes can add stressors during a time of intense personal and relational transition. Abuse has been known to begin or, if already present, to escalate during pregnancy.[34] The prevalence of physical and sexual abuse among pregnant women in general is approximately 3% to 30%, with some research showing higher rates in lower-income groups.[34]

Overall, IPV during pregnancy is considered a significant public health issue, as it is associated with adverse pregnancy outcomes and negative consequences for both mother and child.[34] Pregnant women who are experiencing IPV are twice as likely to delay prenatal care and more likely to experience adverse outcomes including low birth weight, preterm delivery, and placental abruption, although there is also increased risk of miscarriage/abortion, fetal injury, and perinatal maternal death.[34,35] Extremes of violence can also be related to pregnancy: 54.3% of pregnancy-associated suicides involve intimate-partner conflict attributable to the suicide, and 45.3% of pregnancy-associated homicides are associated with IPV.[35]

Like all IPV survivors, pregnant women are vulnerable to potential adverse mental health consequences including depression, anxiety disorders, PTSD, and suicidal ideation. Increased risky behaviors such as perinatal usage of alcohol and illicit drugs and unprotected sex are consistently associated with IPV around the time of pregnancy.[34]

Given these risks, it is important to monitor pregnant interpersonal-violence trauma patients closely for complications that can be life threatening for both mother and child. Care of the pregnant trauma patient presents a unique window of opportunity in which healthcare providers can begin to build a trusting relationship, increasing the likelihood of detection of interpersonal violence and mitigating the related negative consequences to both mother and child (see **Figure 16-3**).[36] For many women, pregnancy is the only time when they maintain regular contact with healthcare providers. Trauma nurses should have a high index of suspicion for IPV in pregnant patients with traumatic injuries, especially when red flags are noted during the physical assessment. For more information on physical assessment of the pregnant trauma patient see Chapter 15, "Special Populations: The Pregnant Trauma Patient."

Drug-Facilitated Sexual Assault

DFSA is associated with the inability of a victim to consent to a sexual act due to incapacitation from drugs and/or alcohol, whether self-administered or covertly slipped to an unsuspecting victim. Agents used in DFSA include many different substances—for example, alcohol and medications such as flunitrazepam, gamma-hydroxybutyrate, ketamine, tetrahydrozoline (Visine), phenobarbital, and promethazine.[37-40] These substances can go undetected when added to food, drink, or another substance. The effects of these drugs include sedation and amnesia, and victims often cannot resist the assault or may not be aware that a sexual act has occurred.[37] Other substances, legal or illicit, such as marijuana, benzodiazepines, cocaine, heroin, and amphetamines, can also be

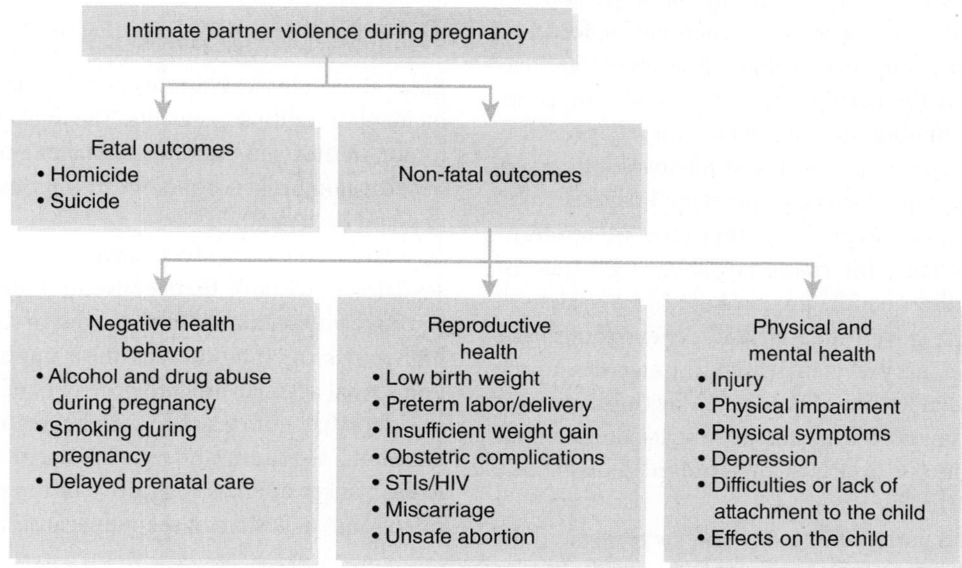

Figure 16-3 *Health outcomes of intimate-partner violence during pregnancy.*

Reproduced from World Health Organization. (2011). Intimate partner violence durng pregnancy (Information sheet). Retrieved from http://apps.who.int/iris/bitstream/handle/10665/70764/WHO_RHR_11.35_eng.pdf; jsessionid=4EC5CBA17EF2F2F32A53A1D7E44BD05C?sequence=1.

associated with sexual violence. DFSA accounts for more than half of sexual assault cases, and incidence rates are increasing in young males as well as females.[38]

Lesbian, Gay, Bisexual, and Transgender Population

Research focused on the lesbian, gay, bisexual, and transgender (LGBT) population has increased considerably in the past decades. The prevalence of IPV among LGBT individuals may be as high as or even higher than that in the general population.[41] LGBT victims encounter the same barriers to seeking assistance as are experienced by the general population. However, additional barriers unique to this population include limitations of state definitions of domestic violence that may exclude LGBT individuals and couples, the availability of LGBT-specific resources, and the personal conflict of "outing" oneself and one's partner when seeking assistance. Healthcare providers who are not aware of LGBT considerations for care can be a barrier as well. The lack of competency, knowledge, or comfort level on how to address LGBT issues can make it difficult for survivors to seek help.

Human Trafficking

Human trafficking is often described as modern-day slavery; it is a crime of exploitation of a person for forced sex or labor.[42] Human trafficking is a complex public health issue whose scope spans the globe. Sex trafficking is the recruitment, harboring, provision, transportation, soliciting, patronizing, or obtaining of a person for commercial sex acts that involves coercion or force, or involves a child younger than than 18 years of age.[4] Labor trafficking is the harboring, recruitment, provision, transportation, or obtaining of a person for labor services by using force, coercion, and fraud for involuntary servitude, debt bondage, slavery, or peonage.[4] An estimated 40.3 million people experience this type of modern-day slavery globally. International labor organizations estimate 19 million people are exploited in a variety of private industry, governmental, and rebel groups. The exact incidence and prevalence are unknown due to the inherently hidden nature of human trafficking, underreporting by survivors, variations in severity of activities, multiple definitions, and lack of standardized tracking databases.[4]

IPV and human trafficking victims can be one and the same person. The perpetrator may have an intimate relationship with the victim, and may even have a child with the victim, but then trafficks the person or both of those individuals for personal gain.[4]

Three-fourths of trafficking victims are women and girls, while 25% are children. One in six runaways in 2016 was reported by the U.S. National Center for Missing and Exploited Children to be a likely sex trafficking victim.[6,43,44]

Emergency nurses caring for trauma patients should understand that IPV and human trafficking survivors will not usually self-identify, but are among the most vulnerable patient populations receiving care in the ED.[45] **Figure 16-4** provides some additional context for understanding human trafficking.[46]

Elder Abuse

Elder abuse is an intentional act or a failure to act by another person or a caregiver that creates or causes a risk of harm to the older adult. According to the Older Americans Act of 1965, an older adult is an individual who is age 60 years or older.[47] Elder abuse is a public health concern because 1 in 10 adults older than the age of 60 years who lives at home experiences exploitation in the form of elder abuse.[47] Hundreds of thousands of elders experience abuse or neglect each year, yet these crimes go underreported. Reasons for underreporting include dementia, culture, language barriers, distrust of law enforcement, fear of losing their present living arrangement, and fear of retribution by the perpetrator.[9,48,49]

According to the Centers for Disease Control and Prevention's (CDC) Injury Center, there are six types of elder abuse: physical abuse, sexual abuse, emotional abuse, neglect, abandonment, and financial abuse.[47] For more information on elder abuse, refer to Chapter 13, "Special Populations: The Geriatric Trauma Patient."

Physical/Sexual Abuse

Elder abuse physical injuries may be the result of a single incident or multiple incidents. The injuries can range from minor, in the form of minor scratches and bruises, to serious, causing broken bones, head injuries, lasting disabilities, and even death.[9,50,51]

Sexual abuse involves engaging an elder person in sexual acts without their consent.[3] Elders in communal settings with memory loss or who are nonverbal are at higher risk of being the victim of unwanted or unsolicited sexual acts. Healthcare providers or family members of elders may notice a change in behavior, wetting undergarments, blood on undergarments, or behavioral problems; bruises in areas suggestive of forced sexual acts; or infections suggestive of sexually transmitted routes.

Emotional (Psychological) Abuse

Emotional abuse is the deliberate attempt to destroy or impair a person's self-esteem or competence. It includes

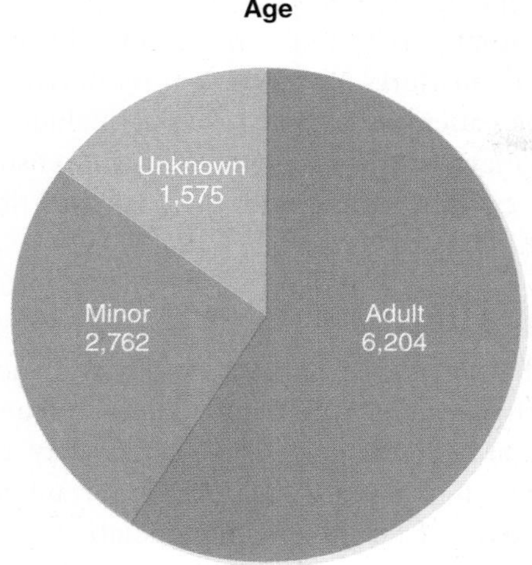

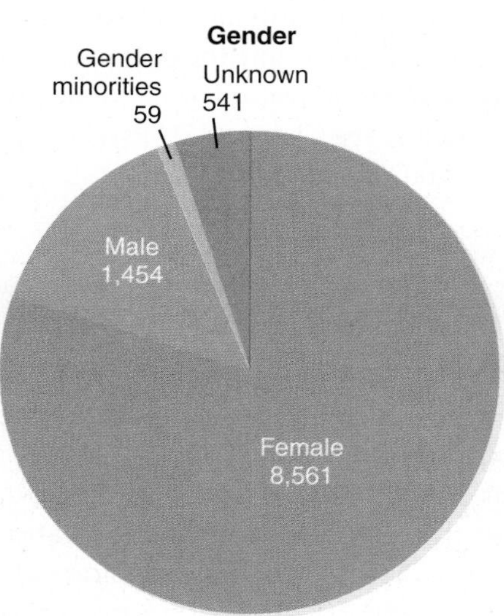

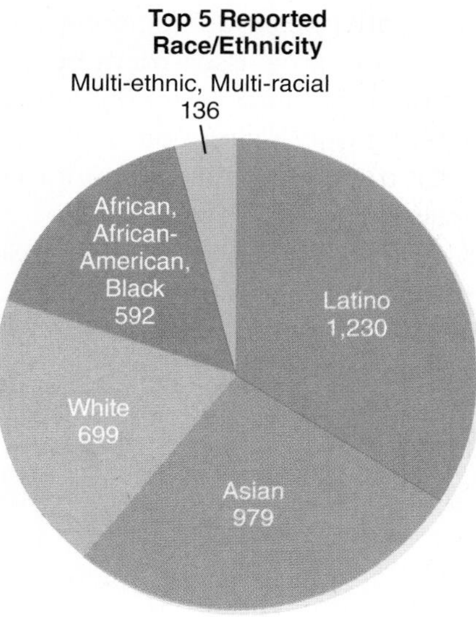

Figure 16-4 *Data from the National Human Trafficking Hotline, 2017.*

Data from Polaris. (n.d.). Share infographics from the National Human Trafficking Hotline. Retrieved form https://act.polarisproject.org/page/21744/action/1.

verbal and nonverbal insults, humiliation, or isolation. Other forms of abuse frequently include some level of emotional abuse.[13] Any persistent or unexplained change in a patient's behavior may be the result of emotional abuse.

Neglect

Neglect is the failure to provide for a person's basic needs, including food, shelter, clothing, education, and medical care, and is one of the most common forms of pediatric and elder maltreatment. Emotional neglect may be suspected, but can be very difficult to substantiate. Physical signs may be nonspecific and healthcare providers can only rely on behavioral indicators to identify a possible abusive situation.

Emotional Neglect

Unlike emotional abuse, emotional neglect occurs when caregivers withhold love and nurturing behavior and fail to meet the victim's emotional and developmental needs, including psychological care. It is particularly seen in children, but may also be seen in the elder population. Fear and passivity can accompany this type of neglect and require careful listening and sensitive probing to uncover. This type of abuse can lead to feelings of depression, hopelessness, and helplessness in individuals. Additionally, caregivers may fail to seek necessary care for an individual with emotional or behavioral problems.

Physical Neglect

Physical neglect is the failure to prevent harm to a person or to provide for that person's basic needs, such as health care, food, shelter, and supervision.[3] It may involve an older adult who is unable to care for themselves and is left unattended. It may also include failure to provide proper nutrition, to ensure seasonally appropriate clothing, or to follow up with necessary medical or dental care. If there is an expectation of care and that care is not provided by a caregiver or facility, it is neglect.

Abandonment

Abandonment occurs when a person who has assumed responsibility for providing care purposefully and permanently deserts the caregiving needs of that individual while neglecting to arrange sufficient care for the duration of the absence. The victim can be an elderly person, a person with disabilities, or a dependent. Symptoms of a victim of abandonment can include poor hygiene, malnourishment, dehydration, or unattended health problems. Victims are commonly abandoned at a hospital, a nursing facility, or even a public place.[52]

Financial Abuse

Financial abuse takes many forms. Financial exploitation commonly involves trusted persons in the life of the victim,[53] but scams and frauds committed by strangers are also common. Financial abuse can be another form of maintaining power and control over the victim (Figure 16-2).[54]

Initial Assessment for Interpersonal Violence

The initial assessment of a trauma patient specifically affected by interpersonal violence must include a trauma-informed care approach starting from the time of notification in preparation and triage. See **Box 16-1**.

Safe Care

Part of providing safe care is ensuring that the patient can receive the appropriate care and resources in a safe environment. Trauma nurses can act to provide the patient with a safe environment while in the ED by initiating security measures if necessary or reinforcing privacy during the patient's stay. Safe care also includes providing the patient with available resources to ensure there is a safe environment awaiting the patient following discharge.

Safe Practice

Due to the prevalence of interpersonal violence, especially in the trauma patient population, trauma team members are increasingly faced with safety concerns when caring for these patients. An important consideration when caring for this patient population is a security plan. Trauma nurses are also entitled to feel safe in their work environment. Identifying and addressing gaps in knowledge or skills regarding the response plan for a violent family member or visitor is vital to the protection of staff and patients. See Chapter 17, "Psychosocial Aspects of Trauma Care," for more information.

BOX 16-1 How Do I Talk to Survivors of IPV?

In talking to survivors of IPV, trauma nurses will follow these guidelines[67]:

- Provide clear explanations of the plan of care, including what to expect in the screening and assessment process.
- Approach the patient in a matter-of-fact, yet supportive manner. Be sensitive to how the patient might hear what you have to say in response to personal disclosures. Patients who have been traumatized may be more reactive even to benign or well-intended questions.
- Respect the patient's personal space. Survivors may have a particular sensitivity about their bodies, personal space, and boundaries.
- Be aware of your own emotional responses to hearing a patient's traumatic history. Hearing about the victim's experience may be very painful and can elicit strong emotions. The patient may interpret your reaction as disinterest, disgust, or some other inaccurate interpretation.
- Elicit only the information necessary. Given the lack of a therapeutic relationship in which to process the information safely, pursuing details of trauma can cause retraumatization.
- Give the patient as much personal control as possible during the assessment by:
  - Explaining the purpose for the interview and its stress-inducing potential, and clarifying that the patient has the right to refuse to answer any and all questions.
  - Providing the option of being interviewed by someone of the gender with which the patient is most comfortable.
- Avoid phrases that imply judgment.
- Allow time for the patient to process their reactions.

Healthcare providers can find negligence, abuse, or intentional injury to vulnerable patient populations extremely difficult to manage both professionally and personally. In these circumstances, a professional approach may conflict with the emotions the trauma nurse is feeling. The trauma nurse and team members are recommended to identify and evaluate their personal emotions, beliefs, values, and past experiences to determine how these perceptions may affect their attitude and care toward these patients and patient care situations. Based on the cases and situations involved, debriefings and counseling may be indicated for all involved. See Chapter 17 for additional information on compassion fatigue and workplace violence.

Specific Considerations for the Care of Patients with Physical Abuse

Special considerations for the care of patients with physical abuse are highlighted in this section.

H: History

The history of all patients looks for the following elements:

- Unreasonable delay in seeking medical attention
- Previous ED visits or hospitalization for an injury or a medical condition that might have been prevented with appropriate care
- Vague, unclear, or changing account of how the injury occurred
- Patient is accompanied by another person who acts controlling in attitude or speaks for the patient
- Poor hygiene and/or inappropriate attire
- Multiple sexually transmitted infections
- Multiple pregnancies and abortions
- Malnourishment or chronic dehydration
- Inactivity or extreme passiveness
- Untreated medical conditions such as dental caries and periodontal disease

Some red flags nurses need to consider for possible human trafficking survivors are the following[4,55,56]:

- The patient arrives at the ED without control of their own identification or no identification.
- The person bringing the patient to the ED for care does not speak the same native language of patient and appears unrelated.
- Sex trafficking survivors frequently are branded or tattooed with a dollar sign ($), the trafficker's name, or a gang name.
- Chips implanted with radiofrequency identification can also be a red flag.[51]
- A female patient has a history of multiple abortions and sexually transmitted infections.
- Migrant workers.[56]
- Workplace injuries involve lack of proper protective gear, working long hours, or heavy physical activities with limited availability of food or drink.
- The patient's pain is consistent with repetitive use injuries. Factory workers and/or sex workers may have back pain, musculoskeletal complaints, and abdominal pain.
- Runaway children are at risk for child sex trafficking, with estimates from 2016 suggesting that 1 out of 6 runaways is endangered and may be exploited.[6] Of those exploited runaway children, 86% are estimated to have run away from foster care or social services care.[6]

Some red flags nurses need to consider for child neglect and abuse are the following[16,17,57]:

- Malnourished, failure to thrive (weight below the fifth percentile), and child's physical appearance inappropriate for age
- Inappropriate reaction to injury for developmental age—for example, infants, toddlers or children failing to cry with pain
- Deficits or delays in emotional and intellectual development, especially language
- Use of self-soothing behaviors such as finger sucking, biting, scratching, or rocking by an older child
- Child who arrives to ED with immunizations incomplete or unknown—suggests neglect or that the person accompanying child is not the primary caregiver
- No explanation for the injury, discrepancy between the caregiver's and patient's accounts, or explanation inconsistent with identified injuries
- History of previous injuries, ingestions, or exposures to toxic substances

- History of being left alone, abandoned, or with inadequate supervision
- Excessive absenteeism from school or other social events or programs
- Isolation from friends and other family members
- Substance misuse
- Delinquency or repeated encounters with law enforcement
- Child in foster care
- Child in an environment characterized by IPV directed at a parent or caregiver—such behavior also puts the child at risk for abuse and is considered a form of child maltreatment

H: Head-to-Toe Assessment

When assessing the patient with suspected physical abuse, inconsistencies between the injury history and the injuries sustained should alert the trauma team to the possibility of abuse as the cause. Examples of the behaviors and injuries are discussed in the following sections.

Head Injuries

Certain types of head injuries can indicate interpersonal violence. For example, skull fractures, intracranial or extracranial bleeds, spotty balding (from hair pulling), retinal hemorrhage, or other eye injuries such as a dislocated lens or corneal laceration and dental injuries. Abusive head trauma is a serious form of child maltreatment that occurs when the child has sustained sudden shaking or other impact injuries. A head injury in an adult that is inconsistent with the history may also be suspicious.

Strangulation

Strangulation occurs when external pressure is placed on the neck, leading to reduced blood flow to the brain and/or airway closure. Occlusion of the jugular veins results in venous congestion and intracranial pressure. Carotid artery obstruction stops blood flow and impedes oxygen delivery to the brain. Pressure on the carotid sinus can cause acute bradycardia and/or cardiac arrest.

Strangulation can result in injuries to the soft tissues of the neck, esophagus, larynx, trachea, cervical spine, and the laryngeal and facial nerves.[58] Other findings include:

- Dysphonia, dysphagia, odynophagia, or dyspnea
- Neck and mastoid: ligature marks, edema, abrasions, erythema, contusions
- Petechiae in the eyelids, periorbital region, face, scalp, neck, ears, or soft palate, or under the tongue
- Subconjunctival or scleral hemorrhage
- Neurologic findings: ptosis, facial droop, unilateral weakness, loss of sensation, paralysis, or seizure
- Lung injuries: aspiration pneumonia, pulmonary edema

Bruises

Bruises are often seen in cases of interpersonal violence. Those intentionally inflicted injuries have distinguishing characteristics that can raise the index of suspicion for maltreatment:

- Unexplained bruises or welts
- Multiple or symmetric bruises or marks
- Bruises and welts to the face, mouth, neck, chest, abdomen, back, flank, thighs, or genitalia
- Bruises and welts with patterns descriptive of an object, such as a looped cord, belt buckle, boot tread, wire hanger, or hand or pinch marks
- Bruises in various stages of healing (indicating serial or repeated injury)

Burns

Correlation of the severity and pattern of the burn injury with the history provides a basis for the identification of inflicted burns.

- Burns to the lips or tongue, especially if surrounded by bruising: This may indicate forcing hot liquids.
- Burns to the rectum or perineum.
- Bilateral burns, such as a stocking-type (on the lower extremities) or glove-type (on the upper extremities) burn, with sharp lines of demarcation, indicate the victim was held down in hot liquid. In contrast, an accidental burn usually has irregular borders and splash burns.
- Sharp lines of demarcation, limited injury to the protected area, and uniform burn depth.
- Burns in the shape of an object such as a cigar or cigarette, cigarette lighter, iron, heating grate, or stove coils.

Bite Injuries

Bite injuries have specific abuse-related patterns as well:

- Ovoid patterns of bruising, abrasions, or lacerations may be indicative of a bite mark, triggering the need for the patient to be screened and evaluated for interpersonal violence.
- Clenched-fist injuries, resulting from a clenched fist striking the teeth of another person, are treated as

bites. Due to the site of injury (the knuckles) and the velocity, there is a higher risk of injury to bone, joint, tendon, or cartilage.
- Bite wounds involving marked tissue destruction have an increased risk for transmission of infection through blood and body fluids.

Skeletal Injuries

Fractures resulting from physical abuse may be single or multiple, recent or old, or a combination of fractures involving both multiple numbers and sites. One of the more commonly injured bones from child abuse is the metaphysis of the humerus, whose fracture is caused by the victim being grasped by the arm and pulled, swung, or jerked. In this injury, a piece of the bone is broken from the growth plate by shearing forces. Other types of suspicious fractures include bilateral or symmetric fractures; transverse, oblique, and spiral shaft fractures; rib fractures; scapular or sternal fractures; dislocations, multiple fractures in various bones; and fractures in different stages of healing.

Abdominal Injuries

Abdominal injuries that may be indicative of interpersonal violence include intestinal perforation, hemorrhage, and laceration; abdominal contusion; or hematoma to the organs of the abdomen and retroperitoneum including the liver, spleen, and kidney due to blunt force trauma. Concurrent findings such as abdominal distention, vomiting, abdominal pain, bruising, fever, hematuria, and shock (septic and hypovolemic) may also be signs of abuse.

Abdominal injuries are commonly seen in the pregnant population. Injuries from sexual violence include genital and rectal trauma as well as vaginal infections.

Psychosocial Impact: Trauma-Informed Care Framework

Emergency nurses need to recognize the profound long-term psychological, biological, neurologic, and interpersonal effects that the traumatic event, or series of events, will have on the patient. The trauma-informed care framework encourages emergency nurses to approach all patients as potential abuse survivors to diminish the retraumatization that the emergency visit may trigger. It involves identifying survivor strengths and resilience, assisting survivor recovery and healing, and working collaboratively with the survivor to develop short- and long-term care plans that support healthy coping mechanisms.

Each survivor needs to, and has a right to, feel safe during care so as to encourage active participation in their recovery. Approach each patient with respect, patience, and empathy. On a practical level, this means sharing information, sharing control, respecting boundaries, and encouraging mutual learning to understand healing stages (Box 16-1). All of these practices show awareness and understanding of interpersonal violence and help both the survivor and the nurse initiate and engage in the recovery process.[4]

Diagnostic Procedures

Diagnostic procedures include the following:

- Imaging studies: Full-body radiographic films are used to determine if there is evidence of previously healed fractures or any missed injuries. If fractures are suspected or confirmed, document these findings with at least two views. Computed tomography (CT) is used to detect intracranial or extracranial injuries such as skull fractures, hemorrhage, or hematoma. CT scan can also document injuries to the solid and hollow abdominal organs. For strangulation injuries, CT angiogram can detect damage to the carotid and vertebral arteries as well as bony structures.[59]
- Laboratory studies: Laboratory studies include a toxicology screen of the patient's blood and urine if there is a suspicion of ingestion or exposure to toxic substances, use of alcohol, or overmedication. Blood and urine are the best samples for collection, as the substance used may have been metabolized and be present only in the urine. A urine or blood pregnancy test should be performed on female trauma survivors. If excessive bruising is discovered, complete blood count, platelet count, and coagulation studies can rule out bleeding disorders.

Considerations for the Care of Patients Who Have Experienced Sexual Violence: National Protocol for Sexual Assault Medical Forensic Examinations

Nurses need to know their facility's protocol, including legal jurisdiction policies and procedures regarding the chain of custody in medico-legal forensic examinations. It is important for the trauma nurse to offer a medical examination and forensic evaluation if the trauma patient has disclosed or is suspected of having been sexually assaulted. Sexual assault medical forensic examinations can be performed up to 5 days after assault, even if survivor has showered, urinated, defecated, and changed clothes.[60]

Forensic technology advancements have enabled the extension of post–sexual assault forensic examinations up to 9 days in some situations with living persons.[60]

Be sure to obtain informed consent for a forensic evaluation. These patients, who have experienced a loss of control during the trauma, need to be provided with choices regarding their care in the ED.[60,61]

Preparation Considerations

Preparation considerations include the following:

- Use a safe, private room for the primary patient consultation and initial law enforcement interviews.
- Offer a waiting area for family members and friends and provide child care if possible.
- Assess and respond to safety concerns, such as threats to the patient or staff.
- Follow facility and jurisdictional procedures, while respecting patients and maximizing evidence preservation.

Triage considerations include the following:

- Due to the time-sensitive nature of the situation, treatment required, and recognition that every minute patients spend waiting to be examined may cause loss of evidence and undue trauma, sexual assault patients are assigned a triage category of Emergency Severity Index 2, or its equivalent in other triage systems. They are considered a priority for care.
- Make all efforts to bring the patient immediately to a private room.
- Triage nurses should be mindful on their questioning techniques. As patients arrive, ask them to share what happened to them and communicate that you are pleased they came to be examined. Incorporate active listening and observation skills to decrease unintentional revictimization during communication.[4]
- Notify specially trained examiners if available.

Personnel with specific training in sexual assault care, forensic evidence collection, and medico-legal documentation and chain-of-evidence requirements should be utilized in these instances if they are an available resource. If the facility does not utilize specially trained forensic examiners, the emergency nurse will likely assist in the forensic examination (**Appendix 16-1**). Specially trained sexual assault personnel may include the following professionals:

- Sexual Assault Nurse Examiners (SANEs) are registered nurses with specialized education to fulfill the didactic and clinical training requirements to properly perform these medical forensic examinations.[62,63]
- Some registered nurses have been certified as SANE-Adult and Adolescent (SANE-AA) and SANE-Pediatric (SANE-P) through the International Association of Forensic Nurses (IAFN).[62,63]
- Other registered nurses fulfill the clinical requirements that quality them as Forensic Nurse Examiners (FNEs), enabling them to collect forensic evidence in a variety of situations, not just in cases of sexual assault. Death investigations, screening and assessment of domestic violence, elder and child abuse, and working in correctional facilities are other examples of the FNE role.[64]
- The designations of Sexual Assault Forensic Examiner (SAFE) and Sexual Assault Examiner (SAE) more broadly describe a healthcare provider (physician, physician assistant, nurse, or nurse practitioner) with special education and demonstrated clinical expertise to perform this examination.
- Victim advocates are able to assist with safety and resource planning and community advocacy for sexual assault and rape victims.[62,63]

History includes the following information:

- A detailed description of the incident, if appropriate, based on facility policy and guidelines. Document everything the patient remembers about the incident. Be as detailed as possible, be objective, and use direct quotes. This record should include the following elements:
  - Date, time, and place of the incident
  - Events surrounding the incident
  - Information regarding all acts committed by the perpetrator, including verbal and physical threats, weapons or restraints used, all sites of penetration and/or ejaculation, and the use or non-use of a condom
  - Injuries associated with the incident
  - Activities by the victim following the incident, such as bathing or showering, wound care, drinking, eating, urination and defecation, and/or changing clothes
- Additional obstetric and gynecologic history for female patients
  - Gravida and para status
  - Date of last menstrual period
  - Current method of birth control and compliance with the method
  - Time of last consensual intercourse (oral, vaginal, anal) routine and recent condom use

- In any suspected drug-facilitated sexual violence, the history may include the following:
    - The patient may report having awakened in strange surroundings with disheveled clothing, unclear memory, or a feeling of being sexually violated.
    - If some memory of the event remains, the patient may describe feeling paralyzed, powerless, or a disassociation of mind and body.
    - The patient may report symptoms similar to the feeling of alcohol intoxication, although the severity may not match the amount consumed.
    - The patient may report the sudden onset of symptoms such as drowsiness, lack of coordination, confusion, impaired memory, or complete lack of memory (amnesia), within 15–20 minutes after consuming a drink.

Mandated Reporting

A mandated reporter is required by law to report suspected maltreatment or abuse of a child or vulnerable adult. This designation may be applied to many professionals, including law enforcement, teachers, clergy, and others. Nurses are mandated reporters in most jurisdictions. As such, they are responsible for raising the question, assessing the patient for signs of maltreatment or abuse, and reporting their suspicions to social services or law enforcement. Nurses are mandated reporters in 48 states of the United States, the District of Columbia, the Northern Mariana Islands, Guam, American Samoa, Puerto Rico, and the U.S. Virgin Islands.[65] All of these entities have statutes regarding both mandated and permissive reporting of suspected child maltreatment.[65]

Trauma nurses should follow jurisdictional policies if children are in the care of the patient who may have experienced interpersonal or domestic violence, as statutes vary in these cases. Many states have adopted legislation to require reporting for suspected elder abuse, IPV, and human trafficking. Procedures for reporting vary by state and facility, so refer to the hospital policies and procedures as needed.

Lethality Assessment

Recognizing a survivor of IPV is not always easy. In fact, such abuse is often missed. The sequelae of a missed opportunity to intervene could place the victim back into a high-risk environment. The Danger Assessment is a lethality screening tool with an accompanying referral protocol that prompts appropriate action based on the results of the screening process.[66] The goal of the Danger Assessment is to prevent domestic violence homicides, serious injury, and reassault through identification and utilization of domestic violence support services. Different versions of the tool are available for victims in same-sex relationships, immigrant victims, and different languages. The Lethality Assessment tool is a shortened version used by law enforcement. A Danger Assessment for clinicians is another shortened version useful in the ED.[28]

Rehabilitation

Persons who personally experience violence or are exposed to interpersonal violence may have hidden long-term consequences. If a victim's psychological traumatic history and related symptoms go undetected, it could lead providers to direct services toward symptoms and disorders that may only partially explain patients' presentations and distress. Universal screening for trauma history and trauma-related symptoms can help practitioners identify individuals at risk of developing more pervasive symptoms of traumatic stress. Screening, early identification, and intervention serves as a prevention strategy.[67]

Every trauma team member needs to incorporate trauma-informed care principles and understanding of the long-term sequelae of interpersonal violence into the care provided to these patients (**Figure 16-5**).[1,4] PTSD changes the survivor's pleasure, self-control, engagement, and trust.[68] Eliminate any practice that is potentially harmful, including seclusion and restraint practices; interactions that are shaming, minimizing, discrediting, or ignoring of the patient's response; labeling intense feelings as pathological; treatment planning without collaboration; and providing medical interventions without privacy.[67]

Emergency nurses need to be aware that survivors of interpersonal violence can experience a wide range of emotions, from anger and rage to terror and withdrawal. Should these responses develop, ensure referral of patients to appropriate follow-up counseling and provide patient teachings from a trauma-informed framework. Innovative programs that utilize neurofeedback, meditation, yoga, sports, and drama to help recovery are available.[4,68] Refer to **Appendix 16-2** and **Appendix 16-3** for available resources.

Prevention

Identification of this patient population is fundamental to the provision of care and improved health outcomes. Screening remains a recommendation of several nursing and physician organizations and should be done by emergency nurses per their facility policy.

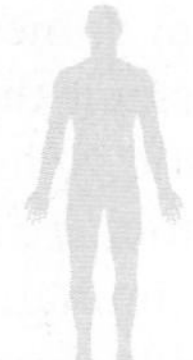
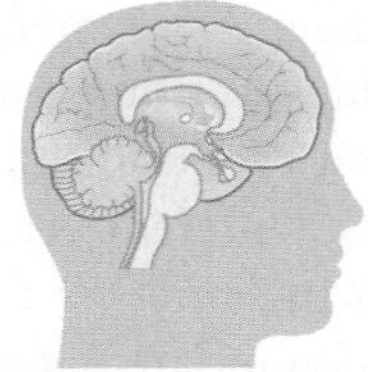
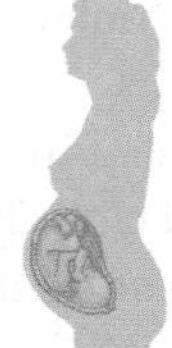
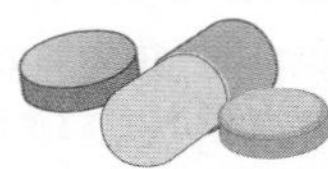

Physical

Abdominal injuries
Thoracic injuries
Brain injuries
Burns/scalds
Fractures
Lacerations
Disability

Mental health and behavioral

Alcohol and drug abuse
Depression and anxiety
Post-traumatic stress disorder
Eating and sleep disorders
Attention deficits
Hyperactivity
Externalizing behavior
Smoking
Suicidal thoughts
Suicidal behavior
Unsafe sex

Sexual and reproductive health

Unintended pregnancy
Pregnancy complications
Unsafe abortions
Gynecological disorders
Complex pain syndromes
Chronic pelvic pain
HIV
Other sexually transmitted infections

Chronic disease

Arthritis and asthma
Cancer
Cardiovascular disorders
Diabetes
Kidney problems
Liver disease
Stroke

Figure 16-5 *Behavior and health consequences of violence.*

Reproduced from World Health Association. (2014). *Global status report on violence prevention 2014*. Geneva: Author. Retrieved from http://apps.who.int/iris/bitstream/10665/145086/1/9789241564793_eng.pdf?ua=1&ua=1.

Effective prevention of interpersonal violence will focus on healthy relationships across the lifespan. Programs and policies must be developed that are responsive to those populations at greatest risk. The causes of interpersonal violence are complex and often the result of multiple individual, familial, community, cultural, and societal factors. Collaboration is essential, including diverse professional perspectives as well as increased community participation to address interpersonal violence within diverse communities. Including law enforcement, nurses, physicians, social workers, advocacy groups, and academic–community collaborative groups in the public response increases efficacy by building comprehensive, well-coordinated policies and procedures that maximize community resources.[35]

Preventive measures for emergency nurses to initiate include distribution of educational materials discussing interpersonal violence, including intimate-partner or domestic violence, child and vulnerable adult maltreatment and abuse, and human trafficking, as well as healthy relationships. ED waiting rooms, treatment rooms, and restrooms are excellent areas for placement of materials that educate the public about this public health epidemic.

Emergency nurses can also become active participants in legislative processes to support and develop prevention programs that address forming healthy relationships and prevention of interpersonal violence. The Emergency Nurses Association (ENA) and IAFN have developed a joint position statement that provides suggestions for nurses regarding interpersonal violence prevention and documentation.[69] The WHO reports that a growing body of research is demonstrating that interpersonal violence can be prevented and its consequences mitigated on a national and international level. Prevention programs and survivor services, along with national action plans, policies, and laws to support prevention and response efforts can begin to address the gaps that are still seen in violence prevention and mitigation in countries around the world.[1]

Summary

Violence in society is a complex, multifaceted problem with many contributing issues. The public health consequences—both physical and psychological—are myriad and far-reaching. Interpersonal violence occurs across all ages, cultures, genders, races, and classes. Trauma patients who have experienced interpersonal violence require special considerations in addition to high-quality trauma care. Trauma nurses should utilize a patient-centered and trauma-informed framework of care that addresses the survivor's physical, medico-legal, and psychosocial needs, thereby facilitating the interpersonal violence survivor's recovery. Recognition is the first step toward care and advocacy for what may often be hidden interpersonal violence situations.

Trauma nurses are in a unique position to effect change not only by effectively and empathetically caring for survivorsofinterpersonalviolenceafterinjuryhasoccurred, but also by advocating for action plans, policies for prevention, and resources at every level—local, national, and global—for this extremely vulnerable patient population.

References

1. World Health Association. (2014). *Global status report on violence prevention 2014.* Geneva: Author. Retrieved from http://apps.who.int/iris/bitstream/10665/145086/1/9789241564793_eng.pdf?ua=1&ua=1
2. National Coalition Against Domestic Violence. (2018). Domestic violence national statistics. Retrieved from www.ncadv.org/statistcs
3. Nielson, M. H. (2018). Abuse and neglect. In V. Sweet (Ed.), *Emergency nursing core curriculum* (7th ed., pp. 36–46). St. Louis, MO: Elsevier.
4. Chisolm-Straker, M., & Stoklosa, H. (2017). *Human trafficking is a public health issue.* Cham, Switzerland: Springer.
5. Violence Prevention Alliance. (2018). *Definition and typology of violence.* Geneva, Switzerland: World Health Organization. Retrieved from http://www.who.int/violenceprevention/approach/definition/en/
6. Polaris Project. (2017). Human trafficking: The facts. Retrieved from https://polarisproject.org/human-trafficking/facts
7. Centers for Disease Control and Prevention. (2018). Population characteristics and environmental health: CDC tracking network. Retrieved from https://ephtracking.cdc.gov/showPopCharEnv
8. Centers for Disease Control and Prevention. (2018). Social Vulnerability Index (SVI) (Factsheet). Retrieved from https://svi.cdc.gov/Documents/FactSheet/SVIFactSheet.pdf
9. Mills, T. J. (2015, February). Elder abuse. *Medscape.* Retrieved from https://emedicine.medscape.com/article/805727-overview
10. Agency for Persons with Disabilities. (2017). Common signs and symptoms of abuse, neglect, and exploitation. Retrieved from http://apd.myflorida.com/zero-tolerance/common-signs/
11. Beal, J. A. (2017). Healthcare of the transgender youth still inadequate . . . still at risk. *Journal of Maternal/Child Nursing, 42*(5), 296. https://doi.org/10.1097/NMC.0000000000000362
12. Tracy, E. E., & Macias-Konstantopoulos, M. (2018, March 16). Human trafficking: Identification and evaluation in the health care setting. *UpToDate.* Retrieved from https://www.uptodate.com/contents/human-trafficking-identification-and-evaluation-in-the-health-care-setting
13. Campana, D. (2018). Hidden in plain sight: Labor trafficking victims in the ED. *ENA Connection, 42*(1), 16–19.
14. National Center on Domestic and Sexual Violence. *Power and control wheel.* Austin, TX: Author. Retrieved from http://www.ncdsv.org/images/powercontrolwheelnoshading.pdf
15. National Coalition Against Domestic Violence. (2015). Dynamics of abuse. Retrieved from https://ncadv.org/dynamics-of-abuse
16. Mikton, C. R., Tanaka, M., Tomlinson, M., Streiner, D. L., Tonmyr, L., Lee, B. X., & MacMillan, H. (2017). Global research priorities for interpersonal violence prevention: A modified Delphi study. *Bulletin of the World Health Organization, 95*(1), 36–48. https://doi.org/10.2471/BLT.16.172965
17. Nagle, J. (2020). Child maltreatment. In D. Brecher (Ed.), *Emergency nursing pediatric course: Provider manual* (5th ed., pp. 129–141). Schaumburg, IL: Emergency Nurses Association.
18. Centers for Disease Control and Prevention. (2017). Child abuse and neglect: Definitions. Retrieved from https://www.cdc.gov/violenceprevention/childabuseandneglect/definitions.html
19. Centers for Disease Control and Prevention. (2016). Violence prevention: Intimate partner violence definitions. Retrieved from https://www.cdc.gov/violenceprevention/intimatepartnerviolence/definitions.html
20. Rodrigues, J. L., Lima, A. P., Nagata, J. Y., Rigo, L., Cericato, G. O., Franco, A., & Paranhos, L. R. (2016). Domestic violence against children detected and managed in the routine of dentistry: A systematic review. *Science Direct, 43,* 34–41. https://doi.org/10.1016/j.jflm.2016.07.006
21. American Society for the Positive Care of Children. (2018). Child maltreatment statistics in the U.S. Retrieved at https://americanspcc.org/child-abuse-statistics/
22. U.S. Department of Health and Human Services, Administration for Children and Families, Administration on Children, Youth and Families, Children's Bureau. (2016). Child maltreatment 2016. Retrieved from https://americanspcc.org/wp-content/uploads/2018/03/2016-Child-Maltreatment.pdf
23. World Health Organization. (2013). *Global and regional estimates of violence against women: Prevalence and health effects of intimate partner violence and non-partner sexual violence* (NLM classification: HV 6625). Geneva, Switzerland: WHO Press.
24. Smith, S. G., Chen, J., Basile, K. C., Gilbert, L. K., Merrick, M. T., Patel, N., Walling, M., & Jain, A. (2017). *The national intimate partner and sexual violence survey: 2010–2012: State report.* Atlanta, GA: National Center for Injury Prevention and Control, Centers for Disease Control and Prevention.
25. Wong, J. Y., Choi, A. W., Fong, D. Y., Choi, E. P., Wong, J. K., So, F. L., . . . Kam, C. (2016). A comparison of intimate partner violence and associated physical injuries between cohabitating and married women: A 5-year medical chart review. *BMC Public Health, 16*(1207), 1–9. https://doi.org/10.1186/s12889-016-3879-y
26. Messing, J. T., Patch, M., Wilson, J. S., Kelen, G. D., & Campbell, J. (2018). Differentiating among attempted, completed, and multiple nonfatal strangulation in women experiencing intimate partner violence. *Women's Health Issues Journal, 28*(1), 104–111. https://doi.org/10.1016/j.whi.2017.10.002
27. Emergency Nurses Association. (2017). ENA topic brief: An overview of strangulation injuries and nursing implications. Retrieved from https://www.ena.org/docs/default-source/resource-library/practice-resources/topic-briefs/overview-of-strangulation-injuries-and-nursing-implications.pdf?sfvrsn=1bc6735a_8
28. Messing, J. T., Campbell, J. C., & Snider, C. (2017). Validation and adaptation of the Danger Assessment-5: A brief intimate partner violence risk assessment. *Journal of Advanced Nursing, 73,* 3220–3230. https://doi.org/10.1111/jan.13459

29. Diez, C., Kurland, R. P., Rothman, E. F., Bair-Merritt, M., Fleegler, E., Xuan, Z., & Siegel, M. (2017). State intimate partner violence-related firearm laws and intimate partner homicide rates in the United States, 1991–2015. *Annals of Internal Medicine, 167*, 536–543. https://doi.org/10.7326/M16-2849
30. Susan B. Anthony Project. (2017). Date and acquaintance rape. Retrieved from https://sbaproject.org/just-for-teens/date-and-acquaintance-rape/
31. Roelofs, K. (2017). Freeze for action: Neurobiological mechanisms in animal and human freezing. *Philosophical Transactions of the Royal Society B: Biological Sciences, 372*(1718). http://doi.org/10.1098/rstb.2016.0206
32. Moller, A., Sondergaard, H. P., & Helstrom, L. (2017). Tonic immobility during sexual assault: A common reaction predicting post-traumatic stress disorder and severe depression. *Acta Obstetricia et Gynecologica Scandinavica, 96*, 932–938. https://doi.org/10.1111/aogs.13174
33. Cuevas, K. M., Balbo, J., Duval, K., & Beverly, E. A. (2018). Neurobiology of sexual assault and osteopathic considerations for trauma-informed care and practice. *Journal of the American Osteopathic Association, 118*(2), e2–e10. http:/doi.org/10.7556/jaoa.2018.018
34. Van Parys, A., Verhamme, A., Temmerman, M., & Verstraelen, H. (2014). Intimate partner violence and pregnancy: A systematic review of interventions. *PLoS One, 9*(1), E85084. https://doi.org/10.1371/journal.pone.0085084
35. Alhusen, J. L., Ray, E., Sharps, P., & Bullock, L. (2015). Intimate partner violence during pregnancy: Maternal and neonatal outcomes. *Journal of Women's Health, 24*(1), 100–106. https://doi.org/10.1089/jwh.2014.4872
36. World Health Organization. (2011). Intimate partner violence during pregnancy (Information sheet). Retrieved from http://apps.who.int/iris/bitstream/handle/10665/70764/WHO_RHR_11.35_eng.pdf;jsessionid=4EC5CBA17EF2F2F32A53A1D7E44BD05C?sequence=1
37. Wiemann, C. M., & Harrykissoon, S. D. (2018, January 11). Date rape: Identification and management. *UpToDate*. Retrieved from https://www.uptodate.com/contents/date-rape-identification-and-management
38. Richer, L. A., Fields, L., Bell, S., Heppner, J., Dodge, J., Boccellari, A., & Shumway, M. (2015). Characterizing drug-facilitated sexual assault subtypes and treatment engagement of victims at a hospital-based rape treatment center. *Journal of Interpersonal Violence, 32*(10), 1524–1542. https://doi.org/10.1177%2F0886260515589567
39. Spiller, H. A., Rogers, J., & Sawyer, T. S. (2007). Drug facilitated sexual assault using an over-the-counter ocular solution containing tetrahydrozoline (Visine). *Legal Medicine, 9*(4), 192–195.
40. Madea, B., & Mußhoff, F. (2009). Knock-out drugs: Their prevalence, modes of action, and means of detection. *Deutsches Ärtzeblatt, 106*(20), 341–347. https://doi.org/10.3238/arztebl.2009.0341
41. Brown, T., & Herman, J. L. (2015). *Intimate partner violence and sexual abuse among LGBT people: A review of existing research.* Los Angeles, CA: UCLA, Williams Institute. Retrieved from https://williamsinstitute.law.ucla.edu/wp-content/uploads/Intimate-Partner-Violence-and-Sexual-Abuse-among-LGBT-People.pdf
42. Office for Victims of Crime. (n.d.). Human trafficking: What is human trafficking? Retrieved from https://ovc.ncjrs.gov/humantrafficking/
43. Rafferty, Y. (2016). Challenges to the rapid identification of children who have been trafficked for commercial sexual exploitation. *Child Abuse & Neglect, 52*, 158–168. https://doi.org/10.1016/j.chiabu.2015.11.015
44. Greenbaum, V. J., Dodd, M., & McCracken, C. (2018). A short screening tool to identify victims of child sex trafficking in the health care setting. *Pediatric Emergency Care, 34*(1), 33–37. https://doi.org/10.1097/PEC.0000000000000602
45. Normandin, P. A. (2017). Child human trafficking: See, pull, cut the threads of abuse. *Journal of Emergency Nursing, 43*(6), 588–590. https://doi.org/10.1016/j.jen.2017.07.014
46. Polaris. (n.d.). Share infographics from the National Human Trafficking Hotline. Retrieved from https://act.polarisproject.org/page/21744/action/1
47. Hall, J., Karch, D. L., & Crosby, A. (2016). Elder abuse surveillance: Uniform definitions and recommendations core data elements. Retrieved from https://www.cdc.gov/violenceprevention/pdf/EA_Book_Revised_2016.pdf
48. Colwell, C. (2017, August 2). Geriatric trauma: Initial evaluation and management. *UpToDate*. Retrieved from https://www.uptodate.com/contents/geriatric-trauma-initial-evaluation-and-management
49. National Center on Elder Abuse. (2017). Research: Statistics/data. Retrieved at https://ncea.acl.gov/whatwedo/research/statistics.html
50. Halphen, J. M., & Dyer, C. B. (2018, May 23). Elder mistreatment: Abuse, neglect, and financial exploitation. *UpToDate*. Retrieved from https://www.uptodate.com/contents/elder-mistreatment-abuse-neglect-and-financial-exploitation
51. Normandin, P. A. (2015). Identifying maternal intimate partner violence in the emergency department. *Journal of Emergency Nursing, 41*(5), 444–446. https://doi.org/10.1016/j.jen.2015.05.011
52. National Center of Elder Abuse. (2017). Frequently asked questions: Abandonment. Retrieved from https://ncea.acl.gov/faq/abusetypes.html#abandonment
53. National Adult Protective Service Association. (2018). Elder financial exploitation. Retrieved from http://www.napsa-now.org/policy-advocacy/exploitation/
54. National Network to End Domestic Violence. (2017). About financial abuse. Retrieved from https://nnedv.org/content/about-financial-abuse/
55. Dadi, F., & Thimsen, K. (2015). Identifying human trafficking in health care settings: Guidance document. Retrieved from https://healtrafficking.org/wp-content/uploads/2017/08/Guidance-doc-on-HT-10-7-2015.pdf
56. International Labour Office. (2017). Global estimates of modern slavery: Forced labour and forced marriage. Retrieved from http://www.ilo.org/global/publications/books/WCMS_575479/lang--en/index.htm

57. Zijlstra, E., Esselink, G., Moors, M. L., LoFoWong, S., Hutschemaekers, G., & Lagro-Janssen, A. (2017). Vulnerability and revictimization: Victim characteristics in a Dutch assault center. *Journal of Forensic and Legal Medicine, 52,* 199–207. https://doi.org/10.1016/j.jflm.2017.08.003
58. International Association of Forensic Nurses. (2017). Nonfatal strangulation documentation toolkit. Retrieved from https://www.forensicnurses.org/page/STAssessment
59. Dunn, R. J., & Smock, W. (2018). Strangulation injuries. Retrieved from https://www.ncbi.nlm.nih.gov/books/NBK459192/
60. U.S. Department of Justice. (2017). *National best practices for sexual assault kits: Multidisciplinary approach*. National Institute of Justice. Retrieved from https://www.ncjrs.gov/pdffiles1/nij/250384.pdf
61. U.S. Department of Justice, Office of Violence Against Women. (2013). *A national protocol for sexual assault forensic examinations: Adults/adolescents* (2nd ed.). Retrieved from https://www.ncjrs.gov/pdffiles1/ovw/241903.pdf
62. Zilkens, R. R., Smith, D. A., Kelly, M. C., Mukhtar, A., Semmens, J. B., & Philips, M. A. (2017). Sexual assault and general body injuries: A detailed cross-sectional Australian study of 1163 women. *Forensic Science International, 279,* 112–120. https://doi.org/10.1016/j.forsciint.2017.08.001
63. National Institute of Justice. (2017). The most important features for an effective sexual assault response team. Retrieved from https://nij.gov/topics/crime/rape-sexual-violence/Pages/important-features-for-sart.aspx
64. International Association of Forensic Nurses. (2017). Areas of forensic nursing practice. Retrieved from https://www.forensicnurses.org/page/AreasFNPractice
65. Child Welfare Information Gateway. (2015). *Links to state and tribal child welfare law and policy*. Washington, DC: U.S. Department of Health and Human Services, Children's Bureau. Retrieved from https://www.childwelfare.gov/topics/systemwide/laws-policies/statutes/resources/
66. Danger Assessment. (2014). Johns Hopkins University. Retrieved from https://www.dangerassessment.org
67. Substance Abuse and Mental Health Services Administration. (2014). *Trauma-informed care in behavioral health services: Treatment improvement protocol (TIP) Series 57* [HHS Publication No. (SMA) 13-4801]. Rockville, MD: Author.
68. Van der Kolk, B. (2014). *The body keeps the score*. New York, NY: Penguin.
69. Emergency Nurses Association, International Association of Forensic Nurses. (2013). Joint position statement: Intimate partner violence. Retrieved from https://www.ena.org/docs/default-source/resource-library/practice-resources/position-statements/joint-statements/intimatepartnerviolence.pdf?sfvrsn=4cdd3d4d_8

APPENDIX 16-1

Forensic Evidence Collection: Maintain Chain of Custody Preservation

Evidence protection and collection[1,2] can be an essential aspect of the care provided to the patient who has experienced interpersonal violence. Consideration is given to the patient's potential life-threatening injuries, their emotional response, as well as the patient's rights. Complete the forensic examination only after the patient's immediate life threats are treated and the patient is stabilized. Consider the following points when collecting evidence:

- Patients are cautioned not to wash, change clothes, urinate, defecate, smoke, drink, or eat until initially evaluated by examiners, unless necessary for treating acute medical needs. If any of this was done by the patient prior to examination, include what and when in documentation.
- Clothing:
  - When cutting to remove the patient's clothing, avoid any areas that appear to be cut or torn by a weapon or projectile, are stained, or have debris, such as gunshot residue
  - Dry and store each item of patient clothing in a separate paper bag. Plastic bags are not recommended for evidence collection because moisture can cause fungal growth, rendering evidence useless.
- Carefully assess all skin surfaces, and ask the patient about areas that hurt or were injured.
- Use body diagrams to identify and describe each injury in detail, using correct terminology as well as direct quotes.
  - As direct quotes are an important aspect of clear and complete documentation, certain terms used by the patient may not reflect medical terminology
  - Documentation includes explanation of the mutually agreed-upon terminology for clarification.
- Forensic photography of injuries:
  - Many jurisdictions have policies on who is qualified to take forensic photographs. Follow the organizational guidelines for forensic photography.
  - Obtain photographs whenever possible before medical treatment.
  - Obtain consent.
  - Use good lighting.
  - Include a patient identifier (date of birth, medical record label) in the photograph.
  - Take a distance shot of the whole body; take a picture at midrange and a close-up of the injury.
  - Include a measuring device, such as a ruler or scale (the American Board of Forensic Odontology scale is recommended).
  - Photograph bite marks for dental forensic analysis.
- Specimen collection:
  - Swabs
    - Moisten the swab with sterile water.
    - Swab the following:
      - Potential areas of retained body fluids, including sites of kissing or licking
      - Bite marks
      - Vagina and external and vaginal vault
      - Penis
      - Anus
    - Label all swabs for the specific site, including the date, patient's name, and name of collector.
    - Allow the swab to dry completely.
    - Scrape under the fingernails (in some jurisdictions, swabbing may be preferred).
  - Comb the patient's hair, both head hair and pubic hair. This step can help investigators differentiate between strands of the patient's hair and that of the perpetrator.
  - Use evidence tape to seal and sign or initial each receptacle once sealed.
  - Place all properly sealed biohazard evidence (sexual assault kit) in a locked refrigerator area.
  - Key to locked evidence refrigerator should be locked in a secured area.
  - Documentation log should be maintained that maintains chain of custody until evidence picked up by law enforcement.
  - Name of person and title who placed the forensic evidence in the locked refrigerator with date and time.
  - In the same log, document transfer of chain of evidence information with name, badge number, and agency of law enforcement person picking up evidence, date, and time collected.

Additional considerations for the patient presenting to the ED following sexual violence include the following:

- Provide emotional support; incorporate the trauma-informed care framework principles.[3]

- Interpersonal violence and human trafficking survivors often develop PTSD, depression, anxiety, and suicidal ideation.
- Contact a survivor advocate to provide services to the patient, if not already done.
- Follow jurisdictional and organizational policies regarding reporting.
- Complete medico-legal documentation to include a description of the events, body maps, diagrams, and photos (as required or allowed). Use direct quotes as appropriate. Do not allow the evidentiary chain of custody to be broken.
- Provide emergency contraceptive prophylaxis.
- Provide sexually transmitted infection prophylaxis, including human immunodeficiency virus prophylaxis.
    - Adhere to the current CDC guidelines.
    - Refer to facility protocols.
- Arrange for follow-up care to address any new infections or other medical issues, monitor both physical and psychological effects of incident and treatment, and arrange post-trauma counseling or other treatments as may be appropriate for the patient's situation.

References

1. U.S. Department of Justice. (2017). *National best practices for sexual assault kits: Multidisciplinary approach.* National Institute of Justice. Retrieved from https://www.ncjrs.gov/pdffiles1/nij/250384.pdf
2. U.S. Department of Justice, Office of Violence Against Women. (2013). *A national protocol for sexual assault forensic examinations: Adults/adolescents* (2nd ed.). Retrieved from https://www.ncjrs.gov/pdffiles1/ovw/241903.pdf
3. Chisolm-Straker, M., & Stoklosa, H. (2017). *Human trafficking is a public health issue.* Cham, Switzerland: Springer.

APPENDIX 16-2

IPV and Human Trafficking: Resources for the Community

Organization	Phone Number/Website
CDC Facebook page on violence prevention	www.facebook.com/vetoviolence
National Domestic Violence Hotline	www.ndvh.org 1-800-799-SAFE (7233), 1-800-787-3224 TTY
National Coalition Against Domestic Violence	www.ncadv.org
National Sexual Violence Resource Center	www.nsvrc.org
Futures Without Violence (formerly Family Violence Prevention Fund)	www.futureswithoutviolence.org
Department of Homeland Security: Human Trafficking	www.dhs.gov/topic/human-trafficking
Human Trafficking—HEAL (Health, Education, Advocacy, and Linkage): nonprofit, public health approach, interprofessional model	https://healtrafficking.org
Polaris Project	www.polarisproject.org
Partners in Prevention	www.enddomesticabuse.org/consulting.html
National Resource Center on Domestic Violence	www.nrcdv.org/dvrn
National Human Trafficking Hotline	www.nhtrc.org www.humantraffickinghotline.org Forced sex? Text "BeFree" to 233-733 or call 1-888-373-7888
National Adult Protective Services Association	www.napsa-now.org
National Center on Elder Abuse	https://ncea.acl.gov/resources/state.html 1-800-677-1116
Love Is Respect: National Dating Abuse Helpline	http://www.loveisrespect.org
National Domestic Violence Hotline › Deaf, deaf-blind, and hard-of-hearing services › LGBT abuse › Pregnancy and abuse	www.thehotline.org

APPENDIX 16-3

IPV and Human Trafficking: Resources for the Healthcare Worker

Organization	Phone Number/Website
National Child Traumatic Stress Network	www.nctsn.org
National Protocol for Sexual Assault Medical Forensic Examinations, Adult/Adolescent (2013): SAFE Protocol	www.ncjrs.gov/pdffiles1/ovw/241903.pdf
U.S. Department of Justice (2017): National best practices for sexual assault kits: multidisciplinary approach	www.ncjrs.gov/pdffiles1/nij/250384.pdf
Healthcare Toolbox: Healthcare Providers' Guide to Traumatic Stress in the Ill or Injured Child: After the ABCs, consider the DEF (Distress, Emotional Support, Family) Protocol for Trauma-Informed Care	www.healthcaretoolbox.org
SOAR free online human trafficking training resources	www.acf.hhs.gov/otip/training/soar-to-health-and-wellness-training www.acf.hhs.gov/otip/resource/soarhealthcare
Recognizing and Responding to Human Trafficking in a Healthcare Context	https://humantraffickinghotline.org/resources/recognizing-and-responding-human-trafficking-healthcare-context
Nation Human Trafficking Hotline Data Report	https://humantraffickinghotline.org/sites/default/files/2016%20National%20Report.pdf
Alliance 8.7	https://www.alliance87.org
2017 Global Estimates of Modern Slavery: Forced Labour and Forced Marriage	https://www.ilo.org/global/publications/books/WCMS_575479/lang--en/index.htm
Substance Abuse and Mental Health Services Administration (SAMHSA): a free in-depth trauma-informed treatment care protocol in behavioral health services that trauma nurses can obtain	www.samhsa.gov 1-877-SAMHSA-7 (1-877-726-4727)
International Association of Forensic Nurses	www.forensicnurses.org
World Health Organization: Strengthening health systems to respond to women subjected to intimate-partner violence or sexual violence: A manual for health managers.	www.who.int/reproductivehealth/publications/violence/vaw-health-systems-manual/en/
Hate Crimes Bureau of Justice Statistics, 2004–2015	www.bjs.gov/content/pub/pdf/hcv0415_sum.pdf
Danger Assessment for Clinicians	www.dangerassessment.org

CHAPTER 17

Psychosocial Aspects of Trauma Care

Cassie A. Lyell, MSN, RN, TCRN

OBJECTIVES

Upon completion of this chapter, the learner will be able to:

1. Describe characteristics of psychological distress resulting from trauma.
2. Indicate interventions related to psychosocial aspects of trauma care.
3. Evaluate the effectiveness of appropriate psychosocial interventions in trauma care.
4. Discuss ethical issues that affect trauma care.

Introduction

Patients who experience a traumatic injury are at risk for suffering long-term physical effects of those injuries. Additionally, many patients and their families experience psychological, emotional, and spiritual effects as a result of trauma.

Caring is at the heart of nursing practice. Evidence suggests that continued exposure to traumatic situations can affect trauma nurses, just as it affects the victims of trauma. Nurses who routinely work with severely injured and traumatized patients may experience physical, psychological, emotional, and behavioral consequences of this ongoing stress.[1,2]

While interventions for life-threatening physical injuries remain the priority in injured patients, focusing on the psychological aspects of trauma patient care, completing a thoughtful assessment, and planning and implementing psychosocial interventions can significantly affect recovery.[3] According to the American College of Surgeons' most recent iteration of "Resources for Optimal Care of the Injured Patient" (2014), approximately 20% to 40% of injured trauma survivors experience acute and chronic stress and/or depressive disorders following discharge from the acute care setting, resulting in a higher incidence of functional impairments, inability to return to work within 12 months after injury, reduced quality of life, and increased healthcare and societal costs.[4] Understanding the human response to injury and disability can provide the nurse with the tools to enhance patient care and increase self-awareness of how repeated exposure to these events may negatively affect one's well-being.

Human Response to Trauma

Traumatic events can be characterized as dangerous, frightening, unpredictable, violent, or uncontrollable threats to life.[5] Although responses to traumatic events vary, support and guidance are needed for patients and their families as they work through the process of coping with trauma.

Various characteristics are common to this human response[6]:

- Intense or unpredictable emotional reactions
- Changes to thought and behavior patterns
- Physical reactions such as increased heart rate, diaphoresis, headache, chest pain, or nausea
- Impaired ability to concentrate or make decisions
- Disrupted sleep and eating patterns
- Increased sensitivity to light, sound, and smell
- Exacerbation of preexisting medical conditions
- Feelings of being overwhelmed or anxious
- Conflict and strain on relationships

The following factors can affect the level of distress experienced by the patient and their family[5,6]:

- The nature of the injury or traumatic event, including the following:
  - Intensity
  - Inescapability
  - Uncontrollability
  - Unexpectedness
  - Prolonged exposure
- Characteristics of the individual exposed to the event, including the following:
  - Previous exposure to trauma
  - History of behavioral health conditions
  - Substance misuse or abuse
  - Support systems
  - Cultural norms
- The reaction or response, including the following:
  - Coping mechanisms
  - Defense mechanisms
  - Availability of resources and access to medical care

These factors influence the experience of injury, loss, and difficult news in the emergency care setting, leading to reactions that can range from stoic acceptance to a tearful response, anger, or even violent outbursts.

Psychosocial Nursing Care of the Trauma Patient

The psychosocial assessment begins after life-threatening injuries have been identified and stabilized. See Chapter 3, "Initial Assessment," for the systematic approach to care of the trauma patient. The aim of the assessment and interventions is to provide patient- and trauma-informed care by understanding the correlation between the present injury and condition and the past psychosocial and trauma history.[7]

Secondary Survey

Secondary survey begins with the history.

H: History

Complete a psychosocial history assessment for the following purposes[8,9]:

- Determine the patient's recollection of the event.
- Monitor the patient's description of and reaction to the incident.
- Identify any previously diagnosed stress disorders or other mental health issues, including substance use.
- Provide a baseline for ongoing reevaluation of status.
- Plan for additional resources that may be needed to cope with the effects of the events.

H: Head-to-Toe Assessment

Complete all necessary assessments to rule out a physiologic cause for behavioral signs and symptoms. Many signs can have either physiologic or emotional causes that can be difficult to differentiate. These signs may vary depending on the physical, cognitive, or emotional reactions to the event[6]:

- Physical: Heart palpitations, tachypnea, hyperventilation, headache, nausea, vomiting, diaphoresis, muscle pain, shaking, feeling jittery, or being easily startled
- Cognitive: Repetitive questioning, forgetfulness, numbness or a blunted affect, intrusive thoughts or repetitive description of events, hyper-alertness, silence, or difficulty with concentration
- Emotional: Silence, generalized fearfulness, tearfulness, anger, disbelief, vulnerability, or fear of being alone or desire to be left alone

Interventions

Repeated reassessments can guide interventions that may help to lessen symptoms. For example, if the patient repeatedly questions events leading to the injury, continue to orient the patient to place, time, and location and provide assurance that they are safe. Present a calm and soothing demeanor to facilitate coping. The RESPOND mnemonic provides an outline for interventions for both the patient and family after a traumatic event[7,8,10]:

- **R**eassure the patient and family that they are safe and well-cared for.
- **E**stablish rapport with the patient and family; introduce yourself and the trauma team. Create a connection between the patient and key trauma team members.
- **S**upport the patient through the initial aftermath of the trauma. Help the patient contact family or friends. Assign a primary support person from the trauma team. Involve the hospital chaplain or bereavement team, if available and if the patient agrees to this support. Encourage a member of the support system to remain with the patient when possible.
  - Patients or family members may prefer to have a social worker, a trusted friend, or advisor from the community fill the role of support.
  - Some patients prefer to be alone or to involve others only when the extent of injury is known or admission is likely. It is important to consider the patient's wishes.
- **P**lan care; manage **p**ain.
  - Explain the plan of care with the patient and family succinctly, clearly, and in simple language.
  - Explain the need for diagnostic procedures to evaluate the extent of injury.
  - Set expectations for changes in the plan of care as a result of assessment or diagnostic findings.
  - Include the patient and family in the planning of care when possible.
  - Update the patient or family regularly so they are apprised of what to expect next in the plan of care.
  - Explain the pain assessment tool upon patient arrival and regularly reassess pain, the response to medication, or need for additional analgesia.
- **O**ffer hope.
  - While one should not offer false hope regarding the extent of injury or the likelihood of survival, it is essential to provide reassurance and support to the patient and family with open, compassionate communication.
  - With the patient's consent, update family members at regular intervals and as changes occur.
- **N**ever deliver news of death or disability alone to the patient or the family.
  - Patients and family members or friends can exhibit various reactions to news of a traumatic event, ranging from withdrawal to outbursts of emotion or violence.
  - Rely upon colleague support when approaching the patient and family with difficult news. For example, conference or three-way calling by the physician and the trauma team is a great option when news of severe disability or death of a patient must be delivered via telephone to family.
- **D**etermine the patient's needs.
  - Encourage the patient and family to express their feelings and needs following a traumatic event.
  - Support patient involvement in the planning of care.
  - Determine the patient's preferences for confidentiality and sharing information with family.
  - Allow the opportunity to express fear, anger, and vulnerability in response to the event.
  - Consider the use of a tool to screen for acute stress disorder (ASD) symptoms and risk of post-traumatic stress disorder (PTSD). Advocate for cognitive-behavioral therapy interventions including education, relaxation, imaginal exposure, and cognitive restructuring of fear-related beliefs.

NOTE

The RESPOND Mnemonic

R: Reassure
E: Establish rapport
S: Support the patient
P: Plan care; manage pain
O: Offer hope
N: Never deliver news of death or disability alone to the patient or the family
D: Determine the patient's needs

Selected Psychosocial Trauma Reactions

This section presents selected psychosocial trauma reactions.

Stress Reaction

Stress reaction is caused by an unusual event—usually an experience that elicits a feeling of dread, fear, helplessness, or threat to life or safety. An acute stress reaction occurs in response to traumatic events and can result in physical or mental distress. The stress reaction is typically short-lived, subsiding within hours or days. An acute stress reaction may be experienced by the injured patient as well as family members and may occur in the absence of any preexisting behavioral health issues.[11]

Crisis

Crisis often occurs following an extraordinary or traumatic event. In this circumstance, the patient's usual coping mechanisms no longer work, and the patient is unable to function normally due to distress. Patients may become anxious and disorganized and may panic or try to escape. They may also revert to less functional behaviors such as violence, substance abuse, and depression.[8] The trauma nurse can apply basic principles of crisis assessment and intervention to these situations (**Table 17-1**).[9,10,12]

If crisis symptoms are sustained longer than 3 days, assessment for acute stress disorder should be considered.[8] An acute stress reaction may improve with a resolution of symptoms; however, if symptoms are sustained and/or worsened, a diagnosis of a stress disorder may result. The goal of the trauma team is to support the patient in their progress toward independent functioning and recovery.[8]

Traumatic Stress Disorders

Involvement with a traumatic event or sustaining an injury has been found to result in increased risk for development of maladaptive behaviors such as ASD or PTSD. Early recognition of these traumatic stress disorders

TABLE 17-1 Assessment and Interventions for Patients in Crisis

Assessment	Intervention
› Assess for the patient's perception of what happened › Assess mental status and risk for harm to self or others	› Assure patient safety › Provide one-to-one observation if the patient is at risk for suicide › Remove any potentially harmful items › Provide reassurance and support › Communicate regularly to relay information throughout the ED stay
› Determine past and present medical history, including medications › Screen for the presence of substances that may alter behavior	› Use a calm and empathetic manner
› Assess for family and social issues	› Establish rapport and trust › Allow for expression of feelings
› Ask about previous, successful coping mechanisms › Inquire about existing support systems	› Focus on problem solving › Offer simple basic choices to promote decision making › Facilitate patient involvement in the plan of care › Monitor for therapeutic communication with visitors and encourage a supportive person to stay with the patient

Data from Burston, A. (2017). Communication helped reduce anxiety for a patient and his family. Nursing Standard, *32*(15), 65. https://doi.org/10.7748/ns.32.15.65.s38; Emergency Nurses Association. (2016). Tips for providing safe structure for adult behavioral health patients [Infographic]. Retrieved from https://www.ena.org/docs/default-source/resource-library/practice-resources/infographics/tips-for-providing-sage-structure-for-adult-behavioral-health-pts-in-the-ed.pdf?sfvrsn=6aefd9fa_4; Emergency Nurses Association & International Nurses Society on Addictions. (2012). Expanded roles and responsibilities for nurses in screening, brief intervention, and referral to treatment (SBIRT) for alcohol use (Joint position statement). Retrieved from https://www.ena.org/docs/default-source/resource-library/practice-resources/position-statements/joint-statements/expandedrolesresponsibilitiesfornursesinsbirt.pdf?sfvrsn=594e67b0_6.

is essential for optimal recovery; thus, nursing assessments and screening are essential during the acute care phase.[7]

ASD and PTSD are diagnoses recognized by the American Psychological Association (APA) in the fifth edition of the *Diagnostic and Statistical Manual of Mental Disorders* (DSM-5, 2103). Although the criteria for these diagnoses are extensive, diagnosis for each requires exposure to one or more traumatic events resulting in a stress reaction. ASD and PTSD symptoms often overlap. PTSD is a more chronic disorder and may not be diagnosed until symptoms are present for longer than 1 month, while ASD symptoms may begin immediately after the trauma and persist at least 3 days.[11,13] Development of ASD increases the risk of developing PTSD.[7] Screening of trauma patients to identify and intervene with those at higher risk for ASD and PTSD is recommended by the U.S. Department of Veteran Affairs.[3] Screening for stress reactions and disorders is part of the post-resuscitative acute care phase as well as the post-acute care phase.

Trauma nurses caring for patients in the acute phase of care following injury are believed to be essential in assessing early symptoms of traumatic stress disorders and advocating for interventions. Although several screening tools are available, the more efficient tools are believed to be the most successful.[11] In the post-acute phase of care, providers may also screen for symptoms of PTSD.

The Primary Care PTSD Screen for DSM-5 (PC-PTSD-5) tool is composed of five questions that correspond to the diagnostic criteria for ASD and PTSD.[14] Patients with a positive screen finding may warrant a further psychological or neuropsychological evaluation and treatment plan.[7] Part of the PC-PTSD-5, the response scale, is shown here:

In the past month, have you . . .

1. Had nightmares about the event(s) or thought about the event(s) when you did not want to?
   YES/NO
2. Tried hard not to think about the event(s) or went out of your way to avoid situations that reminded you of the event(s)?
   YES/NO
3. Been constantly on guard, watchful, or easily startled?
   YES/NO
4. Felt numb or detached from people, activities, or your surroundings?
   YES/NO
5. Felt guilty or unable to stop blaming yourself or others for the event(s) or any problems the event(s) may have caused?
   YES/NO

Fear and Anxiety

After experiencing a traumatic event, patients may be fearful and anxious, demonstrating variable degrees of uneasiness, distress, and worry. The trauma nurse helps the patient to manage and mitigate the negative effects of these emotions (Table 17-1). Overall, the provision of clear information delivered in a thoughtful, consistent manner to patients and families can increase perception of control and diminish fear and anxiety.[15]

Grief, Bereavement, and Mourning

Grief, bereavement, and mourning[16,17] are not static events, but rather processes that are influenced by personality, family, culture, religion, circumstances involving loss, manner of death, and relationship to the deceased person.[9] While the terms "bereavement," "mourning," and "grief" are sometimes used interchangeably, they are actually unique concepts[9]:

- Grief is the personal response to loss.
- Mourning is the individual expression of grief and loss.
- Bereavement is the state of loss and the period in which grief and mourning occur.

Grief has been described as the feelings experienced after loss, while mourning is the active expression of grief. Examples of mourning may include acceptance of the loss, working through the grief, adjusting to a new normal, or withdrawing emotionally. Grief and mourning take place during the period of bereavement.

Loss may include events such as the loss of a child, the loss of a home, or the loss of a feeling of security after a natural disaster.[6] Patients suffer varying dimensions of loss. Some of those include the following:

- *Material*: Loss of a home, vehicle, or other physical objects that have meaning to a person. These can also be items of sentimental value, such as heirlooms or keepsakes.[17]
- *Relationship*: The loss of ability to share experiences and have the physical presence of a person. Whether patients and family members are young or old, they may express the loss of a loved one or of a vital friendship.
- *Intrapsychic or spiritual*: Loss of an aspect of one's self-image or focusing on possibilities of what might have been. For example, the death of a child

may lead to feeling of the loss of the experience of raising a child or the death of spouse may lead to feelings of the loss of growing old with that person.

- *Functional*: Feelings of grief that follow the loss of function of a limb or use of arms, legs, and the body, such as in the case of quadriplegia.
- *Role*: Feelings of loss of a specific role within one's social network. At times, functional loss affects the ability to perform a particular role. For example, the loss of the use of a hand or arm can affect a person's ability to work in a particular profession.

Grief Assessment

The experience of grief has physical, emotional, cognitive, behavioral, and spiritual dimensions.[16-18] While grief may be considered a universal human emotion, not all patients or family members experience grief in the same way. Just as the physiologic response to trauma varies from patient to patient, so individual grief responses vary. Observation of these reactions can guide the trauma nurse in planning and intervention on behalf of the patient and family (**Table 17-2**).[18,19]

TABLE 17-2 Human Responses Following Grief

Dimension of Grief	Behaviors
Somatic expression	› Physical complaints, such as pain, nausea, and headache › Loss of appetite › Overeating or weight gain › Restlessness, sleep disturbances, fatigue
Cognitive expression	› Preoccupation with the loss › Fear and loneliness › Low self-esteem › Inability to concentrate or remember › Helplessness and hopelessness › Situations seem unreal
Affective expression	› Anxiety › Guilt, resentment, and aggression › Depression and despair › Loneliness › Defensiveness or self-blame
Behavioral expression	› Agitation › Fatigue › Crying › Social withdrawal › Most common sign of grief in children

Data from Bugge, K. E., Darbyshire, P., Rokholt, E. G., Sulheim Haugsvedt, K. T., & Helseth, S. (2014). Young children's grief: Parents' understanding and coping. *Death Studies, 38*(1), 36–43. https://doi.org/10.1080/07481187.2012.718037; Ramachandran, V. S. (2012). *Encyclopedia of human behavior* (2nd ed.). London, UK: Academic Press.

Cultural Considerations of Grief

In addition to the individual responses to grief, ethnic and cultural variations exist in response to loss and death. Therefore, providing culturally congruent care is essential. Culturally competent care is described as being sensitive to the patient's cultural background, beliefs, values, and practices.[20] A cultural assessment can be helpful in caring for families dealing with grief and loss.

Grief Interventions

Many of the interventions for patients experiencing stress, fear, worry, and crisis are applicable to the patient experiencing grief. Additionally, it is important that trauma team members provide spiritually sensitive interventions appropriate to each individual's unique responses to grief. Questions related to these interventions include the following:

- Are there preferred rites or rituals?
- Is there a spiritual or family leader to be contacted?
- Can these needs be met or addressed within the emergency setting?
- Is there a support person to be with them?

Support can also be provided as the patient or family prepares to leave the ED. Put together a grief discharge package to include pamphlets and phone numbers of local support groups. A follow-up phone call the next day can identify needs that arise after discharge.

Complicated grief is a more severe and chronic form of grieving characterized by problematic cognitive, behavioral, and emotional symptoms. Long-term management of complicated grief includes interventions to support the integration and acceptance of loss as well as the promotion of recognizing meaning in loss.[17]

Additional Psychosocial Care Considerations

Providing referrals for resources for the continued support of patients who have experienced injury is a fundamental step in the process of recovery. Clear policies and procedures serve to support patients and their families and to address the following needs:

- Communication and provision of interpreter services
- Family-centered care
- Opportunity for family presence during resuscitation and invasive procedures

Communication and Use of Interpreter Services

When language barriers exist, the use of interpretive services assures accuracy of medical information communicated to patients and families. In the United States, the Office of Minority Health issues standards for culturally and linguistically appropriate care. These standards state that healthcare organizations are required to provide interpreters in a timely manner to all patients who need language assistance during all hours of operation.[21]

Communication interventions include the following:

- Determine the patient's preferred language for communication.
- Identify family or friends designated to receive important medical information if the patient cannot speak for themselves.
- Speak slowly and clearly to patients and families, and allow time for questions when delivering clinical findings or sharing the plan of care.
- Use a professional interpreter.
- Refrain from utilizing friends or family as interpreters who may attempt to protect the patient instead of simply translating.
- However, if the patient requests a friend or family member to act as interpreter, the patient's wishes are considered.[21] Follow organizational policy regarding the use of interpreters.

Family-Centered Care

Family-centered care[22] and patient involvement in care are essential components of appropriate, safe, and timely healthcare in the trauma setting. The Health and Medicine Division of the National Academies of Sciences, Engineering, and Medicine (formerly the Institute of Medicine) recommends patient and family involvement in healthcare-related decisions. The Institute for Patient- and Family-Centered Care suggests that hospitals review and revise organizational visitor policies with several key concepts in mind:

- Reconsider the use of the term "visitor" with respect to family members in the language used in hospital policies. Family members and key friends may offer pivotal support in provision of care and should be respected as part of the care team.
- Change the cultural views of families as "visitors" to accept families as "partners." Find practical ways to work together (**Table 17-3**).[23]
- Modify the definition of "family" to include those persons whom the patient considers to be family members.
- Assure patients have the support needed for recovery.
- Collaborate with the trauma care team to support palliative care and end-of-life care across the continuum of care.[24]

TABLE 17-3 Guide for Being PARTNERS with Family

Mnemonic	Description
P	Present yourself and explain you will work together
A	Ask the patient and care partners to participate in decision making when possible
R	Reassure patients and care partners that their input is valued
T	Trust the shared goal—optimal care and outcome for the patient
N	Nurture relations with the care team
E	Encourage input and shared decision making when possible
R	Review plans of care and discharge plans so preferences and goals are recognized
S	Support participation of care partners as team members

Data from Institute for Patient- and Family-Centered Care. (n.d.). *Better together pocket guide for staff.* Bethesda, MD: Author. Retrieved from http://www.ipfcc.org/bestpractices/guides-for-teams.html.

Family Presence During Resuscitation and Invasive Procedures

Family presence during resuscitation and invasive procedures in high-acuity settings such as the ED or the intensive care unit is more likely to be a positive experience when facilities have sound policies and procedures in place that support such a practice.[25,26] Facilitation of family presence is most successful when clear policies are in place, when patient care teams are educated regarding expectations and parameters of such policies, and when a dedicated staff support person is assigned to family members during resuscitative events and throughout invasive procedures.[27] If there is no clear policy in place to support family presence during resuscitative events, the trauma nurse can work with administration to develop policies to support patients, families, and staff in their preferences regarding family presence. In developing policies for family presence, include consideration of patient and staff safety and infection control measures.[25]

Research on family presence during resuscitations has focused on the attitudes of culturally and ethnically diverse patient, family, and provider populations. Studies have concluded that family presence either positively or negatively impacts clinical outcomes for the patient, but the literature is inconclusive on the impacts on families and providers.[28,29]

Psychosocial Aspects of Caring for Agitated Patients and Families

Each ED is a microcosm of the community it serves, and trauma nurses in this setting may be exposed to difficult or even violent behavior. This behavior may be demonstrated by patients or family members under the influence of drugs or alcohol, with psychiatric disorders, and ineffective communication patterns. The ED often serves as a primary entry to the hospital, with public access available 24 hours a day. Trauma patients and families experiencing stress may exhibit escalating behaviors such as agitation, inappropriate communication, hostility, and physical violence. Education regarding the best approach to patients and families, de-escalation techniques, and care of the psychiatric or agitated patient can help the trauma nurse control difficult situations. It is also important to implement a safety response for situations that may become out of control.

Preventing Escalation

Some techniques for preventing escalation include the following:

- Minimize the chaos.
- Have one point-of-contact person for message clarity.
- Talk to families in a designated, quiet, private room.
- Limit environmental stimuli.
- Promote clear communication with support.
- Assess the need for and try to provide personal space.
- Sit and talk on the same level.
- Avoid healthcare jargon and terminology.
- Promote and assist with contacting other family members or support persons.
- Assess the need for spiritual support.
- Make multidisciplinary referrals for support.
- Provide comfort measures (drink, food, phone, quiet room).
- Observe verbal and nonverbal cues as they may indicate family member needs.

De-escalation

If the tension and frustration lead to behavioral escalation, then take the following steps:

- Notify public safety personnel to stand by.
- Remain calm and nonjudgmental.
- Speak in a calm, quiet voice.
- Listen actively and observe the individuals' body language.
- Maintain an exit route; place yourself between the patient or family and the door.
- Set realistic limits and offer choices if possible.

Mitigating Violence

Clinical and safety considerations in the management of violent behavior may include the following:

- Minimize stimulation in the environment.
- Use a low voice and speak calmly and slowly to the patient and family.
- Facilitate a safe environment for patients, families, and staff.
- For a patient who is violent, consider the following:
  - Assess for a physiologic cause for the behavior.
    - Obtain a point-of-care glucose level to assess for hypoglycemia.
    - Assess for oxygen desaturation and other signs and symptoms that suggest hypoxia.

   - Anticipate a head computed tomography scan to rule out neurologic injury.
   - Obtain a toxicology screen to rule out substance abuse.
  - Administer medications as ordered with support from other staff as necessary.
  - If restraints are necessary, apply them and follow the care protocol according to organizational policy.
- If assaulted, after assuring your safety and treatment, report the incident by following your organization's procedures and seek counseling.

The presence of policies and protocols together with education can optimize the trauma nurse's competence and ability to handle these difficult situations.

Ethical Considerations in Trauma

The trauma nurse will encounter ethical dilemmas in practice and may also experience moral distress. The American Nurses Association (ANA) defines moral distress as "the condition of knowing the morally right thing to do, but institutional, procedural or social constraints make doing the right thing nearly impossible; threatens core values and moral integrity."[30(p44)]

According to the Emergency Nurses Association (ENA) Scope and Standards of Practice, the emergency nurse "Delivers care in a manner that preserves and protects healthcare consumer autonomy, dignity, rights, values, and beliefs."[3(p33)] This standard of practice describes the nurse's role as an advocate for all patients and families despite any personal beliefs or values.

Providers have an ethical, legal, and moral duty to provide care and ensure the safety of vulnerable patients; respect the wishes of the family in crisis, including the patients, parents, and surrogate decision makers; determine decision-making authority; and adhere to legal precedent.[31] It is imperative that trauma nurses are familiar with both implied and informed consent. With informed consent, providers have a duty to disclose the risks, benefits, and alternatives for suggested medical care. Implied consent may be presumed in instances where a patient or surrogate decision maker is unable to authorize informed consent. It is not uncommon for injured patients to present to the hospital with conditions that prevent them from exercising self-determination and medical decision-making capacity.

Most states have legislation in place regarding implied consent for emergency care that waives the requirement of informed consent in emergent situations, when death or permanent impairment is impending without medical intervention. For non-emergent care, a surrogate decision maker is required to provide informed consent for minors, prisoners, and patients found to be physically or mentally incapacitated.[32]

Advance Directives

Advance directives may be unavailable when the trauma patient arrives in the ED. If the patient is alert, ask about any particular wishes related to care. If the patient is not alert, ask the family or legal guardian to provide a copy of any advance directive. If there is no advance directive and the patient is not alert, follow organizational policy for care. If information on the patient's preferences is not initially accessible, the trauma team follows the patient's wishes for care once such information becomes available.[33]

Trauma nurses should be familiar with legal statutes and regulations that relate to consent and advance directives and that are specific to the area in which they practice. Legal rules for consent should be used as the guide to determine and assign surrogate decision makers in the event a patient does not have decision-making capacity and does not present an advance directive. In some cases, consent may be legally waived if there is a need for emergency care, including when patients have acute medical or traumatic conditions that without immediate treatment may result in serious jeopardy, serious impairment to bodily functions, serious dysfunction of any bodily organ or part, or death.[34]

Advance directives include living wills and a healthcare power of attorney or proxy. They can include directives such as the following[35]:

- Do not intubate
- Do not resuscitate (DNR)
- Do not defibrillate
- Do not hospitalize
- Comfort care only

Documents and forms can vary, so it is important for the nurse to become familiar with the documents used in their organization and jurisdiction and to understand the implications of each directive.[35]

Advance directives are often signed in the context of a medical illness, and the patient or proxy may wish them to be revoked in the event of a traumatic injury. Clear explanations, when possible, will help the patient or proxy decide if the original criteria surrounding these directives are still relevant in the current situation.[33] Consider the following examples of the patient's right to choose and the patient's right to be informed.

Patient's Right to Choose

An 80-year-old female is hit by a motor vehicle and sustains a fractured femur. She has a history of hypertension and heart failure, and the family brought a signed DNR order from a past hospitalization. The patient is currently living independently in her own home. What is the responsibility of the trauma team in this situation?

Discussion

The trauma nurse examines the hospital policy regarding the use of DNR orders and the circumstances in which they are legal and binding. An order from another facility or an order from a previous hospitalization may not be binding during this hospitalization. In this case, the trauma team educates the patient regarding the meaning of an advance directive and assures that the patient understands the implications of an advance directive within the context of the injury and surgery. With the patient's health history, extubation following surgery may be difficult and carry some risk. It is important to discuss what will be involved during recovery and rehabilitation and to explain that chances for recovery may be very good. The patient and family need to consider all risks and benefits to make decisions for care with this hospitalization.[35]

Right to Be Fully Informed

An 89-year-old woman arrives at the ED following a slip and fall. The options for treatment include a surgical repair or conservative treatment. The patient's daughter states that she wishes for the conservative treatment and requests the staff not discuss it with the patient because it will "just upset her." The patient presents alert and oriented. How should the trauma team manage this situation?

Discussion

Unless there is documentation giving the daughter healthcare power of attorney *and* the mother is unable to make decisions for herself, the daughter is not legally able to make decisions for her mother. In this instance, the patient is alert and oriented. Therefore, she has the right to know all the treatment options and may include her daughter in the decision-making process if she wishes, but the patient must be fully informed.

Organ and Tissue Donation

When death is inevitable, some families may receive comfort from the ability to donate their loved one's organs or tissues. Sensitivity and respect are vital when approaching families for this request. Federal law mandates that all U.S. transplant centers and organ procurement organizations (OPOs) be members of the National Organ Procurement and Transplantation Network so that they will meet the eligibility requirements for Medicare funding and reimbursement.[36]

The OPO determines whether the patient meets the qualifications as a potential donor and whether the patient is medically suitable for donation. Declaration of death, medical examiner approval, notification of the OPO, and consent from next of kin are all prerequisites before organ procurement can take place.[36] The process of organ donation and recovery is a collaborative team effort between the OPO and the patient care team. Increased awareness of that process can help the trauma nurse meet the needs of the donor and their family.

Psychosocial Care of the Trauma Team

The nature of trauma care exposes the trauma nurse to suffering. Repeated exposure to suffering or trauma can lead to compassion fatigue (CF) or secondary traumatic stress (STS).[1] Both CF and STS can impact the trauma nurse's ability to deliver quality, empathetic care.[2,37-40] Contrasting with CF and burnout is the concept of compassion satisfaction (CS). CS is defined as a sense of professional and personal fulfillment experienced by caregivers as a result of helping patients experiencing trauma and traumatic situations.[37,39]

Compassion Fatigue

Although most research regarding traumatic stress has focused on the experience of the injured patient and first responders, traumatic stress has also been found to impact nurse providers indirectly through their caring for injured patients.[2] Numerous studies confirm that nurses witness human suffering and tragic situations; in turn, CF is a serious professional issue that nurses need to address.[37] When it was first studied in the 1980s, CF was described as a natural and disruptive by-product of working with traumatized and troubled clients. Today, CF is defined as a loss of a nurse's ability to empathize and provide compassionate care to patients.[39] CF is the sum of two parts: burnout and secondary traumatic stress.[37,41]

Recognition of CF risk factors as well as formal debriefing, education, and supportive leadership have the potential to reduce the incidence of CF. In particular, interventions focused on raising awareness, recognition,

TABLE 17-4 Symptoms of Compassion Fatigue

Work-Related	Physical	Emotional
› Avoidance or dread of working with certain patients or patient types › Reduced ability to feel empathy toward patients or families › Errors in judgment › Impaired focus › Chronic tardiness › Frequent use of sick days › Decreased sense of purpose	› Chronic fatigue › Headaches › Digestive problems: diarrhea, constipation, upset stomach › Muscle tension › Sleep disturbances: inability to sleep, insomnia, too much sleep › Cardiac symptoms: chest pain/pressure, palpitations, tachycardia › Frequent and lingering illness	› Chronic worry › Depression › Moral distress, stress-related illness › Anxiety › Irritability › Anger and resentment › Detached or disinterested

Data from Henson, J. S. (2017). When compassion is lost. *MedSurg Nursing, 26*(2), 139–142. Retrieved from https://www.highbeam.com/doc/1G1-491949347.html; Lombardo, B., & Eyre, C. (2012). Compassion fatigue: A nurse's primer. *Online Journal of Issues in Nursing, 16*(1), 3. Retrieved from http://www.nursingworld.org/MainMenuCategories/ANAMarketplace/ANAPeriodicals/OJIN/TableofContents/Vol-16-2011/No1-Jan-2011/Compassion-Fatigue-A-Nurses-Primer.html; Sorenson, C., Bolick, B., Wright, K., & Hamilton, R. (2017). An evolutionary concept analysis of compassion fatigue. *Journal of Nursing Scholarship, 49*(5), 557–563. https://doi.org/10.1111/jnu.12312.

prevention strategies, and resiliency tools appear to have the most significant impacts.[1,42] Newer nurses are at higher risk for the development of CF, and more experimental research is needed to identify effective interventions for this condition.[43,44] With increased awareness and understanding, CF can be prevented or its effects can be mitigated.[41] **Table 17-4** describes symptoms associated with CF.[45-47]

Secondary Traumatic Stress

STS is a component of CF that occurs with direct exposure to a stressor in the work environment (workplace violence). It can also occur in response to caring for people who have experienced traumatic events and injuries. In one study, symptoms were reported to occur in three categories: intrusion, avoidance, and arousal (**Table 17-5**).[1,48] STS may manifest as negative feelings driven by fear and work-related trauma.[41]

The prevalence of STS has been reported to be alarmingly high in trauma nurses as well as those working in other similar high-stress areas, such as hospice, critical care, oncology, pediatric, and mental health nursing.[42-45]

Burnout

Burnout is also an element of CF. It occurs over time, with a gradual onset, building to a stress response. Burnout is not unique to healthcare providers but when occurring in these professionals, it may manifest as emotional exhaustion, patient depersonalization, negative attitude toward patients, and diminished feelings of personal and

TABLE 17-5 Secondary Traumatic Stress Symptoms

Category	Symptoms
Intrusion	› Recurring thoughts about patients › Dreams about work and patients › Sense of reliving the disturbing events over and over
Avoidance	› Avoiding certain patients › Staying away from people and crowded places › Inability to remember patient information › Emotionless › Disconnected from others › Inactive
Arousal	› Sleep disturbances › Irritability › Inability to focus › Nervousness and agitation

Data from Cocker, F., & Joss, N. (2016). Compassion fatigue among healthcare, emergency and community service workers: A systematic review. *International Journal of Environmental Research and Public Health, 13*. https://doi.org/10.3390/ijerph13060618; Dominguez-Gomez, E., & Rutledge, D. (2009). Prevalence of secondary traumatic stress among emergency nurses. *Journal of Emergency Nursing, 35*(3), 199–204.

work accomplishments.[37,39] Burnout symptoms may be organized into three categories:

- Emotional exhaustion
- Depersonalization or distancing oneself from the work and others
- Decreased sense of accomplishment

Burnout is also associated with difficulties in dealing with the stress of work or feelings of helplessness and professional inadequacy. **Table 17-6** describes additional symptoms associated with burnout.[2,37,39,49]

A nurse experiencing the effects of burnout may be judgmental of patients or may be easily irritated by patients and colleagues.[49] The nurse with burnout can be easily overwhelmed by routine or ordinary work conditions. Burnout can lead to indifference, disengagement, and withdrawal from patients and the work environment. Ultimately, burnout impacts job satisfaction, productivity, and performance, and may contribute to absenteeism and turnover.[2]

TABLE 17-6 Burnout Symptoms

Burnout Component	Symptoms
Emotional exhaustion	› Headache › Fatigue › Gastrointestinal complaints › Muscle strain and tightness › Increased blood pressure › Respiratory symptoms › Sleep disorders
Depersonalization	› Anxiety › Irritability › Sadness and despair › Hopelessness
Personal accomplishment	› Absenteeism › Frustration › Thinking about quitting › Inefficiency on the job › Decreased satisfaction with the job › Lack of dedication to the job

Data from Beck, C. T. (2011). Secondary traumatic stress in nurses: A systematic review. *Archives of Psychiatric Nursing, 25*(1), 1–10. https://doi.org/10.1016/j.apnu.2010.05.005; Berg, G. M., Harshbarger, J. L., Ahlers-Schmidt, C. R., & Lippoldt, D. (2016). Exposing compassion fatigue and burnout syndrome in a trauma team: A qualitative study. *Journal of Trauma Nursing, 1*, 3–10. https://doi.org/10.1097/JTN.0000000000000172; Hinderer, K. A., VonRueden, K. T., Friedmann, E., McQuillan, K. A., Gilmore, R., & Murray, M. (2014). Burnout, compassion fatigue, compassion satisfaction, and secondary traumatic stress in trauma nurses. *Journal of Trauma Nursing, 21*, 160–169. https://doi.org/10.1097/JTN.0000000000000055; Sacco, T. L., Ciurzynski, S. M., Harvey, M. E., & Ingersoll, G. L. (2015). Compassion satisfaction and CF among critical care nurses. *Critical Care Nurse, 35*(4), 32–42. https://doi.org/10.4037/ccn2015392.

Social Networking

Social networking as an outlet for debriefing after an emotionally distressing shift or incident may be alluring. However, the trauma nurse should recognize the risks involved and take pains to maintain compliance with institutional policies as well as legal and ethical responsibilities to patients. The ENA's position statement for social networking outlines the ethical responsibility of an emergency nurse to follow their employer's institutional policies regarding code of conduct when using a social media platform. Refer to the ENA's position statements for more information on social networking by emergency nurses.[50]

Workplace Violence

Workplace violence in the ED is highly prevalent and believed to be underreported. Studies indicate between 35% and 80% of hospital staff have been physically assaulted at least once, with 46% of the nonfatal assaults being committed against registered nurses.[51] These stressful conditions can have an impact on the trauma nurse, especially with repeated exposure. Among the potential consequences of practicing in a high-stress and potentially dangerous environment are psychological, emotional, and physical effects on the health of the trauma nurse.

In an effort to mitigate workplace violence, the ENA promotes a comprehensive approach including practical measures to prevent, respond to, and report occurrences. Consequences of workplace violence include decreased job satisfaction, turnover, development of stress disorders, and abandonment of the profession.[51,52]

Critical Incidents

A critical incident (CI) is a traumatic event that elicits unusually strong emotional reactions or responses to the event by healthcare team members, which in turn may adversely affect workplace morale. Care for children and adults who have been injured as a result of interpersonal violence, pediatric resuscitation, and care for a dying

TABLE 17-7 Common Responses to a Traumatic Event

Cognitive	Emotional	Physical	Behavioral
Poor concentration	Shock	Nausea	Suspicion
Confusion	Numbness	Light-headedness	Irritability
Disorientation	Disbelief	Dizziness	Arguments with friends and loved ones
Indecisiveness	Anger or short-temperedness	Loss of appetite	Withdrawal
Shortened attention span	Anxiety or fear	Gastrointestinal problems	Increased substance use or abuse
Memory loss	Feeling overwhelmed	Skin rashes	Excessive silence
Unwanted thoughts and images	Depression	Rapid heart rate	Inappropriate humor
Difficulty making decisions	Fear of harm to self and/or loved ones	Tremors	Increased/decreased eating
Nightmares	Feeling nothing	Headaches	Change in sexual desire or functioning
	Feeling abandoned	Grinding of teeth	Increased smoking
	Uncertainty of feelings	Fatigue	
	Volatile emotions	Worsening of chronic health problems	
		Poor sleep	
		Pain	
		Hyperarousal	
		Jumpiness	

Reproduced from Centers for Disease Control and Prevention. (2017, December 18). Coping with a disaster or traumatic event. Retrieved from https://emergency.cdc.gov/coping/index.asp.

colleague may be considered CIs. Additional stressors may be acute, chronic, or cumulative in effect, resulting in changes in both the personal and professional lives of trauma nurses. **Table 17-7** lists common reactions to a traumatic event such as a CI.[53]

Approach to the Care of the Trauma Team

Assessment tools are helpful in caring for the trauma team.

Assessment Tools

Use of the Professional Quality of Life scale and the Maslach Burnout Inventory (MBI) instrument is discussed here.

Professional Quality of Life

The Professional Quality of Life: Compassion Satisfaction and Fatigue Version 5 (ProQOL) is a 30-item instrument used to score responses related to the phenomena of CF, burnout, and CS (**Appendix 17-1**).[41] ProQOL has been useful in identifying nurses' response to traumatic events, their ability to cope,[53] and the possible need for intervention. Nurse leaders can administer this tool to screen for CS and CF. Interventions, support, and programs may then be needed to promote recovery from the effects of traumatic events for the individual nurse and the entire department.

Maslach Burnout Inventory

The MBI is most often used to measure a person's level of burnout.[54,55] In this tool, elements of burnout are divided into six categories:

- Workload: Addressing both quality and quantity
- Control: Having autonomy at work and influence over one's own practice
- Reward: Being recognized by others and having internal job satisfaction
- Sense of community: Being engaged at work and having a supportive work environment

- Fairness: Feeling that decisions are made equitably and fairly
- Values: Having purpose and enthusiasm for the work

An analysis of these factors determined that shorter patient length of stay, which is associated with more work for nurses in fewer hours, with a constant turnover of patients in the ED setting, is often overwhelming for trauma nurses.[54] The results from this tool can be used to develop strategies for preventing the emotional exhaustion, depersonalization, and lack of a sense of accomplishment. More research is needed to identify specific strategies for treating nurse burnout, and to evaluate the effectiveness of existing interventions.

Support and Strategies for the Trauma Team

Support and strategies for the trauma team include developing resilience, promoting self-awareness, and using critical incident stress management (CISM).

Developing Resilience

Resilience comprises a unique set of attributes or protective behaviors that may buffer an individual from the detrimental effects of acute and chronic stress.[56,57] The literature emphasizes that development of personal and professional resilience allows one to cope with the effects of stress and achieve a positive work experience.[58]

Examples of attributes that contribute to resilience include the following[58]:

- Hardiness
- Coping skills
- Self-efficacy
- Optimism
- Patience
- Tolerance
- Faith
- Adaptability
- Self-esteem
- Sense of humor

The American Psychological Association has outlined additional factors associated with a resilient response, based upon learned behaviors[59]:

- The power to make realistic plans and take steps to carry them out
- A positive self-view and confidence in one's strengths and abilities
- Learned communication skills and problem solving
- The self-control to manage strong feelings and impulses

Box 17-1 describes ways to build resilience.[59]

Promoting Self Awareness

Awareness of loss of caring and negative attitude can prevent the development of CF and burnout, including

BOX 17-1 Ten Ways to Build Resilience

1. **Make connections.** Good relationships with close family members, friends, or others are important. Accepting help and support from those who care about you and will listen to you strengthens resilience. Some people find that being active in civic groups, faith-based organizations, or other local groups provides social support and can help with reclaiming hope. Assisting others in their time of need also can benefit the helper.
2. **Avoid seeing crises as insurmountable problems.** You can't change the fact that highly stressful events happen, but you can change how you interpret and respond to these events. Try looking beyond the present to how future circumstances may be a little better. Note any subtle ways in which you might already feel somewhat better as you deal with difficult situations.
3. **Accept that change is a part of living.** Certain goals may no longer be attainable because of adverse situations. Accepting circumstances that cannot be changed can help you focus on circumstances that you can alter.
4. **Move toward your goals.** Develop some realistic goals. Do something regularly—even if it seems like a small accomplishment—that enables you to move toward your goals. Instead of focusing on tasks that seem unachievable, ask yourself, "What's one thing I know I can accomplish today that helps me move in the direction I want to go?"
5. **Take decisive actions.** Act on adverse situations as much as you can. Take decisive actions, rather than detaching completely

from problems and stresses and wishing they would just go away.

6. **Look for opportunities for self-discovery.** People often learn something about themselves and may find that they have grown in some respect because of their struggle with loss. Many people who have experienced tragedies and hardship have reported better relationships, greater sense of strength even while feeling vulnerable, increased sense of self-worth, a more developed spirituality, and heightened appreciation for life.
7. **Nurture a positive view of yourself.** Developing confidence in your ability to solve problems and trusting your instincts helps build resilience.
8. **Keep things in perspective.** Even when facing very painful events, try to consider the stressful situation in a broader context and keep a long-term perspective. Avoid blowing the event out of proportion.
9. **Maintain a hopeful outlook.** An optimistic outlook enables you to expect that good things will happen in your life. Try visualizing what you want, rather than worrying about what you fear.
10. **Take care of yourself.** Pay attention to your own needs and feelings. Engage in activities that you enjoy and find relaxing. Exercise regularly. Taking care of yourself helps to keep your mind and body primed to deal with situations that require resilience.

Reproduced with permission from American Psychological Association. American Psychological Association. (n.d.). The road to resilience. Retrieved from http://www.apa.org/helpcenter/road-resilience.aspx.

the potentially negative mental, emotional, and physical effects of these conditions.[57] ED leaders can support the trauma team with the following interventions[60]:

- Help the trauma nurse develop a personal plan of care.
  - Institute policies and encourage habits that promote a healthy work and personal life balance.
- Encourage the nurse to develop a self-care plan as part of the annual evaluation process.[47]
  - Establish informal follow-up.
  - Check in with team members following a traumatic event or a period of continued high stress.
  - A brief conversation, email, or card can be a quick way to remind the trauma nurse of the importance of self-care.
- Provide private counseling services for the trauma nurse.
  - Most hospitals offer employee assistance programs that support employees in work-related issues.[47]
  - Counseling may provide a venue for self-reflection, identification of stressors, or identification of the need for referral to more comprehensive psychosocial services.
- Develop mentorship support.
  - Mentorship can be useful for the novice and the experienced nurse.
  - A formal mentorship program within the department or referral to a program through a professional organization is a way to provide this support.
  - Perspective and support from others can offer valuable insight into challenges common to trauma nursing practice.
- Provide care for the team.
  - Explore other internal resources, including social work, pastoral care, and chaplaincy.
  - Provide departmental, organizational, and community defusing and debriefing resources. Establish routines for formal debriefing and informal defusing to promote a positive attitude to psychosocial care for the trauma team.

Critical Incident Stress Management

CISM is reported to mitigate the impact of traumatic events and restores adaptive functioning to those exposed to a particular incident.

- *Debriefings* offer a structured response to CIs[56,61]:
  - A formal debriefing is open to voluntary participants within 24 to 72 hours of the CI.
  - It is meant to offer a review of events throughout a given CI and sharing of individual responses.[29]
  - It provides an opportunity to review performance and reflect on areas for improvement.
  - It promotes improved communication and patient safety.
  - It supports the resiliency and perceived psychological safety of team members.
- *Defusings* are more spontaneous or unstructured and are carried out informally within several hours of a traumatic event.

Overall, support following a CI or other traumatic event is not a one-size-fits-all solution. Those affected by the event are invited—not forced—to receive support, and resources are made available to all members of the healthcare team on a consistent, transparent basis.

Emerging Trends and Resources for Trauma Nurses

As more is learned about the lasting secondary effects of trauma, there has been an emergence of resources for patients, families, and providers.

Relationships have been identified between trauma, chronic pain, and psychological disorders, such as PTSD, depression, and substance use.[62,63] It has become imperative for trauma providers to consider the increased risk of these sequelae, especially given current trends in opioid addiction.[64] Clinicians should strive for appropriate use of opioids in pain management while introducing nonpharmacologic techniques to treat chronic pain in patients with or without PTSD.[65] Treatment programs focusing on mindfulness-based stress-reduction tactics and mindfulness-based cognitive therapies are proven effective approaches for treating PTSD and supporting recovery after trauma.[66]

There is growing awareness of the approach to Trauma-Informed Care (TIC) and interventions. TIC is a framework for clinicians that emphasizes physical, psychological, and emotional safety for both patients and providers. Trauma-informed clinicians are those who do the following[67]:

- Realize the widespread impact of trauma
- Recognize the signs and symptoms of trauma in clients, families, and providers
- Respond by integrating knowledge about trauma into procedures and practices
- Actively resist retraumatization

Key principles of the TIC approach include the following:

- Safety
- Trust and transparency
- Peer support
- Collaboration
- Empowerment
- Cultural, historical, and gender issues

Interventions that might be considered consistent with TIC include the following[67]:

- Dialogue and education on recovery expectations
- Awareness of warning signs including depression, anxiety, eating disorders, and substance abuse
- Connecting survivors and families with resources which will support recovery

Hospitals and providers may develop programs on their own or partner with others such as the American Trauma Society's Trauma Survivor Network to adopt practices and access resources that promote recovery.[68]

Caring for caregivers and supporting providers is becoming a priority of healthcare organizations as a means to promote resilience and ability to provide quality care. Schwartz Rounds is an example of a formal program that features interdisciplinary dialogue focused on the human dimension of healthcare and the experiences of healthcare providers.[69] Effective resiliency strategies include formal education programs, social support, and meaningful recognition.[70]

Summary

Provision of competent, safe, and compassionate psychosocial nursing care to those persons suffering sudden, unexpected injury or death remains a cornerstone of emergency and trauma nursing.[3] Understanding the human response to trauma can be key in offering support and guidance to patients and families and plays an important role in the development of assessment skills for the trauma nurse to use not only with patients and families, but also among colleagues and oneself.

Trauma nurses work in a highly stressful environment that often includes exposure to severely injured and dying patients, emotionally laden situations, or violence. STS and burnout can be a natural consequence of that exposure, so it is essential that trauma nurses are aware of and recognize the potential for these conditions to develop. It is important to realize that CF is a predictable, treatable, and preventable consequence of working with suffering people.[45,46,71] Information, education, and selected interventions can be used by the trauma nurse to ameliorate the symptoms and limit maladaptive consequences of acute, chronic, and continual exposure.

References

1. Cocker, F., & Joss, N. (2016). Compassion fatigue among healthcare, emergency and community service workers: A systematic review. *International Journal of Environmental Research and Public Health, 13*. https://doi.org/10.3390/ijerph13060618
2. Berg, G. M., Harshbarger, J. L., Ahlers-Schmidt, C. R., & Lippoldt, D. (2016). Exposing compassion fatigue and burnout syndrome in a trauma team: A qualitative study.

Journal of Trauma Nursing, 1, 3–10. https://doi.org/10.1097/JTN.0000000000000172

3. Emergency Nurses Association. (2017). *Emergency nursing scope and standards of practice* (2nd ed.). Des Plaines, IL: Author.
4. American College of Surgeons. (2014). Resources for optimal care of the injured patient (6th ed.) [Adobe Digital Editions]. Retrieved from https://www.facs.org/~/media/files/quality%20programs/trauma/vrc%20resources/resources%20for%20optimal%20care.ashx
5. Birur, B., Moore, N. C., & Davis, L. L. (2017). An evidence-based review of early intervention and prevention of post-traumatic stress disorder. *Community Mental Health Journal, 53*(2), 183–201. https://doi.org/10.1007/s10597-016-0047-x
6. American Psychological Association. (2013). Recovering emotionally from disaster. Retrieved from http://www.apa.org/helpcenter/recovering-disasters.aspx
7. Frank, C. A., Schroeter, K., & Shaw, C. (2017). Addressing traumatic stress in the acute traumatically injured patient. *Journal of Trauma Nursing, 24*(2), 78–84. https://doi.org/10.1097/JTN.0000000000000270
8. Hiskey, S. (2012). Psychological responses to trauma in older people. *Mental Health Practice, 16*(3), 12–16. Retrieved from https://doi.org/10.7748/mhp2012.11.16.3.12.c9393
9. Emergency Nurses Association, & International Nurses Society on Addictions. (2012). Expanded roles and responsibilities for nurses in screening, brief intervention, and referral to treatment (SBIRT) for alcohol use (Joint position statement). Retrieved from https://www.ena.org/docs/default-source/resource-library/practice-resources/position-statements/joint-statements/expandedrolesresponsibilitiesfornursesinsbirt.pdf?sfvrsn=594e67b0_6
10. Emergency Nurses Association. (2016). Tips for providing safe structure for adult behavioral health patients [Infographic]. Retrieved from https://www.ena.org/docs/default-source/resource-library/practice-resources/infographics/tips-for-providing-sage-structure-for-adult-behavioral-health-pts-in-the-ed.pdf?sfvrsn=6aefd9fa_4
11. TraumaDissociation.com. (2018). Acute stress disorder. Retrieved from http://traumadissociation.com/acutestressdisorder
12. Burston, A. (2017). Communication helped reduce anxiety for a patient and his family. *Nursing Standard, 32*(15), 65. https://doi.org/10.7748/ns.32.15.65.s38
13. U.S. Department of Veterans Affairs. (2015). PTSD: National Center for PTSD. Retrieved from https://www.ptsd.va.gov/public/problems/acute-stress-disorder.asp
14. Prins, A., Bovin, M. J., Kimerling, R., Kaloupek, D. G., Marx, B. P., Pless Kaiser, A., & Schnurr, P. P. (2015). Primary Care PTSD Screen for DSM-5 (PC-PTSD-5) [Measurement instrument]. Retrieved from https://www.ptsd.va.gov/professional/assessment/screens/pc-ptsd.asp
15. Emergency Nurses Association & International Association of Forensic Nurses. (2016). Joint position statement: Adult and adolescent sexual assault patients in the emergency care setting. Retrieved from https://www.ena.org/docs/default-source/resource-library/practice-resources/position-statements/joint-statements/adultandadolescentsexualassaultpatientser.pdf?sfvrsn=234258f1_6
16. Maple, M., Pearce, T., Sanford, R., Cerel, J., Castelli Dransart, D. A., & Andriessen, K. (2017). A systematic mapping of suicide bereavement and postvention research and a proposed strategic research agenda. *Journal of Crisis Intervention and Suicide Prevention*, 1–8. https://doi.org/10.1027/0227-5910/a000498
17. Thimm, J. C., & Holland, J. M. (2017). Early maladaptive schemas, meaning making, and complicated grief symptoms after bereavement. *International Journal of Stress Management, 24*(4), 347–367. https://doi.org/10.1037/str0000042
18. Bugge, K. E., Darbyshire, P., Rokholt, E. G., Sulheim Haugsvedt, K. T., & Helseth, S. (2014). Young children's grief: Parents' understanding and coping. *Death Studies, 38*(1), 36–43. https://doi.org/10.1080/07481187.2012.718037
19. Ramachandran, V. S. (2012). *Encyclopedia of human behavior* (2nd ed.). London, UK: Academic Press.
20. Leininger, M., & McFarland, M. (2006). *Culture care diversity and universality: A worldwide nursing theory* (2nd ed.). Sudbury, MA: Jones and Bartlett.
21. U.S. Department of Health and Human Services, Office of Minority Health. (2016). National CLAS Standards. Retrieved from https://minorityhealth.hhs.gov/omh/browse.aspx?lvl=2&lvlid=53
22. Institute for Patient- and Family-Centered Care. (n.d.). Better together: Partnering with families. Retrieved from http://www.ipfcc.org/bestpractices/better-together.html
23. Institute for Patient- and Family-Centered Care. (n.d.). *Better together pocket guide for staff.* Bethesda, MD: Author. Retrieved from http://www.ipfcc.org/bestpractices/guides-for-teams.html
24. Emergency Nurses Association. (2013). Palliative and end-of-life care in the emergency setting (Position statement). Retrieved from https://www.ena.org/docs/default-source/resource-library/practice-resources/position-statements/palliativeendoflifecare.pdf?sfvrsn=1777bb45_6
25. Kingsnorth-Hinrichs, J. (2010). Family presence during resuscitation. In P. K. Howard & R. A. Steinmann (Eds.), *Sheehy's emergency nursing: Principles and practice* (6th ed., pp. 148–154). St. Louis, MO: Mosby Elsevier.
26. Kingsnorth, J., O'Connell, K., Guzetta, C. E., Eden, J. C., Atabaki, S., Mecherikunnel, A., & Brown, K. (2010). Family presence during trauma activations and medical resuscitations in a pediatric emergency department: An evidence-based practice project. *Journal of Emergency Nursing, 36*(2), 115–121. https://doi.org/10.1016/j.jen.2009.12.023
27. Institute for Patient- and Family-Centered Care. (2012). Changing hospital "visiting" policies and practices: Supporting family presence and participation—executive summary. Retrieved from http://www.ipfcc.org/resources/visiting.pdf
28. Emergency Nurses Association. (2009). *Clinical practice guideline: Family presence during invasive procedures and resuscitation.* Des Plaines, IL: Author. Retrieved from https://www.ena.org/docs/default-source/resource-library/practice-resources/cpg/familypresencecpg3eaabb7cf0414584ac2291feba3be481.pdf?sfvrsn=9c167fc6_12

29. Leske, J. S., McAndrew, N. S., Brasel, K. J., & Feetham, S. (2017). Family presence during resuscitation after trauma. *Journal of Trauma Nursing, 24*(2), 85–96. https://doi.org/10.1097/JTN.0000000000000271
30. American Nurses Association. (2015). *Code of ethics for nurses with interpretive statements.* Silver Spring, MD: Nursesbooks.org.
31. Macrohon, B. C. (2012). Pediatrician's perspectives on discharge against medical advice (DAMA) among pediatric patients: A qualitative study. *BMC Pediatrics, 12*(74). https://doi.org/10.1186/1471-2431-12-75
32. Pozgar, G. D. (2014). *Legal and ethical essentials of health care administration* (2nd ed.). Burlington, MA: Jones & Bartlett Learning.
33. Heilicser, B. (2013). Ethical dilemmas in emergency nursing. In B. B. Hammond & P. G. Zimmerman (Eds.), *Sheehy's manual of emergency care* (7th ed., pp. 43–48). St. Louis, MO: Mosby Elsevier.
34. Texas Civil Practices and Remedies Code, Liability in Tort, Sec. § 74.151, Liability for Emergency Care. Retrieved from https://texas.public.law/statutes/tex._civ._practice_and_remedies_code_section_74.151
35. Somes, J., & Donatelli, N. (2012). Do not intubate/do not resuscitate: Treating the severely ill or injured geriatric patient in the emergency department. *Journal of Emergency Nursing, 38*(3), 283–286. https://doi.org/10.1016/j.jen.2012.03.013
36. Bonalumi, N. (2010). Organ and tissue donation. In P. K. Howard & R. A. Steinmann (Eds.), *Sheehy's emergency nursing: Principles and practice* (6th ed., pp. 155–163). St. Louis, MO: Mosby Elsevier.
37. Sacco, T. L., Ciurzynski, S. M., Harvey, M. E., & Ingersoll, G. L. (2015). Compassion satisfaction and CF among critical care nurses. *Critical Care Nurse, 35*(4), 32–42. https://doi.org/10.4037/ccn2015392
38. van Mol, M. M. C., Kompanje, E. J., Benoit, D. D., Bakker, J., & Nijkamp, M. D. (2015). The prevalence of CF and burnout among healthcare professionals in intensive care units: A systematic review. *PLoS One, 10*(8), 1–22. https://doi.org/10.1371/journal.pone.0136955
39. Hinderer, K. A., VonRueden, K. T., Friedmann, E., McQuillan, K. A., Gilmore, R., & Murray, M. (2014). Burnout, compassion fatigue, compassion satisfaction, and secondary traumatic stress in trauma nurses. *Journal of Trauma Nursing, 21*, 160–169. https://doi.org/10.1097/JTN.0000000000000055
40. Potter, P., Deshields, T., & Rodriguez, S. (2013). Developing a systemic program for compassion fatigue. *Nursing Administration Quarterly, 37*(4), 326–332. https://doi.org/10.1097/NAQ.0b013e3182a2f9dd
41. Stamm, B. H. (2010). *The concise ProQOL manual* (2nd ed.). Pocatello, ID: ProQOL.org.
42. Missouridou, E. (2017). Secondary posttraumatic stress and nurses' emotional responses to patient's trauma. *Journal of Trauma Nursing, 24*(2), 110–115. https://doi.org/10.1097/JTN.0000000000000274
43. Mooney, C., Fetter, K., Gross, B. W., Rinehart, C., Lynch, C., & Rogers, F. B. (2017). A preliminary analysis of compassion satisfaction and compassion fatigue with considerations for nursing unit specialization and demographic factors. *Journal of Trauma Nursing, 24*(3), 158–163. https://doi.org/10.1097/JTN.0000000000000284
44. Newcomb, A. B., & Hymes, R. A. (2017). Life interrupted: The trauma caregiver experience. *Journal of Trauma Nursing, 24*(2), 125–133. https://doi.org/10.1097/JTN.0000000000000278
45. Henson, J. S. (2017). When compassion is lost. *MedSurg Nursing, 26*(2), 139–142. Retrieved from https://www.highbeam.com/doc/1G1-491949347.html
46. Sorenson, C., Bolick, B., Wright, K., & Hamilton, R. (2017). An evolutionary concept analysis of compassion fatigue. *Journal of Nursing Scholarship, 49*(5), 557–563. https://doi.org/10.1111/jnu.12312
47. Lombardo, B., & Eyre, C. (2012). Compassion fatigue: A nurse's primer. *Online Journal of Issues in Nursing, 16*(1), 3. Retrieved from http://ojin.nursingworld.org/MainMenuCategories/ANAMarketplace/ANAPeriodicals/OJIN/TableofContents/Vol-16-2011/No1-Jan-2011/Compassion-Fatigue-A-Nurses-Primer.html
48. Dominguez-Gomez, E., & Rutledge, D. (2009). Prevalence of secondary traumatic stress among emergency nurses. *Journal of Emergency Nursing, 35*(3), 199–204.
49. Beck, C. T. (2011). Secondary traumatic stress in nurses: A systematic review. *Archives of Psychiatric Nursing, 25*(1), 1–10. https://doi.org/10.1016/j.apnu.2010.05.005
50. Emergency Nurses Association. (2018). *Social networking by emergency nurses* (Position statement). Des Plaines, IL: Author. Retrieved from https://www.ena.org/docs/default-source/resource-library/practice-resources/position-statements/socialnetworkingbyernurses.pdf?sfvrsn=5e069b1a_8
51. Emergency Nurses Association. (2010). ENA workplace violence toolkit. Retrieved from https://www.ena.org/docs/default-source/resource-library/practice-resources/toolkits/workplaceviolencetoolkit.pdf?sfvrsn=6785bc04_28
52. Avander, K., Heikki, A., Bjersa, K., & Engstrom, M. (2016). Trauma nurses' experience of workplace violence and threats: Short- and long-term consequences in a Swedish setting. *Journal of Trauma Nursing, 23*(2), 51–57. https://doi.org/10.1097/JTN.0000000000000186
53. Centers for Disease Control and Prevention. (2017, December 18). Coping with a disaster or traumatic event. Retrieved from https://emergency.cdc.gov/coping/index.asp
54. Poghosyan, L., Aiken, L. H., & Sloane, D. M. (2009). Factor structure of the Maslach Burnout Inventory: An analysis of data from large scale cross-sectional surveys of nurses from eight countries. *International Journal of Nursing Studies, 46*(7), 894–902. https://doi.org/10.1016/j.ijnurstu.2009.03.004
55. Maslach, D., & Leiter, M. P. (2007). Burnout. In G. Fink (Ed.), *Encyclopedia of stress* (2nd ed., pp. 368–371). London, UK: Academic Press.
56. Schmidt, M., & Haglund, K. (2017). Debrief in emergency departments to improve compassion fatigue and promote resiliency. *Journal of Trauma Nursing, 24*(5), 317–322. https://doi.org/10.1097/JTN.0000000000000315
57. Schroeter, K. (2017). Ethics in practice: From moral distress to moral resilience. *Journal of Trauma Nursing, 24*(5), 290–291. https://doi.org/10.1097/JTN.0000000000000317

58. Grafton, E., Gillespie, B., & Henderson, S. (2010). Resilience: The power within. *Oncology Nursing Forum, 37*(6), 698–705. https://doi.org/10.1188/10.ONF.698-705

59. American Psychological Association. (n.d.). The road to resilience. Retrieved from http://www.apa.org/helpcenter/road-resilience.aspx

60. Emergency Nurses Association. (2018). Nurse leaders in emergency care settings (Position statement). Retrieved from https://www.ena.org/docs/default-source/resource-library/practice-resources/position-statements/nurseleaders.pdf?sfvrsn=316948d8_12

61. Berg, G. M., Harvey, A. M., Basham-Saif, A., Parsons, D., Acuna, D., & Lippoldt, D. (2014). Acceptability and implementation of debriefings after trauma resuscitation. *Journal of Trauma Nursing, 21*(5), 201–208. https://doi.org/10.1097/JTN.0000000000000066

62. Darnall, B. D. (2019). Depression, anxiety, and posttraumatic stress disorder. In *Psychological treatment for patients with chronic pain* (pp. 49–61). https://doi.org/10.1037/0000104-000

63. U.S. Department of Veterans Affairs. (2015). Chronic pain and PTSD: A guide for patients. Retrieved from https://www.ptsd.va.gov/understand/related/chronic_pain.asp

64. Centers for Disease Control and Prevention. (2018). CDC guideline for prescribing opioids for chronic pain. Retrieved from https://www.cdc.gov/drugoverdose/prescribing/guideline.html

65. Nathoo, T., Poole, N., & Schmidt, R. (2018). *Trauma informed practice and the opioid crisis: A discussion guide for health care and social service providers.* Vancouver, BC: Centre of Excellence for Women's Health. Retrieved from https://preventionconversation.files.wordpress.com/2018/05/opioid-tip-guide_may-2018.pdf

66. Boyd, J. E., Lanius, R. A., & McKinnon, M. C. (2018). Mindfulness-based treatments for posttraumatic stress disorder: A review of the treatment literature and neurobiological evidence. *Journal of Psychiatry & Neuroscience, 43*(1), 7–25. https://doi.org/10.1503/jpn.170021

67. Substance Abuse and Mental Health Services Administration. (2018, April 27). Trauma-informed approach and trauma-specific interventions. Retrieved from https://www.samhsa.gov/nctic/trauma-interventions

68. Trauma Survivors Network. (n.d.). Home page. Retrieved from https://www.traumasurvivorsnetwork.org/pages/home

69. Schwartz Center for Compassionate Healthcare. (n.d.). Supporting caregivers: Schwartz Rounds. Retrieved from http://www.theschwartzcenter.org/supporting-caregivers/schwartz-center-rounds/

70. Kester, K., & Wei, H. (2018). Building nurse resilience. *Nursing Management, 49*(6), 42–45. https://doi.org/10.1097/01.NUMA.0000533768.28005.36

71. Hooper, C., Craig, J., Janvrin, D. R., Westel, M. A., & Reimels, E. (2010). Compassion satisfaction, burnout, and compassion fatigue among emergency nurses compared with nurses in other selected inpatient specialties. *Journal of Emergency Nursing, 36*(5), 420–427. https://doi.org/10.1016/j.jen.2009.11.027

APPENDIX 17-1

The Professional Quality of Life Scale

Professional Quality of Life Scale (ProQOL) Compassion Satisfaction and Fatigue (ProQOL) Version 5 (2009)

When you provide nursing care for people, you have direct contact with their lives. As you may have found, your compassion for those you nurse for can affect you in positive and negative ways. Below are some questions about your experiences, both positive and negative, as a nurse. Consider each of the following questions about you and your current work situation. Select the number that honestly reflects how frequently you experienced these things in the *last 30 days*.

1 = Never	2 = Rarely	3 = Sometimes	4 = Often	5 = Very Often

_____1. I am happy.
_____2. I am preoccupied with more than one person I have cared for.
_____3. I get satisfaction from being able to care for people.
_____4. I feel connected to others.
_____5. I jump or am startled by unexpected sounds.
_____6. I feel invigorated after working with those I care for.
_____7. I find it difficult to separate my personal life from my life as a nurse.
_____8. I am not as productive at work because I am losing sleep over traumatic experiences of a person I care for.
_____9. I think that I might have been affected by the traumatic stress of those I care for.
_____10. I feel trapped by my job as a nurse.
_____11. Because of nursing, I have felt "on edge" about various things.
_____12. I like my work as a nurse.
_____13. I feel depressed because of the traumatic experiences of the people I care for.
_____14. I feel as though I am experiencing the trauma of someone I have cared for.
_____15. I have beliefs that sustain me.
_____16. I am pleased with how I am able to keep up with nursing techniques and protocols.
_____17. I am the person I always wanted to be.
_____18. My work makes me feel satisfied.
_____19. I feel worn out because of my work as a nurse.
_____20. I have happy thoughts and feelings about those I care for and how I could help them.
_____21. I feel overwhelmed because my patient load seems endless.
_____22. I believe I can make a difference through my work.
_____23. I avoid certain activities or situations because they remind me of frightening experiences of the people I care for.
_____24. I am proud of what I can do to for patients.
_____25. As a result of nursing, I have intrusive, frightening thoughts.
_____26. I feel "bogged down" by the system.
_____27. I have thoughts that I am a "success" as a nurse.
_____28. I can't recall important parts of my work with trauma victims.
_____29. I am a very caring person.
_____30. I am happy that I chose to do this work.

What Is My Score and What Does It Mean?

In this section, you will score your test and then you can compare your score to the following interpretation.

Scoring

1. Be certain you respond to all items.
2. Go to items 1, 4, 15, 17, and 29 and reverse your scores. For example, if you scored the item 1, write a 5 beside it. We ask you to reverse these scores because we have learned that the test works better if you reverse these scores.

You Wrote	Change To
1	5
2	4
3	3
4	2
5	1

To find your score on **Compassion Satisfaction,** add your scores on questions 3, 6, 12, 16, 18, 20, 22, 24, 27, and 30.

The Sum of My Compassion Satisfaction Questions Was	So My Score Equals	My Level of Compassion Satisfaction
22 or less	43 or less	Low
Between 23 and 41	Around 50	Average
42 or more	57 or more	High

To find your score on **Burnout**, add your scores on questions 1, 4, 8, 10, 15, 17, 19, 21, 26, and 29. Find your score on the following table.

The Sum of My Secondary Traumatic Stress Questions	So My Score Equals	My Level of Secondary Traumatic Stress
22 or less	43 or less	Low
Between 23 and 41	Around 50	Average
42 or more	57 or more	High

To find your score on **Secondary Traumatic Stress,** add your scores on questions 2, 5, 7, 9, 11, 13, 14, 23, 25, and 28. Find your score on the following table.

The Sum of My Burnout Questions	So My Score Equals	My Level of Burnout
22 or less	43 or less	Low
Between 23 and 41	Around 50	Average
42 or more	57 or more	High

Your Scores on the ProQOL: Professional Quality of Life Screening

Based on your responses, your personal scores are below. If you have any concerns, you should discuss them with a physical or mental health care professional.

Compassion Satisfaction _______

Compassion satisfaction is about the pleasure you derive from being able to do your work well. For example, you may feel like it is a pleasure to help others through your work. You may feel positively about your colleagues or your ability to contribute to the work setting or even the greater good of society. Higher scores on this scale represent a greater satisfaction related to your ability to be an effective caregiver in your job.

The average score is 50 (SD 10; alpha scale reliability .88). About 25% of people score higher than 57 and about 25% of people score below 43. If you are in the higher range, you probably derive a good deal of professional satisfaction from your position. If your scores are below 40, you may either find problems with your job, or there may be some other reason—for example, you might derive your satisfaction from activities other than your job.

Burnout _______

Most people have an intuitive idea of what burnout is. From the research perspective, burnout is one of the elements of compassion fatigue. It is associated with feelings of hopelessness and difficulties in dealing with work or in doing your job effectively. These negative feelings usually have a gradual onset. They can reflect the feeling that your efforts make no difference, or they can be associated with a very high workload or a non-supportive work environment. Higher scores on this scale mean that you are at higher risk for burnout.

The average score on the burnout scale is 50 (SD 10; alpha scale reliability .75). About 25% of people score above 57 and about 25% of people score below 43. If your score is below 18, this probably reflects positive feelings about your ability to be effective in your work. If you score above 57, you may wish to think about what at work makes you feel like you are not effective in your position. Your score may reflect your mood; perhaps you were having a "bad day" or are in need of some time off. If the high score persists or if it is reflective of other worries, it may be a cause for concern.

Secondary Traumatic Stress _____

The second component of compassion fatigue (CF) is secondary traumatic stress (STS). It is about your work-related, secondary exposure to extremely or traumatically stressful events. Developing problems due to exposure to others' trauma is somewhat rare but does happen to many people who care for those who have experienced extremely or traumatically stressful events. For example, you may repeatedly hear stories about the traumatic things that happen to other people, commonly called vicarious traumatization. You may see or provide treatment to people who have experienced horrific events. If your work puts you directly in the path of danger, due to your work as a soldier or civilian working in military medicine personnel, this is not secondary exposure; your exposure is primary. However, if you are exposed to others' traumatic events as a result of your work, such as providing care to casualties or for those in a military medical rehabilitation facility, this is secondary exposure. The symptoms of STS are usually rapid in onset and associated with a particular event. They may include being afraid, having difficulty sleeping, having images of the upsetting event pop into your mind, or avoiding things that remind you of the event.

The average score on this scale is 50 (SD 10; alpha scale reliability .81). About 25% of people score below 43 and about 25% of people score above 57. If your score is above 57, you may want to take some time to think about what at work may be frightening to you or if there is some other reason for the elevated score. While higher scores do not mean that you do have a problem, they are an indication that you may want to examine how you feel about your work and your work environment. You may wish to discuss this with your supervisor, a colleague, or a health care professional.

CHAPTER 18

Disaster Management

Steven F. Jacobson, MSN, MS, MBA, RN, CEN, CFRN, NREMT-P

OBJECTIVES

Upon completion of this chapter, the learner will be able to:

1. Identify the four phases of emergency management and the components involved in an all-hazards approach to emergency preparedness.
2. Discuss the types of illnesses or injuries associated with natural and human-made disasters.
3. Compare conventional triage to mass-casualty triage.
4. Discuss nursing roles and responsibilities related to the all-hazards approach to emergency preparedness.

Introduction

On October 1, 2017, a gunman opened fire from his hotel window into a crowd of concert-goers in Las Vegas. As the event quickly made the news, the active shooter at the Route 91 Harvest Music festival on the Las Vegas Strip left 58 people dead and more than 800 injured. Local healthcare resources were quickly mobilized for the response in an effort to triage, transport, and save as many lives as possible.

The closest hospital, Sunrise Hospital and Medical Center, received a reported 212 victims in the 7 hours after the event.[1] As the victims came flooding into the hospital, the staff quickly set up a process of triage to sort through those victims who were salvageable and to provide the best care to as many wounded victims as possible. This process involved a well-rehearsed plan, not only on the part of Sunrise, but also the University Medical Center of Southern Nevada (UMCSN), Dignity Health, and local paramedics and law enforcement.[2] On a routine night, UMCSN might see 15 or more trauma activations, but on this occasion the number went into the hundreds.[3]

As information was received, unit clerks and support staff quickly called in more staff. Nurses and physicians set up treatment areas, support staff stepped into their designated roles, and the seemingly controlled chaos took over. Management of this disaster relied heavily on implementing an established plan, as the volume of patients quickly exceeded the capacity of all the area hospitals.

Disaster Defined

Disaster has many definitions. The International Federation of Red Cross and Red Crescent Societies defines a disaster as a "sudden, calamitous event that seriously disrupts the functioning of a community or society and causes human, material and economic losses that exceed the community's or society's ability to cope using its own resources."[4] The World Health Organization (WHO) defines a disaster as a "situation or event, which overwhelms local capacity, necessitating a request to national or international level for external assistance."[5] Both definitions describe disaster as a situation in which the demand for support exceeds the normal available resources. Resources affected include the healthcare system, personnel, supplies and equipment, utilities, and structure of the facilities.

It is important to note that every disaster situation is unique and can stress a system at various levels. Multiple-casualty incidents (MCIs) typically occur on a more frequent basis and may have substantial impact at the local level. A multiple-car pileup on a large highway is an example of an MCI. When faced with an MCI, the healthcare system may strain its resources but is not overwhelmed. At the other end of the spectrum, mass-casualty events (MCEs) have a large enough number of casualties to overwhelm and disrupt the healthcare services in the affected community or geographic area.[6] Hurricanes, earthquakes, and wildfires are examples of MCEs.

A disaster is different for every community. Elements such as geographic location, available resources, and community size will all affect the definition of a disaster for these communities. A small community hospital with limited healthcare resources could define a small factory explosion as a major disaster for the community, whereas the resources of a large metropolitan hospital could easily accommodate the number of patients generated by an event. Whether the incident is large or small, however, a disruption of normal operating conditions requires the trauma nurse to be familiar with which actions to take in this situation.

Disasters can be natural or human-made in origin. Although most disasters are natural, the world appears to be facing an increased incidence of human-made disasters. As a result, coordinated response efforts and asset integration focus on emergency management and creating a more resilient infrastructure.[7] This approach integrates an all-hazards approach, but also looks at the various consequences of the disaster on the population.[8]

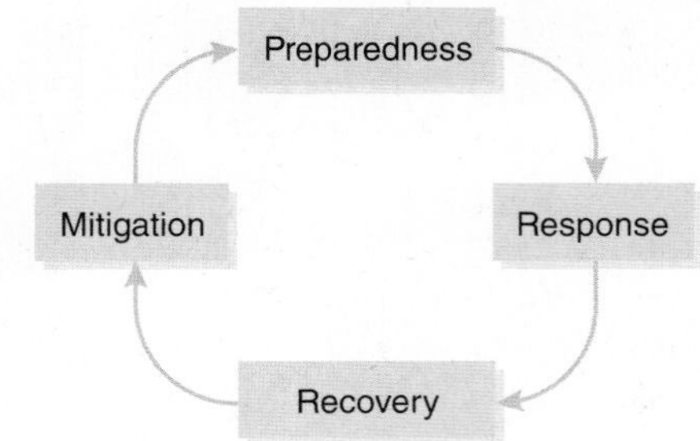

Figure 18-1 *The disaster life cycle.*

Reproduced from Federal Emergency Management Agency, National Earthquake Hazards Reduction Program. (n.d.). Earthquake coordinators web site. Retrieved from https://training.fema.gov/emiweb/earthquake/neh0101220.htm.

The all-hazards approach to emergency management acknowledges that the specific type of disaster that may strike is uncertain and that considering the many different threats and potential hazards is necessary. An organization's emergency management plan or a Hazard Vulnerability Analysis done for that organization should identify specific threats and vulnerabilities, that may be present and plan strategies for prevention, deterrence, or minimization of the impact.[8]

Emergency management is organized into a four-phase, ongoing process known as the disaster life cycle. These four phases are mitigation, preparedness, response, and recovery (**Figure 18-1**).[9]

Mitigation

Mitigation provides a foundation of knowledge to reduce loss of life and property from disaster by limiting or avoiding potential impact and incorporating lessons learned from previous events.[10] Findings from real events and drills are key elements that drive the mitigation process. Lessons learned, deficiencies identified, and areas of improvement provide insights that inform prevention and steps to minimize the potential impact on the facility. By identifying these elements, the facility can take steps such as activating prior arrangements for assets and resources can be implemented as well as engaging effective procedures to minimize the impact of the event.

In a proactive approach, a hazard vulnerability analysis (HVA) is developed as a systematic approach to recognizing and identifying potential hazards that may have an impact on a healthcare facility and its surrounding community. Hazards considered in the HVA include any type of technological, hazardous materials, natural, or human-made hazards. Each hazard is scored based on its potential to affect the facility, the preparedness of the facility, and the external resources available. This tool enables the facility to focus on the high-risk hazards and determine which actions it could take to prevent or lessen their impacts. For example, an HVA could identify a weather-related vulnerability such as flooding that would likely result in water leaks, electrical outages, loss of use of areas, and loss of supplies due to water damage. Steps to mitigate those effects might involve regular inspections by maintenance personnel for leak-prone areas throughout the facility, creation of a defined process for generator use, and identification of alternative locations to store supplies and materials. These procedures and processes identified for mitigation are the components that should then drive the development of an emergency operations plan.

The goal of the mitigation phase is not to prevent the disaster. Instead, infrastructure mitigation efforts are intended to minimize the impact of life and property loss.

Preparedness

Preparedness is built upon the premise that not all disasters can be prevented. To be ready for the situations identified in an HVA, hospitals should have a properly maintained emergency operations plan and all staff should be familiar with the Incident Command System.

Hospital Disaster Preparedness Plans

It is critical for hospitals to develop comprehensive disaster preparedness plans that address all potential hazards and prioritize risks identified in the HVA. Healthcare agencies are required to have a hospital emergency management program that addresses all phases of the disaster cycle—mitigation, preparedness, response, and recovery.[10] The Joint Commission has identified six critical areas in which hospitals must demonstrate proper planning: communication, supplies, security, staff, utilities, and clinical activity.[11] Trauma nurses who have an understanding of the overall plan and how their roles are integrated with the emergency management system will be able to provide the best patient care possible in the face of complex, extreme events.

The hospital emergency operations plan should encompass unit-based response plans as well as expand outward to include coordination with the community. Local, regional, and countywide healthcare coalitions extending to the state level and potentially the federal level are necessary to ensure a more effective response in a disaster.[12] Disaster plans should include the reallocation of supplies/equipment and system process changes as necessary. Additional guidelines for adjusting mandated staffing ratios, assigning role responsibilities, and creating alternative care areas are necessary to ensure safe and legal steps are taken in a disaster. The trauma nurse needs to be aware of their department's emergency response plan and how the department and the individual's role may change during a disaster.

An important aspect of preparedness is conducting disaster exercises. These exercises are beneficial because they ensure that the plans are effective, and because they provide an opportunity for staff to familiarize themselves with how the plans are carried out.

Disaster exercises vary in complexity from simple seminars to full-scale exercises. There are seven types of exercises that are divided into discussion- and operations-based types. Discussion-based exercises focus more on familiarizing staff with, or developing, plans and policies; they include seminars, workshops, tabletop exercises, and games. Operations-based exercises focus more on validating existing plans, identifying gaps, and clarifying roles; they include drills, functional exercises, and full-scale exercises.[13] **Table 18-1** provides more detailed descriptions and examples of each of these exercises. The most challenging endeavor is a full-scale exercise, which often takes months to plan and requires the participation of multiple organizations at one time.[13]

Disaster exercises can serve a variety of purposes, from evaluating current plans to rehearsing for a real event. After the exercise, there are multiple formal and informal steps used to review the results of the exercise. A "hot wash" is an immediate after-action discussion and evaluation of the participants' actions during the exercise. An important document that is constructed post exercise is the after-action report, which reviews the elements of a formal or informal exercise. This retrospective analysis looks at the sequence of events of the exercise and determines whether goals were met and which areas need improvement.

Incident Command System

The approach to disaster response is based on the Incident Command System (ICS), which is a standardized management tool. ICS has its roots in California and came about in the 1970s, after the state experienced a series of severe fires and the involved response agencies recognized there was a failure in communication and coordination that resulted in confusion and improper use of resources. As a result, Congress allocated money to the U.S. Forest Service to create a system to improve the ability to manage multiagency and multijurisdictional responses. After the September 11, 2001, terrorist attacks against the World

TABLE 18-1 Types of Disaster Exercises

Types of Exercises	Description
Seminar	Informal discussion that is designed to orient exercise participants to plans, policies, or procedures.
Workshop	Similar to a seminar, but has the goal of creating a plan or policy.
Tabletop exercise	A simulation in which key personnel discuss and role-play a scenario to assess plans and procedures. This type of exercise resembles a disaster "board game."
Game	A larger-scale simulation of operations involving teams, which is designed to be competitive and includes rules and data in an artificial environment.
Drill	An exercise in which a single department or entity employs a simulated operation or function. Most often thought of as a triage or decontamination drill.
Functional exercise	An exercise in which individuals practice their roles in a simulated disaster, and which often involves multiple agencies and departments. Team members have an opportunity to practice their roles without engaging in an actual or simulated response.
Full-scale exercise	As close to a real scenario as possible. Team members from multiple disciplines and agencies practice an emergency response to a disaster using as much equipment and performing duties as if the simulation were a real scenario.

Data from California Hospital Association. (n.d.). Types of exercises. *Emergency Preparedness*. Retrieved from https://www.calhospitalprepare.org/post/types-exercises.

Trade Center, the Pentagon, and an airline flight that crashed in Pennsylvania, the U.S. Department of Homeland Security was created and subsequently developed the National Incident Management System (NIMS), of which ICS is a key component.[10] NIMS is a nationwide approach that can be used by federal, state, tribal, and local governments as well as nongovernmental organizations. Federal grant funding is tied to the implementation of ICS in many circumstances.

Hospitals, too, have implemented a form of ICS called the Hospital Incident Command System (HICS).[14] Using HICS enables hospitals to standardize the management of an incident within an organizational structure. The trauma nurse should be familiar with the standard terminology, roles, and responsibilities defined in HICS in order to be an effective member of the team during an emergency response.

Response

Often the most highly visible portion of a disaster, the response phase includes elements of warning/evacuation, rescue, triage of victims, aiding victims, damage assessment, and actions to support infrastructure. During the response phase, plans and preparation are put into place to save lives or prevent further loss of life or property. This phase begins when the incident occurs.

The trauma nurse's role in the response phase begins when notification is made to the nurse of the disaster. These notifications can come in many ways, both coordinated and uncoordinated. For example, the trauma nurse may receive an alert from prehospital providers or a governmental organization, see an event unfolding on the news or social media, or in some cases encounter an influx of patients who self-transported to the facility. Whatever the circumstances, the trauma nurse can have many important roles in the response phase of a disaster.

Patient Surge

The immediate aftermath of a disaster often results in increased demands on the capacity and capability of healthcare services, also known as surge capacity. The surge of patients obligates the hospital to expand the use and availability of space, supplies, staff, and the system as a whole. This can be especially difficult in today's environment, when so many hospitals are already operating at or near capacity on a daily basis. Medical surge in the aftermath of a disaster will likely put a significant strain on the healthcare system. Having plans in place for alternative care locations, resource allocation, and security allows for a rapid ramp-up of operations to prepare for incoming victims. Examples of alternative care locations include patient care tents, emergency shelters, or deployable shelters. After receiving notification of an incident, the trauma nurse can expect that activation of the disaster plan will occur before the first influx of victims arrives.[15]

Throughout an incident, patient tracking remains a key component to ensure adequate resources are available for ongoing operations and to minimize loss of life. Alternative forms of tracking will likely be used because of the impact a disaster may have on human resources, infrastructure, and technology. Low technology tools (e.g., dry erase boards or written logs) may be part of the established plan for patient tracking. The trauma nurse should be familiar with the established practices for patient tracking during a disaster. The hospital can take steps to address patient surge, such as by recalling off-duty staff to work or holding over current staff, establishing alternative patient care areas, adjusting staff ratios, changing supply distribution, and expediting discharges of admitted patients or cancellation of elective surgeries or procedures. No matter which method is used, it is essential that the trauma nurse be familiar with the process prior to the initiation of the response phase and be ready to support workflow, manage supplies and equipment, and decompress overwhelmed units during the surge.

Disaster Triage

Triage is a fundamental function in a disaster. The goal of disaster triage is to do "the greatest good for the greatest number"[5]—a notion that operates under a different ethical approach than routine triage in the hospital setting. When healthcare resources are scarce during a disaster, the trauma nurse must function based on the utilitarian ethical theory, according to which the goal is to achieve the greatest good for the most number of people.[16] This approach is contrary to the philosophy that is frequently at the heart of nursing, in which the sickest patients receive the highest priority and heroic efforts are put forth to resuscitate them. In a disaster, the sickest patients may consume too many resources and divert resources away from the larger group of patients who have a better chance of survival given the situation. Thus, disaster triage algorithms assess and sort patients based on their condition, likely prognosis, and the availability of resources (**Appendix 18-1**).

Several methodologies of disaster triage have been developed, including Simple Triage and Rapid Treatment (START) and Sort–Assess–Lifesaving Interventions–Treatment and/or Transport (SALT). It is important for facilities to determine ahead of time which type of disaster triage system they will use, including clinical documentation and patient tracking tools. Other key elements of disaster triage include who will be assigned to each role, locations where groups of patients will be treated, and dissemination of adequate resources to defined areas.[5]

Primary triage is the first step in sorting patients during an MCI or MCE. The START disaster triage system (Appendix 18-1A) relies on four color-coded groups of patients sorted according to the level of care required: red (immediate), yellow (delayed), green (minor), and black (expectant).[5] The patient assessment in START is brief, so as to facilitate rapid sorting, with the assessment elements being respirations, perfusion, and mental status (RPM). START has also been adapted for use with pediatric patients (JumpSTART; Appendix 18-1B).

The SALT triage algorithm (Appendix 18-1C) uses a similar sorting method to sort and assess victims, provide limited lifesaving interventions, and then prioritize treatment and transportation.[17] The algorithm results in the same color-coded outcomes, with patients given black tags being described as deceased or expectant. This group includes those patients who are still alive but have injuries incompatible with life, given the resources available. An important aspect of SALT is to globally sort victims at a scene into walkers, who can walk from the scene; wavers, who make purposeful movement but cannot ambulate; and patients who are still. This sorting quickly identifies those patients who are the highest priority for assessment.

Both the START and SALT methods of sorting disaster victims have merit, and the trauma nurse should be well versed in the method chosen by local organizations. One comparison of the SALT and START triage methods found that SALT was more accurate in identifying higher-priority patients than START.[18] However, healthcare systems have been slow to adopt this method.

Large-scale communicable disease outbreaks that can affect a significant population would be a situation where a triage process is also useful. Communicable disease triage can be based on the Susceptible-Exposed-Infectious-Removed-Vaccinated (SEIRV) (Appendix 18-1D) method, which separates a population into five categories: susceptible, exposed, infectious, removed and vaccinated.[19] While biological events are similar to other MCEs, they include additional considerations such as exposure, duration of the symptom-free period, and infectiousness of the pathogen. The benefits of the SEIRV model include the ability to manage patients as well as control transmission to nonsymptomatic patients.

Overall, these rapid sorting processes assess patients with little to no interventions performed to identify where to use limited resources. It is imperative that the nurse who is performing primary triage be cognizant of the resources available. In a resource-limited environment, patients may not be classified into the deceased or expectant category solely based on physiological assessment. Instead, patients who would otherwise be salvageable by going to surgery, receiving blood, or being placed on a ventilator may be placed into the expectant category because that resource is not available at that point in time. The line between patients who warrant immediate treatment and those who are expectant changes in an MCI—a reality that can be difficult for trauma nurses to accept. To make an even finer distinction, some patients may be classified as expectant because of *wounds,* because they are simply not salvageable under any circumstances. These individuals are given dignity and respect but are not resuscitated. Others may be classified as expectant because of *resources*; that is, they could be treated if more capabilities were available. These patients may be sequestered and held in a basic life support capacity; if and when a more opportune time occurs and resources open up, they could be brought into treatment areas and receive the benefit of lifesaving interventions.

Each disaster situation is dynamic. Reevaluation of the incident and its action plan is ongoing. Secondary triage is typically performed at a casualty clearing area after the initial sorting. Victims are medically reassessed based on their prognosis, condition, and available resources to determine if they need to be recategorized.

Evacuation

In the event that a healthcare facility's structure or functionality is impacted by a natural disaster, and the situation escalates to threaten the health or safety of the facility's patients, visitors, and staff, evacuation may be necessary.[20] Such an incident may include a loss of emergency power, compromise of the heating, ventilation, and air conditioning system, or structural damage as a result of human-made events (e.g., terrorism) or natural disasters (e.g., flooding, earthquake, or tornado). As a part of the emergency operations plan, the decision-making process and responsible party for the evacuation should be clearly defined. The decision-making process can also include options for partial or full evacuation as well as a horizontal evacuation. Depending on the specifics of the event, a partial evacuation may accomplish the desired outcome of ensuring patient safety with a smaller disruption in patient care services.[21] An example of a horizontal evacuation would be moving patients and staff away from the area of danger to another area that is safe to use on the same floor. Larger academic centers with multiple buildings could potentially implement a partial horizontal evacuation in the event that one building becomes damaged or unusable but other areas remain functional.

Once the decision is made to evacuate a hospital, the disaster management team will need to identify transportation resources that are both within and outside the facility. It is necessary to identify the order of evacuation (ambulatory patients before stretcher-carried patients) and the methods of evacuation (stair chairs versus blanket carries). During an evacuation, it is essential to maintain accurate tracking of patient movement. This allows staff to record which patients went to other areas within the facility or community, as well as their locations. Accurate tracking facilitates the continuity of patient care, and the ability to inform families and visitors of the current patient location. Transport of supplies, records, and medications must also be considered. Staff should know which supplies, medications, and records need to go with the patient to maintain an adequate level of care. This process includes protocols and processes for transfer of controlled substances to other care providers and ensuring privacy of patient records. For more information, refer to Chapter 19, "Transition of Care for the Trauma Patient."

Alternative care sites should be identified during the planning process to provide for ongoing safe provision of care for patients, staff, and visitors. Memoranda of understandings are developed ahead of time to address considerations such as facility proximity and the resources needed to meet the healthcare needs of patients based on various care priorities and acuity.

The Joint Commission has developed a guideline for ensuring facility sustainability during a disaster that is known as the Emergency Management 96-Hour Plan. The expectation is that an organization will understand its capabilities and limitations during a declared disaster and recognize how services can be prioritized and maintained for as long as possible. The organization is required to predetermine the progressive curtailment of services and an identified point in time where an evacuation will need to take place within the 96-hour period.[22] The 96-Hour Plan is a useful tool to anticipate initiation of early notification to external resources when assistance with evacuation becomes necessary.

In certain cases, resources from the federal government may be deployed ahead of a storm that is expected to have a significant healthcare impact. One example is a Disaster Medical Assistance Team (DMAT) that can provide a self-sustaining, temporary healthcare system. Additional information on DMAT resources can be found by researching the National Disaster Medical System under the Department of Health and Human Services.

Shelter in Place

In a shelter-in-place situation, staff and patients are evacuated to a safe location(s) inside the facility for a portion or the duration of a disaster. Such a situation may be prompted by a threat from the environment outside the hospital building or even directly outside of the hospital unit, such as in an active shooter situation. To shelter in place, individuals retreat to an interior location until the threat is resolved and an "all clear" signal is sent. To provide for everyone's safety, the location might be placed on lockdown and secured by law enforcement until it is safe to leave the facility. Other examples of events that may require staff and patients to shelter in place include earthquakes, hurricanes, chemical exposures, road closures, or external safety concerns that prevent staff and patients from leaving the facility.

Children in Disasters

In the last few decades, the United States has witnessed the pediatric population evolve from becoming the bystander victims in disasters to becoming the actual targets, particularly in human-made disasters. Unfortunately, most adult hospitals are not prepared to manage a surge of pediatric disaster victims.[23] This challenge is further compounded by the variable availability of pediatric specialty–trained staff, pediatric-sized equipment, pediatric-focused systems, and space available to address pediatric-specific cases.

Children make up approximately one-fourth of the population, and their unique needs and characteristics make them a vulnerable population. In particular, their anatomy and physiology differ from those of adults. Examples include children's larger occiput, larger tongue, higher respiratory rates, higher metabolic rates, and a variable range of cognitive development. It is important to incorporate these special considerations of children into disaster drills and emergency response plans. For more information, refer to Chapter 12, "Special Populations: The Pediatric Trauma Patient."

Types of Disasters

Types of disasters include natural and human-made.

Natural Disasters

It is important to recognize the potential for high-risk natural disasters in the community and their effects on healthcare facilities. Natural disasters can include floods, hurricanes, wildfires, severe temperatures, landslides, volcanoes, and earthquakes.[24] As part of the mitigation and preparedness phases, specific planning considerations unique to each type of natural hazard are taken into account. In addition, the potential for the consequences of one disaster to overlap with another concurrent hazard must be recognized. For example, a large-scale wildfire may be contained but severe rain may follow, causing mudslides and flooding. The trauma nurse can expect the nearby hospital to incur a loss of power, ventilation issues, and possible staffing shortages due to road closures, all while a surge of patients continue to seek medical care.

Natural disasters can be costly and the recovery process impactful to the healthcare facility. For example, Puerto Rico was struck by Hurricane Maria in September 2017 and suffered substantial damage as a result. Incidentally, Puerto Rico was a major supplier of IV normal saline to healthcare facilities. In the aftermath of the hurricane, the Puerto Rican suppliers' operations were curtailed and, consequently, hospitals were faced with shortages of saline.[25] Also during 2017, the United States experienced a historic year of weather and climate disasters. The cumulative damage from these 16 U.S. events during 2017 was $309.5 billion—a new U.S. annual record (**Figure 18-2**).[26] In 2018, Hurricanes Florence and Michael have caused extensive damage.

Pandemic

While an infrequent disaster, pandemics tend to occur in our global society every 10 to 50 years. They pose a substantial threat to our planet, especially with the proliferation of global transportation.[27] Personal hygiene and distancing from potential infectious sources helps reduce transmission of the virus in such a case, but may not eliminate it. Pandemic illnesses can be spread through a variety of vectors, including humans and animals. Over the past decade, the potential for transmission between animals and humans has been seen with the H1N1 swine flu and the H5N1 avian flu. While neither of these pandemics was as devastating as the 1918 Spanish flu, the potential for significant impacts remains.

Trauma nurses should ensure proper hygiene remains their top priority at all times not only to protect themselves, but also to protect other patients and uninfected individuals from getting sick. Appendix 18-1D outlines the SEIRV triage algorithm, which can be used to identify and prioritize care for patients who are victims of an infection disease or pandemic.

Earthquake

Certain areas of the world are more prone to earthquakes, in which a shifting in the Earth's tectonic plates suddenly causes shaking of the planet's surface. Such an event can vary in magnitude but has the potential to

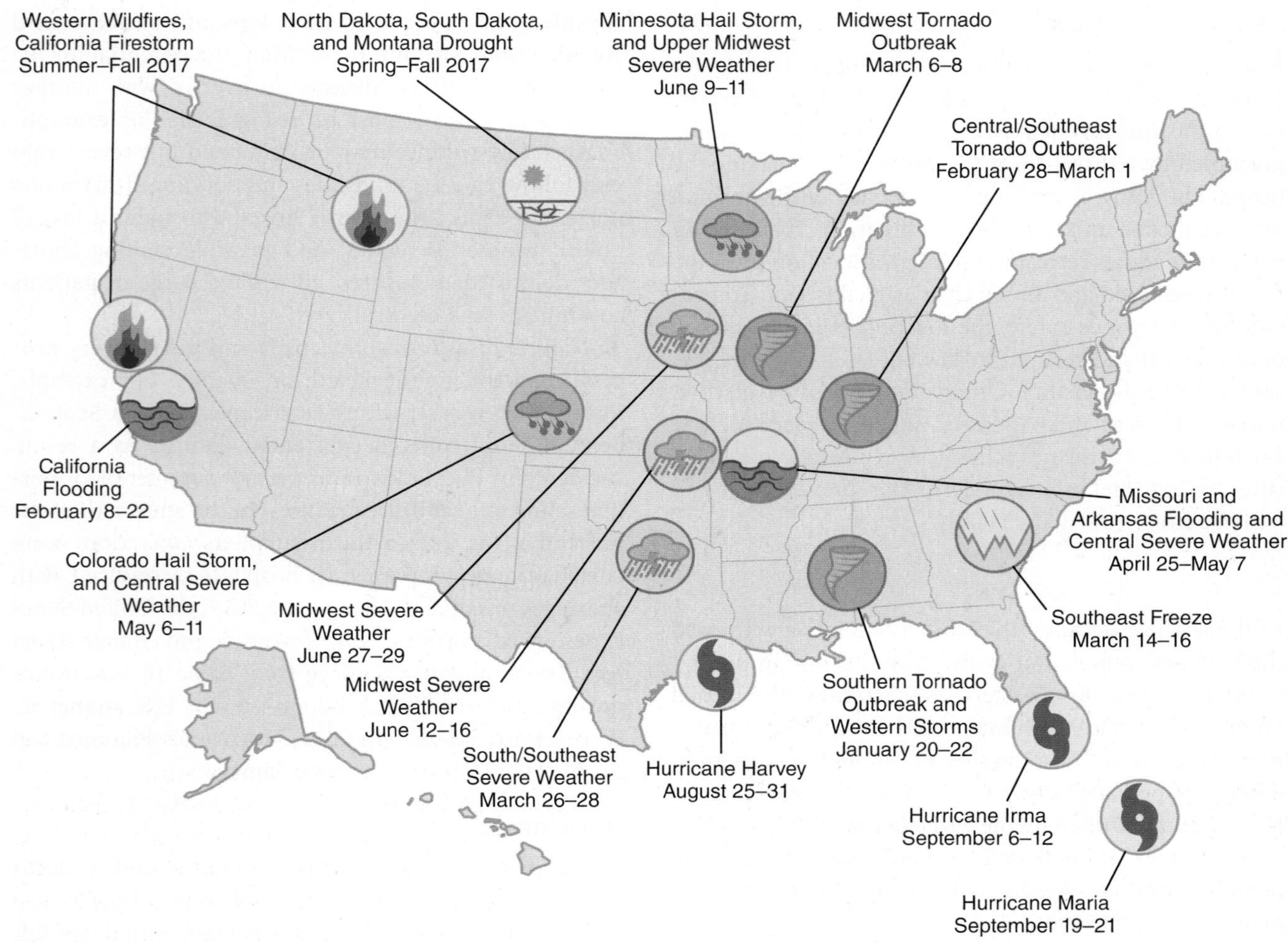

Figure 18-2 *Weather and climate disasters, 2017.*

Reproduced from National Oceanic and Atmospheric Administration, National Centers for Environmental Information. (2018). Billion-dollar weather and climate disasters: Overview. Retrieved from https://www.ncdc.noaa.gov/billions/.

cause widespread damage and destruction. Based on the 9.1 magnitude earthquake that occurred off the coast of Japan in 2011, the U.S. Geological Survey (USGS) determined that it was plausible that an earthquake off the Alaskan peninsula could produce a tsunami with waves greater than 24 feet high and cause devastation as far away as southern California.[28]

Infrastructure such as roads, water resources, and public utilities can be damaged and become unusable when an earthquake strikes, creating new problems for healthcare facilities. Accessibility can become a problem, as patients may not be able to access the healthcare system using standard methods, and established healthcare facilities may be rendered unusable due to damage from the earthquake or after-effects that could include fire, landslide, tsunami, or collapse. Evacuation plans may need to be activated for massive areas with little to no notice. Trauma nurses should be familiar with plans established to protect themselves during such an event, and also seek to maintain a safe area for themselves and the victims of the disaster after the initial earthquake subsides.

In the United States, California and Alaska are well-known seismically active regions, with Alaska being home to 11% of the world's recorded earthquakes, including the second largest earthquake ever recorded.[29] These earthquake-prone regions often have more extensive planning and mitigation efforts in place to prepare for an earthquake, but such disasters can happen anywhere.

Hurricane

Hurricanes are large but slow-moving tropical cyclones that have sustained winds of 74 mph or greater. They most often form around the Atlantic Coast and Gulf of

Mexico, but other areas of the United States are also susceptible to their effects. Due to hurricane's slow-moving nature, there is often lead time prior to a storm reaching land that allows communities to prepare or evacuate if necessary.[30] Despite this warning period, the storm remains unpredictable and can sometimes cause damage in unexpected areas. Hurricanes are dangerous not only because of their winds, but also because of the accompanying storm surge and heavy rain that can cause widespread flooding. Preparedness for a storm impact involves reinforcing known areas of weakness, preparing for a shelter-in-place situation that could last days, and/or evacuating areas vulnerable to wind and water damage. The trauma nurse should anticipate a surge of injured victims in case of hurricane, but also be prepared to receive victims who may not be able to return home and need assistance with temporary shelter.

Tornado

Often associated with the U.S. Midwest, tornados are weather events that can occur anywhere, with little to no warning. While warnings and watches have become more accurate in recent years, the exact timing and location of a tornado remains unpredictable and its emergence may occur with very little lead time.[31] Preparedness includes becoming familiar with the local alerting systems, monitoring for tornado-like activity when weather patterns favor the formation of such a storm, and pre-identification of sheltering locations. Trauma nurses must be prepared to shelter in place or evacuate at a moment's notice depending on the resiliency of the structure in which they are working. Damage to infrastructure has the potential to impact a community beyond just the path of the tornado.

Flood

Flooding may occur from many causes, including heavy rain, snow, coastal storms, and damage to dams or diversionary systems. Certain areas are more prone to flooding—a fact that is recognized by the federal government, which designates those areas as floodplains. Trauma nurses should be aware of which areas are prone to flooding in their communities, and preparedness plans should be in place to ensure that hospital infrastructure is protected. If areas are impacted by high waters, they may need to be evacuated to maintain operations and safety. The dangerous nature of flooded roads creates the potential need to shelter in place due to an inability to gain road access to areas.[32] Specialized rescue teams are necessary to access victims in flooded areas, but their capacity could potentially be overwhelmed during a widespread storm.

> **NOTE**
>
> **The Force of Moving Water**
>
> As little as 6 inches of moving water can create enough force to cause someone walking to fall down and could even carry a vehicle away.

Burn Mass-Casualty Incident

Wildfires are natural disasters that are caused when vegetation burns uncontrollably. While wildfires play an integral role in nature by burning dead or decaying matter, human-caused fires or those that impact population centers have the potential to cause death and injury on a wide scale. Injury patterns extend beyond just burns and can include exacerbation of chronic medical illnesses due to poor air quality or lack of access to normal resources. The wildfires in Southern California in 2018 accounted for the loss of hundreds of thousands of acres of land and more than 11,000 homes and over 70 deaths. As the most devastating wildfire in California history, the Camp Fires struck so fast that many people died in their homes with little warning as high winds and dry terrain enabled the fire to burn up to 10 football-field-sized areas of terrain a minute.[33,34]

Whether it be from wildfires, explosions, transportation-related disasters, or building fires, the trauma nurse should be prepared to receive an influx of patients from such disasters who may overwhelm specialty units. In a burn mass-casualty incident (BMCI), the number of burn victims exceeds the capacity of the local burn center to provide optimal burn care. Capacity in this scenario includes the availability of burn beds, burn surgeons, burn nurses, operating rooms, equipment, and supplies.

Both the American Burn Association (ABA) and the U.S. Department of Health and Human Services recognize that the total number of burn centers in the United States is inadequate for a BMCI. The expectation is that surge capacity plans will incorporate burn centers and non-burn centers into state and local disaster plans. In case of a large-scale BMCI, victims will be transported according to local MCI protocols. The local community hospital is responsible for initial assessment and stabilization until adequate resources become available to transfer patients to a facility with appropriate burn care resources.[35] This arrangement allows for burn centers at the state and federal levels to redistribute the critically ill burn victims, who may be overwhelming the capabilities of the facility closest to the disaster. The ABA provides guidelines for care of burn patients in such dire situations. The trauma nurse can expect to be responsible for the management of these patients for hours to days in some cases.[36]

Human-Made Disasters

Human-made disasters occur suddenly, and their impact is more difficult to predict, which requires a heightened sense of awareness. These disasters can be both intentional and unintentional and include industrial incidents, shootings, and acts of terrorism or mass violence. Human-made disasters can also be related to natural disasters that impair the integrity of an industry or geographic area.

Active Shooter

Over the years 2000–2012, the frequency of active shooter events steadily increased, with each event having a staggering number of casualties. In fact, the number of people both shot and wounded and shot and killed steadily trended upward during that time period.[37] In many recent civilian active shooter events, there has been an increase in the number of fatal wounds occurring as a result of the shooting event. This results in the potential for increased mass fatalities in a mass-casualty incident.[38] The Federal Bureau of Investigation (FBI) has noted a steady rise in mass shootings since 1999, creating a new type of human-made disaster for emergency responders and healthcare professionals with which to contend.[37]

The trauma nurse should be prepared to respond to an active shooter event in the community and within the facility using the principles of disaster triage, ICS, and mass fatality plans. Of course, ensuring the nurse's own safety is paramount to being able to provide for the most good to the greatest number of people. The trauma nurse should be alert to patients with multiple major vascular injuries, hidden blood loss, and injuries incompatible with life. Preparations for dealing with such an event need to include activation of surgical teams and notification and inventory of the blood bank given the potential need for multiple massive transfusions.

If the active shooter occurs in the hospital facility, nurses have three options: run, hide, or fight. It is critical that trauma nurses ensure their own protection before assisting others, which is contrary to the nurse's natural inclination to assist others first. This protection extends to the emergency treatment area as well. The overarching principle is simple: The nurse cannot help anyone if they are affected by the exposure and becomes a victim as well.[39,40] Important steps include staying calm, evacuating away from the path of the shooter (run), turning off lights and items that make noise, keeping the door locked and barricaded with large objects in front of doors or windows (hide), contacting 911 or local emergency responders, and then waiting until it is safe to evacuate. If the trauma nurse cannot run or hide from the shooter, then the last resort, if the nurse is in imminent danger, is to fight. The U.S. Department of Homeland Security recommends that individuals or groups who decide they must fight commit to their actions and act aggressively to defend themselves from the shooter.[40] This can include staging an ambush, using makeshift weapons, and trying to distract or disarm the shooter.

CBRNE

The U.S. Department of Homeland Security reports that reliable chemical, biologic, radiologic, nuclear, and explosive (CBRNE) countermeasures can be used to "protect life, health, property, and commerce."[41] An overview of each of the CBRNE components is important to gain an understanding of potential disaster risk, complete the hazard vulnerability assessment, and create emergency operations plans for events that are most likely to occur in a specific area. Regardless of type, if a CBRNE agent is involved, immediate identification of the agent is not as important as immediate recognition, response, and treatment of any unusual symptoms presenting across various age groups and populations.

Decontamination

When a natural disaster, industrial incident, or human-made event occurs, recognizing the need for adequate decontamination is crucial to ensuring the safety of emergency personnel and minimizing any cross-contamination to other people.[42] Contaminated victims may present with symptoms following a chemical, biological, or radiologic incident. Mass-casualty decontamination is a public health intervention that is most often performed with soap and water to remove contaminants from the skin surface. As much as 95% of hazardous material can be decontaminated by removing the patient's clothing and immediately washing the skin.[42]

NOTE

Exposure versus Contamination versus Infection

Exposure to a chemical, biological, or radiologic substance occurs when the body surfaces are introduced to a contaminant. Radioactive material, for example, gives off a form of energy that travels in waves or particles.[43] CT scans and x-rays are examples of exposure to radiation. With infectious material, the contaminant can be exposed to the body, but the body does not become contaminated unless the pathogen has a source of entry into the body. Exposure does not require decontamination, nor is it transmittable.

Contamination of a patient, when exposed to a chemical, biological, or radiologic substance, can be external or internal. External contamination occurs when a contaminant comes in contact with skin, hair, or other external structure. Decontamination is required to remove the particles to minimize their transmission. Internal contamination can occur when contaminants are breathed in, are swallowed, or enter the body through an open wound. Internal contamination will manifest with symptoms, for which medical treatment is required. Decontamination is necessary with chemical, biological, and external radiologic contamination to reduce the risk of transmission. Internal radiologic contaminants, such as shrapnel, may require only decontamination of the site of injury.[43]

Infection is the presence of a microorganism, such as a virus or bacteria, within the body tissues that causes damage. An inflammatory response follows introduction of the pathogen. Contamination or exposure does not necessarily lead to infection but if the contaminant consists of an infectious organism, there is potential for infection. Control of contamination and exposure is key to reducing transmission.

Decontamination is typically employed by emergency responders in the field. However, experience with many mass-casualty incidents has shown that most victims do not wait for emergency response personnel to receive field decontamination, but rather transport themselves to the hospital via privately owned vehicles.[44] The trauma nurse must be prepared to identify patients presenting to the hospital after a chemical, biological, or nuclear disaster who may have bypassed scene decontamination and proceed to decontaminate the victims according to hospital protocols. To minimize any potential adverse effects, only basic lifesaving measures are completed in the hot or warm zone of a decontamination area so as to minimize delays in the decontamination process. An example of a typical decontamination design is seen in **Figure 18-3**. Recommended practices for decontamination involve several steps that have been shown to be effective and are part of evidence-based protocols. **Table 18-2** outlines the best practices and rationales for each step in the process of victim decontamination.[42]

Personal Protective Equipment

Emergency responders have a variety of personal protective equipment (PPE) available to protect them from different types of hazards. Such equipment includes fully encapsulating suits that provide splash protection and respiratory protection of various levels. Correct use of PPE requires ongoing training and, at some levels, certification for use.

Disasters may bring a number of hazards, which could include infectious, radioactive materials, or chemicals. Identifying the specific hazardous substance is important but not required. If the substance is unknown, the trauma nurse should increase their index

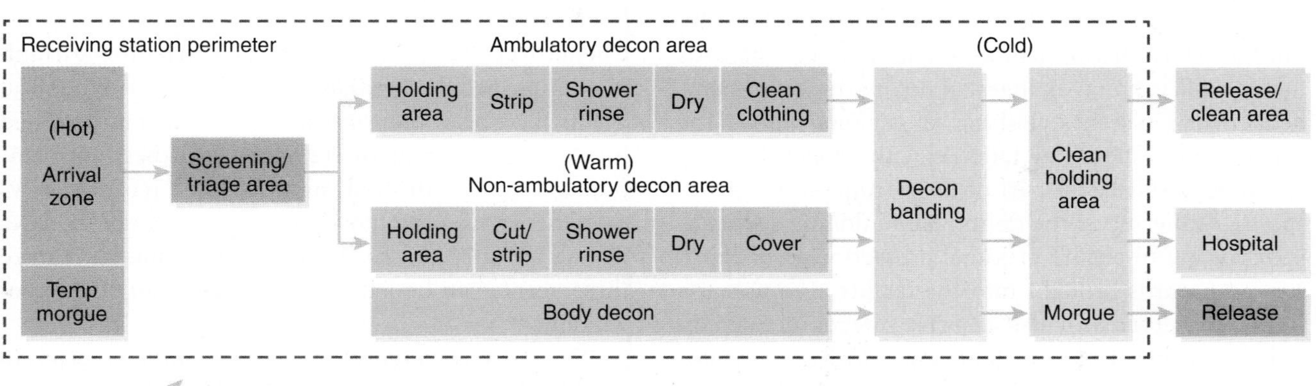

Figure 18-3 *Example decontamination design.*

TABLE 18-2 Primary Response Incident Scene Management (PRISM) Processes

Best Practice	Description	Rationale
Evacuation	Casualties should be evacuated from the scene of a hazardous chemical release.	Self-evacuation halts continued exposure or worsened contamination.
Disrobe	Remove all clothing, jewelry, and other inanimate objects on each person as soon as possible and before showering.	Limits transfer of contaminants to skin and prevents secondary contamination through off-gassing from clothing. Eliminates 90% or more of contaminants after an incident.
Improvised decontamination	Can be dry or wet, where the victim immediately wipes or rinses off the skin.	Removes visible contamination from exposed skin rapidly after the incident, further decreasing ongoing exposure.
Gross decontamination	The use of standard equipment to grossly decontaminate a large number of victims with copious water. Can utilize large-diameter water discharges from fire apparatus or hydrants.	Copious amounts of water from a fire truck ladder pipe system, decontamination corridor, or decontamination trailer is an effective way to remove remaining contaminants from skin.
Active drying	Victims use a dry towel or other material following any form of wet decontamination.	Dry towels remove small portions of contaminants that may remain following other forms of decontamination.
Technical decontamination	Thorough manual decontamination focused on reducing contamination to an acceptable level. This is the step where soap should be used if determined to be necessary.	A more time-consuming and in-depth process that is used to decontaminate victims to a higher degree or those who are not ambulatory.

Data from Chilcott, R. P., & Amlôt, R. (2015). Strategic guidance for mass casualty disrobe and decontamination. In *Primary Response Incident Scene Management (PRISM) guidance for chemical incidents* (Vol. 1). Retrieved from https://www.medicalcountermeasures.gov/media/36872/prism-volume-1.pdf.

of suspicion and potentially increase their level of PPE until a determination can be made. Potential hazards include off-gassing of ingested toxins or toxins embedded in a patient's clothing or personal items. The trauma nurse should be familiar with proper donning and doffing of PPE as part of the decontamination response. Adhering to the donning and doffing sequence is important to ensure maximal protection from exposure to hazards brought into the facility. The use of a trained observer provides an extra safeguard. Such an individual monitors for compliance with PPE protocols, guides and corrects any deviations from the appropriate process, and assists trauma nurses in properly protecting themselves.

Chemical Agents

Chemical exposures have the potential to harm the health of multiple people simultaneously. Historically, chemical agents have been used in warfare, but chemical-related incidents in the modern era have largely been unintentional, such as industrial mishaps. Most recently, however, there have been more intentional chemical releases during terrorist attacks. Trauma nurses must recognize these agents can be lethal, with a very short treatment window.

The *2016 Emergency Response Guide* is used to quickly identify the specific or generic class of the materials involved in an incident.[45] *National Institute for Occupational Safety and Health (NIOSH) Pocket Guide to Chemical Hazards* has general information on several hundreds of chemicals.[46] In addition to those immediately available resources, these guides include contact information for manufacturers and specialists on chemical agents. Important resources for dealing with specific hazardous chemical agents include the Poison Control Center as well as Safety Data Sheets (SDS), which are required by Occupational Safety and Health Administration (OSHA) to be available at all worksites with potentially hazardous chemicals. The most prominent chemical agents considered in terrorist incidents include nerve agents, which enter the body either percutaneously or through inhalation and affect the cholinergic nervous system. Asphyxiants are chemicals that interfere with the ability of the body to perform aerobic metabolism. Pulmonary agents affect the lungs and can cause symptoms such as pulmonary edema and permanently damage the lung tissue. Vesicants cause blistering and redness to the exposed area and are associated with pain. If the exposure is to the lungs, patients will experience respiratory distress. Riot control agents, or more commonly, tear gases, are lacrimators that cause painful irritation to the eyes and skin. **Appendix 18-2** lists these common chemical agents and describes their known signs and symptoms in more detail.[6,47]

Biologic Agents

Biologic agents can consist of bacteria, viruses, or toxins. Potential disease transmission vectors include person-to-person, contact, inhalation, and ingestion routes. Natural unintentional outbreaks include Ebola, severe acute respiratory syndrome, and influenza.

Deliberate release of a biologic agent, also known as bioterrorism, has the general goal to cause illness or death in people, animals, and plants. Bio-agents are typically found in nature but can be altered to increase their ability to cause disease, modified to increase their resistance to medications, or weaponized to spread into the environment. The release of these agents may not be immediately recognized because of the delay between exposure to the agent and illness onset. In many cases the presenting symptoms can closely resemble those which occur naturally.[48] Indications of intentional release of a biologic agent include an unusual temporal or geographic clustering of illness as well as an unusual age distribution for common diseases. Increased sharing of information and vigilance on the part of the trauma nurse will promote improved public health preparedness and early response.[49] Biological agents that could cause a communicable disease disaster include anthrax, botulism, plague, tularemia, and smallpox.[50] are discussed in more detail in **Appendix 18-3**.

Radiologic/Nuclear Events

Ionizing radiation is electromagnetic energy, or energy containing particles emitted from a source. In living things, it causes damage to the cells by denaturation of the DNA. Both nuclear and radiologic risks are recognized as threats, including use of radiological dispersal devices (dirty bombs) and nuclear irradiation (such as a bomb or reactor leak).

The two major types of ionizing radiation are electromagnetic radiation (gamma and x-rays) and particle radiation (alpha and beta particles). Exposure after a radiologic event can lead to external exposure that is either localized or generalized as well as internal contamination. Differentiating between patients who are contaminated versus those who are only exposed is an important part of appropriate victim management during a radiologic event. A patient is contaminated when a radioisotope that was released into the environment is ingested, inhaled, or deposited onto the patient's body surface. A patient who is exposed to an external source and whose body absorbs penetrating radiation is not radioactive or contaminated once removed from the radiation source. **Figure 18-4** provides an algorithm for the initial evaluation of patients with contamination and/or exposure.[43]

Three basic elements determine the amount of exposure: time, distance, and shielding (**Figure 18-5**). The risk of acute radiation illness is minimized by a shorter duration of exposure, a greater distance from the nucleus of the explosion, and a greater amount of shielding between the person and the explosion. Symptoms of acute radiation syndrome begin with nausea, vomiting, headache, and diarrhea. These symptoms then progress—depending on the duration, mechanism, and type of radiation exposure—to include poor appetite, fatigue, fever, and skin damage. **Appendix 18-4** describes acute radiation syndrome in more detail, while **Figure 18-6** illustrates the penetrating ability of various types of radiation.[51]

Radiologic and nuclear events are not isolated to radiation exposure. In particular, the trauma nurse should be prepared to handle victims who have experienced thermal and blast injuries concurrent to radiation exposure.

Explosives

Explosions—either intentional or unintentional—have the greatest likelihood of the various types of disasters of occurring in any community. Intentional acts may involve bombs, acts of terrorism, and improvised explosive devices. Examples of unintentional acts include industrial incidents and transportation-related incidents.

In mass-casualty situations, explosions cause a blast wave that can affect victims over a wide area. This over-

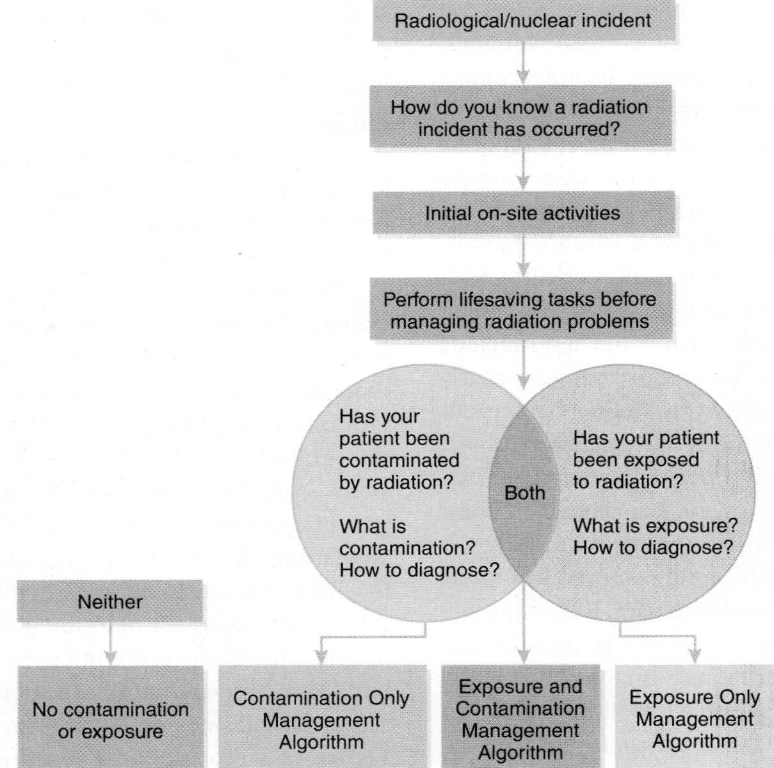

Figure 18-4 *Delineation between contamination and exposure.*

Reproduced from U.S. Department of Health and Human Services. (2018). Choose appropriate algorithm: Evaluate for contamination and/or exposure. *Radiation Emergency Medical Management.* Retrieved from https://www.remm.nlm.gov/EvalContamExp.pdf.

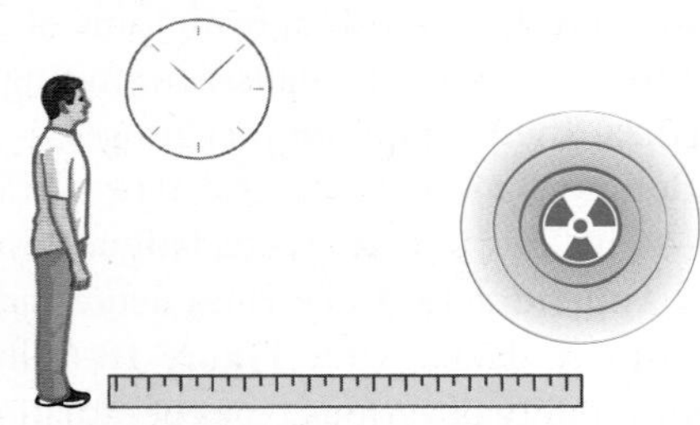

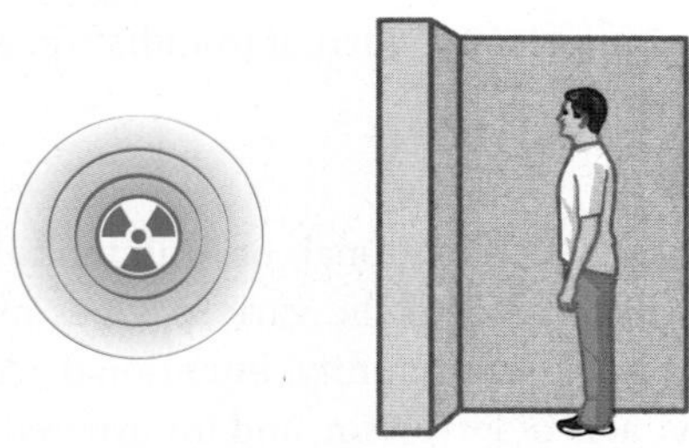

Figure 18-5 *Radiation exposure reduction techniques.*

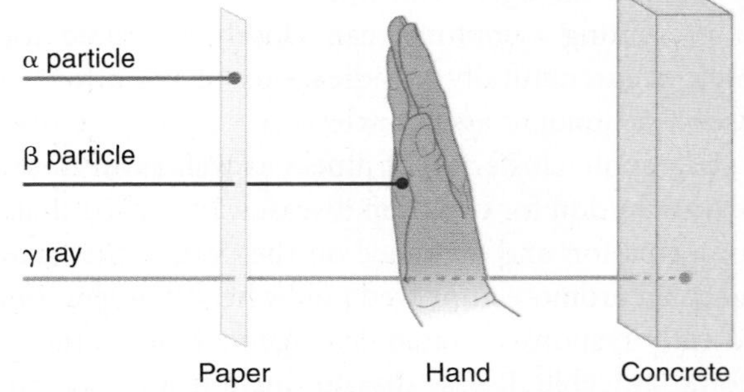

Figure 18-6 *Penetrating abilities of various types of radiation.*

pressurization shock wave can cause multiple levels of injury. Organ rupture can occur at air–fluid interfaces, along with secondary and tertiary blast injuries from flying objects or collision of the victim with another object.[6] See Chapter 2, "Biomechanics, Kinematics, and Mechanisms of Injury," for information on injuries related to explosions and blasts.

The explosives used in a mass-casualty situation can cause life-threatening hemorrhage on a large scale. Typically, bystanders are often present before the arrival of first responders. In recent mass-casualty explosive events, interventions such as tourniquets placed by bystanders have been found effective in preventing the loss of life. The "Stop the Bleed" campaign trains laypersons in how to stop profuse bleeding and save lives.[52] See Chapter 10, "Musculoskeletal Trauma," for more information on tourniquet application.

Recovery

Disasters are known to have significant impacts on communities and their infrastructure long after the response phase has ended. In the recovery phase, a continuity of operations plan for healthcare organizations is essential in ensuring financial and operational recovery once the acute phase of a disaster has resolved. Within the trauma and emergency services realm, operational ability in the aftermath of a disaster needs to be maintained because regular patient volume will continue to be present. The emergency response plan addresses the immediate needs for minimal operation, such as repair of damages to the facility, restoration of services, restocking of supplies, and accounting for any equipment damaged or lost during the event. Continuity of operations, by contrast, focuses on restoration of the facility to its normal day-to-day function. This is important not just to restart clinical operations, but also for logistical and financial accounting. Many organizations have a business continuity plan.

Mass-Fatality Incidents

Traditional emergency management plans focus on the preservation of life and property; however, these plans must also take into account the possibility of a mass-fatality disaster. While emergency responders, hospitals, and law enforcement routinely train for multiple- and mass-casualty incidents, none of them respond to or practice responses to disasters where many or all of the victims suffer fatal injuries.[53] In the process of triaging victims, the trauma nurse should be cognizant that an incident with a large number of fatalities can overwhelm a system's resources in the same manner as a large number of sick and injured patients. The remains of these victims will need to be recovered and stored for identification and for medicolegal authorities' later investigation. Incidents where there is high fragmentation of remains presents an additional challenge, as identification may be possible only using DNA testing. This is especially important given that the severity and frequency of civilian mass-shooting incidents is on the rise and the injury patterns associated with these events tend to lead to more fatal wounds.[38] The trauma nurse can expect that social services, the coroner's office, and local mortuary services will be involved in the planning and response phases of a mass-fatality incident. Federal Government resources like a Disaster Mortuary Operational Response Team (DMORT) can provide tracking and a variety of funeral services during an event where the number of fatalities exceeds local resources. Additional information on DMORT resources can be found by researching the National Disaster Medical System under the Department of Health and Human Services.

Family Reunification

Immediately after an incident where multiple people are separated, injured, or killed, family members will arrive or call the hospital, requesting information about their loved ones. The trauma nurse can also anticipate that not all incoming victims of a disaster will have a medical issue; that is, many victims of a disaster may present with a social or psychological need. Children, for example, may have lost or been separated from a parent, caregiver, or family member. Elderly or unconscious victims may not have identification or the ability to contact family themselves. The trauma nurse can expect that family members or victims themselves will come through the emergency department (ED) requesting assistance, essentially overcrowding the department.[54]

Family information centers (FICs) staffed with support personnel are useful tools to deal with this cohort of victims and should be included throughout the response and recovery phase of an event. Setup of a FIC is most beneficial when it is located away from the ED, so as to minimize overcrowding of the ED. FICs are typically organized by the facility's social work and spiritual care departments and can provide family members with resources for family reunification, spiritual care, bereavement, and child care.[54]

Psychological Triage

Disasters may produce both psychological and physiological traumas to members of the community and professional responders who were a part of the incident.

Early identification of psychological needs can promote a return to adaptive function and can identify those persons at risk for serious mental health outcomes, allowing for intervention before the trauma becomes a permanent part of their lives. The PsySTART mental health triage[55] is a method that individuals who are part of the affected population can use to measure their exposure to severe traumatic events after a disaster and prioritize crisis intervention resources. Examples of serious traumatic events include death of an immediate family member, a friend, or pet; a situation in which there was a direct threat to the individual's life; witnessing loss of life; a missing family member; loss of the home; or a child isolated from all caretakers. These severe events would trigger crisis intervention resources, clinical providers, and trauma-focused cognitive-behavioral therapy. Moderate risk categories include family members separated but accounted for, history of mental health needs, having been decontaminated after an exposure, or health concerns related to a possible exposure; such risks would trigger secondary screening and monitoring as a part of a community unit (i.e., schools). Low-risk individuals are those without any identified risk factors; they would be connected with community resources as needed.

Long after patients have been treated for physical injuries related to a disaster, the psychological effects may persist, among both patients and healthcare professionals. If trauma nurses are aware of the risk factors associated with traumatic events, they will be in a position to assist traumatized patients as well as any colleagues who were affected.[56] See Chapter 17, "Psychosocial Aspects of Trauma Care," for additional information.

Emerging Trends

Personal preparedness of the trauma nurse is essential to mount an effective overall response to a disaster. If the nurse is experiencing concerns about the welfare of their own family or suffered a personal loss related to the disaster, it is likely the nurse may not be able to perform the duties required of him or her. Personal preparedness at home can include establishing communication methods with family and stores of emergency supplies. Food, water, and special diets or medications for each family member should be stockpiled for at least 3 days in the case of extended work periods. Options for home evacuation or relocation and a method to reunite with loved ones should be identified in case family members become separated or the disaster subsides. This type of preparedness puts trauma nurses in a better situation to manage their duties in the hospital with the reassurance that concerns at home are managed.[57] Ready.gov has multiple resources for setting up a personal preparedness plan.[8]

Examining past disasters is useful for predicting future events and gaining experience with the planning, preparedness, response, and recovery phases of the disaster life cycle. Future implementations of disaster resiliency entail an expansion of psychological first aid, family resource centers, and other long-term approaches to disaster aid in promoting recovery and return to adaptive functioning. Triage methods, including SALT and SEIRV are expanding on the original algorithms to create better strategies for responding to disaster and minimizing loss of life.

Emergency management agencies are including new strategies for disaster management and response. Communication methodologies are expanding to include mass notification systems within hospitals, school systems, and cities. Social media have features to disseminate information as well as to gather information related to disasters. As an event is unfolding, emergency management professionals are beginning to embrace the opportunity to disseminate information to the public and clarify inaccuracies while also gathering together the live feeds that many individuals post on their social media pages. The increasing availability of satellites, drones, and connectivity allows for images, video, and commentary about an incident to be made available in real time, oftentimes before field responders or the formal news media arrive.

Cyber-security is assuming an increasingly important role in preparing for major disasters, as cyber-terrorism can compound the disruptions that occur after a natural or human-made disaster or can be the disaster itself. Ransomware and malware have the potential to disrupt infrastructure on a global scale, paralyzing governments, businesses, and other organizations. A single click on a malicious email can precipitate an event in which file-encrypting malware compromises a healthcare organization's electronic medical record system or network access.[58] Such a compromise may lead to exposure of patient health information, render medical devices dysfunctional, and compromise processes that affect patient safety. Trauma nurses must also be familiar with backup systems, or "downtime procedures," in the event a cyber-attack attempts to infiltrate and interrupt the healthcare system's infrastructure.

A key trend in disaster management is the ability to review incidents and responses and plan for the future based on the lessons learned. Instead of subsidizing bad behavior, prevention and preparedness programs are increasing, with a proactive approach. Primary examples included the availability of government-subsidized flood insurance and requirements for retrofit of buildings for earthquake compliance. By adopting these approaches, communities can use the lessons from the past to build resilient and sustainable communities instead of inviting the same disaster scenario to repeat itself. Communities and schools are participating in active shooter drills with increasing frequency to familiarize individuals with the options-based response (i.e., run, hide, fight) when a lockdown is not simply enough. This trend of taking a proactive approach to disasters is applicable with floods, earthquakes, wildfires, terrorism, and any number of other historical events that can be evaluated and scrutinized.

Summary

Disasters continue to occur more frequently and affect more people. A disaster can happen anywhere, at any time. Although most disasters are natural, it is important for trauma nurses to be aware of and familiar with human-made disasters. Understanding the basic foundation of a hospital's emergency operations plan and the department's response plan will help prepare nurses and their departments to handle all hazards while ensuring patients and the community at large are provided with the greatest care possible for the greatest number of people.

References

1. Woods, A. (2017, October 30). "Is this real": Seven hours of chaos, bravery at Las Vegas Hospital after mass shooting. *Azcentral, The Republic*. Retrieved from https://www.azcentral.com/story/news/nation/2017/10/30/seven-hours-chaos-bravery-las-vegas-sunrise-hospital-after-mass-shooting/796410001/
2. Welch, A. (2017, November 13). Inside the ER the night of the Las Vegas shooting. *CBS News, CBS Interactive*. Retrieved from https://www.cbsnews.com/news/inside-the-er-the-night-of-the-las-vegas-shooting/
3. Obert, D., Scherr, S., & Murawsky, J. (2018). How Las Vegas hospitals responded to nation's deadliest mass shooting. *Relias*. Retrieved from https://www.ahcmedia.com/articles/141697-how-las-vegas-hospitals-responded-to-nations-deadliest-mass-shooting
4. International Association of Red Cross and Red Crescent Societies. (n.d.). *What is a disaster?* Retrieved from http://www.ifrc.org/en/what-we-do/disaster-management/about-disasters/what-is-a-disaster/
5. World Health Organization. (n.d.). *Environmental health in emergencies*. Retrieved from http://www.who.int/environmental_health_emergencies/en/
6. American College of Surgeons (2018). *Advanced trauma life support: Student course manual* (10th ed.). Chicago, IL: Author.
7. Prevention Web. (2018). *The knowledge platform for disaster risk reduction*. Retrieved from https://www.preventionweb.net/english/
8. U.S. Department of Homeland Security. (n.d.). *Planning*. Retrieved from https://www.ready.gov/planning
9. Federal Emergency Management Agency, National Earthquake Hazards Reduction Program. (n.d.). Earthquake coordinators web site. Retrieved from https://training.fema.gov/emiweb/earthquake/neh0101220.htm
10. Federal Emergency Management Agency. (2018, January 16). *National Incident Management System*. Retrieved from http://www.fema.gov/national-incident-management-system
11. The Joint Commission. (2016). *Emergency management standards supporting collaboration planning*. Retrieved from https://www.jointcommission.org/assets/1/6/EM_Stds_Collaboration_2016.pdf
12. Robert Wood Johnson Foundation. (2016). *When disaster strikes*. Retrieved from https://www.rwjf.org/en/library/research/2016/05/when-disaster-strikes.html
13. California Hospital Association. (n.d.). Types of exercises. *Emergency Preparedness*. Retrieved from https://www.calhospitalprepare.org/post/types-exercises
14. California Emergency Medical Services Authority. (2014). *Hospital incident command system: Guidebook and appendices*. Retrieved from http://www.emsa.ca.gov/disaster-medical-services-division-hospital-incident-command-system/
15. California Department of Public Health. (2016). *15 'til 50*. Retrieved from http://cdphready.org/wp-content/uploads/2016/01/15-til-50-MCI-Guide.pdf
16. Wagner, J. M., & Dahnke, M. D. (2015). Nursing ethics and disaster triage: Applying utilitarian ethical theory. *Journal of Emergency Nursing, 41*(4), 300–306. https://doi.org/10.1016/j.jen.2014.11.001
17. Lerner, E. B., Cone, D. C., Weinstein, E. S., Schwartz, R. B., Coule, P. L., Cronin, M., . . . Hunt, R. C. (2011). Mass casualty triage: An evaluation of the science and refinement of a national guideline. *Disaster Medicine and Public Health Preparedness, 5*(2), 129–137. https://doi.org/10.1001/dmp.2011.39
18. Silvestri, S., Field, A., Mangalat, N., Weatherford, T., Hunter, C., McGowan, Z., . . . Papa, L. (2017). Comparison of START and SALT triage methodologies to reference standard definitions and to a field mass casualty situation. *American Journal of Disaster Medicine, 12*(1), 27–33. https://doi.org/10.5055/ajdm.2017.0255
19. Burkle, F., & Burkle, C. (2015). Triage management, survival, and the law in the age of Ebola. *Society for Disaster Medicine and Public Health, 9*(11), 38–43. https://doi.org/10.1017/dmp.2014.117
20. McGinty, M. D., Burke, T. A., Resnick, B., Barnett, D. J., Smith, K. C., & Rutkow, L. (2017). Decision processes and determinants of hospital evacuation and shelter-in-place during Hurricane Sandy. *Journal of Public Health Management and Practice, 23*(1), 29–36. https://doi.org/10.1097/PHH.0000000000000404
21. Chen, W., Guinet, A., & Ruiz, A. (2015). Modeling and simulation of a hospital evacuation before a forecasted flood.

Operations Research for Health Care, 4, 36–43. https://doi.org/10.1016/j.orhc.2015.02.001

22. The Joint Commission. (2016). Emergency management 96-hour plan. In *The Joint Commission standards interpretation.* Retrieved from https://www.jointcommission.org/standards_information/jcfaqdetails.aspx?StandardsFaqId=1187&ProgramId=46
23. Goodhue, C. J., Lin, A. C., Burke, R. V., Berg, B. M., & Upperman, J. S. (2013). Consider the children: Pediatric disaster planning. *Journal of Nursing Management, 44*(11), 44–51. https://doi.org10.1097/01.NUMA.0000432222.09629.df
24. Centers for Disease Control and Prevention. (2018, October 10). National disasters and severe weather. Retrieved from https://www.cdc.gov/disasters/index.html
25. Scutti, S. (2018). IV bags in short supply across U.S. after Hurricane Maria. *CNN.* Retrieved from https://www.cnn.com/2018/01/16/health/iv-bag-shortage/index.html
26. National Oceanic and Atmospheric Administration, National Centers for Environmental Information. (2018). Billion-dollar weather and climate disasters: Overview. Retrieved from https://www.ncdc.noaa.gov/billions/
27. Xu, J., & Peng, Z. (2015). People at risk of influenza pandemics: The evolution of perception and behavior. *PLoS One, 10*(12). https://doi.org/10.1371/journal.pone.0144868
28. Wilkey, R. (2013). Alaskan earthquake could destroy California coast: U.S. Geological Survey. *Environment.* Retrieved from https://www.huffingtonpost.com/2013/09/05/alaska-earthquake-california_n_3875015.html
29. Department of Natural Resources, Division of Geological and Geophysical Surveys. (2018). Earthquakes in Alaska. *Alaska Seismic Hazards Safety Commission.* Retrieved from http://seismic.alaska.gov/earthquake_risk.html
30. Occupational Safety and Health Administration. (n.d.). *Hurricane preparedness and response.* Retrieved from https://www.osha.gov/dts/weather/hurricane/preparedness.html
31. Occupational Safety and Health Administration. (n.d.). *Tornado preparedness and response.* Retrieved from https://www.osha.gov/dts/weather/tornado/index.html
32. Ready. (2017). *Floods.* Retrieved from https://www.ready.gov/floods
33. National Geographic. (n.d.). Climate 101: Wildfires. Retrieved from https://www.nationalgeographic.com/environment/natural-disasters/wildfires/
34. Fagan, K., Tucker, J., & McBride, A. (2018, November 19). Camp Fire: What we know about the deadly blaze that destroyed Paradise. *San Francisco Chronicle.* Retrieved from https://www.sfchronicle.com/california-wildfires/article/What-we-know-about-the-deadly-Camp-Fire-13401383.php
35. Kearns, R. D., Conlon, K. M., Matherley, A. F., Chung, K. K., Bebarta, V. S., Hansen, J. J., . . . Palmieri, T. L. (2016). Guidelines for burn care under austere conditions: Introduction to burn disaster, airway and ventilator management, and fluid resuscitation. *Journal of Burn Care and Research, 37*(5), e427–e439. http://doi.org/10.1097/BCR.0000000000000304
36. Kearns, R. D., Holmes, J. H., Alson, R. L., & Cairns, B. A. (2014). Disaster planning: The past, present, and future concepts and principles of managing a surge of burn injured patients for those involved in hospital facility planning and preparedness. *Journal of Burn Care & Research, 35*(1), e33–e42. https://doi.org/10.1097/BCR.0b013e318283b7d2
37. Blair, J. P., Martaindale, M. H., & Nichols, T. (2014, January 7). Active shooter events from 2000 to 2012. *Law Enforcement Bulletin.* Retrieved from https://leb.fbi.gov/articles/featured-articles/active-shooter-events-from-2000-to-2012
38. Smith, E. R., Shapiro, G., & Sarina, B. (2016). The profile of wounding in civilian public mass shooting fatalities. *Journal of Trauma and Acute Care Surgery, 81*(1), 86–92. https://doi.org/10.1097/TA.0000000000001031
39. Yale University. (2018). Emergency management: Shelter in place. Retrieved from https://emergency.yale.edu/be-prepared/shelter-place
40. Federal Emergency Management Agency. (2018). *How to prepare for an active shooter* (FEMA Publication V-1000, Catalog No. 17233-1). Retrieved from https://www.fema.gov/media-library-data/1523561958719-f1eff6bc841d56b7873e018f73a4e024/ActiveShooter_508.pdf
41. U.S. Department of Homeland Security. (2017). Science and technology: National strategy for chemical, biological, radiological, nuclear, and explosives standards. Retrieved from https://www.dhs.gov/national-strategy-chemical-biological-radiological-nuclear-and-explosives-cbrne-standards
42. Chilcott, R. P., & Amlôt, R. (2015). Strategic guidance for mass casualty disrobe and decontamination. In *Primary Response Incident Scene Management (PRISM) guidance for chemical incidents* (Vol. 1). Retrieved from https://www.medicalcountermeasures.gov/media/36872/prism-volume-1.pdf
43. U.S. Department of Health and Human Services. (2018). Choose appropriate algorithm: Evaluate for contamination and/or exposure. *Radiation Emergency Medical Management.* Retrieved from https://www.remm.nlm.gov/EvalContamExp.pdf
44. Carter, H., Amlôt, R., Williams, R., Rubin, G. J., & Drury, J. (2016). Mass casualty decontamination in a chemical or radiological/ nuclear incident: Further guiding principles. *PLoS Currents.* http://doi.org/10.1371/currents.dis.569a83b893759346e511a070cb900d52
45. U.S. Department of Transportation. (2016). *Emergency response guide.* New York, NY: Skyhorse Publishing.
46. U.S. Department of Health and Human Services. (2007). *NIOSH pocket guide to chemical hazards* (DHHS Publication No. 2005-149). Retrieved from https://www.cdc.gov/niosh/docs/2005-149/pdfs/2005-149.pdf
47. Centers for Disease Control and Prevention. (2016). Emergency preparedness and response: Chemical emergencies. Retrieved from https://emergency.cdc.gov/chemical/index.asp
48. Kwo, J., & Johnson, D. W. (2018). Disaster medicine, bioterrorism and Ebola. In P. E. Parsons, J. P. Wiener-Kronish, R. D. Stapleton, & L. Berra (Eds.), *Critical care secrets* (6th ed., pp. 457–464). Philadelphia, PA: Elsevier.
49. Lall, R., Abdelnabi, J., Ngai, S., Parton, H. P., Saunders, K., Sell, J., . . . Mathes, R. W. (2017). Advancing the use of emergency department syndromic surveillance data, New York City,

2012–2016. *Public Health Reports, 132*(1), 23S–30S. https://doi.org/10.1177/0033354917711183

50. Centers for Disease Control and Prevention. (2017). Emergency preparedness and response: Bioterrorism agents/diseases. Retrieved from https://emergency.cdc.gov/agent/agentlist-category.asp
51. Libretexts. (2016). The interaction of nuclear radiation with matter. Retrieved from https://chem.libretexts.org/Textbook_Maps/General_Chemistry/Map:_Chemistry_(Averill_and_Eldredge)/20:_Nuclear_Chemistry/20.3:_The_Interaction_of_Nuclear_Radiation_with_Matter
52. U.S. Department of Homeland Security. (2015). Stop the bleed. Retrieved from https://www.dhs.gov/stopthebleed
53. Carroll, E., Johnson, A., DePaolo, F., Adams, B. J., Mazone, D., & Sampson, B. (2017). Trends in United States mass fatality incidents and recommendations for medical examiners and coroners. *Academic Forensic Pathology, 7*(3), 318–329. https://doi.org/10.23907/2017.029
54. Los Angeles County Emergency Medical Services. (2013). *Family information center: Planning guide for healthcare entities.* Retrieved from https://www.calhospital.org/sites/main/files/file-attachments/readytoreunify_handout1of1_0.pdf
55. Sylwanowicz, L., Schreiber, M., Anderson, C., Gundran, C. P. D., Santamaria, E., & Lopez, J. C. F. (2018). Rapid triage of mental health risk in emergency medical workers: Findings from typhoon Haiyan. *Disaster Medicine and Public Health Preparedness, 12*(1), 19–22. https://doi.org/10.1017/dmp.2017.37
56. Centers for Disease Control and Prevention. (2017). Emergency preparedness and response: *Coping with a disaster or traumatic event.* Retrieved from https://www.emergency.cdc.gov/coping/index.asp
57. Raveis, V. H., VanDevanter, N., Kovner, C. T., & Gershon, R. (2017). Enabling a disaster-resilient workforce: Attending to individual stress and collective trauma. *Journal of Nursing Scholarship, 49*, 653–660. https://doi.org/10.1111/jnu.12340
58. Jalali, M. S., & Kaiser, J. P. (2018). Cybersecurity in hospitals: A systematic, organizational perspective. *Journal of Medical Internet Research, 20(*5), e10059. https://doi.org/10.2196/10059

APPENDIX 18-1

Triage Methods

A. START Adult Triage

Simple Triage and Rapid Treatment (START) triage is a quick and rapid method to identify and sort patients in a situation in which the number of patients overwhelms current resources available. Patients are sorted in a manner that allows the trauma nurse to provide the most good to the greatest number of patients.[1]

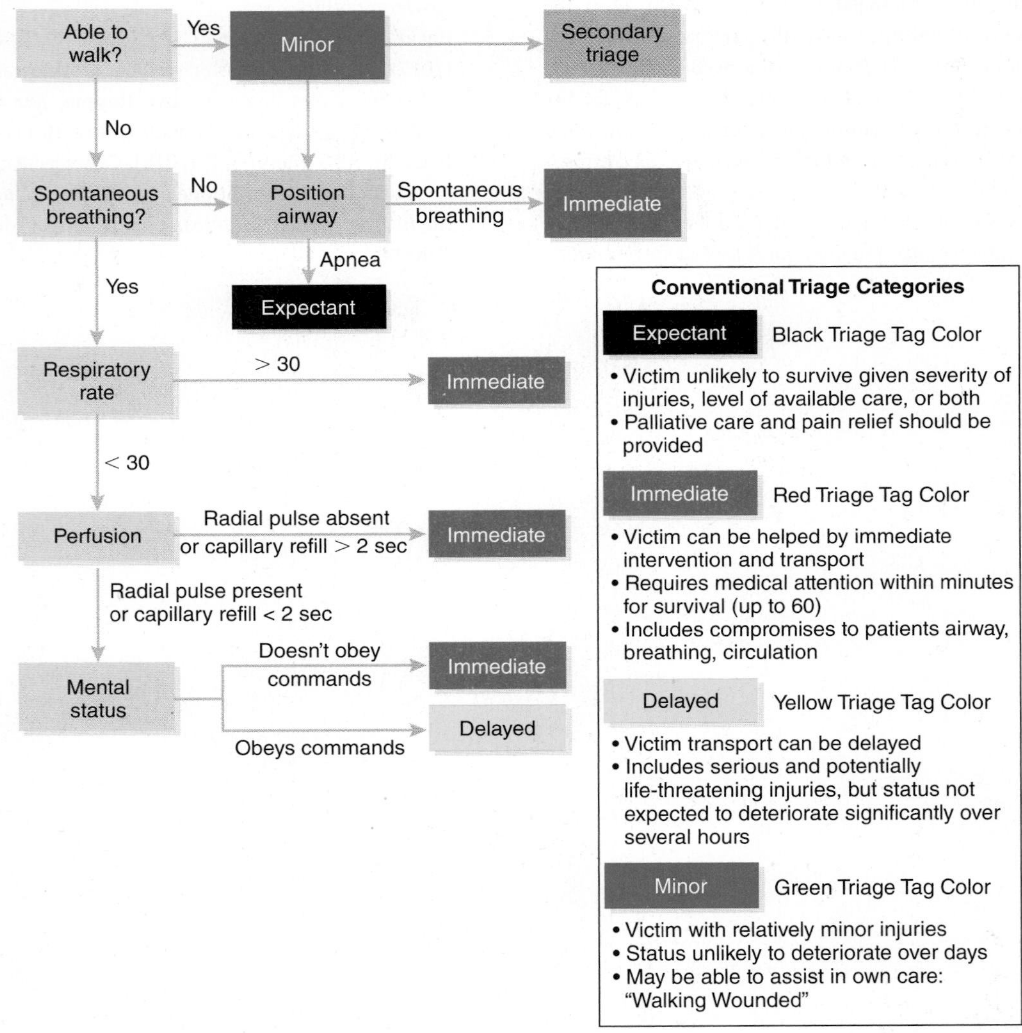

Reproduced from U.S. Department of Health and Human Services. (2013, February 22). START adult triage algorithm. Retrieved from http://chemm.nlm.nih.gov/startadult.htm.

B. JumpSTART Pediatric Multiple Casualty Incident Triage

JumpSTART is a modified version of START triage that takes into account the differences in the pediatric population. JumpSTART provides for limited interventions to the nonbreathing patient appropriate for the pediatric population, but the overall premise is the same as with the START triage algorithm.[2]

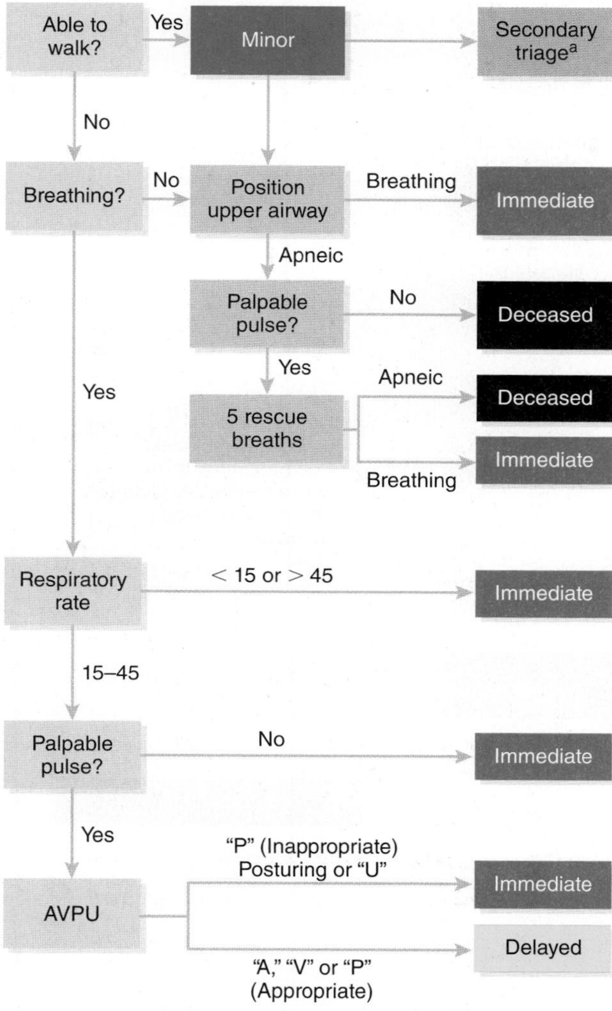

[a] Non-ambulatory children (infants who cannot walk yet, children with pre-existing conditions) are evaluated beginning with breathing.[3]

Reproduced from U.S. Department of Health and Human Services. (2017). JumpSTART pediatric triage algorithm. Retrieved from https://chemm.nlm.nih.gov/startpediatric.htm.

C. SALT Triage

Sort–Assess–Lifesaving Interventions–Treatment and/or Transport (SALT) uses a similar sorting method as START triage to sort and assess victims, provide limited lifesaving interventions, and then prioritize treatment and transportation. SALT has been found to be more accurate in identifying higher-priority patients than START, but health care systems have been slow to adopt this method. Trauma nurses should be aware of the standard used by their health care facility.[4]

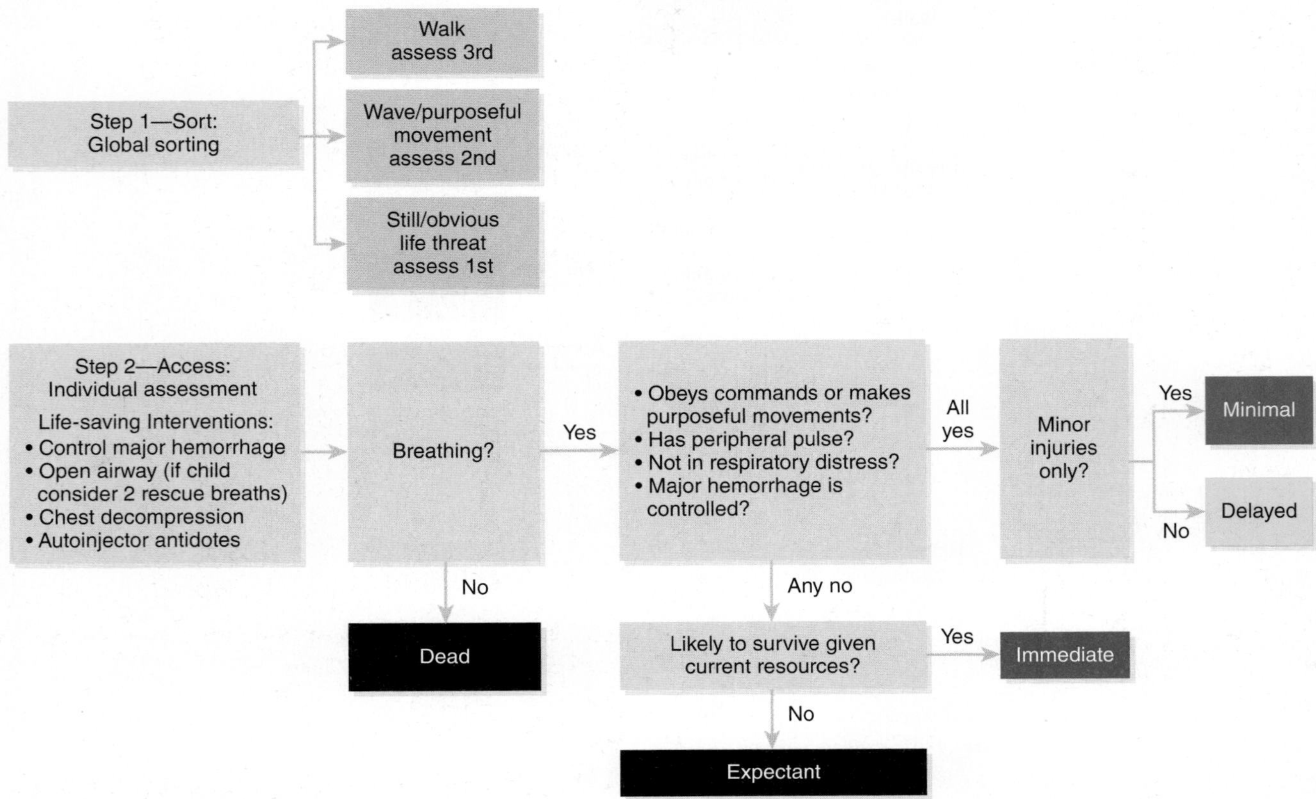

Reproduced from SALT Mass Casualty Triage: Concept Endorsed by the American College of Emergency Physicians, American College of Surgeons Committee on Trauma, American Trauma Society, National Association of EMS Physicians, National Disaster Life Support Education Consortium, and State and Territorial Injury Prevention Directors Association. (2008). *Disaster Medicine and Public Health Preparedness, 2*(4), 245–246. https://doi.org/10.1097/DMP.0b013e31818d191e.

D. SEIRV Triage

Susceptible-Exposed-Infectious-Removed-Vaccinated (SEIRV) is a triage sorting method that can be used to sort patients during a biological or pandemic-like event.[5]

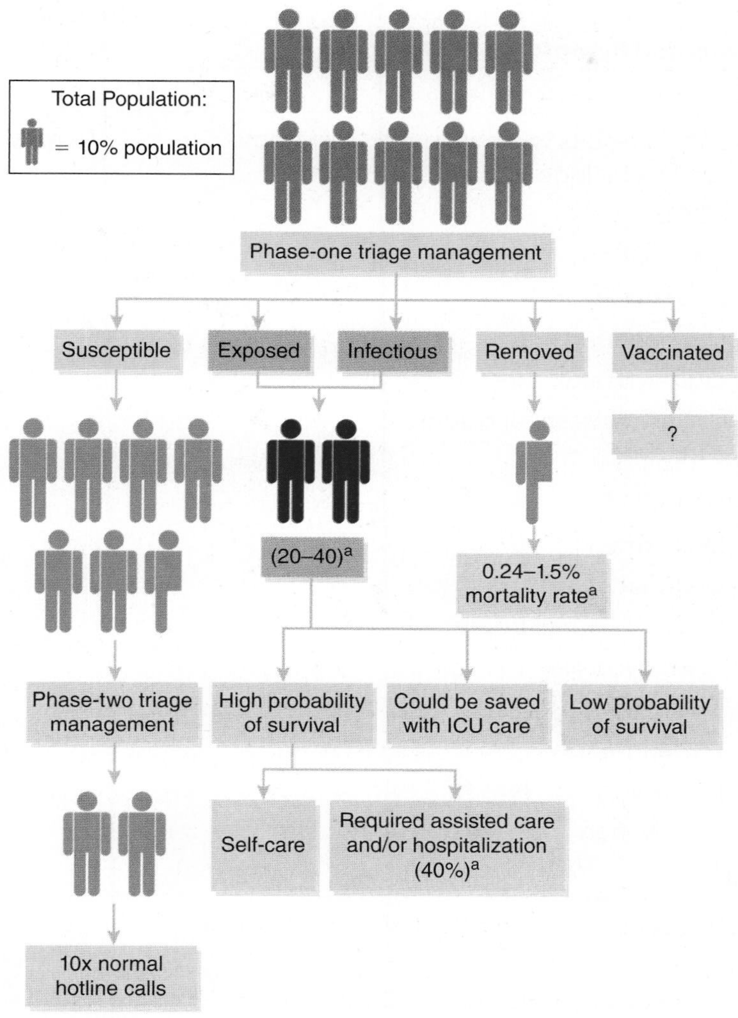

[a] Percentages based on influenza and severe acute respiratory syndrome outbreak data.

Reproduced from Burkle, F. M. (2006). Population-based triage management in response to surge-capacity requirements during a large-scale bioevent disaster. *Journal of Academic Emergency Medicine, 13*(11), 1118–1129.

References

1. U.S. Department of Health & Human Services. (2013, February 22). START adult triage algorithm. Retrieved from http://chemm.nlm.nih.gov/startadult.htm
2. U.S. Department of Health and Human Services. (2017). Jump-START pediatric triage algorithm. Retrieved from https://chemm.nlm.nih.gov/startpediatric.htm.
3. Illinois Department of Public Health and Illinois Emergency Medical Services for Children. (2016). Pediatric disaster triage training scenarios: Utilizing the JumpSTART Method. Retrieved from https://ssom.luc.edu/media/stritchschoolofmedicine/emergencymedicine/emsforchildren/documents/disasterpreparedness/otherresources/mcitriage/emscjumpstarttrainingprogramandmaterials/JumpSTART%20Training%20Scenarios%202016%20final(2).pdf
4. SALT Mass Casualty Triage: Concept Endorsed by the American College of Emergency Physicians, American College of Surgeons Committee on Trauma, American Trauma Society, National Association of EMS Physicians, National Disaster Life Support Education Consortium, and State and Territorial Injury Prevention Directors Association. (2008). *Disaster Medicine and Public Health Preparedness, 2*(4), 245–246. https://doi.org/10.1097/DMP.0b013e31818d191e
5. Burkle, F. M. (2006). Population-based triage management in response to surge-capacity requirements during a large-scale bioevent disaster. *Journal of Academic Emergency Medicine, 13*(11), 1118–1129.

APPENDIX 18-2

Chemical Agents

Agent	Signs and Symptoms	Decontamination and Treatment
Nerve Agents		
Tabun (GA) Sarin (GB) Soman (GD) Cyclosarin (GF) V Agents (VX)	Exposure results in a cholinergic toxidrome. Acronyms include SLUDGE: S: Salivation L: Lacrimation U: Urination D: Diarrhea G: Gastrointestinal distress E: Emesis DUMBBELLS: D: Diarrhea U: Urination M: Miosis (small pupils) B: Bradycardia E: Emesis L: Lacrimation L: Lethargy S: Salivation	› Remove contaminated clothing › Flush with a soap and water › Treat with atropine, 2-PAM, Mark I Kit/Duodote autoinjector
Vesicants (Blister Agents)		
Sulfur mustard (HD) Nitrogen mustard (HN)	Acts first as a cellular irritant, then as a cellular poison Conjunctivitis, reddened skin, blisters, nasal irritation, inflammation of throat and lungs Usually not fatal	› Remove contaminated clothing › Flush with soap and water › Supportive care (no antidote)
Lewisite (L)	Immediate pain with blisters later Readily absorbed through skin and moist tissue	
Pulmonary Agents		
Phosgene oxime (CX)	Cough, burning, and immediate pain, with blisters later Necrosis equivalent to full- and partial-thickness burns	› Leave area of exposure and get to fresh air › Remove clothing and double-bag it in plastic bags to contain off-gassing

Agent	Signs and Symptoms	Decontamination and Treatment
Chlorine	Coughing; chest tightness; burning sensation to nose, throat, and eyes; watery eyes; blurry vision; nausea and vomiting; shortness of breath or difficulty breathing; burning pain, redness, or blisters on skin	› Flush with soap and water, irrigate eyes if affected
Chemical Asphyxiants (Blood Agents)		
Hydrogen cyanide (AC) Cyanogen chloride (CK) Arsine (SA)	Cherry red skin or approximately 30% cyanosis May appear to be gasping for air Seizures prior to death Effect is similar to asphyxiation but is more sudden	› Remove contaminated clothing › Decontaminate patient skin with a soap and water solution

Data from Centers for Disease Control and Prevention. (2016). Emergency preparedness and response: Chemical emergencies. Retrieved from https://emergency.cdc.gov/chemical/index.asp.

APPENDIX 18-3

Biologic Agents

Agent	Symptoms	Transmission	Treatment
Anthrax (*Bacillus anthracis*) Incubation usually less than 7 days but can be up to 60 days	Cutaneous: Intense itching with raised bump initially; progresses to ulcerated blister with necrotic center and scabs Inhalation: Initially, nonspecific flu-like illness characterized by fever, myalgia, headache, nonproductive cough, and mild chest discomfort; followed by marked high fever, dyspnea, stridor, cyanosis, and shock	Person-to-person spread extremely unlikely	Multiple antibiotics including doxycycline, ciprofloxacin, fluoroquinolones, and others; effective for both types
Botulism (*Clostridium botulinum*) Incubation usually 12–36 hours (range of 6 hours to 2 weeks)	Double vision, blurred vision, drooping eyelids, slurred speech, difficulty swallowing, and dry mouth	Not spread person-to-person	Antitoxin effective if diagnosed early; supportive care
Plague (*Yersinia pestis*) Incubation usually 2–4 days	Fever, chills, headache, severe debilitation, rapidly developing shortness of breath, and chest pain	Person-to-person (Airborne and droplet precautions recommended)	Early treatment is crucial Streptomycin, doxycycline; gentamicin when streptomycin is not available
Smallpox (*Variola major*) Incubation usually 7–17 days	Initially, high fever, fatigue, headache, and backaches Rash usually develops 2–3 days after onset of symptoms; rash appears first on the mouth, face, and extremities, then spreads inward to the trunk of the body	Person-to-person (Airborne and droplet precautions recommended)	Supportive therapy; antibiotics to treat secondary infections
Tularemia (*Francisella tularensis*) Incubation usually 3–5 days	Insect bite: Slow-healing sore and swollen lymph nodes Inhalation: High fever, chills, headache, fatigue, cough, and chest pain Ingestion: Sore throat, abdominal pain, diarrhea, and vomiting	Not spread person-to-person	Streptomycin; gentamicin also effective

Agent	Symptoms	Transmission	Treatment
Viral hemorrhagic fevers (VHF) Incubation usually 4–21 days	Fever, fatigue, dizziness, muscle aches, loss of strength, and exhaustion Severe cases often show signs of bleeding under the skin, in internal organs, or from body orifices Severely ill patients may also experience shock, nervous system malfunction, coma, delirium, and seizures Some types of VHF are associated with renal failure	Person-to-person (Follow the CDC's infection control recommendations)	Antibiotics for secondary infections, blood transfusions and supportive care; some types respond to antiviral medication

Data from Centers for Disease Control and Prevention. (2017). Emergency preparedness and response: Bioterrorism agents /diseases. Retrieved from https://emergency.cdc.gov/agent/agentlist-category.asp.

APPENDIX 18-4

Acute Radiation Syndromes

Syndrome	Dose[a]	Prodromal	Latent Stage	Manifest Illness Stage	Recovery
Hematopoietic (bone marrow)	> 0.7 Gy (> 70 rads) (Mild symptoms may occur from exposure as low as 0.3 Gy or 30 rads)	Symptoms are anorexia, nausea, and vomiting Onset occurs 1 hour to 2 days after exposure Stage lasts for minutes to days	Stem cells in bone marrow are dying, although the patient may appear and feel well Stage lasts 1–6 weeks	Symptoms are anorexia, fever, and malaise Drop in all blood cell counts occurs for several weeks Primary cause of death is infection and hemorrhage Survival decreases with increasing dose Most deaths occur within a few months after exposure	In most cases, bone marrow cells will begin to repopulate the marrow There should be full recovery for a large percentage of patients from a few weeks up to 2 years after exposure Death may occur for some patients at 1.2 Gy (120 rads) The LD50/60[b] is about 2.5–5 Gy (250–500 rads)
GI	> 10 Gy (> 1,000 rads) (Some symptoms may occur from exposure as low as 6 Gy or 600 rads)	Symptoms are anorexia, severe nausea, vomiting, cramps, and diarrhea Onset occurs within a few hours after exposure Stage lasts about 2 days	Stem cells in bone marrow and cells lining the GI tract are dying, although the patient may appear and feel well Stage lasts less than 1 week	Symptoms are malaise, anorexia, severe diarrhea, fever, dehydration, and electrolyte imbalance Death is due to infection, dehydration, and electrolyte imbalance Death occurs within 2 weeks of exposure	The LD100[c] is about 10 Gy (1,000 rads)

Syndrome	Dose[a]	Prodromal	Latent Stage	Manifest Illness Stage	Recovery
CV/CNS	> 50 Gy (5,000 rads) (Some symptoms may occur from exposure as low as 20 Gy or 2,000 rads)	Symptoms are extreme nervousness and confusion; severe nausea, vomiting, and watery diarrhea; loss of consciousness; and burning sensations of the skin Onset occurs within minutes of exposure Stage lasts for minutes to hours	Patient may return to partial functionality Stage may last for hours but often is shorter	Symptoms include return of watery diarrhea, convulsions, and coma Onset occurs 5–6 hours after exposure Death occurs within 3 days of exposure	No recovery is expected

Abbreviations: CNS, central nervous system; CV, cardiovascular; GI, gastrointestinal; LD, lethal dose.

[a] The absorbed doses quoted here are "gamma equivalent" values. Neutrons or protons generally produce the same effects as gamma radiation, beta radiation, or radiographs, but at lower doses. If the patient has been exposed to neutrons or protons, consult radiation experts on how to interpret the dose.

[b] The LD50/60 is the dose that can kill 50% of the exposed population in 60 days.

[c] The LD100 is the dose that can kill 100% of the exposed population.

Reproduced from Centers for Disease Control and Prevention. (2017). A brochure for physicians: Acute radiation syndrome. Retrieved from https://emergency.cdc.gov/radiation/pdf/ars.pdf.

CHAPTER 19

Transition of Care for the Trauma Patient

Jennifer Radtke, MSN, RN, CEN, TCRN, CIC

OBJECTIVES

Upon completion of this chapter, the learner will be able to:

1. Describe trauma patient characteristics that may require specialized or a higher level of care.
2. Recognize national, state, and/or provincial laws and regulations in place to protect patients and to facilitate the improvement of outcomes and transport for trauma patients with complex injuries.
3. Examine the risks and benefits of both intrafacility and interfacility trauma transport.
4. Discuss transport modes and qualifications of transport team members.
5. Identify concepts that promote communication for intrafacility and interfacility transport.

Introduction

Patients who experience traumatic injury require rapid assessment and stabilization of life-threatening injuries and transport to a facility capable of providing definitive care. The American College of Surgeons (ACS) recommends that certain injured patients be transported to a verified trauma center with sufficient number and types of resources.[1] Time to treatment has also been identified as crucial to optimal patient outcomes, particularly the time from injury to definitive care.[1] Timely and definitive care is related to decreased morbidity and mortality from traumatic injury.[1]

As the patient moves through the trauma care continuum, multiple transfers and hand-offs occur. These may take place within the hospital (intrafacility) or to a different facility (interfacility). It is essential for each trauma care provider to assure safe transport and provide essential information regarding the care of the patient to the next care provider using a standardized format. To do so effectively, the trauma nurse needs to be aware of the resources available at their facility as well as local and regional policies, procedures, and laws, in particular those regarding transport.

Trauma Systems and Classification of Trauma Centers

Trauma care provided in the emergency setting is only one phase of the trauma care continuum. That continuum begins with injury prevention and involves each phase of the patient's progress from the point of injury through rehabilitation and reintegration into the community. Although trauma systems vary from jurisdiction to jurisdiction, the guidelines and standards published by the ACS incorporating injury prevention, acute care, and rehabilitation are widely used.

Since trauma nurses are involved in trauma patient transport, whether it is to send or receive the injured patient, it is beneficial to understand the trauma system and the methods used to define and classify trauma centers. The American College of Surgeons Committee on Trauma (ACS-COT) describes capabilities and resources for four levels of trauma centers.[2] Hospitals may apply to the ACS to participate in a rigorous on-site survey and review process through which they can achieve verification by the ACS as a trauma center. A brief description of each trauma center level is provided in **Table 19-1**.[2]

TABLE 19-1 American College of Surgeons Committee on Trauma Levels of Trauma Centers

Trauma Center	Description of Trauma Center
Level I	› A regional trauma center is a tertiary care facility. › Capable of providing leadership and total care for every aspect of injury from prevention to rehabilitation. › Commonly is a university-based teaching hospital with residency and postgraduate programs. › Research, injury prevention programs, education, and systems planning are essential components.
Level II	› Provides trauma resuscitation and initial definitive trauma care, regardless of the severity of the injury. › Clinically equivalent to a Level I facility, but capabilities do not include the comprehensive services and specialty care that are provided by Level I trauma centers. › In many areas without access to a Level I facility, the Level II trauma center will take accountability to provide education, prevention, and community outreach. › May be involved in trauma research.
Level III	› Provides the trauma patient with prompt assessment, resuscitation, stabilization, and emergency surgery as necessary. › Uses accepted trauma triage criteria and ACS transfer guidelines for definitive care of the trauma patient. › Generally does not accept incoming trauma transfers. › A Level III trauma center may take accountability to provide education and system leadership in remote areas.
Level IV	› Provides initial assessment, interventions, and resuscitation of the patient with advanced trauma life support, initial assessment, and intervention. › Exists in a remote area and may be a clinic without an in-house physician. › Provides 24-hour emergency coverage by a physician or mid-level provider. › Has a transfer agreement with and provides care under the direction of a Level I or II trauma center. › Provides advanced trauma life support until patients can be transferred to a higher level of trauma care. › Uses ACS trauma triage and transport criteria. › Generally does not accept incoming transfers.

Data from American College of Surgeons, Committee on Trauma. (2014). *Resources for optimal care of the injured patient*. Chicago, IL: Author. Retrieved from https://www.facs.org/~/media/files/quality%20programs/trauma/vrc%20resources/resources%20for%20optimal%20care.ashx.

Initial Care and the Emergency Medical Treatment and Active Labor Act

In the United States, the federal Emergency Medical Treatment and Active Labor Act (EMTALA) requires that all patients who present to an emergency department (ED) receive a medical screening examination, resuscitation, and stabilization of any identified emergency condition, regardless of their ability to pay. If the patient's condition warrants treatment beyond the capabilities and resources of the initial facility and the patient needs to be transferred, EMTALA requires that the following conditions be met prior to transfer[3]:

- Medical screening examination and necessary stabilizing interventions (within the capacity of the facility)
- Informed consent
- Accepting physician at the receiving facility
- Available bed and resources to deliver appropriate care at the receiving facility
- Patient report provided to the receiving facility
- All available medical records, laboratory, radiographic, and other related information or copies provided to receiving facility or transferred with the patient
- Appropriate transfer personnel

Although these requirements are only pertinent to those U.S. facilities that receive government funding, they are widely considered the standard of care.

Characteristics of Trauma Patients Who Require Transport

When the patient's care needs exceed the available resources at the initial facility, transport to a facility that can provide the necessary specialized or higher level of care is recommended. In an organized trauma system, severely injured trauma patients are transferred to the closest facility with appropriate resources, preferably a verified trauma center. ACS-COT has established guidelines to help identify those patients most at risk who would benefit from being transported to a trauma center (**Table 19-2**).[2]

TABLE 19-2 American College of Surgeons' Criteria for Consideration of Transfer

A. Critical Injuries Considered for Transfer to Level I or Highest Regional Trauma Center
› Carotid or vertebral arterial injury
› Torn thoracic aorta or great vessel
› Cardiac rupture
› Bilateral pulmonary contusion with PaO_2:FiO_2 ratio less than 200 mm Hg
› Major abdominal vascular injury
› Grade IV or V liver injuries requiring more than 6 units RBC transfusion in 6 hours
› Unstable pelvic fracture requiring more than 6 units RBC transfusion in 6 hours
› Fracture or dislocation with loss of distal pulses
B. Life-Threatening Injuries Considered for Transfer to Level I or Level II Trauma Center
› Penetrating injury or open fracture of the skull
› GCS score less than 14 or lateralizing neurologic signs
› Spinal fracture or spinal cord deficit
› Complex pelvis/acetabulum fractures
› More than two unilateral rib fractures or bilateral rib fractures with pulmonary contusion
› Significant torso injury with advanced comorbid disease (coronary artery disease, chronic obstructive pulmonary disease, type 1 diabetes mellitus, or immunosuppression)

Abbreviations: GCS, Glasgow Coma Scale; RBC, red blood cell.

Note: It may be appropriate for an injured patient to undergo operative control of ongoing hemorrhage before transfer if a qualified surgeon and operating room resources are promptly available at the referring hospital.

Data from American College of Surgeons, Committee on Trauma. (2014). *Resources for optimal care of the injured patient.* Chicago, IL: Author. Retrieved from https://www.facs.org/~/media/files/quality%20programs/trauma/vrc%20resources/resources%20for%20optimal%20care.ashx.

Decision to Transport

The decision to transport a patient to a specialized or higher level of care rests solely with the physician responsible for the patient's care at the initial receiving facility. Directly after the primary survey, a reevaluation decision point emphasizes early consideration for patient transfer. At the end of the secondary survey, there is another reevaluation point when all patient assessment findings can be summarized and a determination made of the need for transfer. Timeliness is key in making this decision. Factors for transfer consideration include the following:

- Knowledge of facility resources, capabilities, and limitations to provide the necessary care for that trauma patient
- Availability of specialty or higher level of trauma centers to provide definitive care (Level I trauma center, burn centers, pediatric trauma centers, acute brain and spinal cord injury referral centers, reimplantation centers, high-risk obstetric centers)
- Available transportation services (e.g., ground, air)
- Team configuration and type of equipment required to accomplish the transport
- Risks and benefits to the patient (the patient's reaction to transport and/or the mode of transport selected)
- Policies, procedures, protocols, and transfer agreements in place

Once the decision to transport the patient to another facility is made and the patient is accepted by the receiving facility, transportation arrangements are determined and the sending and receiving physicians collaborate to choose the most appropriate mode of transport. Considerations include the availability of equipment, workspace needs, qualifications of the transport personnel, weather and road conditions or other environmental factors, as well as the patient's or family's preference. Familiarity with existing procedures, protocols, and interfacility transfer agreements, along with the regulatory requirements pertinent to the jurisdiction, help to guide the interfacility transfer process.

Modes of Transport

The most frequently used interfacility modes of transport are described in **Table 19-3**.[4-11]

Transport Team Composition

Transport team composition can be analyzed in terms of whether an intrafacility or interfacility transport is being undertaken.

Intrafacility

Intrafacility transport may involve multiple transfers to various departments: radiology, special procedures, angiography, surgery, inpatient unit, rehabilitation, or other areas within the hospital. Typically, the trauma nurse prepares, coordinates, and carries out these intrafacility transports. Respiratory therapists, additional nurses, and other personnel may assist. Having an adequate number of personnel with appropriate skills to accomplish the transport is essential.[12,13]

Interfacility

In interfacility transports, the sending physician is responsible for the care of the patient until the patient's arrival at the receiving facility. This physician makes decisions regarding the appropriate level of care and method of transport.

The composition of the transport team used during interfacility transport is determined based on the patient's condition and required level of care.[14] Depending on the nature and severity of the injuries, personnel trained in critical care or specialized teams may be required.[15] Interfacility transport teams should consist of, at a minimum, two patient care providers and a vehicle operator.[15]

NOTE

Certification for Transporting Patients

Nurses who specialize in transporting patients may be certified as either a Certified Transport Registered Nurse (CTRN), for those who specialize in ground transport nursing, or a Certified Flight Registered Nurse (CFRN), for those who specialize in aeromedical transport.

- If ground transportation is used, the transferring facility may send personnel and equipment with the patient:
  - This usually requires a nurse who is experienced in the care of trauma patients, as well as other qualified transport team members.[15]
  - In some instances, specialty trauma centers may send ground transport with their own specially trained personnel.
  - It is important to have facility policies in place before the actual transfer becomes necessary.
- Air transportation usually involves a critical care team:
  - Air-medical transport teams usually include two clinical care providers in various combinations of roles, plus the pilot.
    - Nurse and paramedic is a common combination.

TABLE 19-3 Modes of Patient Transportation

Mode of Transport	Benefits	Drawbacks
Ground	› Readily available › May have space for family members › Weather less of a factor › Fewer restrictions on the weight of the team, patient, and equipment	› Longer travel time › Traffic and road conditions › Risk of collision
Helicopter	› Rapid transport within short distances › Improved survival rates when initiated from the field › Usually a dedicated team with advanced skills › Improves access to Level I and II trauma centers for patients in rural areas	› Restricted use in certain weather conditions › Expensive › Risk of crash › Noise and vibration › Physiologic changes from altitude › Space and weight restrictions › Not all hospitals are equipped with a helipad › No clear evidence that the time benefit for interfacility air transport improves patient outcomes
Fixed-wing aircraft	› Able to handle longer distances than a helicopter › May be pressurized	› Prolonged transport times with transition to and from hospital to airfield

Data from Boackle, P. C. (2012). Stabilization and transport. In *Emergency nursing pediatric course provider manual* (4th ed., pp. 383–387). Des Plaines, IL: Emergency Nurses Association; Borst, G. M., Davies, S. W., Waibel, B. H., Leonard, K. L., Rinehart, S. M., Newell, M. A., . . . Toschlog, E. A. (2014). When birds can't fly: An analysis of interfacility ground transport using advanced life support when helicopter emergency medical service is unavailable. *Journal of Trauma and Acute Care Surgery, 77*(2), 331–337. https://doi.org/10.1097/TA.0000000000000295; Galvagno, S. M., Haut, E. R., Zafar, S. N., Millin, M. G., Efron, D. T., . . . Haider, A. H. (2012). Association between helicopter vs ground emergency medical services and survival for adults with major trauma. *Journal of the American Medical Association, 307*(15), 1602–1610. https://doi.org/10.1001/jama.2012.467; Malekpour, M., Younus, J. M., Jaap, K., Neuhaus, N., Widom, K., Rapp, M., . . . Wild, J. (2017). Mode of transport and clinical outcome in rural trauma: A helicopter versus ambulance comparison. *American Surgeon, 83*(12), 1413–1417; Mathison, D. J., Berg, E., & Beaver, M. (2013). Variations in interfacility transport: Approach to call intake, team composition, and mode of transport. *Clinical Pediatric Emergency Medicine, 14*(3), 193–205. https://doi.org/10.1016/j.cpem.2013.08.004; Meyer, M. T., Gourlay, D. M., Weitze, K. C., Ship, M. D., Drayna, P. C., Werner, C., & Lerner, E. B. (2016). Helicopter interfacility transport of pediatric trauma patients: Are we overusing a costly resource? *Journal of Trauma & Acute Care Surgery, 80*(2), 313–317. https://doi.org/10.1097/TA.0000000000000904; Swearingen, C. (2018). Transport physiology. In R. S. Holleran, A. C. Wolfe Jr., & M. A. Frakes (Eds.), *Patient transport: Principles and practice* (55th ed., pp. 274327–274343). St. Louis, MO: Mosby Elsevier; Werman, H. A., Darbha, S., Cudnik, M., & Caterino, J. (2017). Do trauma patients age 55 and older benefit from air medical transport? *Prehospital Emergency Care, 21*(4), 461–465. https://doi.org/10.1080/10903127.2016.1269223.

    - At times, the team may include a physician, respiratory therapist, or some combination of these.[15]
- Air transport teams are trained for and qualified to monitor and respond to altitude-related hazards in addition to caring for traditional trauma conditions and complications.[15]

Risks of Transport

Any transport of trauma patients, regardless of whether it is interfacility or intrafacility, involves risk. It is the responsibility of the team caring for the patient to ensure that the transport is accomplished in a manner that is efficient, yet safe for both the patient and the transport team. The trauma nurse anticipates the potential for, and prepares to manage, the following risks of transport:

- Loss of airway patency
- Displaced or obstructed tubes, lines, or catheters
- Dislodged splinting devices
- Need to replace or reinforce dressings

- Deterioration in patient status; change in vital signs or level of consciousness
- Injury to the patient and/or team members

Nursing Considerations for Transport

Multiple factors can affect the outcome of patient transport, so planning is essential. Nursing considerations include assisting with the medical screening examination and required resuscitation and/or stabilizing interventions, within the capabilities of the sending facility. Other considerations that the transferring nurse should anticipate include the following:

- Patient consent
    - Assist with and support the process to assure that the patient and/or family are aware of the need for, as well as the risks and benefits of, transport, so they can make an informed decision regarding transport and sign the consent for transfer.
- Transfer requirements
    - Ensure that the sending physician has received acceptance for the transfer from the receiving hospital.
    - Arrange for the transport team.
    - Provide a patient report to the receiving nurse.
    - Send copies of all available medical records, laboratory, radiographic, and other related reports.[3]
- Patient care
    - Ensure definitive airway control.
    - Suction the airway and endotracheal tube as needed.
    - Maintain breathing and provide assisted ventilations.
    - Ensure patency and flow rate of intravenous (IV) infusions.
    - Continually reassess the patient's neurologic status.
    - Secure all monitoring devices and equipment, such as chest tubes.
- Family and patient preparation
    - Explain the logistics of the transport to the patient, family, and assistive staff.
    - Ensure that the family has information regarding where the patient is being taken and directions to that location.
    - Ensure that the family has seen the patient prior to departure, if possible.
- Transport team
    - Give a report to the transporting personnel as necessary.
    - Provide the team with copies of documentation as needed.
- Follow-up
    - Call the receiving facility to notify it of the patient's departure time and the estimated time of arrival.
    - Fax or send electronically any additional laboratory or radiographic reports that become available after the patient has departed.

Equipment for Transport

The trauma nurse caring for the patient is responsible for ensuring the availability of proper equipment needed during transport. Depending on the status of the patient, equipment may include the following:

- Airway equipment
    - Suction devices
    - Oral airways
    - Endotracheal tubes
    - Laryngoscope blades and handles
    - Supplies to secure the endotracheal tube
    - Failed-airway equipment, such as a supraglottic device
    - Bag-mask device
    - Ventilator
- Medications
    - Pain medications
    - Sedation agents
    - Vasoactive medications
    - Resuscitation medications
- IV access supplies
- IV fluids
- Cardiac monitor/defibrillator
- Equipment to monitor vital signs, including oxygen saturation and capnography
- Equipment to perform a needle thoracostomy
- Restraints

Emergency Department Boarding

Once initial assessment and stabilization of the trauma patient has been completed and the decision to transfer the patient to another facility or to admit has been made, it is essential that the patient be moved from the ED to an inpatient unit as quickly as possible for the next phase in the continuum of care.[16-18] If an inpatient bed is not readily available, post-resuscitation care of the trauma patient may be provided in the ED. ED staff may be required to perform inpatient care, or inpatient nursing staff may be redirected to the ED to care for boarding patients. It is important that EDs have policies and procedures in place related to the nursing care of the critically ill trauma patient while they are being held (boarded) in the ED. Such a patient must receive the same standard of care that would be provided on the assigned inpatient unit.

Emerging Trends

ED crowding and boarding may adversely affect patient outcomes, including increased mortality, rates of medical errors, and length of stay.[19,20] Many organizations have developed performance improvement teams to address the challenges that accompany patient boarding in the ED. Uncovering the root cause of the crowding is imperative to finding solutions. As organizations across the United States have struggled with crowding and boarding, some initiatives in these areas have shown promise, including the following:

- Developing an area in the ED designed similarly to a nursing unit, with consistent scheduling of regular non-ED RNs[21]
- Improving hospital discharge time to drive ED throughput[22]
- Triaging critical care beds[21]
- Use of supplemental (float) ED RN staffing to enable one-to-one care of critical patients

Summary

A majority of trauma patients who present to the ED will require transport or patient hand-off during their care—whether intrafacility to another department such as radiology or the inpatient unit, or interfacility to a trauma or specialized center of care. Using a standardized approach for care and communication, the trauma nurse ensures safe and appropriate transitions of care, regardless of how and where patients are being transported. All patient transports must follow the pertinent institutional, regional, and federal laws, guidelines, policies, and procedures. The level of trauma care a patient receives should progressively improve as the patient moves from the field to definitive care,[1] then continue at the same level of care during intrafacility transitions. The goal of the trauma teams at both the sending and receiving facilities is to provide high-quality, safe care for patients, protecting them from further injury, and to ensure safe practice for the trauma team.

References

1. American College of Surgeons. (2018). *Advanced trauma life support: Student course manual* (10th ed.). Chicago, IL: Author.
2. American College of Surgeons, Committee on Trauma. (2014). *Resources for optimal care of the injured patient.* Chicago, IL: Author. Retrieved from https://www.facs.org/~/media/files/quality%20programs/trauma/vrc%20resources/resources%20for%20optimal%20care.ashx
3. Centers for Medicare and Medicaid Services. (2009, May 29). *Revision to Appendix V, "Emergency Medical Treatment & Active Labor Act (EMTALA) interpretive guidelines."* Retrieved from http://www.cms.gov/Regulations-and-Guidance/Guidance/Transmittals/downloads/R46SOMA.pdf
4. Borst, G. M., Davies, S. W., Waibel, B. H., Leonard, K. L., Rinehart, S. M., Newell, M. A., . . . Toschlog, E. A. (2014). When birds can't fly: An analysis of interfacility ground transport using advanced life support when helicopter emergency medical service is unavailable. *Journal of Trauma, 77*(2), 331–337. https://doi.org/10.1097/TA.0000000000000295
5. Boackle, P. C. (2012). Stabilization and transport. In *Emergency nursing pediatric course provider manual* (4th ed., pp. 383–387). Des Plaines, IL: Emergency Nurses Association.
6. Galvagno, S. M., Haut, E. R., Zafar, S. N., Millin, M. G., Efron, D. T., . . . Haider, A. H. (2012). Association between helicopter vs ground emergency medical services and survival for adults with major trauma. *Journal of the American Medical Association, 307*(15), 1602–1610. https://doi.org/10.1001/jama.2012.467
7. Malekpour, M., Younus, J. M., Jaap, K., Neuhaus, N., Widom, K., Rapp, M., . . . Wild, J. (2017). Mode of transport and clinical outcome in rural trauma: A helicopter versus ambulance comparison. *American Surgeon*, *83*(12), 1413–1417.
8. Mathison, D. J., Berg, E., & Beaver, M. (2013). Variations in interfacility transport: Approach to call intake, team composition, and mode of transport. *Clinical Pediatric Emergency Medicine, 14*(3), 193–205. https://doi.org/10.1016/j.cpem.2013.08.004
9. Meyer, M. T., Gourlay, D. M., Weitze, K. C., Ship, M. D., Drayna, P. C., Werner, C., & Lerner, E. B. (2016). Helicopter interfacility transport of pediatric trauma patients: Are we overusing a costly resource? *Journal of Trauma & Acute Care Surgery, 80*(2), 313–317. https://doi.org/10.1097/TA.0000000000000904
10. Swearingen, C. (2018). Transport physiology. In R. S. Holleran, A. C. Wolfe Jr., & M. A. Frakes (Eds.), *Patient transport: Principles and practice* (55th ed., pp. 274327–274343). St. Louis, MO: Mosby Elsevier.
11. Werman, H. A., Darbha, S., Cudnik, M., & Caterino, J. (2017). Do trauma patients age 55 and older benefit from air medical transport? *Prehospital Emergency Care, 21*(4), 461–465. https://doi.org/10.1080/10903127.2016.1269223
12. Beachley, M. (2009). Evolution of the trauma cycle. In K. A. McQuillan, M. B. Flynn Makic, & E. Whalen (Eds.), *Trauma nursing from resuscitation through rehabilitation* (4th ed., pp. 1–18). St. Louis, MO: Saunders Elsevier.
13. Fitzpatrick, M. K., & McMaster, J. (2009). Performance improvement and patient safety in trauma care. In K. A. McQuillan, M. B. Flynn Makic, & E. Whalen (Eds.), *Trauma nursing from resuscitation through rehabilitation* (4th ed., pp. 29–43). St. Louis, MO: Saunders Elsevier.
14. Von Rueden, K. T. (2009). Nursing practice through the cycle of trauma. In K. A. McQuillan, M. B. Flynn Makic, &

E. Whalen (Eds.), *Trauma nursing from resuscitation through rehabilitation* (4th ed., pp. 136–160). St. Louis, MO: Saunders Elsevier.

15. Commission on Accreditation of Medical Transport Systems. (2015, October). *Tenth edition accreditation standards of the Commission on Accreditation of Medical Transport Systems*. Anderson, SC: Author. Retrieved from http://69.89.31.68/~camtsorg/wp-content/uploads/2017/06/10th_Standards_Free_-_021017.pdf
16. Mowery, N. T., Dougherty, S. D., Hildreth, A. N., Holmes, J. H., Chang, M. C., Martin, R. S., . . . Miller, P. R. (2011). Emergency department length of stay in an independent predictor of hospital mortality in trauma activation patients. *Journal of Trauma, 70*(6), 1317–1325. https://doi.org/10.1097/TA.0b013e3182175199
17. Intas, G., Stergiannis, P., Chalari, E., Tsoumakas, K., & Fildissis, G. (2012). The impact of ED boarding time, severity of illness, and discharge destination on outcomes of critically ill ED patients. *Advanced Emergency Nursing Journal, 34*(2), 164–169. https://doi.org/10.1097/TME.0b013e318251515f
18. American College of Emergency Physicians. (2017). Boarding of admitted and intensive care patients in the emergency department. Retrieved from https://www.acep.org/patient-care/policy-statements/boarding-of-admitted-and-intensive-care-patients-in-the-emergency-department/#sm.000irp8m7rz6dnd11bh29rs29mrr4
19. Emergency Nurses Association. *Position statement: Crowding, boarding and patient throughput*. Des Plaines, IL: Author. Retrieved from https://www.ena.org/docs/default-source/resource-library/practice-resources/position-statements/crowdingboardingandpatientthroughput.pdf?sfvrsn=5fb4e79f_4
20. Clark, K., & Normile, L. B. (2002). Delays in implementing admission orders for critical care patients associated with length of stay in emergency departments in six mid-Atlantic states. *Journal of Emergency Nursing, 28*(6), 489–495. https://doi.org/10.1067/men.2002.128714
21. Bornemann-Shepherd, M., Le-Lazar, J., Makic, M. B., DeVine, D., McDevitt, K., & Paul, M. (2015). Caring for inpatient boarders in the emergency department: Improving safety and patient and staff satisfaction. *Journal of Emergency Nursing, 41*(1), 23–29. https://doi.org/10.1016/j.jen.2014.04.012
22. El-Eid, G. R., Kaddoum, R., Tamim, H., & Hitti, E. A. (2015). Improving hospital discharge time: A successful implementation of Six Sigma methodology. *Medicine, 94*(12), e633. http://doi.org/10.1097/MD.0000000000000633

CHAPTER 20

Post-Resuscitation Care Considerations

Kyndra P. Holm, MSN, RN, CEN, TCRN

OBJECTIVES

Upon completion of this chapter, the learner will be able to:

1. Recognize potential and actual patient outcomes as a result of injuries and resuscitation efforts.
2. Discuss assessment modalities for the trauma patient during post-resuscitative care.
3. Identify potential consequences of injury and care rendered by anticipating the pathophysiologic changes for the trauma patient during post-resuscitative care.
4. Plan appropriate interventions for the trauma patient during post-resuscitative care.
5. Evaluate the effectiveness of nursing interventions for the trauma patient during post-resuscitative care.
6. Understand important quality measures in the emergency department care of the trauma patient.
7. Recognize emerging trends in post-resuscitation care of the trauma patient.

Introduction

Trauma happens quickly, yet the consequences of injury can take hours, months, or years to overcome. Care of the injured patient may begin with activation of emergency medical services or arrival into the emergency department (ED), but the continuum of care for the trauma patient does not end with the initial resuscitation. The goal of trauma care is to return the patient to his or her full potential within the community, and trauma care continues until that potential is reached.

Post-Resuscitation Care

Post-resuscitation care takes place in many environments. It may begin in the ED or prehospital environment but continues in the intensive care unit (ICU), operating room, medical or surgical unit, rehabilitation unit, and the patient's home after discharge. Multiple clinicians are involved in every step of the process of trauma care, making coordination of care and communication critical. Ideally, the trauma patient will move quickly from the initial assessment and stabilization phase in the

ED to definitive care; however, that is not always possible. Often, the trauma patient will remain in the ED past the post-resuscitation phase of care.

The trauma nurse and the trauma patient are both impacted by hospital overcrowding. ED overcrowding and boarding admitted patients in the ED are widely associated with poorer patient outcomes, increased hospital length of stay, delayed or missed injuries, higher rates of mortality, and increased rates of nursing burnout and staff turnover.[1-4] Even care of the most seriously injured patients who require aggressive resuscitation and blood product administration is negatively impacted by ED overcrowding.[5]

The trauma patient who is boarded in the ED loses the benefit of specialized nursing care in units where staff are familiar with the post-resuscitation care of injured patients. Instead, the trauma patient continues to receive care from the ED nurse, who has a broad, generalized knowledge base and skill set.[1] Different solutions to this problem are being tried in hospitals around the United States, including the increased use of float/resource nurses or dedicated trauma nurses, increased use of point-of-care (POC) testing, and even attempts at streamlining patient throughput from the computed tomography (CT) scanner directly to the ICU.[6] Ultimately, the issue of ED overcrowding and hospital throughput are complex issues that will not be quickly or easily solved.[7]

The trauma patient can be especially challenging. With such a patient, the trauma nurse will need to care for multiple injuries to multiple body systems, recognize the natural evolution of identified injuries and sequelae of resuscitative interventions, and be alert for commonly missed injuries. See **Table 20-1** for additional information about delayed presentation of injuries and commonly missed injuries.[8,9]

An orderly, systematic process of assessment and intervention for the priorities of airway, breathing, circulation, disability and exposure/environmental (ABCDE) control helps to direct the resuscitative efforts for the trauma patient in the ED. In turn, post-resuscitation care reflects the same organized and systematic approach as the initial resuscitation. The trauma nurse begins by reevaluating the ABCDE parameters to note any change from the initial assessment and subsequent stabilization. Trauma nurses will anticipate and be able to recognize injury evolution and its likely consequences, so they can be prepared with appropriate interventions no matter where they work, whether in the ED, ICU, post-anesthesia care unit, telemetry/intermediate care unit, or surgical care floor. Frequent, ongoing monitoring can help the trauma nurse to recognize changes in patient status and to intervene quickly.

Airway

Airway management continues to be the priority in trauma patients during post-resuscitation care. If the patient does not have a definitive airway, continuous monitoring and reassessments will alert the trauma nurse to potential compromise and identify the need for a definitive airway. See Chapter 4, "Airway and Ventilation," for additional information.

Tube Displacement or Obstruction

Endotracheal tubes (ETT) can easily become displaced or obstructed, particularly during transport to tests or between units.[10] This requires diligent observation to assure the tube remains properly placed and patent. Use of the DOPE mnemonic can help the trauma nurse to resolve these issues; see Chapter 4 for more information. Additional considerations include the following:

- If the patient has a definitive airway, careful and continuous monitoring assures correct tube placement, adequate oxygenation, and ventilation.
- Informing other providers that an airway was difficult to place can prevent early extubation and enable proper planning and preparation for extubation.
  - Use of a difficult airway identifier, such as an armband, or sticker on the ETT, a chart sticker, or progress note, can communicate this information.

Breathing and Ventilation

Patients with multiple injuries will benefit from the administration and titration of oxygen (see Chapter 4 for more information). Oxygen concentration and delivery is guided by monitoring arterial blood gases (ABGs), end-tidal carbon dioxide ($ETCO_2$), pulse oximetry (SpO_2), and frequent reassessment of the quality of the patient's respiratory rate and effort, changes in breathing patterns, lung sounds, and overall appearance. Trauma patients may be at higher risk for impaired breathing and inadequate ventilation from many factors.

- Injuries that impact respiratory effort:
  - Central nervous system (CNS) depression
  - High cervical spinal cord injury (SCI)—above C3 or C4
- Patients with difficult, fast, or shallow respirations:
  - Thoracic injuries (including rib fractures, hemothorax, pneumothorax)
  - Under deep sedation
  - Prescribed analgesia

TABLE 20-1 Delayed Presentations and Responses and Commonly Missed Injuries

System	Delayed Presentations and Responses	Commonly Missed Injuries
Respiratory	› Pneumothorax/hemothorax › Flail chest/rib fractures › Pulmonary contusion › Diaphragmatic laceration › Acute respiratory distress syndrome acute lung injury, aspiration › Fat or pulmonary embolism	› Pneumothorax/hemothorax › Pneumomediastinum › Rib injuries
Cardiovascular	› Cardiogenic shock › Sepsis	
Neurologic/spinal	› Intracranial hematoma › Secondary brain injury › Alcohol/substance withdrawal	› Spinal subluxations › Spinal cord syndromes
Abdominal	› Hollow viscus injury › Intestinal rupture › Compartment syndrome › Splenic rupture	› Liver injuries › Intestinal injuries › Renal injuries
Musculoskeletal	› Compartment syndrome › Rhabdomyolysis	Fractures of the: › Face › Extremities › Clavicle/scapula › Tibial plateau › Vertebrae

Data from Buduhan, G., & McRitchie, D. I. (2000). Missed injuries in patients with multiple trauma. *Journal of Trauma, 49*, 600–605; Montmany, S., Navarro, S., Rebassa, P., Hermoso, J., Hidalgo, M., & Canovas, G. (2007). A prospective study on the incidence of missed injuries in trauma patients. *Cirugía Española, 84*, 32–36.

Circulation

Circulation care includes fluid management and use of hypertonic solutions.

Fluid Management

Controlling hemorrhage and treating shock with appropriate volume resuscitation is a basic principle in caring for the trauma patient.[11] While lab values including lactate, ABGs, and base deficit help direct resuscitation efforts for the patient in shock, urine output remains a reliable indicator of resuscitation status.[11] Most clinicians aim for a urine output of 0.5–1.0 mL/kg/hr.

Rapid and copious administration of isotonic crystalloids used in the treatment of hypovolemic shock can result in fluid overload, capillary leak syndrome, and fluid shifts to the interstitial space. With ongoing research and a greater understanding of the physiologic response, better alternatives to large-volume administration of isotonic fluid have been instituted, including balanced resuscitation and massive transfusion protocols (MTPs; see Chapter 5, "Shock," for more information).

Use of Hypertonic Solutions

Hypertonic solutions, such as hypertonic saline, have been considered potential adjuncts in resuscitation of the trauma patient to raise the intravascular circulating volume without requiring the administration of large volumes of fluid. The long-held assumption has been that hypertonic solutions draw water into the vasculature because of higher osmotic pressure. Relatively small volumes of 3% saline have been shown to have up to a four-fold increase in intravascular volume.[12] In addition to the osmotic effects on intravascular volume, recent research has shown that 3% saline may increase cardiac contractility and improve cardiac output.[13] Most trauma nurses are familiar with hypertonic saline (3% sodium chloride) solutions for the management of increased intracranial pressure (ICP) (see Chapter 6, "Head Trauma"). While this treatment is consistently used in ICP management, the potential benefit of hypertonic solutions in volume expansion is a topic of ongoing research in trauma care, and current practice standards do not advocate hypertonic solution administration during trauma resuscitation.

Disability (Neurologic Status)

Close attention should be given to the patient with known or suspected neurologic injury, as brain injuries evolve with time.[14,15] Brain injuries range from mild traumatic brain injury (TBI) to severe hypoxic ischemic encephalopathy. In the patient with brain injury, the CT scan may initially appear normal but then progress as the injury evolves. Patients with brain injury also require careful monitoring of laboratory values—such as coagulation measures and sodium levels—and careful temperature regulation to avoid hypothermia or fever greater than 38°C (100.4°F).[16-19]

TBI progression may be complicated by factors such as age, use of antiplatelet or anticoagulant medications, or chronic alcohol use. Subdural hematomas may develop over time and are most common in the older adult or patient who chronically uses alcohol.[20] In these patients, brain atrophy produces a larger space between the dura mater and the skull where blood has space to accumulate before symptoms occur. Observe the patient over time for subtle neurologic changes that may identify increasing ICP or developing subdural hematoma. These patients may present with a history of several remote falls and a recent change in mental status that could be a layering of an acute condition on a chronic subdural hematoma. Trauma nurses caring for the pediatric patient with TBI should monitor blood pressure (BP) carefully to prevent hypotension and subsequent secondary brain injury.[16]

SCI—especially contusions and hematoma—may also evolve with time and require the nurse to closely monitor for symptom progression, respiratory compromise, or the development of hypotension.[21] See Chapter 9, "Spinal Trauma," for additional information. Steroids are no longer recommended for the treatment of spinal cord contusion.[22]

Exposure and Environmental Control

The key exposure and environmental control concerns are hypothermia and hyperthermia.

Hypothermia

Temperature monitoring is important not just in the immediate resuscitation period, but remains a concern throughout the care of the trauma patient. Continue to maintain a warm ambient temperature in the trauma room, use warming interventions as needed, and monitor the patient's temperature to avoid overheating. Prevent heat loss during transport to other departments with warmed blankets or other techniques. Hypothermia has been associated with the following complications[23]:

- Development of coagulopathy
- Delayed wound healing
- Increased surgical-site infections
- Prolonged hospitalization
- Increased myocardial complications
- Increased blood loss and need for blood transfusion
- Delayed recovery from anesthesia and increase in postoperative discomfort

Hypothermia in the trauma patient can be a particularly deadly issue. Hypothermia—defined as a core temperature of less than 35°C (95°F)—is highly associated with both early and late mortality in the trauma patient.[24] One of the most serious complications of trauma is the deadly triad of hypothermia, acidosis, and coagulopathy. Because of this risk, prevention of hypothermia is vital to the hypovolemic trauma patient.[25]

Therapeutic hypothermia—that is, cooling the patient's core body temperature to between 32°C and 36°C (89.6°F and 96.8°F)—is a common intervention in the post–cardiac arrest patient with return of spontaneous circulation to help preserve neurologic function. While recommended as part of the 2015 Advanced Cardiac Life Support (ACLS) care, therapeutic hypothermia has not been demonstrated to improve outcomes for the trauma patient with severe TBI and should not be used.[26]

Hyperthermia

Trauma patients can be at risk of hyperthermia due to the nature of their injuries. Hyperthermia syndromes are rare in the initial phase of severe trauma care, but temperature elevation from systemic inflammatory response may begin early.

Once the trauma patient is successfully resuscitated, his or her temperature and metabolic rate may increase.[27] This increase is a natural result of stimulation of the immune system, wound healing, tissue remodeling, and functional recovery.[28] Thermoregulation may be impaired in patients after TBI, causing fever.[29] Like hypothermia, early fever (i.e., temperature greater than 38.3°C [100.9°F]) is associated with worse outcomes for the trauma patient.[30] While some degree of temperature elevation may be expected, the cause of the hyperthermia should be vigorously investigated, as additional treatment may be necessary to address it.

Acidosis

Acidosis is a common complication of multiple traumatic injuries. An acidotic environment can affect all body systems, as it changes cellular function. Specifically, in the bloodstream, acidosis can affect oxygenation, making it more difficult for hemoglobin to bind with oxygen, and thereby decreasing oxygen delivery and cellular ability to use oxygen. Acidosis in combination with hypothermia intensifies the adverse effects on coagulation and worsens clotting times.[31,32] Acidosis can occur via two separate routes: respiratory or metabolic.[33]

Respiratory Acidosis

The respiratory route to acidosis involves the following mechanisms:

- Respiratory acidosis occurs because of inadequate ventilation and retained carbon dioxide (CO_2).
- Hypoventilation in patients with pain, a change in mental status, signs of a developing pneumothorax, or weakening chest muscles, or in those receiving analgesia or sedation, may result in respiratory acidosis.
- Treatment includes improving ventilation by assisting with a bag-mask device or adjusting ventilator settings and providing pain relief to increase respiratory rate and improve air exchange.

Metabolic Acidosis

The metabolic route to acidosis involves the following mechanisms:

- A by-product of tissue hypoperfusion, metabolic acidosis is associated with hemorrhagic shock in the trauma patient.
- When tissues are deficient in oxygen, cells shift to anaerobic metabolism, which produces lactic acid and leads to acidosis.
- Kidney hypoperfusion leads to the development of acute kidney injury (AKI), and the kidney loses its ability to excrete hydrogen ions, resulting in acidosis.
- Acidosis can result in vasodilation, hypotension, and worsened coagulopathy.
- Restoration of tissue perfusion is needed to correct metabolic acidosis. Hypoperfusion may be prevented by hemorrhage control and early balanced resuscitation with blood products and intravenous (IV) fluids.

Monitoring

Acidosis can be detected by monitoring ABGs, serum lactate levels, and base deficit. New, noninvasive technology using near-infrared spectroscopy to monitor tissue oxygen delivery and shock is being used increasingly in EDs and ICUs.[34] See Chapter 5 for more information.

Coagulopathy

The final component of the "deadly trauma triad" is coagulopathy. Trauma patients may develop coagulopathy because of the combination of injury and overzealous crystalloid resuscitative efforts, or they may have been on anticoagulation therapy prior to their injury, making the goal of achieving hemostasis more challenging for the trauma team. The trauma nurse should be alert for the possible presence of medications that would impair platelet function, such as aspirin and clopidogrel, or other anticoagulant medications, such as warfarin, rivaroxaban, dabigatran, apixaban, and enoxaparin, and communicate that information to the rest of the trauma team.[31]

Nearly all trauma patients with multiple injuries will develop some degree of coagulopathy that is worsened by hypothermia and acidosis.[35] MTPs with prescribed blood, platelet, and plasma administration and the use of tranexamic acid (TXA) are linked to improved patient outcomes in adult trauma patients.[36] Traditional methods of monitoring clotting ability, including prothrombin/international normalized ratio and partial thromboplastin time, address only the early steps in clot formation, but do not monitor later steps of clot evolution and lysis.[36] POC testing for thromboelastometry and rotational elastometry are increasingly being used to help guide fluid resuscitation and coagulopathy management in real time.[31] See Chapter 5 for more information.

Post-Resuscitation Care of Selected Injuries

Post-resuscitation care of selected injuries is covered in this section.

Rib Fractures

Rib fractures are one of the most common thoracic injuries, found in approximately 20% of patients who sustain blunt chest trauma, and are commonly associated with underlying pulmonary contusion or pneumothorax.[37] Rib injury associated with pulmonary contusion is an independent risk factor for the development of pneumonia and increased mortality. Aggressive pain management for trauma patients with rib fractures is recommended to prevent atelectasis and improve functional residual and vital capacity. Effective pain management also promotes mobility, deep breathing, productive coughing, and the ability to clear secretions.[38] Aggressive pain management, in combination with early mobilization and pulmonary toilet (or pulmonary hygiene), are important strategies to prevent complications of pneumonia and even death in the patient with blunt chest trauma and associated rib fractures. Although the patient will want to take shallow breaths and will be reluctant to cough, such measures are critical in helping to prevent pneumonia. Use of an incentive spirometer can encourage deep breathing—thereby opening atelectatic alveoli and recruiting collapsed airways for gas exchange. Deep breathing has the added benefit of often provoking a cough as mucus in the airways moves and alveoli open. The combination of deep breathing and coughing will not be popular with the patient, but can be lifesaving for the patient with multiple rib fractures.

Flail Chest

Patients with flail chest may require more aggressive interventions to prevent complications and death.[37] As the number of ribs fractured increases, the risk of severe complications increases.[39] Patients older than age 65 and those with higher Injury Severity Scores (ISS) are at higher risk,[40] with the risk of mortality increasing by as much as 19% for each additional rib that is fractured.[39] Open reduction and internal fixation of the rib fractures has also been included as a treatment for flail chest.[37,41] See Chapter 7, "Thoracic and Neck Trauma," for more information.

Pulmonary Contusion

Pulmonary contusions often occur concomitantly with rib fractures[36] and are associated with respiratory failure that develops over time, rather than immediately following the chest injury. Clinical symptoms—such as respiratory distress with hypoxemia and hypercarbia—peak 72 hours after injury. Management of a pulmonary contusion may change over time as the patient's condition worsens and fluid shifts into the contused area. Significant hypoxia on room air is an indication for elective intubation and ventilation. Management for the patient with pulmonary contusion is largely supportive until the resolution of symptoms occurs, but patients may have long-term respiratory compromise due to fibrosis of the contused area.[42]

Pneumothorax

Insertion of a chest tube is indicated in many patients with a pneumothorax. Positive-pressure mechanical ventilation can worsen pneumothoraces. If it goes undetected, the pneumothorax can progress to tension pneumothorax. Nurses must be vigilant to assess equality of breath sounds, ventilator airway pressures, and hemodynamic stability for intubated patients to identify pneumothorax development or a worsening condition.

Hemothorax

A hemothorax is usually characterized by decreased or absent lung sounds and hypotension. The initial treatment is aimed at restoration of systemic intravascular blood volume and drainage of blood within the chest cavity. Initial drainage of 1,500 mL in adults, continual blood loss of 200 mL/hr for 4 hours, or a need to transfuse blood to maintain hemodynamic stability may be an indication for a thoracotomy.[43] Autotransfusion would be considered when appropriate (i.e., no evidence of diaphragmatic perforation and contamination of bowel contents into chest cavity).

Blunt Cardiac Injury (Formerly Myocardial Contusion)

Myocardial injury after blunt chest trauma can be a challenge to diagnose. Patients with a blunt cardiac injury will complain of chest discomfort, which might erroneously be attributed to a rib fracture or chest wall contusion. An electrocardiogram (ECG) is performed on any patient suspected of a cardiac injury, and complete serial ECGs over a period of 4 to 6 hours can help to detect changes in rhythm and conduction or reveal myocardial infarction (MI).[43,44] Premature ventricular contractions are the most common dysrhythmias in patients with blunt cardiac trauma. The leading cause of death for patients with a blunt cardiac injury is related to the development of ventricular fibrillation.[44]

Management of the patient with a suspected blunt cardiac injury starts with monitoring for hemodynamic changes. Patients with preexisting cardiac risk factors, multiple chest injuries, and abnormal ECG findings are commonly admitted and observed on continuous cardiac monitoring for at least the first 24 hours.

Cardiac Tamponade

The assessment findings related to cardiac tamponade due to an atrial rupture may be slow to develop and may not be evident until after the initial trauma survey and resuscitation.[43] Cardiac tamponade can occur slowly, without complaint of symptoms, or suddenly, with an exaggerated inspiratory decrease in systolic BP, shortness of breath, chest tightness, and dizziness. Diagnosis for cardiac tamponade can be made with focused assessment with sonography for trauma (FAST). In such a case, the nurse would anticipate that the patient would undergo a pericardiocentesis or an expedited trip to the operating room for a pericardial window depending on the setting.

Ruptured Diaphragm

Traumatic diaphragmatic injuries are frequently missed during the initial evaluation of trauma patients. Generally, injuries to the diaphragm are difficult to evaluate with a CT scan and may require surgical intervention for definitive identification of diaphragmatic rupture.[45-47] Diaphragmatic ruptures or tears are more commonly diagnosed when they occur on the left side due to the potential for the liver to conceal or protect the defect on the right side. Evidence of an elevated diaphragm on a chest radiograph as well as bowel sounds over the thorax can indicate a possible diaphragmatic injury and warrants investigation.[43]

Deep Vein Thrombosis

Trauma patients are at substantially increased risk for developing deep vein thrombosis (DVT), with some estimates indicating that incidence is as high as 63% in trauma patients.[48] When considering DVT, note the classic triad that leads to venous thrombosis[49]:

- Stasis
- Endothelial damage
- Hypercoagulability

Numerous risk factors can influence the development of DVT in the trauma patient, including altered hemodynamics (hypotension), increasing age, obesity, prolonged immobility, existing malignancy, pregnancy, and certain medications.[48] Once the risk is identified, the goal is to limit clot development and prevent pulmonary embolism (PE). Low-molecular-weight heparin (e.g., enoxaparin), compression stockings, and intermittent pneumatic compression devices are also useful in the prevention of DVT.[48]

Pulmonary Embolism

PE is the third leading cause of death in trauma patients who survive the first 24 hours following initial injury and do not receive DVT prophylaxis.[50] Research has shown that as many as 24% of PEs occur within the first 4 days after injury and may even occur on day 1.[51] Therefore, prevention of venous stasis and early evaluation for signs of a DVT are critical. An acute PE occurs abruptly, and the symptoms exhibited depend on the size of the embolism. Additional considerations include the following:

- Anxiety may occur.
- PEs can develop early or late; assess the patient who presents even days after the injury for signs of PE.[51]
- Massive PE will cause hemodynamic instability such as hypotension.[52]
- Pulmonary infarction and ischemia may result from complete disruption of blood flow.
- Massive PE may cause right ventricular failure and death shortly after onset of symptoms.[52]

Assessment findings of a PE include the following:

- Abrupt onset of pleuritic chest pain
- Dyspnea
- Hypoxemia (often refractory to supplemental oxygen)
- Hemoptysis
- Cough
- Orthopnea
- Adventitious lung sounds:
    - Wheezing
    - Crackles
- Decreased lung sounds
- Jugular vein distention
- Hypotension

Studies to confirm or exclude a PE include a ventilation–perfusion lung scan, CT pulmonary angiography (CTA), magnetic resonance imaging, or pulmonary angiography. The CTA is essentially the gold standard in diagnosing a pulmonary embolus.[52]

Fat Embolism

During manipulation of long bones for fracture fixation, embolic marrow, including lipid microemboli, can become dislodged, resulting in a fat embolism.[53] Nearly all orthopedic patients who have multiple fractures experience intravasation of bone marrow fat.[54] A fat embolism can travel to the pulmonary vasculature, causing obstruction and subsequent ischemia. Most instances of fat embolism are asymptomatic, but symptomatic patients demonstrate a classic triad presentation[55]:

- Decreased mental status, starting with restlessness and agitation
- Respiratory distress, including dyspnea and hypoxia
- Petechial rash on the head, neck, anterior thorax, conjunctivae, buccal mucous membranes, and axillae[54,55]

Presentation can occur as early as 12 hours following injury or as late as 2 weeks after a precipitating event; however, most fat emboli occur within 24 to 72 hours after long bone fractures.[56] A helical thoracic CT scan and chest radiographs are the most beneficial imaging for diagnosis. Patchy pulmonary infiltrates may be seen on the chest radiograph.[38] ABGs assist in the evaluation and guide treatment of problems with ventilation, acid–base balance, and hypoxia. Fat emboli can contribute to the development of acute respiratory distress syndrome (ARDS).[54] In as many as 5% to 15% of patients, fat emboli are fatal.[56] Treatment is supportive, including oxygenation and ventilation and promoting hemodynamic stability.[57]

Acute Lung Injury/Acute Respiratory Distress Syndrome

Acute lung injury (ALI) is a syndrome resulting in alveolar damage or collapse and pulmonary edema that is not attributable to a cardiovascular origin.[58,59] ALI develops 24 to 48 hours after injury or onset of illness, and is stimulated by the inflammatory process.[58-60] In the trauma patient, ALI can be associated with fluid shifts from the intravascular space to the interstitial space and into the alveoli. ARDS, the most severe form of ALI, was originally known as *shock lung* because of the effects of massive fluid resuscitation with subsequent fluid shift on the lungs.[58-60] Diagnostic criteria for ALI/ARDS include the following[60]:

- Partial pressure of oxygen/fraction of inspired oxygen ratio of less than 200 mm Hg (ARDS) or less than 300 mm Hg (ALI)
- Pulmonary artery occlusion pressure of 18 mm Hg
- No clinical evidence of left atrial or ventricular dysfunction

Risk factors for ALI/ARDS include the following[60]:

- Aspiration
- Pulmonary contusion or other thoracic trauma
- Fat embolism
- PE
- Near-drowning
- Inhalation injury
- Nonthoracic trauma
- Massive transfusion
- Oxygen toxicity
- Disseminated intravascular coagulation (DIC)
- Shock
- Pneumonia or sepsis

Treatment for ALI/ARDS includes supportive care and ventilation strategies meant to recruit atelectatic alveoli. Positive end-expiratory pressure (PEEP) ventilation with lower tidal volumes has been shown to reduce airway pressure and barotrauma.[59]

- PEEP decreases intrapulmonary shunting and increases lung compliance.
- At high levels, PEEP can also cause barotrauma, decrease cardiac output, and increase intrathoracic pressure.
- Optimal PEEP is between 10 and 15 mm Hg.[61]
- More advanced strategies are generally deferred to after admission in the critical care unit and include prone positioning, high-frequency ventilation, and extracorporeal membrane oxygenation.[58-61]

Pneumonia and Aspiration

Pneumonia occurs in as many as 25% of mechanically ventilated patients.[62] Ventilator-associated pneumonia (VAP) develops more than 48 hours after mechanical ventilation has started.[63] One of the most critical risk factors for VAP is colonization of the oral cavity by respiratory pathogens.[64] Patients with poor dental hygiene are at higher risk of having distinctive oral bacteria present; when patients develop VAP, the bacteria in their lung secretions may originate from these oral bacteria.[59]

Secretions that adhere to the ETT provide a direct route for bacteria to migrate into the lower airways. Sinus and gastric colonization can also lead to VAP. Although the patient may not develop pneumonia for 48 hours, oral care provided early after intubation, even in the ED, may impact the development of pneumonia. Risk factors that can affect the development of pneumonia include the following[62,64]:

- Aspiration
- Depressed protective reflexes (gag reflex)
- Elevated gastric pH levels
- Preexisting pulmonary disease
- Immunosuppression
- Malnutrition

VAP prevention includes the following interventions[64]:

- Elevating the head of the bed to 45 degrees
  - This step limits the risk of aspiration.
  - Early in the trauma process, this may be difficult if the patient's spine has not been cleared or if the patient is hypotensive. Facilitate timely removal or employ a reverse Trendelenburg position as tolerated.
- Chlorhexidine oral care to decontaminate the mouth[62-64]
  - Intubated patients can benefit from early chlorhexidine oral care once ETT placement is verified, even in the ED.[62]

- Subglottic suctioning
  - Oral secretions pool above the ETT cuff, enabling contaminated fluid to leak down into the lower airway.[62]
  - Biofilm forms on the surface of an ETT when bacteria adhere to the tube surface, allowing for aspiration of bacteria into the lungs.
- Endotracheal suctioning
  - Using an inline, closed-system suction device to prevent opening the ETT to contamination is also beneficial.

Begin treatment with a broad-spectrum antibiotic as soon as possible, continuing this therapy until an antibiotic can be prescribed that will match the microorganism. Timely antibiotic administration can make a difference in overall mortality. Early diagnosis and treatment is important because VAP leads to ALI and ARDS and carries a high rate of mortality.[63]

Abdominal Trauma

Hemorrhage is the second most common cause of death following trauma, and is the leading cause of death from preventable injury.[65] Missed abdominal injuries are often the cause of late mortality in patients who survived the early post-injury period.[65] Even a serious abdominal injury may not display obvious assessment findings, especially in blunt trauma.[66] Evaluating the abdomen can be difficult for a variety of reasons. In the patient with a decreased level of consciousness, the clinical examination can be unreliable, and some injuries may be missed. The seat belt sign in the lower abdomen can develop slowly and may be overlooked in light of more pressing injuries. External bruising indicative of retroperitoneal hemorrhage may not appear for hours or days.[67] Awareness of these signs in the patient who seeks care days after the traumatic event or continued, serial assessments can help to identify subtle changes as they develop once the patient is admitted in the hospital. See Chapter 8, "Abdominal and Pelvic Trauma," for more information.

Splenic Injury

Management of patients with a splenic injury has evolved toward nonoperative management, with good success realized with this approach.[68] Initial bleeding from the spleen may or may not be identified on the FAST examination. Patients with assessment findings of splenic injury who are deemed appropriate candidates for nonoperative management are generally admitted for observation, including serial laboratory evaluation of hemoglobin and hematocrit levels to identify ongoing or worsening bleeding and clinical abdominal assessments for change in tenderness, pain, or rigidity.[68]

Hepatic Injury

Delayed hemorrhage, hepatic abscess, and hemobilia are complications associated with hepatic trauma that may develop following initial resuscitation. Additional laboratory studies to detect these conditions include liver enzymes and coagulation studies.

Pancreatic Injury

Because of its position in the abdomen, the pancreas can be compressed against the spine with a direct blow during trauma. Pancreatic injuries are rare but can be associated with significant complications, including fistula development and sepsis.[69] Assessment findings with pancreatic injuries may be similar to those found with retroperitoneal hemorrhage, including abdominal pain, nausea and vomiting, diminished or absent bowel sounds, and periumbilical ecchymosis. Studies useful in diagnosing and monitoring pancreatic injuries include CT scan, FAST, and laboratory studies. Current recommendations for treating pancreatic injuries involve monitoring and nonoperative management for most lower-grade injuries.[69]

Bowel Injuries

Bowel injuries may occur either immediately or over time, with resulting contusions, edema, rupture, or infarction. Continued abdominal assessment is valuable in early recognition of delayed or occult complications of abdominal trauma. It is important for the nurse to reevaluate all patients with abdominal trauma when nonoperative management is chosen and to alert the team promptly when signs of deterioration begin to occur.

Shock

Specific assessments and interventions in the post-resuscitation period are unique to each of the types of shock.

Obstructive Shock

Assessment and intervention considerations for obstructive shock include the following:

- Trending the patient's cardiopulmonary status can identify subtle changes that may indicate slowly accumulating pericardial fluid or pneumothoraces.
- FAST can be useful to identify cardiac tamponade or a pneumothorax.
  - Both may be present initially or develop slowly over time with a delayed presentation.
- Treatment should be directed at relieving the obstruction.

Cardiogenic Shock

Assessment and intervention considerations for cardiogenic shock include the following:

- Patients with blunt chest trauma or MI can experience cardiogenic shock.
- This type of shock may not be evident at the time of trauma resuscitation, but can develop following volume replacement when contractility is inadequate to handle the preload.
- For the patient experiencing an MI, early reperfusion therapy is the goal of treatment.
- Percutaneous coronary intervention in the cardiac catheterization laboratory is the definitive treatment.
- Inotropic support may be useful until bleeding is controlled.[70]

Distributive (Neurogenic) Shock

Assessment and intervention considerations for distributive (neurogenic) shock include the following:

- Onset of neurogenic shock can occur soon after the injury or as late as 1 to 2 days later.[71]
- Neurogenic shock is generally associated with SCIs at T6 and above.[71]
- Treatment of hypovolemia is usually the first step, but medications aimed at reestablishing vascular tone and heart rate, including vasopressors and atropine, are more appropriate for use to restore organ perfusion.[72]

Distributive (Anaphylactic) Shock

Assessment and intervention considerations for distributive (anaphylactic) shock include the following:

- The risk of anaphylactic shock as a result of an allergic reaction to a medication may be higher in the trauma patient if allergy information is unavailable upon arrival. As soon as possible, seek out records or sources of possible allergies.
- Signs of anaphylactic shock include hives or an urticarial rash, respiratory distress and stridor, angioedema, and signs of shock.[73]
- Treatment includes intramuscular epinephrine, bronchodilators or racemic epinephrine, IV crystalloids, histamine blockers, and steroids.

Distributive (Septic) Shock

Assessment and intervention considerations for distributive (septic) shock include the following:

- Septic shock due to infection immediately after a traumatic injury is uncommon; its onset is usually delayed.
- Septic patients can be clinically difficult to distinguish from those in hypovolemic shock since both groups have tachycardia, peripheral vasoconstriction, decreased urinary output, and decreased BP with a narrowed pulse pressure.[11]
- An elevated temperature is often associated with septic patients; however, trauma patients may be febrile due to the inflammatory response to injury.
- Prophylactic antibiotic therapy may be indicated with open or contaminated injuries.

Disseminated Intravascular Coagulopathy

DIC begins when the body's clotting system is overwhelmed, such as in cases of multiple trauma. In the patient with multiple trauma, platelets, plasma, and other vital components of the clotting cascade are lost to hemorrhage and dilution, and clotting factors become depleted through diffuse microvascular clot formation as a result of the inflammatory response to injury.[74] Hypothermia may directly interfere by slowing the activity of coagulation and fibrinogen synthesis.[74] Acidosis as a result of tissue hypoperfusion and hypoxia accelerates fibrinolysis, contributing to the development of DIC.[74]

Box 20-1 describes the laboratory findings in DIC.[74] Treatment is aimed at rectifying the cause, though DIC is best treated by prevention. Administration of platelets and fresh frozen plasma can help control bleeding in the trauma patient and may limit the severity for the trauma patient with DIC.[75] While DIC will not be present upon trauma presentation, the treatments and interventions completed during the initial assessment can have a dramatic effect on its development.

Abdominal Compartment Syndrome

Abdominal compartment syndrome is a potentially lethal complication in trauma that was first identified

BOX 20-1 Laboratory Trends in Disseminated Intravascular Coagulation

- Decreased platelet count
- Decreased fibrinogen
- Elevated fibrin degradation product
- Elevated D-dimer
- Prolonged prothrombin time
- Prolonged partial thromboplastin time

Data from Gando, S., Sawamura, A., & Hayakawaa, M. (2011). Trauma, shock, and disseminated intravascular coagulation: Lessons from the classical literature. *Annals of Surgery, 254*(1), 10–19. https://doi.org/10.1097/SLA.0b013e31821221b1.

approximately 25 years ago.[76] With this condition, massive interstitial edema within the abdomen from aggressive volume resuscitation or hematoma formation causes an abnormal increase in intra-abdominal pressures, causing intra-abdominal hypertension (IAH).[76] IAH causes decreased blood flow to the kidneys and abdominal viscera, impaired ventilation, and reduced cardiac output.[76] When combined, these effects contribute to progressive ischemia and multiple-organ dysfunction, which have a high mortality.[76]

Abdominal pressure is 2 to 7 mm Hg in healthy patients and varies inversely with intrathoracic pressure in normal breathing.[76] IAH is diagnosed with pressure greater than 12 mm Hg, and pressure greater than 20 mm Hg in the context of new organ dysfunction is considered to be abdominal compartment syndrome.[76] The risk for IAH is greater in patients who are morbidly obese, have chronic ascites, or are pregnant. Efforts to reduce the volume of crystalloid given during resuscitation have reduced the incidence of abdominal compartment syndrome.[76]

IAH can affect nearly all major body systems.

Abdominal Effects

Abdominal effects of IAH include the following:

- Intra-abdominal bleeding from the spleen, liver, or mesentery is the most common cause of primary IAH. The distended abdomen acts like a pressure dressing, compressing the organs within its compartment. Secondary IAH can occur with massive blood loss from extra-abdominal sites, followed by resuscitation with large-volume crystalloid solution, leading to fluid shifts and peritoneal edema.[76]
- As blood volume increases, so does intra-abdominal pressure (IAP) compressing abdominal structures and organs. This compression results in diminished perfusion and ischemia, acidosis, leaking capillaries, intestinal swelling, and splanchnic translocation.[76]
- Decreased blood flow leads to poor healing. Hepatic hypoperfusion impairs liver function, glucose metabolism, and lactate clearance.[76]

Cardiovascular Effects

Cardiovascular effects of IAH include the following[76]:

- The cardiovascular system is affected as increased IAP pushes up on the diaphragm and increased intrathoracic pressures compress the heart and major vessels.
    - Measurement of central venous pressure may be falsely elevated due to increased intrathoracic pressure.
    - The patient may appear well hydrated or even fluid overloaded in the presence of volume depletion.
- The increased intrathoracic pressure can cause a decrease in venous return, resulting in a decreased preload and loss of cardiac output.
- Rising intrathoracic pressure increases pulmonary vascular resistance and right ventricular afterload, which in turn increases the workload of the right ventricle and decreases left ventricular preload. Greater myocardial oxygen demand results in increased work of the heart.
- The femoral veins are compressed, causing venous stasis and increasing the risk of DVT.

Respiratory Effects

Respiratory effects of IAH include the following[76]:

- Increased thoracic pressure affects the pulmonary system.
- One of the first signs of abdominal compartment syndrome is pulmonary dysfunction.[76]
    - Decreased lung expansion, limited respiratory excursion, and decreased tidal volume are all a result of increased intrathoracic pressure.
    - The result is hypoxemia and hypercarbia with respiratory acidosis.
- Atelectasis, ALI, or ARDS may develop.[76]

Neurologic Effects

Neurologic effects of IAH occur when increased intrathoracic pressure causes pressure on the jugular veins, which decreases the drainage of cerebrospinal fluid and blood from the head, increasing ICP.[76]

Assessment Findings

Assessment findings for IAH and abdominal compartment syndrome include the following[76]:

- IAP measurement
    - One indirect method of monitoring IAP is measurement of urinary bladder pressure. A partially filled bladder accurately reflects IAP. Methods used to monitor urinary bladder pressure include the following[76]:
        - A transducer technique includes attaching a pressurized transducer and tubing to the urine specimen port of a urinary catheter.
        - A bladder scanner is a noninvasive alternative to confirm adequate urine volume prior to pressure measurement.
            - This limits the risk of contamination with backflow into the bladder.

    - Position the patient supine, with zero level established at the symphysis pubis.
  - In addition to bladder pressure, abdominal girth may be beneficial as a trending device, although increased girth is not necessarily present with IAH.[76]
- Low urinary output and hypotensive shock unresponsive to fluid resuscitation
- Tense, rigid, abdomen (distention may or may not be present)
- Increased peak airway pressures without thoracic injury
- Increased ICP without head injury[76]
- Increased IAP (treatment recommended when IAP exceeds 30 mm Hg and the patient is symptomatic)[76]

Rhabdomyolysis

Rhabdomyolysis is most commonly seen in patients with crush injuries or burns. Damage to tissues results in cellular destruction, which in turn releases myoglobin into the circulation. Myoglobin, an intracellular protein, obstructs renal perfusion and glomerular filtration. Sloughing of the renal tubular epithelium, myoglobin cast formation, and myoglobin in the urine produce the distinctive dark red– or brown-colored urine. AKI results from obstruction and decreases in renal blood flow and glomerular filtration; this condition occurs in 24% of patients with rhabdomyolysis.[77]

Hyperkalemia is a life-threatening complication of rhabdomyolysis.[77–80] It occurs when cell destruction releases intracellular potassium into the extracellular space, causing serum potassium levels to rise dramatically; the result can be ECG changes and cardiac irritability.

Treatment for possible rhabdomyolysis begins with IV hydration. Fluid volume increases renal perfusion, prevents cast formation, and prevents additional ischemic kidney damage.[81] Volume aids in correction of acidosis as a result of hypoperfusion.

- Begin with aggressive fluid management to produce urine output of 100 to 300 mL/hr in adults.[78–80]
- Alkalization of the urine (urine pH > 8.0), through the use of bicarbonate and osmotic diuretics, has been used, although evidence of its benefits has not been clearly established.[77–80]
- Patients who develop renal failure may require hemodialysis, peritoneal dialysis, or renal replacement therapy. See Chapter 10, "Musculoskeletal Trauma," for more information.
- Severe hyperkalemia should be treated with calcium gluconate, insulin, glucose, or nebulized beta-agonist.[81]
  - Substances that shift potassium from extracellular to intracellular spaces are only temporarily effective.[78]
  - Calcium does not affect potassium levels, but protects against the cardiotoxic effects of hyperkalemia.
  - Other interventions may be necessary for definitive treatment[78]:
    - Diuresis
    - Intestinal potassium binders, such as sodium polystyrene sulfonate
    - Dialysis

Systemic Inflammatory Response Syndrome

Systemic inflammatory response syndrome (SIRS) is a generalized response to injury or illness that occurs because of an infection, trauma, or ischemia. If two or more of the following assessment findings are present, the patient meets the criteria for SIRS[82]:

- Fever greater than 38°C (100.4°F) or less than 36°C (96.8°F)
- Heart rate greater than 90 beats/minute
- Respiratory rate greater than 20 breaths/minute or $PaCO_2$ less than 32 mm Hg
- White blood cells greater than 12,000 cells/mcL or less than 4,000 cells/mcL or if there are greater than 10% band forms

The only difference between SIRS and sepsis is that sepsis has an identified source of infection and SIRS does not.[82]

Sepsis

In addition to the normal inflammatory process caused by trauma, patients can be at risk for developing an infection or sepsis. Sepsis is the presence of a systemic response, rather than a localized reaction or isolated infection.[82] Patients with a variety of presenting issues may be at risk for developing infection and sepsis, including the following groups:

- Patients with penetrating injuries, or open, or contaminated wounds
- Those with blunt abdominal trauma, or contamination of the peritoneal cavity by intestinal contents (bowel perforation or splanchnic translocation)
- Those experiencing surface or burn trauma with loss of the skin's protective barrier

Sepsis can produce widespread vascular damage:

- Endotoxin release leads to capillary leakage, shifting of fluid into the interstitial space, and edema.
- Increased viscosity of blood leads to clotting in the microcirculation and the development of coagulopathy.
- Tissue hypoxia can affect every organ and, if untreated or extreme, may cause multiple-organ dysfunction to develop.

Early recognition allows for goal-directed therapy, including timely initiation of antibiotic therapy, and improved patient outcomes.

Increased Intracranial Pressure

Cervical collars and flat, supine positioning may exacerbate ICP in the patient with head injuries.[83] Methods for decreasing ICP include the following:

- Remove the cervical collar once the cervical spine is cleared.
- Elevate the head of bed.
- Maintain the patient's head in a neutral, midline position.
- Treat the patient for pain or anxiety.
- Promote diuresis, if any shock state has been controlled.
- Maintain normocarbia.
- Maintain normothermia.
- Reduce external stimuli by dimming lights, limiting noise, and clustering interventions.

Alcohol Withdrawal

Between 30% and 50% of trauma patients report having ingested some form of intoxicant prior to injury.[84] Studies have shown that one in four to five patients admitted to the hospital has some degree of alcohol abuse or dependence.[85] Nevertheless, it is not always easy to identify which patients are at risk for or experiencing alcohol withdrawal. Symptoms of withdrawal can appear within 6 hours after the last drink or may take days to emerge.[84,86] Since alcohol is a CNS depressant, findings related to withdrawal usually indicate CNS stimulation. The first clinical assessment findings of alcohol withdrawal include the following:

- Autonomic hyperactivity
- Hand tremors
- Nausea or vomiting
- Psychomotor agitation
- Anxiety or restlessness

Additional assessment findings include the following:

- Insomnia
- Transient hallucinations
- Generalized tonic–clonic seizure

The Clinical Institute Withdrawal Assessment for Alcohol (CIWA-Ar) tool is a widely used instrument to assess patients for evidence of alcohol withdrawal.[87] The CIWA-Ar tool assesses for presence of nausea or vomiting, tremors, sweating, anxiety, tactile disturbances, auditory disturbances, visual disturbances, headache, and orientation, with the maximum score being 67. Hospitals generally stratify the CIWA protocols for high-risk and low-risk patients, with the dosing of benzodiazepines to manage the symptoms of acute alcohol withdrawal based on the risk stratification and the CIWA-Ar score. The trauma nurse should be alert to the possibility of the trauma patient developing alcohol withdrawal and be ready to intervene appropriately to reduce the risk for the patient.

Treatment of alcohol withdrawal is individualized. Interventions include fluid and electrolyte replacement, supplemental thiamine, glucose, and multiple vitamins. Benzodiazepines to prevent delirium tremens may be prescribed to blunt the effects of withdrawal on the CNS.

Musculoskeletal Trauma

Despite careful assessment, specific fractures that may remain undiagnosed after the initial assessment include the following[88]:

- Femoral neck fractures
- Facial fractures
- Radial head fractures
- Fractures of the scaphoid
- C7 vertebral fractures
- Nondisplaced fractures of the pelvis
- Fractures of the odontoid process

Consequences related to fractures can occur immediately, early, or late. Bones are highly vascular and prone to bleeding. In addition, sharp bone ends can damage surrounding muscle or blood vessels. A broken rib may result in a pneumothorax or lacerated liver. Early consequences related to fractures include the following:

- Infection
- Pneumonia
- DVT/PE
- Compartment syndrome (see Chapter 10)
- Fat embolism
- Pressure ulcers

Missed and Delayed Injuries

Although emergency and trauma physicians and nurses are trained to perform systematic and thorough assessments of trauma patients, the nature and variety of injury severity may not always allow providers the opportunity to fully assess patients and to identify all injuries at the time of admission. Understanding the mechanism of injury (MOI) is useful for the trauma nurse, since different MOIs produce differing injury patterns with predictable associated underlying injuries and injury progression. See Chapter 2, "Biomechanics, Kinematics, and Mechanisms of Injury," for more information.

Missed Injuries

Evaluating a trauma patient with multiple injuries is a challenge even for the most experienced clinician. Multiple factors may contribute to missed injuries, including equivocal radiologic results, inadequate or incomplete studies, simultaneous presentation of multiple patients, complicated patient presentation, or clinically inexperienced staff.[89] The presence of comorbid conditions can also produce a challenging injury assessment. Diseases such as hypertension and diabetes create pathophysiologic factors that may not be evident early in the course of trauma. Diabetes may alter the sensation of an injury due to neuropathy.

Although different institutions have different definitions for a missed injury, generally a missed injury is considered to be an injury that was not found during the initial assessment phase and is discovered when it begins to cause clinical symptoms, such as pain when a non-ambulatory patient begins to walk for the first time after the injury.[90] It may become clinically significant when the injury contributes to morbidity or mortality and results in a delay in treatment. Patients with missed injuries experience higher ISS and longer hospital and ICU stays.[89]

The use of a tertiary survey has been shown to reduce missed injuries by 35%.[90] This survey consists of a complete examination performed following the primary and secondary surveys and within 24 hours after trauma to identify any injuries missed during the initial assessment.[91] The tertiary survey includes a review of initial radiology studies, any additional indicated studies, standardized reevaluation of laboratory studies, and clinical assessment for the effective detection of hidden injuries.

Delayed Injuries

There is a distinct difference between missed injuries and delayed effects of injury. Missed injuries are present upon arrival to the ED, but are not identified then. Delayed effects of injury may not be present upon arrival, but develop over time as a result of the initial injury and should be considered part of the natural progression of the injury. It is absolutely critical to note new findings and identify deterioration in previous findings.

Monitoring Adjuncts

Monitoring adjuncts include mechanical ventilators, capnography, and measurement of central venous pressure.

Mechanical Ventilators

Mechanical ventilators have advanced in recent years, with a variety of new modes and strategies designed to prevent barotrauma and syndromes such as post-ventilation emphysema being introduced. Closed-loop mechanical ventilation regularly monitors respiratory parameters including the patient's intrinsic rate, tidal volume, pulmonary resistance and compliance, and oxygen saturation.[92,93] Based on this information, the ventilator is able to adjust the settings to provide for added or reduced pressure support or oxygen.[92,93] The use of such optimal settings promotes timely weaning and extubation.[92,93] This technology is used more often in the ICU, but it is useful for the trauma nurse to be aware of fluctuations in ventilator settings so as to evaluate the status of the mechanically ventilated patient.

Capnography

$ETCO_2$ measures the level of exhaled CO_2, which can be a marker of metabolic acidosis, dehydration, or tissue perfusion.[81] Post resuscitation, monitoring the $ETCO_2$ level can be helpful in patients who are receiving sedation and analgesia or mechanical ventilation, as it is a valuable marker of hypoventilation and apnea.[91] Interpretation of capnography includes three components: the numeric value, the waveform, and the gradient.[91,94,95]

- Numeric value
  - The partial pressure of $ETCO_2$ ($PETCO_2$) reveals some information regarding ventilation.
  - Changes in $PETCO_2$ identify ventilatory issues before SpO_2 (**Table 20-2**).[91,94,95]
- Waveform
  - The waveform is divided into three phases of the respiratory cycle. Each phase reveals different information.
    - Phase I: During the beginning of expiration, the waveform reflects exhalation of air in the anatomic dead space where there should be no CO_2.

TABLE 20-2 Conditions Associated with Changes in $PETCO_2$

Causes of Abnormal $PETCO_2$	Increase in $PETCO_2$	Decrease in $PETCO_2$
Metabolic	Malignant hyperthermia	Hypothermia
	Thyroid storm	Metabolic acidosis
	Severe sepsis	
Circulatory	Carbon dioxide rebreathing	Pulmonary embolism
	Treatment of acidosis	Profound hypovolemia/shock
		Cardiogenic shock
Respiratory	Hypoventilation	Hyperventilation
	Chronic obstructive pulmonary disease	Intrapulmonary shunt
	Asthma	Pulmonary edema
Technical	Exhausted carbon dioxide absorber	Disconnection
	Contamination of the monitor	Blockage in tubing

Data from Eipe, N., & Doherty, D. R. (2010). A review of pediatric capnography. *Journal of Clinical Monitoring and Computing, 24*(4), 261–268. https://doi.org/10.1007/s10877-010-9243-3; Kodali, B. S. (2013). Capnography outside the operating rooms. *Anesthesiology, 118*(1), 192–201. https://doi.org/10.1097/ALN.0b013e318278c8b6; Ortega, R., Connor, C., Kim, S., Djang, R., & Patel, K. (2012). Monitoring ventilation with capnography. *New England Journal of Medicine, 367*(19), e27–e34. https://doi.org/10.1056/NEJMvcm1105237.

- Phase II: As CO_2 is exhaled, the waveform rises sharply.
- Phase III: This phase encompasses the majority of the expiratory cycle, where the waveform plateaus. The end of this phase is where the $ETCO_2$ is measured.

- The waveform can reveal a great deal of information to those who know how to interpret it.
  - Loss of waveform indicates a misplaced or occluded ETT or a disconnected circuit.
  - A positive waveform with each compression shows effective cardiopulmonary resuscitation.
  - A change in the shape of the waveform may be an indication of bronchospasm, obstruction, or ventilation/perfusion mismatch.
- $PETCO_2$: $PaCO_2$ gradient
  - A changing gradient can mean hemodynamic instability or decreasing lung compliance.

Central Venous Pressure

Measurements of central venous pressure have been traditionally used to evaluate volume status in patients with hypovolemia. Central venous pressure changes minimally in early shock, however, and is a poor identifier of adequate resuscitation.[96]

Quality Measures and the Trauma Nurse

Data and quality metrics are a way of life for the modern healthcare practitioner. The Trauma Quality Improvement Program (TQIP) reviews the care delivered by trauma centers and has been implemented to "elevate the quality of care for trauma patients" in more than 800 trauma centers across the United States.[97] Care initiated by nurses in the ED—such as timely IV antibiotic administration for open fractures—will positively impact the patient and can demonstrate compliance with benchmarked standards, leading to better outcomes for trauma patients.

Emerging Trends

Modern healthcare is ever changing, as both science and technology evolve at increasingly faster rates. Trauma nurses should be aware of emerging trends related to the care of the injured patient.

Nonoperative Management

Although trauma is considered a surgical disease by the American College of Surgeons, increasingly trauma surgeons are moving toward nonoperative management to manage these patients' injuries. Adult trauma surgeons have begun to follow the lead of pediatric trauma surgeons by employing selective nonoperative management of splenic and hepatic injuries, as well as some pancreas, bowel, and renal injuries.[98] Additionally, options such as interventional radiology, endovascular injury repair, and increased training and use of ultrasound mean that trauma patients may spend less time in the OR in coming years.

Venous Thromboembolism Screening and Prophylaxis

Managing bleeding and blood clotting remains a challenge in the trauma population, and that challenge is only expected to increase as the population ages. Massive transfusion and anticoagulation-reversal guidelines have helped to address the issue of bleeding, and TXA is a useful tool in preventing clot degradation. Even so, trauma patients remain at increased risk of venous thromboembolism (VTE) formation.

The Caprini score for VTE stratifies risk of VTE in surgical patients and is finding favor in trauma programs to help guide VTE prophylaxis. The Caprini score has been validated for both medical and surgical patients (**Table 20-3**).[99-101] The Caprini score is calculated by adding the scores of all factors present in the patient and is interpreted as follows:

- Score of 0–1: Low risk of VTE
- Score of 2: Moderate risk of VTE
- Score of 3–4: High risk of VTE
- Score ≥ 5: Highest risk for VTE

TABLE 20-3 Caprini Scale

5 Points	3 Points	2 Points	1 Point
› Stroke[a] › Fracture of the hip, pelvis, or leg › Elective arthroplasty › Acute SCI[a]	› Age greater than 75 years › Prior episodes of VTE › Family history of VTE › Prothrombin 20210A › Factor V Leiden › Lupus anticoagulants › Anticardiolipin antibodies › Elevated blood levels of homocysteine › History of heparin-induced thrombocytopenia › Other congenital or acquired thrombophilia	› Age 61–74 years › Arthroscopic surgery › Laparoscopy or general surgery lasting more than 45 minutes › Cancer › Plaster cast › Bed rest for more than 72 hours › Central venous access	› Age 41–60 years › BMI > 25 kg/m^2 › Minor surgery › Edema in the lower extremities › Varicose veins › Pregnancy › Postpartum › Oral contraceptives › Hormone therapy › Unexplained or recurrent abortion › Sepsis[a] › Serious lung disease such as pneumonia[a] › Abnormal pulmonary function tests › Acute myocardial infarction › Congestive heart failure[a] › Bed rest › Inflammatory bowel disease

Abbreviation: BMI, body mass index; SCI, spinal cord injury; VTE, venous thromboembolism.

[a] Occurring in the last month.

Data from Caprini, J. A. (2005). Thrombosis risk assessment as a guide to quality patient care. *Disease-a-Month, 51*(2–3), 70–78. https://doi.org/10.1016/j.disamonth.2005.02.003.

Ventilator-Associated Pneumonia/ Ventilator-Associated Events

Nurses caring for patients who require mechanical ventilation are familiar with the care bundles to help prevent VAP—including keeping the head of bed elevated, providing oral care, and performing subglottic suctioning. While great attention has been paid to decreasing VAP in the United States, clearly defining VAP remains a challenge. Currently, even the most widely used VAP criteria and definition lack adequate specificity and sensitivity.[102] To establish more objective surveillance criteria, the Centers for Disease Control and Prevention shifted its use of terminology from VAP to ventilator-associated events (VAEs). VAE surveillance is able to detect a broader range of issues and classifies events in three tiers: ventilator-associated conditions, infection-related ventilator-associated complications, and possible/probable VAP.

Nursing interventions suggested to prevent VAE include continuing the components of the traditional VAP bundle (elevating the head of bed, oral care, subglottic suctioning, and peptic ulcer disease prophylaxis), but also incorporating steps such as low-volume tidal-volume ventilation and using the proposed ABCDEF bundle.[103] The ABCDEF bundle components include the following:

- *A: Assess, prevent, and manage pain.* The Pain, Agitation and Delirium (PAD) guideline released in 2013 recognizes that poor pain control is a risk factor for nosocomial infection and prolonged mechanical ventilation. Additionally, inadequate pain control may precipitate delirium.[104,105]
- *B: Both spontaneous awakening trials and spontaneous breathing trials.* Spontaneous awakening and spontaneous breathing trials have been shown to reduce the duration of mechanical ventilation and VAP.[105]
- *C: Choice of analgesia and sedation.* While sedation is important in facilitating mechanical ventilation, caution should be used to maintain the lightest level of sedation possible for the patient and to avoid benzodiazepines.[106]
- *D: Delirium—assess, prevent, and manage.* Delirium is a frequent consequence of mechanical ventilation, with as many as 81% of ventilated patients experiencing some degree of delirium. It is also associated with prolonged mechanical ventilation, longer length of stay in the ICU, increased morbidity and mortality, and long-term cognitive impairment.[103] Daily monitoring for delirium, promoting uninterrupted sleep at night, early mobilization, and benzodiazepine avoidance are steps that the trauma nurse can take to help prevent delirium in trauma patients.
- *E: Exercise and Early mobility.* The PAD guidelines also recommend early exercise and mobility when possible to help prevent neuromuscular weakness associated with critical illness and mechanical ventilation.[103]
- *F: Family engagement and empowerment.* The patient's family can be useful to help promote patient well-being and the other components of the ABCDEF bundle. Educating family members about the need to keep the head of bed elevated, behavioral manifestations of pain, and even ways to provide oral care can help both the patient and the family recover from critical illness.

A final trend in trauma care is the move toward caring more holistically for the patient and family. Just as the screening, brief intervention, and referral to treatment tool is being used to evaluate patient alcohol use, so the American College of Surgeons is moving toward more comprehensive screening and intervention for post-traumatic stress disorder in trauma patients. Additionally, trauma survivor networks are working with trauma patients, families, and communities to help patients thrive after traumatic injury. Watch for these trends to expand as their benefits to trauma patients become more widely recognized.

Summary

Trauma care does not end with the initial assessment. Ongoing monitoring and observation are vital aspects to care of the trauma patient after resuscitation and stabilization. Many complications may develop early in the post-resuscitative period and the prepared trauma nurse will anticipate them, intervening proactively. Even if the initial assessment is inconclusive, a high index of suspicion will help the trauma nurse identify subtle changes based on predicted injuries and MOI. Assessment and reassessment are important for identified injuries and for potential and worsening injuries. The conditions described in this chapter and their consequences may or may not manifest while the trauma patient remains in the ED, ICU, or surgical care floor, but knowledge of potential outcomes can be a valuable factor in the critical thinking and decision making of the trauma nurse. Review of admission orders and knowledge of care pathways will promote early treatment and limit the risk of negative consequences, making the transition to definitive care smooth and efficient.

References

1. Emergency Nurses Association. (2017). *Topic brief: System-wide strategies to reduce emergency department boarding*. Des Plaines, IL: Author. Retrieved from https://www.ena.org/docs/default-source/resource-library/practice-resources/topic-briefs/system-wide-strategies-to-reduce-emergency-department-boarding.pdf?sfvrsn=1eb2b7c5_2
2. Wu, D., Zhou, X., Ye, L., Gen, J., & Zhang, M. (2015). Emergency department crowding and the performance of damage control resuscitation in major trauma patients with hemorrhagic shock. *Academic Emergency Medicine, 22*(8), 915–921. https://doi.org/10.1111/acem.12726
3. Richards, J. R., van der Linden, M. C., & Derlet, R. W. (2014). Providing care in emergency department hallways: Demands, dangers and deaths. *Advances in Emergency Medicine*, Article 495219. https://doi.org/10.1155/2014/495219
4. Salaway, R. J., Valenzuela, R., Shoenberger, J. M., Mallon, W. K., & Viccellio, A. (2017). Emergency department (ED) overcrowding: Evidence-based answers to frequently asked questions. *Revista Medica Clicia Las Condes, 28*(2), 213–219. https://doi.org/10.1016/j.rmclc.2017.04.008
5. DiMaggion, C. J., Avraham, J. B., Lee, D. C., Frangos, S. G., & Wall, S. P. (2017). The epidemiology of emergency department trauma discharges in the United States. *Academic Emergency Medicine, 24*(10), 1244–1256. https://doi.org/10.1111/acem.13223
6. Fuentes, E., Shields, J. F., Chirumamilla, N., Martinez, M., Kaafarani, H., Ye, D. D., . . . Lee, J. (2016). "One-way-street" streamlined admission of critically ill trauma patients reduces emergency department length of stay. *Journal of Internal and Emergency Medicine, 12*, 1019–1024. https://doi.org/10.1007/s11739-016-1511-x
7. Harmohammadian, M. H., Rezaei, F., Haghshenas, A., & Tavakoli, N. (2017). Overcrowding in emergency departments: A review of strategies to decrease future challenges. *Journal of Research in Medical Sciences, 22*, 23. https://doi.org/10.4103%2F1735-1995.200277
8. Buduhan, G., & McRitchie, D. I. (2000). Missed injuries in patients with multiple trauma. *Journal of Trauma, 49*, 600–605.
9. Montmany, S., Navarro, S., Rebassa, P., Hermoso, J., Hidalgo, M., & Canovas, G. (2007). A prospective study on the incidence of missed injuries in trauma patients. *Cirugía Española, 84*, 32–36.
10. Knight, P. H., Maheshwari, N., Hussain, J., Scholl, M., Hughes, M., Papadimos, T. J., . . . Latchana, N. (2015). Complications during intrahospital transport of critically ill patients: Focus on risk identification and prevention. *International Journal of Critical Illness and Injury Science, 5*(4), 256–264. https://doi.org/10.4103/2229-5151.170840
11. American College of Surgeons. (2018). Shock. In *Advanced trauma life support: Student course manual* (10th ed., pp. 42-61). Chicago, IL: Author.
12. Han, J., Renn, H.-Q., Zhao, Q.-B., Woo, Y.-I., & Qiao, Z.-Y. (2015). Comparison of 3% and 7.5% hypertonic saline in resuscitation after traumatic hypovolemic shock. *Shock—Injury, Inflammation and Sepsis: Laboratory and Clinical Approaches, 43*(3), 244–249. https://doi.org/10.1097/SHK.0000000000000303
13. Frithiof, R., Ramchandra, R., Hood, S. G., & May, C. N. (2011). Hypertonic sodium resuscitation after hemorrhage improves hemodynamic function by stimulating cardiac, but not renal sympathetic nerve activity. *American Journal of Physiology—Heart and Circulatory Physiology, 300*(2), H685–H692. https://doi.org/10.1152/ajpheart.00930.2010
14. Geeraets, T., Velly, L., Abdennour, L., Asehnoune, K., Audibert, G., Bouzat, P., . . . Payen, J.-P. (2017). Management of severe traumatic brain injury (first 24 hours). *Anesthesia, Critical Care and Pain Medicine, 37*(2), 171–186. https://doi.org/10.1016/j.accpm.2017.12.001
15. Carnevale, J. A., Segar, D. J., Powers, A. Y., Shah, M., Doverstein, C., Drapcho, B., . . . Assad, W. F. (2018, January 5). Blossoming contusions: Identifying factors contributing to the expansion of traumatic intracerebral hemorrhage. *Journal of Neurosurgery*, 1–12. [Epub ahead of print]. https://doi.org/10.3171/2017.7.JNS17988
16. American College of Surgeons Trauma Quality Improvement Program. (2015). *ACS TQIP best practices in the management of traumatic brain injury*. Chicago, IL: Author.
17. Brain Trauma Foundation. (2016). *Guidelines for the management of severe traumatic brain injury* (4th ed.). New York, NY: Author.
18. Winkelmann, M., Soechtig, W., Macke, C., Schroeter, C., Clausen, J. D., Zeckey, C., . . . Mommsen, P. (2018). Accidental hypothermia as an independent risk factor with poor neurological outcome in older multiply injured patients with severe traumatic brain injury: A matched pair analysis. *European Journal of Trauma and Emergency Surgery*, 1–7 https://doi.org/10.1007/s00068-017-0897-0
19. Andrews, H., Rittenhouse, K., Gross, B., & Rogers, F. B., (2017). The effect of time to international normalized ratio reversal on intracranial hemorrhage evolution in patients with traumatic brain injury. *Journal of Trauma Nursing, 24*(6), 381–384. https://doi.org/10.1097/JTN.0000000000000330
20. Marsh, J. D., & Banasik, J. L. (2013). Acute disorders of brain function. In L. E. Copstead & J. L. Banasik (Eds.), *Pathophysiology* (5th ed., pp. 898–921). St. Louis, MO: Elsevier Saunders.
21. Bauman, M., & Russo-McCourt, T. (2016). Caring for patients with spinal cord injuries. *American Nurse Today, 11*(5), 18–22. Retrieved from https://www.americannursetoday.com/caring-patients-spinal-cord-injuries/
22. Stein, D. M., & Sheth, K. N. (2015). Management of acute spinal cord injury. *Continuum, 21*(1), 159–187. https://doi.org/10.1212/01.CON.0000461091.09736.0c
23. Qadan, M., Gardner, S. A., Vitale, D. S., Lominadze, D., Joshua, I. G., & Polk, H. (2009). Hypothermia and surgery: Immunologic mechanisms for current practice. *Annals of Surgery, 250*(1), 134–140. https://doi.org/10.1097/SLA.0b013e3181ad85f7
24. Balvers, K., Van der Horts, M., Grauman, M., Boer, C., Binnerkade, J. M., Goslings, J. C., & Juffermans, J. P. (2016). Hypothermia as a predictor for mortality in trauma patients at

admittance to the intensive care unit. *Journal of Emergencies, Trauma and Shock, 9*(3), 97–102. https://doi.org/10.4103%2F0974-2700.185276

25. Martini, W. Z. (2009). Coagulopathy by hypothermia and acidosis: Mechanisms of thrombin generation and fibrinogen availability. *Journal of Trauma, 67*(1), 202–208. https://doi.org/10.1097/TA.0b013e3181a602a7
26. Andrews, P., Sinclair, H. L., Rodriguez, A., Harris, B. A., Battison, C. G., Rhode, J. K. J., & Muarrya, G. D. (2015). Hypothermia for intracranial hypertension after traumatic brain injury. *New England Journal of Medicine, 373*, 2403–2412. https://doi.org/10.1056/NEJMoa1507581
27. McIlvoy, L. (2012). Fever management in patients with brain injury. *AACN Advanced Critical Care, 23*(2), 204–211. https://doi.org/10.1097/NCI.0b013e31824db1c6
28. Mizushima, Y., Ueno, M., Idoguchi, K., Ishikawa, K., & Matsuoka, T. (2009). Fever in trauma patients: Friend or foe? *Journal of Trauma, 67*(5), 1062–1065. https://doi.org/10.1097/TA.0b013e3181b848fc
29. Zawadska, M., Szmuda, M., & Mazurkiewicz-Beldzinska, M. (2017). Thermoregulation disorders of central origin: How to diagnose and treat. *Anesthesiology Intensive Therapy, 49*(3), 227–234. https://doi.org/10.5603/AIT.2017.0042
30. Hinson, H., Rowell, S., Morris, C., Lin, A. L., & Schreiber, M. A. (2018). Early fever after trauma: Does it matter? *Journal of Trauma and Acute Care Surgery, 84*(1), 19–24. https://doi.org/10.1097/TA.0000000000001627
31. Katrancha, E. D., & Gonzalez, L. S., III. (2014). Trauma-induced coagulopathy. *Critical Care Nurse, 34*(4), 54–63. https://doi.org/10.4037/ccn2014133
32. Keane, M. (2016). Triad of death: The importance of temperature monitoring in trauma patients. *Emergency Nurse, 24*(5), 19–23. https://doi.org/10.7748/en.2016.e1569
33. Felver, L. (2013). Acid–base homeostasis and imbalances. In L. E. Copstead & J. L. Banasik (Eds.), *Pathophysiology* (5th ed., pp. 539–548). St. Louis, MO: Elsevier Saunders.
34. Mitchel, C. (2016). Tissue oxygen monitoring as a guide for trauma resuscitation. *Critical Care Nurse, 36*(3), 12–70. https://doi.org/10.4037/ccn2016206
35. Napolitano, L., Cohen, M., Cotton, B., Schreiber, M. A., & Moore, E. E. (2013). Tranexamic acid in trauma: How should we use it? *Journal of Trauma and Acute Care Surgery, 74*(6), 1575–1586. https://doi.org/10.1097/TA.0b013e318292cc54
36. Nunn, M., Fischer, P., Sing, R., Templin, M., Avery, M., & Britton, A. (2017). Improvement of treatment outcomes after implementation of a massive transfusion protocol: A Level I trauma center experience. *American Surgeon, 83*(4), 394–398.
37. De Moya, M., Nirula, R., & Biffl, W. (2017). Rib fixation: Who, what, when? *Trauma Surgery and Acute Care Open, 2*(1), 1–4. https://doi.org/10.1136/tsaco-2016-000059
38. Jensen, C. D., Stark, J. T., Jacobson, L. L, Powers, J. M., Joseph, M. F., Kinsella-Shaw, J. M., & Denegar, C. R. (2017). Improved outcomes associated with the liberal use of thoracic epidural analgesia in patients with rib fractures. *Pain Medicine, 18*(9), 1787–1794. https://doi.org/10.1093/pm/pnw199
39. Unsworth, A., Curtis, K., & Asha, S. E. (2015). Treatments for blunt chest trauma and their impact on patient outcomes and health service delivery. *Scandinavian Journal of Trauma, Resuscitation and Emergency Medicine, 23*, 17. https://doi.org/10.1186%2Fs13049-015-0091-5
40. Battle, C. E., & Evans, P. A. (2015). Predictors of mortality in patients with flail chest: A systematic review. *Journal of Emergency Medicine, 32*(12), 961–965. https://doi.org/10.1136/emermed-2015-204939
41. Kasotakis, G., Hasenboehler, E. A., Streib, E. W., Patel, N., Patel, M., Alcaron, L., . . . Como, J. J. (2017). Operative fixation of rib fractures after blunt trauma: A practice management guideline from the Eastern Association for the Surgery of Trauma. *Journal of Trauma and Acute Care Surgery, 82*(3), 618–628. https://doi.org/10.1097/TA.0000000000001350
42. Stewart, D. (2014). Blunt chest trauma. *Journal of Trauma Nursing, 21*(6), 282–284. https://doi.org/10.1097/JTN.0000000000000079
43. American College of Surgeons. (2018). Thoracic trauma. In *Advanced trauma life support: Student course manual* (10th ed., pp. 62–81). Chicago, IL: Author.
44. Mullins, J., & Harrahill, M. (2010). Blunt cardiac trauma. *Journal of Emergency Nursing, 36*(6), 597–598. https://doi.org/10.1016/j.jen.2010.07.019
45. Stein, D. M., York, G. B., Boswell, S., Shanmuganathan, K., Hanna, J. M., & Scalea, T. M. (2007). Accuracy of computed tomography (CT) scan in the detection of penetrating diaphragm injury. *Journal of Trauma, 63*(3), 538–543. https://doi.org/10.1097/TA.0b013e318068b53c
46. Lopez, P. P., Arango, J., Gallup, T. M., Cohn, S. M., Myers, J., Corneille, M., & Dent, D. L. (2010). Diaphragmatic injuries: What has changed over a 20-year period? *American Surgeon, 76*(5), 512–516.
47. Fair, K. A., Gordon, N. T., Barbosa, R. R., Rowell, S. E., Walters, J. M., & Schreiber, M. A. (2015). Traumatic diaphragmatic injury in the American College of Surgeons National Trauma Data Bank: A new examination of a rare diagnosis. *American Journal of Surgery, 209*(5), 864–869. https://doi.org/10.1016/j.amjsurg.2014.12.023
48. Paydar, S., Sabetien, G., Khalill, H., Fallahi, J., Tahami, M., Ziaian, B., . . . Ghahramani, Z. (2016). Management of deep vein thrombosis (DVT) prophylaxis in trauma patients. *Bulletin of Emergency and Trauma, 4*(1), 1–7.
49. Mackman, N. (2012). New insights into the mechanisms of venous thrombosis. *Journal of Clinical Investigation, 122*(7), 2331–2336. https://doi.org/10.1172/JCI60229
50. Gay, S. E. (2010). An inside view of venous thromboembolism. *Nurse Practitioner, 35*(9), 32–39. https://doi.org/10.1097/01.NPR.0000387141.02789.c5
51. Menaker, J., Stein, D. M., & Scalea, T. M. (2007). Incidence of early pulmonary embolism after injury. *Journal of Trauma, 63*, 620–624. https://doi.org/10.1097/TA.0b013e31812f60aa
52. Headley, C. M., & Melander, S. (2011). When it may be a pulmonary embolism. *Nephrology Nursing Journal, 38*(2), 127–137, 152.

53. Whelan, D. B., Byrick, R. J., Mazer, C. D., Kay, C., Richards, R. R., Zdero, R., & Schemitsch, E. (2010). Posttraumatic lung injury after pulmonary contusion and fat embolism: Factors determining abnormal gas exchange. *Journal of Trauma, 69*(3), 512–518. https://doi.org/10.1097/TA.0b013e3181ec484f
54. Blankstein, M., Byrick, R. J., Richards, R. R., Mullen, J. B., Zdero, R., & Schemitsch, E. H. (2010). Pathophysiology of fat embolism: A rabbit model. *Journal of Orthopaedic Trauma, 25*(11), 674–680. https://doi.org/10.1097/BOT.0b013e318206ed30
55. Sara, S., Kenyhertz, G., Herbert, T., & Lundeen, G. A. (2011). Fat emboli syndrome in a nondisplaced tibia fracture. *Journal of Orthopaedic Trauma, 25*(3), e27–e29. https://doi.org/10.1097/BOT.0b013e31820bbafb
56. Tzioupis, C. C., & Giannoudis, P. V. (2011). Fat embolism syndromes: What have we learned over the years? *Trauma, 13*(4), 259–281. https://doi.org/10.1177%2F1460408610396026
57. Carlson, D. S., & Pfadt, E. (2011). Fat embolism syndrome. *Nursing, 41*(4), 72. https://doi.org/10.1097/01.NURSE.0000395312.91409.7f
58. Benson, A. B., & Moss, M. (2009). Trauma and acute respiratory distress syndrome: Weighing the risks and benefits of blood transfusions. *Anesthesiology, 110*(2), 216–217. https://doi.org/10.1097%2FALN.0b013e3181948ac0
59. Maxwell, R. A., Green, J. M., Waldrop, J., Dart, B. W., Smith, P. W., Brooks, D., . . . Barker, D. E. (2010). A randomized prospective trial of airway pressure release ventilation and low tidal volume ventilation in adult trauma patients with acute respiratory failure. *Journal of Trauma, 69*(3), 501–511. https://doi.org/10.1097/TA.0b013e3181e75961
60. Dechert, R. E., Haas, C. F., & Ostwani, W. (2012). Current knowledge of acute lung injury and acute respiratory distress syndrome. *Critical Care Nursing Clinics of North America, 24*(3), 377–401. https://doi.org/10.1016/j.ccell.2012.06.006
61. Stacy, K. M. (2011). Pulmonary disorders. In L. D. Urden, K. M. Stacy, & M. E. Lough (Eds.), *Priorities in critical care nursing* (6th ed., pp. 283–311). St. Louis, MO: Mosby.
62. Grap, M. J., Munro, C. L., Hamilton, V. A., Elswick, R. K., Jr., Sessler, C. N., & Ward, K. R. (2011). Early, single chlorhexidine application reduces ventilator-assisted pneumonia in trauma patients. *Heart & Lung, 40*(5), e115–e122. https://doi.org/10.1016/j.hrtlng.2011.01.006
63. Tseng, C. C., Liu, S. F., Wang, C. C., Tu, M. L., Chung, Y. H., Lin, M. C., & Fang, W. F. (2012). Impact of clinical severity index, infective pathogens, and initial empiric antibiotic use on hospital mortality in patients with ventilator-assisted pneumonia. *American Journal of Infection Control, 40*(7), 648–652. https://doi.org/10.1016/j.ajic.2011.08.017
64. O'Grady, N. P., Murray, P. R., & Ames, N. (2012). Preventing ventilator-associated pneumonia: Does the evidence support the practice? *Journal of the American Medical Association, 307*(23), 2534–2539. https://doi.org/10.1001/jama.2012.6445
65. Jansen, J., Yule, S., & Loudon, M. (2008). Investigation of blunt abdominal trauma. *British Medical Journal, 336,* 938–942. https://doi.org/10.1136/bmj.39534.686192.80
66. Blank-Reid, C. (2007). Abdominal trauma: Dealing with the damage. *Nursing 2018, 37*(4 supp), 4–11. Retrieved from https://www.nursingcenter.com/journalarticle?Article_ID=712384&Journal_ID=54016&Issue_ID=712383
67. Schroeppel, T., & Croce, M. A. (2007). Diagnosis and management of blunt abdominal solid organ injury. *Current Opinion in Critical Care, 13*(4), 399–404. https://doi.org/10.1097/MCC.0b013e32825a6a32
68. Wisner, D. H. (2013). Injury to the spleen. In K. L. Mattox, E. E. Moore, & D. V. Feliciano (Eds.), *Trauma* (7th ed., pp. 561–580). New York, NY: McGraw-Hill.
69. Ho, V. P., Patel, N. J., Bokhari, F., Madbak, F. G., Hambley, J. E., Yon, J. R., . . . Como, J. J. (2017). Management of adult pancreatic injuries: A practice management guideline from the Eastern Association for the Surgery of Trauma. *Journal of Trauma and Acute Care Surgery, 82*(1), 185–199. https://doi.org/10.1097/TA.0000000000001300
70. Reynolds, H. R., & Hochman, J. S. (2008). Cardiogenic shock: Current concepts and improving outcomes. *Circulation, 117,* 686–697. https://doi.org/10.1161/CIRCULATIONAHA.106.613596
71. Mallek, J. T., Inaba, K., Branco, B. C., Ives, C., Lam, L., Talving, P., & Demetriades, D. (2012). The incidence of neurogenic shock after spinal cord injury in patients admitted to a high-volume Level I trauma center. *American Surgeon, 78*(5), 623–626.
72. Calder, S. (2012). Shock. In B. B. Hammond & P. G. Zimmerman (Eds.), *Sheehy's manual of emergency care* (7th ed., pp. 213–221). St. Louis, MO: Mosby Elsevier.
73. Campbell, R. L., & Kelso, J. M. (2018, January 5). Anaphylaxis: Acute diagnosis. *UpToDate*. Retrieved from https://www.uptodate.com/contents/anaphylaxis-acute-diagnosis
74. Gando, S., Sawamura, A., & Hayakawaa, M. (2011). Trauma, shock, and disseminated intravascular coagulation: Lessons from the classical literature. *Annals of Surgery, 254*(1), 10–19. https://doi.org/10.1097/SLA.0b013e31821221b1
75. Wada, H., Matsumato, T., & Yamashita, Y. (2014). Diagnosis and treatment of disseminated intravascular coagulation (DIC) according to four DIC guidelines. *Journal of Intensive Care, 2,* 15. https://doi.org/10.1186/2052-0492-2-15
76. Sugrue, M. (2017). Abdominal compartment syndrome and the open abdomen: Any unresolved issues? *Current Opinion in Critical Care, 23*(1), 73–78. https://doi.org/10.1097/MCC.0000000000000371
77. Elsayed, E. F., & Reilly, R. F. (2010). Rhabdomyolysis: A review, with emphasis on the pediatric population. *Pediatric Nephrology, 25*(1), 7–18. https://doi.org/10.1007/s00467-009-1223-9
78. Bosch, X., Poch, E., & Grau, J. M. (2009). Rhabdomyolysis and acute kidney injury. *New England Journal of Medicine, 361,* 62–72. https://doi.org/10.1056/NEJMra0801327
79. de Wolff, J. F. (2012). Rhabdomyolysis. *British Journal of Hospital Medicine, 73*(Suppl. 2), C30–C32. https://doi.org/10.12968/hmed.2012.73.Sup2.C30
80. Cervellin, G., Comelli, I., & Lippi, G. (2010). Rhabdomyolysis: Historical background, clinical, diagnostic, and therapeutic features. *Clinical Chemistry and Laboratory Medicine, 48*(6), 749–756. https://doi.org/10.1515/CCLM.2010.151
81. Luck, R. P., & Verbin, S. (2008). Rhabdomyolysis: A review of clinical presentation, etiology, diagnosis, and management.

Pediatric Emergency Care, 24(4), 262–268. https://doi.org/10.1097/PEC.0b013e31816bc7b7

82. Kaplan, L. J. (2018, May 7). Systemic inflammatory response syndrome. *Medscape.* Retrieved from http://emedicine.medscape.com/article/168943-overview
83. Schouten, R., Albert, T., & Kwon, B. (2012). The spine-injured patient: Initial assessment and emergency treatment. *Journal of the American Academy of Orthopaedic Surgeons, 20*(6), 336–346. https://doi.org/10.5435/JAAOS-20-06-336
84. Eastes, L. E. (2010). Alcohol withdrawal syndrome in trauma patients: A review. *Journal of Emergency Nursing, 36*(5), 507–509. https://doi.org/10.1016/j.jen.2010.05.011
85. Elliott, D. Y., Geyer, C., Lionetti, T., & Doty, L. (2012). Managing alcohol withdrawal in hospitalized patients. *Nursing 2018, 42*(4), 22–30. https://doi.org/10.1097/01.NURSE.0000412922.97512.07
86. Desy, P., Howard, P. K., Perhats, C., & Li, S. (2010). Alcohol screening, brief intervention, and referral to treatment conducted by emergency nurses: An impact evaluation. *Journal of Emergency Nursing, 36*(6), 538–545. https://doi.org/10.1016/j.jen.2009.09.011
87. Sullivan, J. T., Sykora, K., Schneiderman, J., Naranjo, C. A., & Sellers, E. M. (1989). Assessment of alcohol withdrawal: The revised Clinical Institute Withdrawal Assessment for Alcohol scale (CIWA-Ar). *British Journal of Addiction, 84,* 1353–1357. https://doi.org/10.1111/j.1360-0443.1989.tb00737.x
88. Whiteing, N. L. (2008). Fractures: Pathophysiology, treatment and nursing care. *Nursing Standard, 23*(2), 49–57. https://doi.org/10.7748/ns2008.09.23.2.49.c6671
89. Zamboni, C., Yonamine, A. M., Faria, M. A., Christian, R. W., & Mercadante, M. T. (2014). Tertiary survey in trauma patients: Avoiding neglected injuries. *Injury, 45*(Suppl. 5), S14–S17. https://doi.org/10.1016/S0020-1383(14)70014-2
90. Podolnick, J. D., Donovan, D. S., & Alanda, A. W., Jr., (2017). Incidence of delayed diagnosis of orthopedic injury in pediatric trauma patients. *Journal of Orthopedic Trauma, 31*(9), e281–e287. https://doi.org/10.1097/BOT.0000000000000878
91. Eipe, N., & Doherty, D. R. (2010). A review of pediatric capnography. *Journal of Clinical Monitoring and Computing, 24*(4), 261–268. https://doi.org/10.1007/s10877-010-9243-3
92. Lellouche, F., Bojmehrani, A., & Burns, K. (2012). Mechanical ventilation with advanced closed-loop systems. *European Respiratory Monograph, 55,* 217–218. https://doi.org/10.1183/1025448x.10002911
93. Chatburn, R. L., & Mireles-Cabodevila, E. (2011). Closed-loop control of mechanical ventilation: Description and classification of targeting schemes. *Respiratory Care, 56*(1), 85–102. https://doi.org/10.4187/respcare.00967
94. Kodali, B. S. (2013). Capnography outside the operating rooms. *Anesthesiology, 118*(1), 192–201. https://doi.org/10.1097/ALN.0b013e318278c8b6
95. Ortega, R., Connor, C., Kim, S., Djang, R., & Patel, K. (2012). Monitoring ventilation with capnography. *New England Journal of Medicine, 367*(19), e27–e34. https://doi.org/10.1056/NEJMvcm1105237
96. Marik, P. (2007). Noninvasive hemodynamic monitoring in the intensive care unit. *Critical Care Clinics, 23*(3), 383–400. https://doi.org/10.1016/j.ccc.2007.05.002
97. American College of Surgeons. (2018). Trauma Quality Improvement Program. Retrieved from https://www.facs.org/quality-programs/trauma/tqp/center-programs/tqip
98. Stawicki, S. P. (2017). Trends in nonoperative management of traumatic injuries: A synopsis. *International Journal of Critical Illness & Injury, 7*(1), 38–57. https://doi.org/10.4103/IJCIIS.IJCIIS_7_17
99. Grant, P. J., Greene, M. T., Chopra, V., Bernstein, S. J., Hofer, T. P., & Flanders, S. A. (2016). Assessing the Caprini score for risk assessment of venous thromboembolism in hospitalized medical patients. *American Journal of Medicine, 129*(5), 528–535. https://doi.org/10.1016/j.amjmed.2015.10.027
100. Pannucci, C. J., Bailey, S. H., Dreszer, G., Fisher, C., Zumsteg, J. W., Jaber, R. M., . . . Wilkins, E. G. (2011). Validation of the Caprini Risk Assessment Model in plastic and reconstructive surgery patients. *Journal of the American College of Surgeons, 212*(1), 105–112. https://doi.org/10.1016/j.jamcollsurg.2010.08.018
101. Caprini, J. A. (2005). Thrombosis risk assessment as a guide to quality patient care. *Disease-a-Month, 51*(2–3), 70–78. https://doi.org/10.1016/j.disamonth.2005.02.003
102. Centers for Disease Control and Prevention. (2018). Ventilator-associated event (VAE). Retrieved from https://www.cdc.gov/nhsn/PDFs/pscManual/10-VAE_FINAL.pdf
103. Health Research and Educational Trust. (2018). *Preventing ventilator-associated events change package: 2018 update.* Chicago, IL: Author. Retrieved from http://www.hret-hiin.org/Resources/vae/18/preventing-ventilator-associated-events-change-package.pdf
104. Puntillo, K., Pasero, C., Li, D., Mularski, R. A., Grap, M. J., Erstad, B. L., . . . Sessler, C. N. (2009). Evaluation of pain in ICU patients. *Chest Journal, 135*(4), 1069–1074. https://doi.org/10.1378/chest.08-2369
105. Dale, C. R., Kannas, D. A., Fan, V. S., Daniel, S. L., Deem, S., Yanez, N. D., III, . . . Treggian, M. M. (2014). Improved analgesia, sedation, and delirium protocol associated with decreased duration of delirium and mechanical ventilation. *Annals of the American Thoracic Society, 11*(3), 367–374. https://doi.org/10.1513/AnnalsATS.201306-210OC
106. Frimppong, K., Stollings, J. L., Carolo, M. E., & Ely, E. W. (2015). ICU delirium viewed through the lens of the PAD guidelines and the ABCDEF implementation bundle. In M. Balas, T. Clemmer, & K. Hargett (Eds.), *ICU Liberation* (pp. 79–88). Mount Prospect, IL: Society of Critical Care Medicine.

© Antishock/iStock/Getty Images Plus

CHAPTER 21

Global Trauma Considerations

Tiffiny Strever, BSN, RN, CEN, TCRN, FAEN, Liz Cloughessy, AM, MHM, RN, FAEN, MACN, Darcie Goodman, BSN, MPA, Tracey Taulu, BScN, RN, MHS, Heather Wong, BSN, MHS, RN, Peggy Wun Man Lee, RN, Joop Breuer, RN, CEN, CCRN, FAEN, Theo Lighthelm, MPA, B Soc Sc (Hons), RN, René C. Grobler, RN, FANSA, Agneta Brandt, MSN, RN, CRNA, Gabrielle Lomas, BSc (Hons), RN, and Jill Windle, MSc, BA, RN, FRCN

OBJECTIVES

Upon completion of this chapter, the learner will be able to:

1. Define trauma.
2. Review multinational epidemiologic characteristics associated with trauma.
3. Describe injury prevention program outcome strategies to decrease injuries.

Introduction

Trauma is defined as an injury to living tissue caused by an extrinsic agent.[1] Regardless of the mechanism of injury (MOI), trauma creates stressors that exceed the tissue's or organ's capability to compensate. Epidemiology is the field that studies those factors that determine and influence the frequency and distribution of injury, disease, and other health-related events and their causes in a defined human population.[2] These data are then used to establish prevention programs to control the incidence and prevalence of injury and disease factors.

Traumatic events are, in some capacity, preventable. Even after a traumatic event occurs, the injuries themselves may be avoided or the degree of injury lessened with safety measures. A traumatic incident may be classified as intentional (assault or suicide) or unintentional (falls or collisions).

Trauma is also universal. Epidemiologic statistics from the selected group of countries reported on in this chapter bear that statement out.

United States

Unintentional injury remains the fifth leading cause of death across people of all ages in the United States and the leading cause of death for people age 1 to 44 years.[3] In 2016, 65% of injury-related deaths were from poisoning, motor vehicle collisions (MVCs), and falls. When death attributed to firearms (suicide or homicide) are added to that total, the percentage of deaths attributable to injury rises to 82%.[4] Additionally, traumatic brain injuries

(TBIs) factor into 30% of all injury-related deaths annually in the United States.[5] This equates to more than 150 persons dying from this cause every day.

The majority of injuries do not result in death, though they do impact the community and the healthcare system in its entirety. This impact starts in the prehospital setting and runs through hospitalization to rehabilitation and beyond. In 2015, 28.4% of all emergency department (ED) visits were injury related.[6] In all age categories, from birth to age 65 and older, with the notable exception of ages 15 to 24, falls are the leading cause for nonfatal injuries that require ED visits.[7]

Human Characteristics

Epidemiology is based on the study of factors that influence a particular disease state—in this case, the injuries that affect trauma. When looking at traumatic injuries, certain human characteristics link populations to particular mechanisms of injury, including age, gender, and substance use. This information is important in developing injury prevention programs. Community programs can target those at greatest risk or the most influential factor.

Age

Different MOIs are more common in different age groups. For example, falls are the leading cause of injury-related death for individuals older than 65 years.[4] For people age 5 to 24 years, MVCs are the leading causes of death, whereas poisoning is the leading cause of death for people age 25 to 64 years.[4]

Aging significantly impacts injuries and their effects in older patients. Decreases in vision, hearing, and mobility as well as cognitive changes are age-related factors affecting the older adult. Comorbidities, along with these age-related factors, place this population at a higher risk for morbidity and mortality from trauma. Older adults are more likely to experience complications from and die as a result of their injuries than are younger patients. Adults who are 75 years or older experience the highest rates of hospitalization and death related to TBIs.[5] Older adults are also cited as an at-risk group for fire-related injuries, especially death in home fires.[8] See Chapter 13, "Special Populations: The Geriatric Trauma Patient," for more information.

Gender

Injury and death rates differ between genders, in part due to factors such as cultural norms, occupation, risk-taking activities, and MOIs. Fall data reveal that older men are more likely to die from a fall, whereas older women are twice as likely to sustain a fracture. When looking specifically at hip fractures, women experience three-fourths of all hip fractures.[9] Among those who died from unintentional poisoning in 2016, men had higher death rates than women.[10] Men account for almost 80% of new spinal cord injuries.[11] The death rate involving pedestrians is more than double for men compared to the rate for women.[12] In contrast, women have higher rates of injury and death from interpersonal violence.

Substance Abuse

Substance abuse in the United States includes abuse of alcohol, tobacco, and other substances.

Alcohol

Alcohol affects trauma in two ways: It contributes to the event, and it affects the evaluation of the injured patient. In 2013, nearly one-third of all traffic-related deaths in the United States involved alcohol.[13] The financial impact from alcohol abuse was $44 billion in 2013.[14] Alcohol was involved in 48% of all U.S. traffic crashes that resulted in pedestrian fatalities and was often detected at some level in both drivers and pedestrians.[12] Pedestrians had blood alcohol levels greater than 0.08% over twice as often as the drivers (34% and 15%, respectively).[12]

Smoking Tobacco

Smoking has a two-fold impact on trauma and traumatic injury. First, smoking is the leading cause of fire-related deaths in homes.[8] Second, tobacco use contributes to health issues that can increase morbidity and mortality in the trauma patient.

Other Substances

Substances other than alcohol (legal and illegal) are involved in approximately 16% of all MVCs.[15] Alcohol and these substances are often used simultaneously, adding to the complexity of assessing the person with a traumatic injury. Substance use also contributes to morbidity and mortality and additional health issues, such as pulmonary issues and liver failure.

The risk of substance abuse is not limited to the adult population. In a 2014 survey, 11% of respondents age 16 or older admitted to driving under the influence (DUI) of alcohol, and 4.1% used illicit drugs.[16] Substance abuse is not a benign condition. It can be life altering, particularly when it results in trauma.

Violence

Homicide, assault, interpersonal violence, and abuse (sexual, physical, and psychological) are just a few of the many types of violence that lead to traumatic injury. Whatever form it takes, violence is a public health issue.

Homicide is one of the top five causes of injury-related death for individuals age 1 to 44 years, the second leading cause of death for those younger than age 1, and the third leading cause for individuals age 15 to 34 years.[4] Data from U.S. crime reports indicate that, on an annual basis, 16% of murders are by an intimate partner.[17]

One in four women has been the victim of severe physical violence by an intimate partner, compared with one in seven men.[17] Due to lack of reporting, clear data are lacking on the number or percentage of elderly individuals who are abused. As of 2008, it was estimated one in 10 suffered some sort of abuse.[18] In 2012, Child Protective Services estimated that 686,000 children (9.2/1,000) in the United States were victims of maltreatment.[19] It is also estimated that 1,640 deaths occurred from such maltreatment in that year.[19] For more information see Chapter 16, "Special Populations: The Interpersonal-Violence Trauma Patient."

Injury Prevention

Injury prevention is an important step in reducing the financial burden of injury—not only the loss of property, but also the loss of productivity by the injured individual. The aim of injury prevention is to reduce the number of injury events, whereas injury control considers the number of events and the severity of injuries when they do occur.

Injury prevention interventions can be applied to three different phases of the injury event process: primary, secondary, and tertiary. Each phase has a separate focus and set of goals, but the ultimate endpoint remains injury reduction or elimination:

- Primary: Prevention of the occurrence of the injury
- Secondary: Reduction in the severity of the injury that has occurred
- Tertiary: Improvement of outcomes related to the traumatic injury

Whether a hospital has one program focusing on injury prevention or a department that implements many programs, the process shares common components. Assessment of the problem is the first step in development of any injury prevention program. The following injury prevention model describes the basic principles of injury control:

- Define the problem.
- Identify risk and protective factors.
- Develop and test prevention strategies.
- Assure widespread adoption.[20]

In addition, incorporation of the three E's of injury control is important:

- *Engineering:* This aspect relates to technological interventions such as, in the case of MVCs, side-impact air bags, automated alarms alerting drivers to vehicles in their blind spots, and ignition lock devices for those persons convicted of DUI. For playgrounds and sports, engineering involves placement of surface material under playground equipment and use of athletic safety gear. Another intervention is improved use of smoke alarms in fire prevention.
- *Enforcement and legislation:* These efforts include laws at all jurisdictional levels regarding driving while intoxicated, booster seats, primary seat belt use, and distracted driving. For sports, they include rules regarding illegal hits, examination after impact, and return-to-play requirements after a head injury.
- *Education:* These programs can take the form of community-based initiatives such as public service announcements for improved seat belt use, education regarding risks of distracted driving, programs to commit to no texting while driving, and promotions for bicycle helmet giveaways with instructions for proper use.

The trauma nurse can have an impact when it comes to the legislative process by advocating for stronger laws and more consistent enforcement. Nurses may provide data, expert testimony, and education to legislators, community leaders, and citizens. They can present programs in schools, to parent groups, or in senior centers, and educate patients and families every day in their practice environment. Many programs and information for community education opportunities are available at little or no cost. Resources for injury prevention are included in **Table 21-1**.

Substance Use Education

Healthcare providers can engage in nonjudgmental conversations about substance use. Screening, brief intervention, and referral to treatment (SBIRT) is an effective, evidence-based approach to identifying patients at high risk for complications from substance use. With SBIRT, a routine screening identifies at-risk individuals who might benefit from an in-depth evaluation. Personalized feedback and the ability to modify harmful alcohol- or drug-related behaviors are provided through a brief intervention. Appropriate referrals are provided for further evaluation and treatment depending on the individual's substance abuse risk level. In one study, patients who underwent SBIRT experienced 20% fewer ED visits, 33% fewer nonfatal injuries, 37% fewer hospitalizations, 46% fewer arrests, and 50% fewer MVCs.[21]

Summary

Unintentional injury is a leading cause of death across all age groups in the United States. For those injuries that

TABLE 21-1 Injury Prevention Web Resources for Nurses

Organization	Website
Centers for Disease Control and Prevention	http://www.cdc.gov/injury/ http://www.cdc.gov/Violence Prevention/index.html http://www.cdc.gov/motor vehiclesafety/index.html
Emergency Nurses Association	https://www.ena.org
National Council on Aging	http://www.ncoa.org
National Highway Traffic Safety Administration	http://www.nhtsa.gov http://www.nhtsa.gov/road-safety
SafeKids Worldwide	http://www.safekids.org/worldwide/
STOP Sports Injuries	http://www.stopsportsinjuries.org
U.S. Department of Health and Human Services	http://www.healthypeople.gov
World Health Organization	http://www.who.int/violence_injury_prevention/en/

do not result in death, the community and healthcare settings experience an impact at the economic and social levels. Human characteristics such as age, gender, race, and substance use play a role in the rate of injury and type of injuries seen in the U.S. population. Taking these into consideration, injury prevention strategies can be used to reduce the incidence of traumatic injury through public awareness and education campaigns. Trauma nurses play a role by providing discharge education, working in their communities, and advocating for legislation that can affect injuries related to trauma.

Australia

Data collected on injury and traumatic deaths in Australia has improved since 2012 with the establishment of the Australian Trauma Quality Improvement Program (AusTQIP) and the Australian Trauma Registry (ATR), which brought together Australia's 26 designated trauma centers to assist in the collection of national data.[22] However, the Australian Bureau of Statistics publishes the most recent epidemiologic information on the health status of the Australian population.[23]

Incidence

Injury is a major contributor to overall morbidity and permanent disability. As many as 12,000 people die because of trauma and nearly half a million people are hospitalized because of this cause in Australia each year.[24] Most injuries requiring hospitalization are a result of falls (40%) and land transport incidents (13%),[24] while most deaths are from falls and suicide.[25]

The overwhelming cause of injury in Australia, between 2013 and 2015, was blunt trauma, with 44% of those injuries coming from road traffic accidents (38% "on-road" and 6% "off-road").[26] Second to road trauma as a cause of injury during this period were falls, with most of them occurring in the home, followed by falls in residential institutions. There was also an increase in falls among the elderly population.[26]

Head injury, with or without other injury, was seen in 44% of injury cases. The second largest incidence was injury to multiple body systems, including burns, but excluding head injury.[26]

Males accounted for 70% of all major trauma cases, with the incidence of major trauma in the older than age 75 group rising steadily between 2013 and 2015. Major trauma cases had an overall mortality rate of 11.4%, with females having a higher mortality rate than males (13.8% versus 10.07%).[26]

Between 2014 and 2016, land transport accidents were the most common cause of death in individuals age 1 to 14 (12%), while suicide was the leading cause of death in individuals age 15 to 24 (34%), followed by land transport accidents (21%). In the 25 to 44 age group, most deaths were from suicide (21%), followed by accidental poisoning (12%) and then road accidents.[27]

For all external causes of death, Aboriginal and Torres Strait Islanders had an incidence twice that of other Australians.[25]

Suicide

Suicide-related deaths increased with the death rate in 2017, accounting for 12.6 deaths per 100,000. Suicide was the leading cause of death among people age 15 to 44 years and the second leading cause of death among people age 45 to 54 years. Death by suicide was three times higher in males than females.[28] There has been a decrease in suicide within the 75 to 79 age group, especially in the male population, with mortality from this cause falling from 21.4 deaths per 100,000 in 2016 to 15.5 deaths per 100,000 in 2017.[22] The suicide-related death rates among Aboriginal and Torres Strait Islanders were twice that of other Australians.[24]

Falls

From 2002–2003 to 2014–2015, in the 65 years and older group, the rates of falls increased by 3% per year for males and 2% per year for females.[29] The rate of hip fractures decreased by 2% per year over the same period, while the rate of head injuries increased by 7% per year.[29]

Approximately 30% of adults older than age 65 experience at least 1 fall per year. In this age group, falls account for 40% of all injury-related deaths and 1% of total deaths. Depending on the population under study, between 22% and 60% of older people suffer injuries from falls, with 10–15% sustaining serious injuries, 2–6% sustaining fractures, and 0.2–1.5% sustaining hip fractures.[30]

Females of all ages fall more than males, and the rate of falls increases with age.[29] Most falls (58%) occur at home or in nursing homes (10%). They typically involve slip or trip incidents from the same level or from less than 1 meter in height.[29] The most common injuries from falls are fractures (30%), head injuries (15%), hip fractures (11%), and forearm fractures (9%).[29]

Transport-Related Collisions

In 2014–2015 in Australia, 57,000 people were hospitalized because of land transport crashes. "On-road" incidents numbered 36,000 (65%), while 14,000 (26%) incidents were "off-road" events.[31]

The group with the highest hospitalization rate was males age 15 to 24 who experienced nonfatal MVCs (321 per 100,000). Children younger than 5 years of age had the lowest rates, at 21 per 100,000.[31] For motor cyclists, the male:female ratio per 100,000 was 64%:8%; for cyclists, it was 46%:12% respectively.[31] The most common injuries were to the trunk (26%), shoulder and upper arm (25%), and head (19%).[31]

In 2014, land transport collisions accounted for 45% of all deaths in the 17 to 25 age group, costing Australia $27 billion.[32] Total transport deaths in 2016 numbered 1,295—an increase of 7.5% from 2015, but 19.2% lower than that number of such deaths 10 years earlier (an annual reduction of 2.9%).[33]

Work-Related Injuries

In the 13 years from 2003 to 2015, 3,207 workers were killed in work-related incidents, and two-thirds of these involved a vehicle of some description. Also, 60% of bystander fatalities were due to a vehicle collision. A further 16% of such fatalities involved being struck by moving objects.[34]

In 2015, 195 workers were fatally injured at work, a number that was 37% lower than the highest number in that 12-year period. In 2016, there were 182 deaths, representing a rate of 1.5 per 100,000, with 50% of the fatalities involving transport, postal and warehouse injuries, agriculture, forestry and fishing.[34]

Data collected through Safe Work Australia identifies that work-related fatalities have decreased by 49% since the peak in 2007.[35]

Violence

In 2014–2015, 20,000 people in Australia were hospitalized because of some form of assault (239 per 100,000). The majority of those assaulted were male, and 54% of the patients were between 15 and 44 years of age. Of those assaulted, 60% were assaulted by bodily force (unarmed brawl or fight), 12% by a sharp object, and 14% by a blunt object.[25] Of assaults on men and boys that involved sharp objects, 55% of the attacks were by knives and 18% were by glass of some kind.[36]

The most common injuries sustained were fractures (40%), and 94% were to the upper body, especially the head and neck. Blunt injuries to the head and neck accounted for 71% of injuries.[37]

Firearm-Related Injuries

In 2012–2013, 338 persons were hospitalized in Australia because of firearm-related injuries, and there were 209 deaths from this cause. These rates represent 1.5 hospitalizations per 100,000 population and 0.9 death per 100,000 population, respectively. For both deaths and hospital visits, more than 90% of the victims were male.[38]

For more than 33% of those patients with firearm-related injuries admitted to the hospital, the incident involved unintentional injury. Approximately 33% were assaulted, and in 19% of cases, the intent was undetermined. Of those who died, 79% died from intentional self-harm (suicide) and 17% were from homicide.

For those patients admitted to a hospital, 76% were in the 15 to 44 age group; for those who died. 62% were 45 years or older. In remote and very remote areas, rates for hospitalized cases and deaths were 4 to 6 times higher than the corresponding rates in major cities.[38]

Human Characteristics

Human characteristics important to understanding trauma in Australia are age, alcohol usage, and submersion/drowning.

Children

In Australia, more children die from injury than from cancer and asthma combined. Each year, more than 150 children between 0 and 14 years of age are killed, while 68,000 are hospitalized. Unintentional injury accounts for approximately 88% of all trauma-related deaths.[39]

Children are admitted to hospital at a rate of 1,489 per 100,000—a rate that has not decreased in the last 10 years despite extensive prevention strategies developed at the national, state, and territory levels.[40] The most frequent cause of accidental injury is falls (38.4%), often from playground equipment. The most common activity being carried out at the time of injury is a sporting event (19.9%). Most injuries are sustained in the home (24.5%), and fractures are the most likely injury (41.9%).[40]

Older Adults

Older Australians generally experience injuries requiring hospitalization at a rate lower than other age groups until ages 70 to 74, when women start to become injured more frequently than men, with that trend increasing through age 89.[41] All older adults are more likely to die because of their injuries than are younger adults.[42] As noted previously, they are at higher risk of death due to falls.

Alcohol

Recent studies have identified that injury and death related to trauma are often a consequence of alcohol use. Examples of incidents that may involve alcohol include the following: vehicle, cycling, and pedestrian accidents; falls; drowning; assault and violence; and intentional self-harm. Alcohol is associated with 44% of fire injuries, 34% of falls and drownings, 30% of car accidents, 47% of assaults, 34% of homicides, 32% of suicides, 16% of child abuse incidents, and 7% of industrial machine accidents.[43]

According to the Australian Institute of Health and Welfare (2016), more than 1 in 4 Australians age 14 years and older was the victim of an alcohol-related incident in 2013.[44]

Drowning

The death rate from drowning increased across Australia by 3% in the period from July 1, 2016, to June 30, 2017. There were 291 drowning deaths during this period, an increase of 9 deaths from the previous year's data. The largest number of drowning deaths occurred in the 25- to 34-year age group (43), who accounted for 15% of all such deaths. Drowning rates for children age 0 to 4 years (29) increased by 4%.[45]

Prevention

Australia places a great deal of importance on the multifaceted areas of injury prevention. Indeed, injury is considered a major cause of preventable death and disability in Australia.[46]

The Australasian Injury Prevention Network (AIPN) is the top national body with the role of advocating for injury preventions and safety promotion. In 2017, AIPN extended its activities to include New Zealand. According to the AIPN, with 26 Australians killed through injury and 1,200 people hospitalized every day, preventive strategies are essential, as "injury is no accident."[47]

The Royal Australasian College of Surgeons, in its 2015 position paper *Road Trauma Prevention*, supported all evidence-based initiatives that might assist in the prevention of road trauma and the reduction of the devastating effects of injury. Initiatives such as speed control, air bags, seat belt reminder systems, electronic stability control, and countermeasures for alcohol and driver distraction are endeavors proposed to make a difference in reducing the road toll.[48]

Canada

Preventable injury continues to be the leading cause of death for Canadians between the ages of 1 to 44 and is a leading cause of hospitalization for Canadians of any age.[49] In 2017, nearly 2 million Canadians visited an ED because of an injury.[50]

Cost

The financial cost of preventable injury continues to rise in Canada and is considered unsustainable. The total cost of injury is separated into direct costs (healthcare costs arising from injuries) and indirect costs (costs related to reduced productivity from hospitalization, disability, and premature death). The direct cost of injury is approximately $26.8 billion Canadian and includes more than 3.5 million visits to the ED.[49] The indirect costs of injury are catastrophic, with 43 Canadians dying each day and 16,000 injury deaths occurring annually.[49] Additionally, injury results in more than 60,000 people experiencing some form of disability following injury.[49] Unintentional injury accounts for 82% of all injury costs.[49]

Incidence

In 2017, the leading causes of major injury among all hospital-admitted cases were as follows[50]:

1. Unintentional falls: 57.9%
2. Intentional injury (homicide, suicide, assault): 10.9%
3. MVCs, which have seen a decrease in incidence: 9.4% of inpatient admissions across Canada[51]

Unintentional Falls

Unintentional falls are the leading cause of injury across Canada, accounting for 32% of all reported ED visits for injury and trauma.[50] The information reported by the Canadian Institute for Health Information aligns with data from the National Trauma Data Bank[52] in the United States, showing that falls have eclipsed MVCs as the leading cause of unintentional injury in North America. Slipping, tripping, and stumbling are the main causes of falls, with nearly 33,000 falls resulting in admission to hospital in 2017. Most falls occur in the home (**Figure 21-1**),[51] with such events resulting in more than 114,000 ED visits in 2017. Females have a higher incidence of falling compared to males.

Intentional Injury

Intentional injury results from interpersonal violence as well as self-directed violence. Intentional self-harm remains the leading cause of intentional injury in Canada.[51]

Interpersonal Violence

From 2016 to 2017, 2.7% of all injury hospitalizations in Canada were due to interpersonal violence. The most commonly specified means of interpersonal violence was assault by bodily force (11.7%), sharp objects (6.1%), assault with a blunt object (2.3%), and firearms (1.1%).[51]

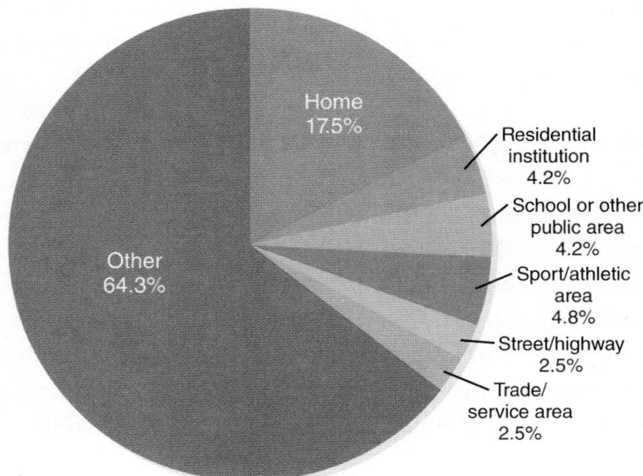

Figure 21-1 *Emergency department visits for unintentional falls, 2016–2017.*

Data from Canadian Institute for Health Information. (2018, July 5). Injury and trauma emergency department and hospitalization statistics, 2016–2017. Retrieved from https://www.cihi.ca/sites/default/files/document/2016-2017-injury-and-trauma-quick-stats-en-web.xlsx.

Self-Directed Violence

From 2016 to 2017, 8.1% of all injuries were from suicide, self-inflicted injury, or self-directed violence. Of the nearly 22,000 hospitalizations for intentional self-injury, poisoning was the leading cause of hospitalization (82.7%). Injury with a sharp object (7.8%) and hanging/strangulation (2.8%) were the other main causes of self-harm.

Motor Vehicle Collisions

Increases in vehicle safety and reductions in impaired driving due to alcohol have resulted in a decreased incidence of MVCs. Trends show a consistent decline in the number of fatalities related to impaired driving in Canada over the past 10 years.[53] Between 2000 and 2014, Canada experienced a 40.8% decline in the number of alcohol-related road fatalities in MVCs[53]; in direct contrast, there have been marginal increases in the number of fatalities involving use of alcohol when operating off-road vehicles.

Distracted driving has become an increased public health concern, with deaths related to distracted driving now surpassing those from impaired driving.[53] Across Canada, distracted driving fatalities are more likely to be female victims and between the ages of 20 and 34 or among individuals 65 and older.[54] Enforcement of distracted driving laws competes with other road safety priorities and challenges related to human and financial resources in law enforcement.[53]

Injuries related to substance use are similar nationally, with drug-impaired driving becoming an increasing concern across Canada. Data show that alcohol use is reported by 77% of Canadians age 15 and older, with 22% using psychoactive pharmaceutical drugs, 12% using cannabis, and 12% using illicit drugs (excluding cannabis).[55] Despite decreases in alcohol-related injuries, 42.4% of drivers fatally injured tested positive for drugs in 2014, with 44.7% of those drivers testing positive for cannabis.[53] A renewed focus on impaired driving emerged in 2017, in relation to the Canadian federal government legalizing the possession, growing, selling, and consumption of cannabis.[53] Increased incidents of positive drug-impaired driving have increased demands on law enforcement with limited access to drug recognition evaluators.[53]

Distinct differences exist in the timing of substance-related MVCs. Whereas alcohol-related collisions typically occur on weekends and between the hours of 11 p.m. and 4 a.m., drug-impaired driving incidents have unpredictable timelines.[53] Variations in substance use patterns necessitate differences in enforcement and cannot solely overlap with current alcohol-impaired driving enforcement initiatives.

Factors Associated with Unintentional and Intentional Injury

Many causative factors contribute to unintentional and intentional injury, including alcohol, firearms, and toxic products.[56] Alcohol consumption is associated with many unintentional injuries, ranging from drownings to traffic injuries.[56] Additionally, alcohol consumption is associated with various forms of violence among youth, intimate-partner violence, sexual assault, and suicide.[56]

Studies suggest that the presence of firearms in the home can increase the risk of homicide three times and the risk of suicide five times for individuals who reside in a home with firearms.[56] Toxic products or medications are associated with suicide and unintentional injury among children from 0 to 4 years of age.[56]

Human Characteristics

Important human characteristics in Canadian trauma epidemiology include age and frailty, gender, socioeconomic status (SES), and Indigenous status.

Frailty

"Frailty is a common condition that impacts the quality of life of older adults, their unpaid caregivers, and the sustainability of health care systems."[57(p5)] Frailty places Canadian seniors at risk for functional impairment, progressive loss of function, falls, hospitalization, long-term care use, and death in relation to stress from a minor illness, injury, or infection.[57] Each year, nearly 400,000 independent-living seniors sustain injuries that limit their functional mobility.[58] Once hospitalized, for minor injuries, these seniors can experience a functional decline of 15–18% 6 months post injury.[58] Early identification of frailty directly contributes to improved health outcomes and quality of life; it also indirectly contributes to the sustainability of health and social care resources.[57]

Gender

From 2016 to 2017, females accounted for 52.8% of all injury hospitalizations (**Table 21-2**).[51] By comparison, males age 18 to 64 accounted for 24.3% of all injury hospitalizations.[51]

TABLE 21-2 Injury Hospitalizations by Age and Sex, Canada, 2016–2017

Age Group (Years)	Female	Male	Total
0–4	2,632	3,540	**6,172**
5–17	7,906	8,983	**16,889**
18–64	44,796	63,985	**108,781**
65–84	46,484	33,003	**79,487**
85 and older	37,381	15,126	**52,507**
Total	**139,199**	**124,637**	**263,836**

Data from Canadian Institute for Health Information. (2018, July 5). Injury and trauma emergency department and hospitalization statistics, 2016–2017. Retrieved from https://www.cihi.ca/sites/default/files/document/2016-2017-injury-and-trauma-quick-stats-en-web.xlsx.

Socioeconomics and the Social Determinants of Injury

Although injury rates have been declining across all income levels, a significant gap still exists between the richest and poorest Canadians. Several studies of hospitalizations in 2008 observed that decreases in SES are associated with increased rates of fatal and serious injuries. As SES increases, rates of injury decline. The Canadian Institute for Health Information reports that the poorest Canadians experience injury at a rate 1.3 times higher than the wealthiest.[59]

Indigenous Peoples

Injury is a leading cause of death and is a serious public health concern among Indigenous peoples in Canada.[60] Data from three provinces show higher injury hospitalization rates among Indigenous peoples living on and off reserves in Western Canada compared to the general population.[60] These rates of injury in Indigenous communities may be due to many complex social and economic determinants of health, such as high rates of poverty, social exclusion, poor housing quality and housing shortages, lower levels of education and employment, and a younger population.[60]

Researchers specifically studying rates of suicide among Indigenous communities found that rates were lowest in those with certain characteristics relevant to enhancing cultural continuity, such as self-governance, education, health and emergency services, cultural facilities, and land claims resolution.[61] Within Canada, initiatives such as Brighter Futures (established in 1992) and the development of an injury curriculum specific to Indigenous peoples are aimed at actively engaging and supporting a decrease in injury rates among this unique population.

National Injury Prevention Strategy

Canada has made great strides in the creation of a national strategy and unified voice for injury prevention through the 2012 development of Parachute—Leaders in Injury Prevention (an amalgamation of four national organizations: Safe Communities Canada, Safe Kids Canada, SMARTRISK, and ThinkFirst Canada). This group

TABLE 21-3 National Injury Databases

Organization	Website
Public Health Agency of Canada	https://www.canada.ca/en/public-health.html
Canadian Hospitals Injury Reporting and Prevention Program	http://www.phac-aspc.gc.ca/injury-bles/chirpp/injrep-rapbles/
Canadian Institute for Health Information	http://www.cihi.ca
Statistics Canada	http://www.statcan.gc.ca
Canadian Red Cross	http://www.redcross.ca
Canadian Agricultural Injury Reporting	http://www.cair-sbac.ca
Canadian Motor Vehicle Traffic Collision Statistics from Transport Canada	http://www.tc.gc.ca/eng/roadsafety/tp-1317.htm
First Nations and Inuit Health Information System	http://www.hc-sc.gc.ca/fniah-spnia/services/home-domicile/index-eng.php

works with federal and various provincial governments, along with Canadian companies, to focus injury prevention efforts on individuals of all ages and on both intentional and unintentional injuries.

In addition, representatives from provincial injury prevention centers and the leading national injury prevention organizations serve on the Canadian Collaborating Centres for Injury Prevention (CCCIP), which has developed the Canadian Injury Prevention Curriculum and Canadian Injury Research Network. The CCCIP provides an opportunity for groundbreaking injury prevention researchers and leaders to collaborate, share knowledge and experiences, and support individual and collective projects, policies, and research.[62]

Table 21-3 lists national databases that provide data on injuries occurring in Canada.

Hong Kong

In Hong Kong, there is no centrally based data collection system for recording morbidity and mortality related to trauma. This makes it difficult to maintain accurate figures and injury data, although the five trauma centers in Hong Kong do collect data for the purposes of service evaluation. In 2017, these trauma centers recorded 3,696 major trauma cases.[63] Among those cases, 594 required inpatient treatment in intensive care units and 632 in high-dependency units.[63] The mean hospitalization length of stay was 11.65 days.[63]

Incidence

External causes of morbidity and mortality were the fifth leading cause of death in Hong Kong in 2016.[64] Following the implementation of public injury prevention and education programs by the Hong Kong government, universities, and other organizations, the number of registered deaths decreased from 27.5 per 100,000 in 2001 to 24.7 per 100,000 in 2016.[64]

Focusing on major trauma, in 2017 the three most common MOIs were (1) falls of 2 meters or less (38.5%), (2) MVCs (23.8%), and (3) struck by or collision with object/person (14%). Blunt trauma (85.8%) was the most common type of traumatic injury, followed by burns (7.6%) and penetrating trauma (6.6%).[63]

Human Characteristics

The major human characteristics related to trauma epidemiology in Hong Kong include age and gender. This section also discusses the characteristics of those persons involved in MVCs.

Age

In keeping with the general trend of aging of the population in Hong Kong,[65] the median age of a patient with major trauma increased from 46 years of age in 2011 to 51.52 years in 2017. In a local single center study, the 30-day mortality rate was 7.5% for those age 55 to 70 and 17.7% for those older than age 70.[66] This suggests the specific need to focus on trauma management and injury prevention in the geriatric trauma population in Hong Kong.

Gender

Gender differences exist in injury rates, depending on the causes of the traumatic injury.[63] Exposure to the injury-producing event, amount of risk involved, occupation, and cultural norms are possible reasons for these gender differences.

From 2016 to 2017, the overall death rate for fall injuries for men was twice as high as that for women.[67] A similar picture exists in the major trauma population. In 2017, the male to female ratio for major trauma was 2.15:1.0.

Motor Vehicle Collisions

In Hong Kong, the most commonly injured patients in MVCs are pedestrians (366), followed by drivers (143), motorcyclists (142), bicyclists (130), and passengers (97).[67] Data from the Hong Kong Transport Department show the number of casualties involved in MVCs peaked in 1982 at 24,222.[68] That number then decreased steadily to 19,888 in 2017. Among these fatalities, only 26 (0.13%) casualties were related to alcohol and drug use by the driver.[68]

Netherlands

The Netherlands is one of the smaller countries in Europe, about the size of the state of Maryland, but it is densely populated. It has 17 million inhabitants (1,259 inhabitants/square mile).[69]

Epidemiology

The Dutch are a generally healthy population, with a life expectancy of 80.6 years for males and 83.3 years for females.[70] The number one cause of death is cancer, followed by heart and vascular disease. In terms of non-natural causes of death in the Netherlands (35 deaths/100,000 inhabitants), suicide is listed as the number one non-natural cause of death, followed by traffic-related incidents, falls, and domestic incidents.[70]

The roadways are relatively safe in the Netherlands. In 2016, the country had 4.7 traffic-related deaths per billion kilometers (by comparison, the U.S. rate was 7.3 traffic-related deaths per billion kilometers).[71] The total number of traffic-related deaths decreased from nearly 1,000 deaths per year in 1990 to 623 in 2017.[70] As bicycles are one of the most frequently used forms of transportation in the Netherlands, they are involved in nearly 30% of all transportation-related deaths. Wearing a helmet while riding a bicycle is not mandatory for adults and children, and only a few people wear a helmet while cycling.

Healthcare

The Netherlands has 114 general hospitals, 93 of which have an ED. Eleven hospitals are granted the status of Trauma Centre, comparable to a Level 1 trauma center in the United States.[72,73]

Every citizen of the Netherlands has compulsory healthcare insurance. For a nominal fee of around 130 euros/month (approximately $150), everyone is insured for healthcare. As the cost of healthcare in the Netherlands rises, public discussion is also increasing about the healthcare system. As it is based on mutual responsibility, everyone—old, young, healthy, chronically ill—pays the same amount. Dutch healthcare is ranked among the best on the various world healthcare indices.[74-76]

South Africa

More than two decades ago, trauma in South Africa was described as a "malignant epidemic." Unfortunately, the situation has not changed significantly, as the trauma numbers remain a major area of concern.[77] At the same time, there has been increased interest in and support for an effective and coordinated trauma system and improvements in the availability of advanced emergency medical services.

Incidence

Trauma is a major contributor to Africa's triple burden of disease: death due to injuries, pretransitional causes related to poverty, and the emerging chronic disease burden. For example, in terms of South African mortality and morbidity, 7.5% of deaths were from injuries versus 6.5% from tuberculosis, and human immunodeficiency virus/acquired immunodeficiency syndrome (HIV/AIDS) remains a concern.[78] In 2016, 88.8% of deaths were due to natural causes and 11.2% due to non-natural causes.[78] Of these non-natural deaths, 66.5% were caused by accidental injury, 14.8% were caused by assaults, and 12.5% were transport related.[78]

South Africa experiences more than 48,000 trauma deaths annually.[78] The World Health Organization (WHO) has estimated that injuries will increase to become the second major contributor to African mortality by 2020.[79]

Injury Type

The majority of the injuries presenting to the EDs of a private hospital group in South Africa were blunt trauma, followed by penetrating injuries, and then burn-related injuries (**Figure 21-2**).[79] In state hospitals, the opposite presentation was observed, with 90% of injuries involving penetrating trauma and only 10% blunt trauma.

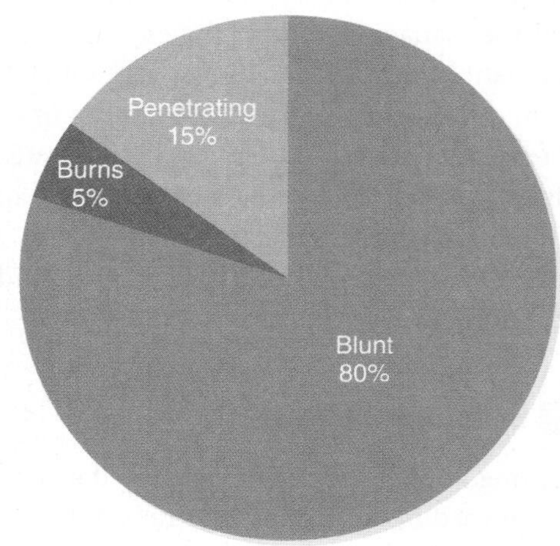

Figure 21-2 *Injury types.*

Data from Medibank Trauma Data Registry: Netcare Private Hospital Group South Africa. (2016). *National trauma epidemiology report 2016*. Pretoria, South Africa: Author.

Injury Priority

The highest percentage of injuries seen in the private hospital group was priority 2 (seriously ill) patients. Men were more likely to present as priority 1 (critically ill) than were women.[79]

Human Characteristics and Behavior

Age, gender, and the use of alcohol and substances are all human characteristics that affect trauma in South Africa. Approximately 1.8% of all deaths in South Africa are caused by assaults or self-harm.[78] The constitutional court in South Africa legalized the use of cannabis in private house settings in September 2018, but the effect of this decision and its long-term influence on trauma incidents have yet to be seen.

Age

In 2017, 4.9 million people in South Africa were older than 60 years—a number that equates to 8.7% of the country's total population of 56.5 million people.[80] Healthcare problems that place the elderly at increased risk for injuries include dementia (which affects 7% of the elderly population[81]) and limitations in eating, bathing, dressing, getting in and out of bed, or using the toilet (which affects 38.4% of the population age 65 to 74 and 49.2% of those older than age 75).

WHO reports that by 2050 the geriatric population in South Africa will have doubled in number. The link between chronic disease and old age means an increase in the already rapidly growing burden of chronic disease, with a concomitant increasing burden on the health system. An area of growing concern is the abuse of elderly people residing in care facilities (retirement homes, frail care centers).[82]

Different mechanisms of injury are common among the pediatric population. The highest percentage of transport-related deaths (15.1%) occurs in the age group 1 to 14 years, and 75.6% of deaths due to accidental injury also occur in the 1- to 14-years age group.[78]

Gender

The ratio of male-to-female trauma cases at state hospitals is almost 4:1. Analysis of the total non-natural causes of death in 2016 revealed that 77.9% of these deaths involved male victims.[78]

Studies have shown that 4% of female trauma cases admitted to state facilities were injured during pregnancy.[83] More than 50% of those injuries were due to assault, resulting in fetal loss in more than 33% of the cases.[84]

Alcohol Use

In South Africa, the legal standard for intoxication is a blood alcohol concentration of 0.05%. Alcohol is the most widely abused drug in South Africa. It is the third-largest contributor to death and disability, after interpersonal violence and sexually transmitted diseases.[85,86]

Types of Injuries

The most frequent injuries involve MVCs, violence, burns, suicide, and drowning.

Motor Vehicle Collisions

The Automobile Association (AA) in South Africa showed an alarming jump in 2016 road fatalities and recorded the highest number of road deaths in the past 10 years during that year. According to the AA, 2016 saw 14,071 people die on South Africa's roads—a significant increase (9%) from the 12,944 deaths recorded in 2015 (an additional 1,120 deaths on a year-on-year basis) (**Figure 21-3**). These numbers represent the highest annual road death toll since 2007, when 14,920 people died on South African roads.[87]

The Road Traffic Management Cooperation (RTMC) in South Africa found that the total cost of MVCs on the country road's network for 2015 amounted to an estimated R142.95 billion ($10.29 billion)—equivalent to 3.4% of South Africa's gross domestic product. Its report also mentions that of the 12,944 road fatalities, 10,613 of them were recorded by the RTMC as MVCs.[88] Human casualty costs represented 69.3% of the total road traffic collision (RTC) cost of R142.95 billion ($10.29 billion), with vehicle repair accounting for 14.9% of the total, and incident costs 15.8%.[88,89]

A study conducted in 2016 found that determinant factors in the causes of MVCs include the following[90]:

- Speed
- Driver capabilities
- Vehicle condition
- Environmental conditions
- Human error

Violence

A 2014 study found that interpersonal violence remains a significant concern in South Africa, accounting for 58.2% of trauma deaths.[77]

Burns

An estimated ZAR262 million ($18.86 million) is spent annually in South Africa for the care of patients with kerosene (paraffin) stove burns. Indirect costs—lost wages, prolonged care for deformities, emotional trauma, and

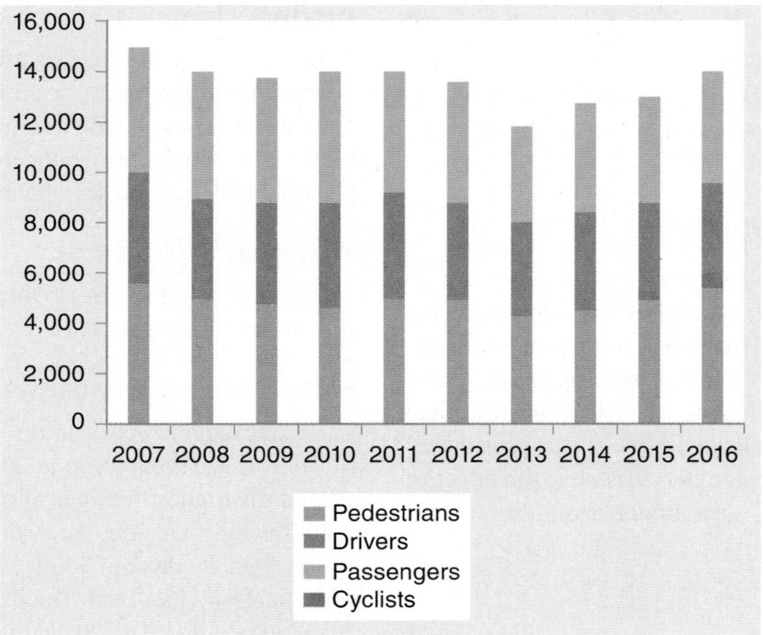

Figure 21-3 *South African road fatalities, 2007–2016.*

Data from South Africa's shocking road death numbers at highest level in 10 years. (2017, June 9). *BusinessTech*. Retrieved from https://businesstech.co.za/news/monitoring/178275/south-africas-shocking-road-death-numbers-at-highest-level-in-10-years.

commitment of family resources—add significantly to the socioeconomic impact of burn injuries on patients and their families.[91]

There is limited access to quality burn care in Africa. The systems that do exist struggle with financial restraints, large numbers of patients, and acute shortages of adequately trained staff and facilities to render burn services.[92]

South Africa has the second largest economy in Africa (after Nigeria), and it is estimated that 3.2% of the population sustains a burn injury each year. The majority of these burns are minor and moderate (1.6 million injuries), with less than 10% being severe (3,200 injuries) and needing specialized care. Admission numbers collected from burn units in the country indicate there are 8,800 admissions per year. Poorly managed burns result in high morbidity and an increased number of burn-related deaths. A 2016 study reported that there are 23 burn "units" in South Africa exhibiting considerable variation in leadership, capacity, and functioning. All can generally render acute emergency care, with a limited number rendering comprehensive care.[92]

Suicide

The Medical Research Council of South Africa evaluated postmortem data to estimate suicidal (self-harm) deaths as part of its 2012 burden of disease study (the most recent available). It placed the number of deaths by suicide at 6,133 in 2012. The majority of suicide victims in South Africa are male. In 2012, 5,095 men of all ages died due to suicide—equaling nearly 14 people each day. The study also reported that suicide was the fourth leading cause of death for young people age 15 to 24 in South Africa in 2012.[93]

Drowning

According to the Princess Charlene of Monaco Foundation, drowning is the second leading cause of accidental death in South Africa, after road accidents. The foundation reports that approximately half of drowning accidents occur in and around the home in buckets, bathtubs, and swimming pools.[94] A large number of children in low-socioeconomic areas do not know how to swim or be water safe.

In 2018, a need was identified for detailed drowning surveillance to monitor national trends and identify risk factors in all South African communities.[95]

Injury Prevention

In South Africa the social and scientific responses to the containment and prevention of injuries remain inadequate. This inadequacy is attributed to the lack of quality national data indicative of the precise extent of the problem, inadequate resources, and the unbalanced attention to criminal justice responses and the burden of chronic diseases.[96]

Several well-established injury prevention and awareness practices are in place for the prevention of passengers' and cyclists' deaths, such as the use of child seats, seat belts, and cycling helmets. However, no single intervention is completely effective. Thus, prevention should include pedestrian skills programs, parent education, education on distractive lifestyles, legislation of environmental modifications, and vehicle changes at the regional, provincial, and national levels.

The Netcare Private Hospital group recognizes such injury prevention groups in South Africa that are addressing specific areas—for example, the Burns Society for burns, the Road Safety Association for road safety, and interest groups for the prevention of drowning. The Netcare Trauma Injury Prevention (NTIP) program was launched in 2012. This program embraces all age groups—expecting parents, caregivers, educators, children, and adults–geriatrics—in its approach to injury prevention and health promotion topics. The NTIP has been implemented in all Netcare hospitals nationally (46 hospitals). Most of the programs and activities start with the pediatric age group in an effort to develop a change in behavior during early childhood development that will lead to responsible adults who will do (or not do) specific actions due to their change of behavior as a young child.[97]

Road Safety Changes and Initiatives

The South African Department of Transport—the lead agency for road safety in South Africa—has developed a road safety strategy through an informed and coordinated effort to improve education and enforcement regarding poor road use behavior. This strategy is in line with international best practice and recommendations from WHO for developing countries.

South Africa is also supporting the Decade of Action for Road Safety, which will emphasize international measures to reduce the effect of poor road safety (particularly in sub-Saharan Africa) through the focusing on five road safety pillars. This strategy will lead multisectoral efforts within the private and public sectors to reduce road carnage through concentration on the highest risk factors: alcohol (driver and pedestrian), seat belt compliance, moving violations including speed, creation of a safe environment for pedestrians, education in schools, public relations concentrated on achievements to gain the support of the public, and creating an awareness of risks as well as improvement in the vehicle and road environment (including reduction in fraud and corruption) and improvement of after-crash care to reduce the number of deaths and disabling injuries.[98]

Sweden

Sweden is a country of more than 10.1 million people, of whom 8.6 million live in towns and other urban areas. Population density is highest around the capital Stockholm, in western parts (Gothenburg) and in southern parts (Malmoe/Lund) of the country. Average life expectancy in Sweden in 2018 is 84.0 years for women and 80.3 years for men.[99]

Statistics from the National Board of Health and Welfare regarding injuries, poisonings, and other external causes are based on a mortality register, a patient register, and the Injury Data Base in Sweden.[99]

Incidence

Trauma is a serious threat to the well-being of Swedish inhabitants. It is the fourth leading cause of death, after heart and vascular disease, respiratory organ disease, and cancer. Young healthy people are often involved in trauma, which causes a loss of their productive years.[100]

According to the Injury Data Base, 94,000 people were admitted to a hospital as a result of an accident in 2017, a total that is 4,000 less than the number for 2016. Approximately 7,600 people were admitted to a hospital after a road accident. The decline in road accidents has occurred over the past 10 years and is mostly found among young people. Taking the increase in population into account, these accidents have decreased by more than 40% since the beginning of the 2000s.[100]

As in previous years, falls are by far the most common cause of injury resulting in admissions to hospital. Falls account for two-thirds of all accidents, which corresponds to approximately 67,000 people—39,000 women (58%) and 28,000 men (42%).[100]

Human Characteristics

Important human characteristics related to trauma include age, gender, alcohol, suicide, and violence.

Age

Most injuries leading to death caused by trauma occur between the ages of 15 and 44 years. Most of the deaths between 16 and 64 years of age are associated with suicide and traffic collisions.[100]

Gender

For men up to the age of 45 years, trauma is the most common cause of death; in women up to the age of 45 years, it is the second most common cause of death. Men tend to be involved in more MVCs and suicide, whereas women sustain falls more often than men do.[100]

Alcohol

Each week in Sweden, 2 people die in alcohol-related traffic accidents; of all those who die in traffic accidents, 30% do so with alcohol in their bloodstream. When considering the number of single-car accidents, that percentage is nearly 50%. Every third drunk driver is between 18 and 24 years old. Young and middle-aged men are prominent in this group: Approximately 90% of people who are affected are men.[101]

Suicide

In 2016, there were 1,129 deaths as a result of suicide in Sweden. From an international perspective, Sweden's suicide rate is roughly at the same level as the European Union (EU) average. Over the last 15 years, the number of suicides has declined by approximately 20% in Sweden, in keeping with the trends in large parts of the EU.

However, this positive trend does not apply to youths and young adults, for whom suicide rates have been at approximately the same level for a long period of time. Suicide is the most common cause of death among women 15 to 29 years and the second most common cause of death among men in the same age group.[102]

Violence

In 2017, approximately 1,600 people were admitted to a hospital as a result of assault. Taking the increase in population into account, the number of people hospitalized for violence-related injuries has almost been cut in half over the past 10 years. Hospitalization due to violence is most common for men age 15 to 24, but it is also among that age group that the biggest decrease has occurred.[100]

Costs

In Sweden, the total societal costs for unintentional injuries are approximately $9.1 billion each year, and falls and traffic collisions account for nearly 75% of this figure. These costs do not reflect the suffering and impact on health and well-being for affected individuals and families.[103]

Prevention

The Baltic Everyday Accident, Disaster Prevention and Resilience Project (BaltPrevResilience) is an EU project that includes countries around the Baltic Sea and started in 2014. Its overall goal is to contribute to the prevention and reduction of the consequences of everyday accidents and disasters or crises. A key element in the accident prevention and consequence reduction effort is improved learning from accidents and disasters, preferably from minor, everyday accidents. Secondary goals are bridging gaps between everyday accident prevention and emergency management and promoting intersectoral collaboration on safety and security matters.[104]

Sweden has, for a long time, been proactive in injury prevention. In 2005, the country enacted a law that made it mandatory for all children younger than 15 years to wear a helmet when on a bicycle. Various studies have shown that wearing a helmet reduces the risk for concussion. Since 1975, Sweden has also required all motorcycle and moped riders to wear a helmet.[105]

Seat belts are mandatory in all cars and buses (except local buses in cities). Use of a three-point belt reduces the risk of severe injury in a collision by approximately 50%. Since 1986, law have required that all passengers use seat belts in a car and that children younger than 7 years are protected with special safety arrangements.[106]

In 1997, the Swedish Parliament developed "Zero Vision," which aims to eliminate severe injury or death from RTCs. The goal is to minimize mechanical injury so as to avoid severely harmful and deadly injuries. This program places the responsibility on the individual to follow road traffic laws and regulations, such as following speed limits and using safety devices, but also includes engineering developments, such as creating barriers between traffic lanes, pedestrians, and wild animals.[107]

Since 2014, Sweden has been conducting an ongoing national review of trauma care in the direction of the county council's mutual insurance company. This nationwide peer-review project aims to raise both quality and safety in the treatment of trauma patients. The project has already given rise to national guidelines on topics such as alarm criteria, spinal movement limitation, trauma computed tomography, and more.[108]

United Kingdom and Ireland

Formal trauma systems were introduced across England beginning in 2012 and are well established. In August 2018, the National Health Service (NHS) England reported an additional 1,600 lives had been saved among patients with severe injuries since use of major trauma centers commenced. The NHS data also showed patients spent fewer days in hospital and had improved quality of life after receiving critical care.[109]

Great progress has also been made in the development and implementation of trauma systems in Northern Ireland, Scotland, Wales, and Ireland.

Incidence in the United Kingdom

In the United Kingdom, data on morbidity and mortality are collected in various ways across England, Northern Ireland, Scotland, and Wales. Consequently, it is difficult to obtain accurate national statistics on injury figures. The Trauma Audit and Research Network (TARN) is the independent monitor of trauma care in England, Wales, and Ireland,[110] while the Scottish Trauma Audit Group (STAG) collates similar information from hospitals in Scotland.[111]

The TARN is committed to making a real difference in the delivery of care to the injured. The data collected are used to promote improvements in care through a national comparative clinical audit that seeks to inform and improve trauma care across the United Kingdom.

Every year across England and Wales, 12,500 people die after being injured. Trauma is the leading cause of death among children and young adults, 44 years and younger. In addition, many thousands of people are left severely disabled from trauma.[110] The TARN reported the following common causes of traumatic death in 2017[110]:

- Falls from less than 2 meters (64.4%)
- Falls from greater than 2 meters (13%)
- MVCs (11.8%)
- Assaults (2.9%)
- Shootings and stabbings (1.6%)
- All other traumatic events (4.3%)

NOTE

All tables included in this section are provided by the TARN and cover the year 2017. The authors would like to acknowledge the TARN group, United Kingdom, for providing the relevant data.

Table 21-4 shows the distribution of life-threatening injuries according to body system. Head injuries remain the leading cause of death, with more than half of all trauma deaths attributed to these injuries (57.8%). Chest injuries are the next most common presentation (31.2%), followed by spinal injuries (24.4%) and abdominal injuries (6.7%).

Human Characteristics

Human characteristics of note are age, gender, and alcohol use.

Age

Although the greatest number of trauma injuries occurs in people age 15 to 54, the highest death rate is for those older than the age of 75 (**Table 21-5**). The elderly population is less likely to recover from injury, with comorbidities playing a part in the poor outcomes for many of these patients.[110]

When analyzing deaths by age and mechanism of injury, the leading cause of death for people age 15 to 44 remains RTCs. However, in the 75-years-plus age group, the most common mechanism is falls of less than 2 meters (Table 21-5).

Gender

Differences in male and female death rates are apparent depending on the cause of the injury. Overall, the death rate from injuries is twice as high for males as for females.[110] Exposure to the injury-producing event, the amount of risk involved, occupation, and cultural norms are possible reasons for the gender differences.

Alcohol

In 2016, there were 7,327 alcohol-specific deaths in the United Kingdom, an age-standardized rate of 11.7 deaths per 100,000 population. The U.K. alcohol-specific deaths rate has remained unchanged since 2013. However, since 2001, rates of alcohol-specific deaths among males have been an average of 55% higher than those observed among females. For both sexes, rates of alcohol-specific deaths were highest among individuals age 55 to 64 years in 2016.[112]

TARN data from 2017 demonstrate that alcohol-related causes accounted for 10.4% of trauma patients and 7.3% of the deaths from trauma (**Table 21-6**).[110] There are strict alcohol limits for drivers in the United Kingdom, but the limits in Scotland were reduced in 2014, resulting in non-uniform levels across the United Kingdom (**Table 21-7**).[113]

Substance Misuse

There is growing recognition that the use of illegal substances, either with or without alcohol ingestion, is a

TABLE 21-4 Frequency of Abbreviated Injury Scale (AIS) Ratings, United Kingdom, 2017

		AIS: 3 + Injury *n* (% of Total)			
Group	**Total**	**Head**	**Chest**	**Abdomen**	**Spine**
All patients	64,670	19,005 (29.4%)	16,248 (25.1%)	3,846 (5.9%)	14,719 (22.8%)
Deaths	4,616	2,668 (57.8%)	1,441 (31.2%)	311 (6.7%)	1,126 (24.4%)

Note: Patients may appear in more than one category, so rows may add up to more than 100%.

TABLE 21-5 Death by Age Cohort and Mechanism, United Kingdom, 2017

		Mechanism *n* (% of Total)					
Age	**Total**	**Motor Vehicle Collision**	**Fall > 2 m**	**Fall < 2 m**	**Shooting/ Stabbing**	**Blow(s)**	**Other**
<1	15	1 (6.7%)	0 (0%)	2 (13.3%)	0 (0%)	4 (26.7%)	8 (53.3%)
1–4	18	6 (33.3%)	2 (11.1%)	0 (0%)	0 (0%)	2 (11.1%)	8 (44.4%)
5–14	32	12 (37.5%)	2 (6.3%)	1 (3.1%)	2 (6.3%)	1 (3.1%)	14 (43.8%)
15–24	170	78 (45.9%)	19 (11.2%)	2 (1.2%)	31 (18.2%)	5 (2.9%)	35 (20.6%)
25–34	163	76 (46.6%)	14 (8.6%)	9 (5.5%)	17 (10.4%)	9 (5.5%)	38 (23.3%)
35–44	152	39 (25.7%)	25 (16.4%)	22 (14.5%)	13 (8.6%)	15 (9.9%)	38 (25%)
45–54	250	59 (23.6%)	43 (17.2%)	87 (34.8%)	5 (2%)	17 (6.8%)	39 (15.6%)
55–64	336	46 (13.7%)	76 (22.6%)	171 (50.9%)	5 (1.5%)	9 (2.7%)	29 (8.6%)
65–74	545	65 (11.9%)	113 (20.7%)	342 (62.8%)	0 (0%)	6 (1.1%)	19 (3.5%)
75–84	1,139	90 (7.9%)	151 (13.3%)	876 (76.9%)	0 (0%)	6 (0.5%)	16 (1.4%)
85+	1,796	74 (4.1%)	155 (8.6%)	1,554 (86.5%)	0 (0%)	0 (0%)	13 (0.7%)

TABLE 21-6 Frequency of Alcohol Use Noted at the Point of Injury, United Kingdom, 2017

		Alcohol *n* (% of Total)	
Group	**Total**	**At Incident**	**As Pre-Existing Medical Conditions**
All patients	64,670	6,752 (10.4%)	4,751 (7.3%)
Deaths	4,616	339 (7.3%)	338 (7.3%)

TABLE 21-7 Alcohol Limits for U.K. Drivers

Level of Alcohol	**England, Wales, and Northern Ireland**	**Scotland**
mcg/100 mL of breath	35	22
mg/100 mL of blood	80	50
mg/100 mL of urine	107	67

factor related to trauma deaths. The true picture of deaths as a result of substance abuse is difficult to capture and calculate. Since March 2015, police in England have been able to carry out random roadside drug testing as a routine feature of traffic policing.[113]

Suicide

In 2017, the Office of National Statistics reported there were 5,821 suicides registered in the United Kingdom, an age-standardized rate of 10.1 deaths per 100,000 population.[114] The U.K. male suicide rate of 15.5 deaths per 100,000 was the lowest since the time series began in 1981; for females, the U.K. rate was 4.9 deaths per 100,000, which is consistent with the rates seen in the last 10 years. Males accounted for three-fourths of suicides registered in 2017 (4,382 deaths), which has been the case since the mid-1990s.The highest age-specific suicide rate was 24.8 deaths per 100,000 among males age 45 to 49 years; for females, the age group with the highest rate was 50 to 54 years, at 6.8 deaths per 100,000.

Scotland had the highest suicide rate in Great Britain, with 13.9 deaths per 100,000 persons; England had the lowest rate, 9.2 deaths per 100,000.[114]

Violence

Violence in British society would appear to be on the increase. However, according to TARN data, only 3.2%

TABLE 21-8 Breakdown of Trauma Injuries by Intent, United Kingdom

		Injury Intent *n* (% of Total)			
Group	**Total**	**Nonintentional**	**Alleged Assault**[a]	**Suspected Self-Harm**	**Other, Including Sports**
All	64,670	56,092 (86.7%)	3,766 (5.8%)	1,010 (1.6%)	3,802 (5.9%)
Dead	4,616	4,099 (88.8%)	147 (3.2%)	202 (4.4%)	168 (3.6%)

[a] Including non-accidental injury.

of trauma deaths are attributed to violent episodes, including penetrating trauma, knife/gunshot wound, and non-accidental injury (**Table 21-8**). The increasing incidence of violence in the United Kingdom is a cause for concern among both the general public and the government. The risks and predetermining factors that need to be investigated include gang culture, lack of nonviolent male role models, drug culture, and unemployment.

Injury Prevention

Across the United Kingdom, there are well-established safety intervention practices to ensure cycle safety, especially for children, including courses on road safety and promotion of helmet wearing. Seat-belt wearing has been mandatory since 1983. Children must use the appropriate child restraint for their weight when traveling in the front or back seat of any car, van, or goods vehicle. "Child restraint" means any baby seat, child seat, booster seat, or booster cushion. Children can use an adult belt when they reach 135 cm or their 12th birthday, whichever comes first.[115]

Safe Drive Stay Alive

Approximately 1 in 4 road deaths in the United Kingdom occurs among drivers age 17 to 24.[116] Young drivers are much more likely to be involved in a collision on the roads, often due to inexperience and a lack of knowledge of the risks. Since 2004, the number of people younger than the age of 25 killed in car collisions has fallen by nearly three-fourths, but there is still more to do.

The Safe Drive Stay Alive initiative is produced by a road safety partnership including police forces, hospitals, local councils, and emergency services. Each partner has been working for years to reduce the number of people dying on the roads, with an estimated 220,000 young people having attended a Safe Drive presentation by the end of 2017. Through a combination of roads policing, road safety education, engineering measures, and speed-limit enforcement, MVC victims killed or seriously injured fell to an all-time low by the end of 2014. A disproportionate number of these remain young, inexperienced drivers, which is why the Safe Drive Stay Alive campaign focuses on reaching new and pre-drivers, in an emotive and hard-hitting way, influencing behavior and attitude on the roads.[117]

References

1. *Merriam-Webster.* (n.d.). Trauma. Retrieved from http://www.merriam-webster.com/medical/trauma?show=0&t=1358537715
2. *Merriam-Webster.* (n.d.). Epidemiology. Retrieved from http://www.merriam-webster.com/medical/epidemiology
3. National Center for Health Statistics. (n.d.). *10 leading causes of death by age group, United States—2016.* Retrieved from https://www.cdc.gov/injury/wisqars/pdf/leading_causes_of_death_by_age_group_2016-508.pdf
4. National Center for Health Statistics. (n.d.). *10 leading causes of injury deaths by age group highlighting unintentional injury deaths, United States—2016.* Retrieved from https://www.cdc.gov/injury/wisqars/pdf/leading_causes_of_injury_deaths_highlighting_unintentional_injury_2016-508.pdf
5. Centers for Disease Control and Prevention. (2017, April 27). TBI: Get the facts. Retrieved from https://www.cdc.gov/traumaticbraininjury/get_the_facts.html
6. Centers for Disease Control and Prevention. (2017, May 3). Emergency department visits. Retrieved from https://www.cdc.gov/nchs/fastats/emergency-department.htm
7. National Center for Health Statistics. (n.d.). *National estimates of the 10 leading causes of nonfatal injuries treated in hospital emergency departments, United States—2015.* Retrieved from https://www.cdc.gov/injury/wisqars/pdf/leading_causes_of_nonfatal_injury_2015-a.pdf
8. National Fire Protection Association. (2017, December). *Fact sheet: Research.* Retrieved from https://www.nfpa.org/-/media/Files/News-and-Research/Fire-statistics-and-reports/Fact-sheets/FireOverviewFactSheet
9. Centers for Disease Control and Prevention. (2016, September 20). Hip fractures among older adults. Retrieved from http://www.cdc.gov/HomeandRecreationalSafety/falls/adulthipfx.html
10. Centers for Disease Control and Prevention. (2018, March 30). Overdose deaths involving opioids, cocaine, and psycho stimulants—United States, 2015–2016. *Morbidity and Mortality Weekly Report, 67*(12), 349–358. Retrieved from https://www.cdc.gov/mmwr/volumes/67/wr/mm6712a1.htm?s_cid=mm6712a1_w

11. National Spinal Cord Injury Statistical Center. (2016). *Spinal cord injury facts and figures at a glance.* Retrieved from https://www.nscisc.uab.edu/Public/Facts%20and%20Figures%20-%202018.pdf
12. National Highway Traffic Safety Administration. (2017). *Traffic safety facts: 2015 data.* Retrieved from https://crashstats.nhtsa.dot.gov/Api/Public/Publication/812375
13. Centers for Disease Control and Prevention. (2015). Alcohol-impaired driving among adults—United States, 2012. *Morbidity and Mortality Weekly Report, 64*(3), 814–817. Retrieved from https://www.cdc.gov/mmwr/preview/mmwrhtml/mm6430a2.htm?s_cid=mm6430a2_w
14. Centers for Disease Control and Prevention. (2015, December 14). State-specific cost of motor vehicle crash deaths. Retrieved from https://www.cdc.gov/motorvehiclesafety/statecosts/
15. Centers for Disease Control and Prevention. (2017, June 16). Impaired driving: Get the facts. Retrieved from http://www.cdc.gov/motorvehiclesafety/impaired_driving/impaired-drv_factsheet.html
16. Lipari, R. N., Hughes, A., & Bose, J. (2016, December 27). *Driving under the influence of alcohol and illicit drugs: 2014.* Substance Abuse and Mental Health Administration. Retrieved from https://www.samhsa.gov/data/sites/default/files/report_2688/ShortReport-2688.html
17. Centers for Disease Control and Prevention. (2017, August 22). Intimate partner violence: Prevention strategies. Retrieved from https://www.cdc.gov/violenceprevention/intimatepartnerviolence/prevention.html
18. Centers for Disease Control and Prevention. (2016). *Understanding elder abuse* (Fact sheet). Retrieved from https://www.cdc.gov/violenceprevention/pdf/em-factsheet-a.pdf
19. Centers for Disease Control and Prevention. (2014). *Child maltreatment: Facts at a glance* (Fact sheet). Retrieved from https://www.cdc.gov/violenceprevention/pdf/childmaltreatment-facts-at-a-glance.pdf
20. Centers for Disease Control and Prevention. (2018, August 15). Injury prevention and control: Our approach. Retrieved from https://www.cdc.gov/injury/about/approach.html
21. SAMHSA–HRSA Center for Integrated Health Solutions. (n.d.). *SBIRT: Screening, brief intervention, and referral to treatment.* Retrieved from https://www.integration.samhsa.gov
22. Australian Trauma Quality Improvement (AusTQIP) Collaboration. (2018). *Australian Trauma Registry: Management of the severely injured in Australia annual report 1 July 2016 to 30 June 2017.* Melbourne, Victoria: Alfred Health. Retrieved from https://www.dropbox.com/s/xa1i07r0av0dzf0/ATR_Annual%20Report_16-17.pdf?dl=0
23. Australian Bureau of Statistics. (2018). Statistics. Retrieved from http://www.abs.gov.au/browse?opendocument&ref=topBar
24. Australian Institute of Health and Welfare. (2018). Injury. Retrieved from https://www.aihw.gov.au/reports-data/health-conditions-disability-deaths/injury/overview
25. Australian Institute of Health and Welfare. (2018). Trends in hospitalized injury, Australia 1999–00 to 2014–15. *Injury research and statistics series no. 110.* Cat. no. INJCAT 190. Canberra, Australia: Author. Retrieved from https://www.aihw.gov.au/getmedia/03743fe9-1ed1-4fe8-9a66-0808405be319/aihw-injcat-190.pdf.aspx?inline=true
26. Ford, J. (2016). Australian Trauma Registry consolidated report 1/1/2013–30/6/2015. Australian Trauma Quality Improvement Program. Retrieved from https://static1.squarespace.com/static/569ce2937086d768fdf7aeac/t/59585ccf4c8b03b8a582b1f2/1498963171223/Australian+Trauma+Quality+Improvement+Program+including+the+Australian+Trauma+Registry+%28AusTQIP-ATR%29+Report+January+2013+-+June+2015.pdf
27. Australian Institute of Health and Welfare. (2018, July 18). Deaths in Australia. Retrieved from https://www.aihw.gov.au/reports/life-expectancy-death/deaths-in-australia/contents/leading-causes-of-death
28. Australian Bureau of Statistics. (2018). 3303.0: Causes of death, Australia, 2017: Intentional self-harm, key characteristics. Retrieved from http://www.abs.gov.au/ausstats/abs@.nsf/Lookup/by%20Subject/3303.0~2017~Main%20Features~Intentional%20self-harm,%20key%20characteristics~3
29. Kreisfeld, R., Pointer, S., & Bradley, C. (2017, October 25). *Trends in hospitalisations due to falls by older people, Australia 2002–03 to 2012–13. Injury research and statistics series no. 106.* Cat. no. INJCAT 182. Canberra, Australia: Australian Institute of Health and Welfare. Retrieved from https://www.aihw.gov.au/getmedia/5f84eadd-6f25-4429-82fc-5e9072278335/aihw-injcat-182.pdf.aspx?inline=true
30. Australian and New Zealand Falls Prevention Society. (n.d.). Info about falls. Retrieved from http://www.anzfallsprevention.org/info/
31. Australian Institute of Health and Welfare. (2018). *Hospitalised injury due to land transport crashes. Injury research and statistics series no. 115.* Cat. no. INJCAT 195. Canberra, Australia: Author. Retrieved from https://www.aihw.gov.au/getmedia/2c2bb67a-4a4a-4b45-a030-aaa977c7292c/aihw-injcat-195.pdf.aspx?inline=true
32. Australian Academy of Science. (n.d.). Australian road statistics (Infographic). Retrieved from https://www.science.org.au/curious/australian-road-statistics
33. Bureau of Infrastructure, Transport and Regional Economics. (2017). Road trauma Australia: 2016 statistical summary. Canberra, Australia: Author. Retrieved from https://bitre.gov.au/publications/ongoing/files/Road_Trauma_Australia_2016_Web.pdf
34. Safe Work Australia. (2016). Work-related traumatic injury fatalities, Australia 2016. Retrieved from https://www.safeworkaustralia.gov.au/system/files/documents/1702/work-related-traumatic-injury-fatalities.pdf
35. Safe Work Australia. (2017). Key work health and safety statistics Australia 2017: Work-related injury fatalities. Retrieved from https://www.safeworkaustralia.gov.au/system/files/documents/1709/em17-0212_swa_key_statistics_overview_0.pdf
36. Australian Institute of Health and Welfare. (2018). Hospitalised assault injuries among men and boys. Retrieved from https://www.aihw.gov.au/getmedia/695ba12d-b0c6-4639-9b9a-db63b92890e1/aihw-injcat-196.pdf.aspx?inline=true

37. Australian Institute of Health and Welfare. (2018). Assaults 2014–15. Retrieved from https://www.aihw.gov.au/search?%7B%22SearchText%22:%22Assault%22%7D
38. Australian Institute of Health and Welfare. (2017). Firearms, injuries and deaths (Fact sheet). Retrieved from https://www.aihw.gov.au/getmedia/fd06f3d6-eac7-47d3-a187-4d0e0f188b27/20368-firearm-injuries-deaths.pdf.aspx?inline=true
39. Kidsafe Australia. (n.d.). Statistics. Retrieved from http://kidsafe.com.au/statistics-2/
40. Mitchell, R., Curtis, K., & Foster, K. (2017). *A 10-year review of the characteristics and health outcomes of injury-related hospitalisations of children in Australia.* Sydney, Australia: Day of Difference Foundation, University of Sydney. Retrieved from http://www.paediatricinjuryoutcomes.org.au/wp-content/uploads/2017/06/Australian-child-injury-report_FINAL-070617.pdf
41. Australian Institute of Health and Welfare. (2018). Trends in hospitalised injury, Australia 1999–00 to 2015–15. Retrieved from https://www.aihw.gov.au/getmedia/03743fe9-1ed1-4fe8-9a66-0808405be319/aihw-injcat-190.pdf.aspx?inline=true
42. Australian Institute of Health and Welfare. (2018, October 9). Trends in injury deaths 1999–00 to 2014–15. Retrieved from https://www.aihw.gov.au/reports/injury/trends-injury-deaths-1999-00-to-2014-15/contents/summary
43. Australian Government, Department of Veteran Affairs. (n.d.). Alcohol and injury. Retrieved from https://www.therightmix.gov.au/factsheets/alcohol-and-injury
44. Australian Institute of Health and Welfare. (2018). *Impact of alcohol and illicit drug use on the burden of disease and injury in Australian: Australian Burden of Disease Study 2011. Australian Burden of Disease Study.* Canberra, Australia: Author. Retrieved from https://www.aihw.gov.au/reports/burden-of-disease/impact-alcohol-illicit-drug-use-on-burden-disease/related-material
45. Royal Life Saving Society—Australia. (2017). Royal Life Saving national drowning report 2017. Retrieved from https://www.royallifesaving.com.au/__data/assets/pdf_file/0010/20260/RLS_NDR2017_ReportLR.pdf
46. Australia Government, Department of Health. (n.d.). Injury prevention in Australia. Retrieved from http://www.health.gov.au/internet/main/publishing.nsf/content/health-pubhlth-strateg-injury-index.htm
47. Australasian Injury Prevention Network. (n.d.). Welcome to the Australasian Injury Prevention Network. Retrieved from https://aipn.com.au
48. Royal Australasian College of Surgeons. (2013). Road trauma prevention (Position paper). Ref. No. FES-FEL-046. Retrieved from https://www.surgeons.org/media/297093/2015-09-09_pos_fes-fel-046_road_trauma_prevention.pdf
49. Parachute Canada. (2015). The cost of injury in Canada. Retrieved from http://www.parachutecanada.org/downloads/research/Cost_of_Injury-2015.pdf
50. Canadian Institute for Health Information. (2018). Watch your step! Falls are sending more Canadians to the hospital than ever before. Retrieved from https://www.cihi.ca/en/watch-your-step-falls-are-sending-more-canadians-to-the-hospital-than-ever-before
51. Canadian Institute for Health Information. (2018, July 5). Injury and trauma emergency department and hospitalization statistics, 2016–2017. Retrieved from https://www.cihi.ca/sites/default/files/document/2016-2017-injury-and-trauma-quick-stats-en-web.xlsx
52. Adams, S. D., & Holcomb, J. B. (2015). Geriatric trauma. *Current Opinion in Critical Care, 21*(6), 520–526. https://doi.org/10.1097/MCC.0000000000000246
53. Robertson, R. D., Brown, S. W., Valentine, D., & Vanlaar, W. G. M. (2018). Status of alcohol impaired driving in Canada. Retrieved from http://tirf.ca/wp-content/uploads/2018/07/Status-of-alcohol-impaired-driving-in-Canada-11.pdf
54. Robertson, R. D., Bowman, K., & Brown, S. (2015). Distracted driving: A national action plan. Retrieved from http://tirf.ca/wp-content/uploads/2017/02/Distracted-Driving-A-National-Action-Plan-Full-Report-12.pdf
55. Rao, D. P., Abramovici, H., Crain, J., Do, M. T., McFaull, S., & Thompson, W. (2018). The lows of getting high: Sentinel surveillance of injuries associated with cannabis and other substance use. *Canadian Journal of Public Health, 109*, 155–163. Retrieved from https://link.springer.com/content/pdf/10.17269%2Fs41997-018-0027-8.pdf
56. Pike, I., Richmond, S., Rothman, L., & Macpherson, A. (2015). *Canadian injury prevention resource.* Toronto, Canada: Parachute. Retrieved from http://www.parachutecanada.org/downloads/research/Canadian_Injury_Prevention_Resource-LR.pdf
57. National Institute on Ageing. (2018). *We can't address what we don't measure consistently: Building consensus on frailty in Canada.* Toronto, ON: National Institute on Ageing. Retrieved from https://www.ryerson.ca/nia/white-papers/frailty-paper.pdf
58. Canadian Frailty Network. (2016). Discharging elders from ED to community: What you need to know? Retrieved from http://www.cfn-nce.ca/news-and-events-overview/webinars/discharging-elders-from-ed-to-community-what-you-need-to-know/
59. Canadian Institute for Health Information. (2010). Injury hospitalizations and socio-economic status. Retrieved from https://secure.cihi.ca/free_products/Injury_aib_vE4CCF_v3_en.pdf
60. Bougie, E., Fines, P., Oliver, L. N., & Kohen, D. E. (2014). Unintentional injury hospitalizations and socio-economic status in areas with a high percentage of First Nations identity residents. *Health Reports, 25*(2), 3–12. Retrieved from https://www150.statcan.gc.ca/n1/en/pub/82-003-x/2014002/article/11902-eng.pdf?st=glDAT37p
61. Atlantic Collaborative on Injury Prevention. (2011). *Social determinants of injury.* Retrieved from http://www.parachutecanada.org/downloads/research/reports/ACIP_Report_SDOI.pdf
62. Canadian Collaborating Centres for Injury Prevention. (n.d.). Home page. Retrieved from http://www.cccip.ca
63. Central Committee on Trauma Service. (2018). *Trauma statistical annual report 2017.* Hong Kong: Hospital Authority.

64. Centre for Health Protection. (2018, September 21). Death rates by leading causes of death, 2001–2017. Retrieved from https://www.chp.gov.hk/en/statistics/data/10/27/117.html
65. Census and Statistics Department. (2018). 2016 population by-census results reveal latest demographic trends. Retrieved from https://www.bycensus2016.gov.hk/en/bc-snapshot.html
66. Hung, K. K., Yeung, J. H. H., Cheung, C. S. K., Leung, L. Y., Cheng, R. C. H, Cheung, N. K., & Graham, C. A. (2018). Trauma team activation criteria and outcomes of geriatric trauma: 10 year single centre cohort study. *American Journal of Emergency Medicine*. [Epub ahead of print]. https://doi.org/10.1016/j.ajem.2018.06.011
67. Hospital Authority. (2017). Hospital Authority statistical report 2016–2017. Retrieved from http://www.ha.org.hk/haho/ho/stat/HASR16_17.pdf
68. Transport Department. (2011). Figure 1.7: Road traffic casualties by casualty contributory factor and degree of injury 2011. Retrieved from https://www.td.gov.hk/filemanager/en/content_4909/f1.7.pdf
69. Centraal Bureau voor de Statistiek. (2018, April 25). StatLine: Bevolking; sleutelfiguren. Retrieved from https://opendata.cbs.nl/statline/#/CBS/en/dataset/37296eng/table?ts=1537535468769
70. Centraal Bureau voor de Statistiek. (2018, April 25). StatLine: Overledenen; doden als gevolg van verkeersongeval in Nederland, provincie. Retrieved from https://opendata.cbs.nl/statline/#/CBS/nl/dataset/71426ned/table?ts=1537227991226
71. International Transport Forum. (2018). *Road safety annual report*. Paris, France: Author. Retrieved from https://www.itf-oecd.org/sites/default/files/docs/irtad-road-safety-annual-report-2018_2.pdf
72. Volksgezondheidenzorg.info. (n.d.). Volksgezondheidenzorg.info: Cijfers en achtergronden. Retrieved from https://www.volksgezondheidenzorg.info/
73. vand den Berg, B., Breur, J., van der Boon, D., & van de lint, L. (2014). Going Dutch: Emergency nursing in the Netherlands. *Journal of Emergency Nursing*, *40*(5), 500–504. https://doi.org/10.1016/j.jen.2014.05.014
74. GBD 2016 Healthcare Access and Quality Collaborators. (2018). Measuring performance on the Healthcare Access and Quality Index for 195 countries and territories and selected subnational locations: A systematic analysis from the Global Burden of Disease Study 2016. *Lancet*, *391*(10136), 2236–2271. https://doi.org/10.1016/S0140-6736(18)30994-2
75. Schneider, E. C., Sarnak, D. O., Squires, D., Shah, A., & Doty, M. W. (2017). *Mirror, mirror 2017: International comparison reflects flaws and opportunities for better U.S. health care*. New York, NY: Commonwealth Fund. Retrieved from https://interactives.commonwealthfund.org/2017/july/mirror-mirror/
76. Miller, L. J., & Lu, W. (2018, September 19). These are the economies with the most (and least) efficient health care. *Bloomberg*. Retrieved from https://www.bloomberg.com/news/articles/2018-09-19/u-s-near-bottom-of-health-index-hong-kong-and-singapore-at-top?srnd=premium
77. Moodley, N. B., Aldous, C., & Clarke, D. J. (2014). An audit of trauma-related mortality in a provincial capital in South Africa. *South African Journal of Surgery*, *52*(4), 101–104. Retrieved from http://sajs.redbricklibrary.com/index.php/sajs/article/view/1863/630e
78. Statistics South Africa. (2017). Mortality and causes of death in South Africa, 2016: Findings from death notification. Retrieved from http://www.statssa.gov.za/publications/P03093/P030932016.pdf
79. Medibank Trauma Data Registry: Netcare Private Hospital Group South Africa. (2016). *National trauma epidemiology report 2016*. Pretoria, South Africa: Author.
80. Statistics South Africa. (2017). Mid-year population estimates 2017. Retrieved from http://www.statssa.gov.za/publications/P0302/P03022017.pdf
81. Health-E News. (2018, August 22). No suitable care for SA's elderly population. Retrieved from https://www.health-e.org.za/2018/08/22/no-suitable-care-for-sas-elderly-population/
82. Samson Institute for Ageing Research. (n.d.). Putting older people on the agenda in South Africa. Retrieved from https://www.sifar.org.za/news/201701/putting-older-people-agenda-south-africa
83. Wall, S., Figueiredo, F., & Laing, G. (2014). The spectrum and outcome of pregnant trauma patients in a metropolitan trauma service in South Africa. *Injury*, *45*(8), 1220–1223. https://doi.org/10.1016/j.injury.2014.04.045
84. Nel, D. (2018). The pregnant trauma patient. *South African Journal of Anaesthesia and Analgesia*, *24*(3 Suppl. 1), S21–S24. Retrieved from http://www.sajaa.co.za/index.php/sajaa/article/view/2095
85. Matzopoulos, R. G., Truen, S., Bowman, B., & Cornigall, J. (2014). The cost of harmful alcohol use in South Africa. *South African Medical Journal*, *104*(2), 127–132. Retrieved from http://www.scielo.org.za/scielo.php?script=sci_arttext&pid=S0256-95742014000200023
86. Schuurman, N., Cinnamon, J., Walker, B. B., Fawcett, V., Nicol, A., Hameed, S. M., & Matzopoulos, R. (2015). Intentional injury and violence in Cape Town, South Africa: An epidemiological analysis of trauma admission data. *Global Health Action*, *8*(1), 27016. https://doi.org/10.3402/gha.v8.27016
87. South Africa's shocking road death numbers at highest level in 10 years. (2017, June 9). *BusinessTech*. Retrieved from https://businesstech.co.za/news/monitoring/178275/south-africas-shocking-road-death-numbers-at-highest-level-in-10-years
88. This is how much money the average car crash cost in South Africa. (2016, November 1). *BusinessTech*. Retrieved from https://businesstech.co.za/news/finance/141937/this-is-how-much-money-the-average-car-crash-costs-in-south-africa/
89. Labuschagne, F. J. J. (2016). *Cost of crashes in South Africa: Research and development report*. Pretoria, South Africa: Road Traffic Management Corporation. Retrieved from https://www.arrivealive.co.za/documents/Cost-of-Crashes-in-South-Africa-RTMC-September-2016.pdf
90. Prince, Z. N., Priviledge, C., & Khobela, P. S. (2016). Road accident fatalities trends and safety management in South Africa. *Problems and Perspectives in Management*, *14*(3), 627–633. http:// doi.org/10.21511/ppm.14(3-3).2016.05

91. World Health Organization. (n.d.). Burns (Fact sheet). Retrieved from http://www.who.int/news-room/fact-sheets/detail/burns
92. Allorto, N. L., Zoepke, S., Clarke, D. L., & Rode, H. (2016). Burn surgeons in South Africa: A rare species. *South African Medical Journal, 106*(2), 186–191. https://doi.org/10.7196/SAMJ.2016.V106I2.9954
93. Msemburi, W., Pillay-van Wyk, V., Dorrington, R. E., Neethling, I., Nannan, N., Groenewald, P., . . . Bradshaw, D. S. (2016). *Second national burden of disease study for South Africa: Cause of death profile. South Africa 1997–2012.* Cape Town, South Africa: South African Medical Research Council.
94. Fisher, S. (2017). Drowning: Second leading cause of accidental death in SA. *Eyewitness News.* Retrieved from https://ewn.co.za/2017/09/09/drowning-second-leading-cause-of-accidental-death-in-sa
95. Saunders, C. J., Sewduth, D., & Naidoo, N. (2018). Keeping our heads above water: A systematic review of fatal drowning in South Africa. *South African Medical Journal, 108*(1), 61–68. https://doi.org/10.7196/SAMJ.2017.v108i1.11090
96. Pongoma, L. (2013, January 6). Festive road carnage bill costs billions. *The New Age.* Retrieved from https://www.raf.co.za/Media-Center/Documents/Festive%20road%20carnage%20costs%20billions%20-%20The%20NewAge%20-%206%20January%202013.pdf
97. Netcare. (2015). Netcare reaches over 270 000 people in their efforts to prevent trauma injury. Retrieved from http://www.netcare911.co.za/Articles/ArticleID=231
98. National Road Safety Strategy 2011–2020. (n.d.). Decade of Action and Arrive Alive. Retrieved from https://www.arrivealive.co.za/documents/Road%20Safety%20Strategy%20for%20South%20Africa%202011.pdf
99. Statistics Sweden. (n.d.). *Home page.* Retrieved from http://www.scb.se
100. National Board of Health and Welfare. (2018). *Statistics on hospitalizations due to injuries and poisonings in 2017.* Stockholm, Sweden: Author.
101. Korkort Sweden. (2018). Accidents and statistics related to alcohol in traffic. Retrieved from https://www.korkortsverige.se/a/olyckor_statistik_alkohol_trafiken
102. Public Health Agency of Sweden. (2018). Suicide prevention. Retrieved from https://www.folkhalsomyndigheten.se/the-public-health-agency-of-sweden/living-conditions-and-lifestyle/suicide-prevention/
103. Swedish Transport Administration. *Road traffic injuries.* Borlänge, Sweden: Author.
104. Swedish Civil Contingencies Agency. (2018). EU project: BaltPrevResilience. Retrieved from https://www.msb.se/baltprevresilience
105. Bicycle Research Foundation. (n.d.). Helmet laws: Sweden. Retrieved from http://www.cyclehelmets.org/1017.html
106. National Society for Road Safety. (n.d.). Cars: Seat belt. Retrieved from https://ntf.se/konsumentupplysning/bilar/skyddssystem/bilbalte/
107. Swedish Transport Administration. (2017). *This is Vision Zero.* Retrieved from https://www.trafikverket.se/en/startpage/operations/Operations-road/vision-zero-academy/This-is-Vision-Zero/
108. County Council's Mutual Insurance Company. (2018). Säker trauma. Retrieved from https://lof.se/?s=s%C3%A4ker+trauma
109. NHS England. (2018). More than 1,600 extra trauma victims alive today says major new study. Retrieved from https://www.england.nhs.uk/2018/08/more-than-1600-extra-trauma-victims-alive-today-says-major-new-study/
110. Trauma Audit and Research Network. (n.d.). Welcome. Retrieved from https://www.tarn.ac.uk
111. Scottish Trauma Audit Group. (2017). What is STAG? Retrieved from http://www.stag.scot.nhs.uk/index.htm
112. Office for National Statistics. (2016). Alcohol-related deaths in the United Kingdom, registered in 2016. Retrieved from https://www.ons.gov.uk/peoplepopulationandcommunity/healthandsocialcare/causesofdeath/bulletins/alcoholrelateddeathsintheunitedkingdom/registeredin2016/pdf
113. Department for Transport. (2014). Drink driving. *Think!* Retrieved from https://www.think.gov.uk/road-safety-laws/#drink-driving
114. Office for National Statistics. (2017). Suicides in the UK: 2017 registrations. Retrieved from https://www.ons.gov.uk/peoplepopulationandcommunity/birthsdeathsandmarriages/deaths/bulletins/suicidesintheunitedkingdom/2017registrations
115. Department for Transport. (n.d.). Child car seats: The law. *RoSPA Child Care Seats.* Retrieved from https://www.childcarseats.org.uk/the-law/
116. Department for Transport. (2018). Reported road casualties in Great Britain: 2017 annual report. Retrieved from https://assets.publishing.service.gov.uk/government/uploads/system/uploads/attachment_data/file/744077/reported-road-casualties-annual-report-2017.pdf
117. Safe Drive Stay Alive. (n.d.). Home page. *Safe Drive Stay Alive Tour.* Retrieved from http://www.safedrive.org.uk

APPENDIX

A

Overview of Skill Stations

OBJECTIVES

Upon completion of the skill stations, the learner will be able to:

1. Apply the trauma nursing process (TNP) to the care of patients with various traumatic injuries and provide appropriate interventions.
2. Discuss, observe, and demonstrate the use of a variety of skills associated with steps in the TNP.

Introduction

Each of these stations gives the learner the opportunity to discuss trauma concepts and observe and practice trauma skills in a simulated, case-based learning environment. This portion of the *Trauma Nursing Core Course* (TNCC) is intended to promote active and collaborative learning. Each learner is expected to contribute to the discussion and to demonstrate and describe assessments and interventions as indicated within the case or selected skill.

During actual patient care, all personnel with direct contact with the patient or the patient's bodily fluids must wear personal protective equipment (PPE). In the skill stations, care is simulated and the use of PPE is optional. Any mention of a certain brand of equipment or supply does not constitute endorsement of that product. It is recommended that each learner and instructor become familiar with brands and products used in their own institutions.

The centerpiece of the TNCC is the TNP skill station—that is, an active performance of a scenario-driven initial assessment of a simulated trauma patient, integrating chapter content, classroom learning, and critical thinking. Throughout the scenario, the learner demonstrates the appropriate assessment techniques of inspection, auscultation, and palpation.

The four types of *TNP behaviors* are the foundation for the steps outlined in the skill station:

- Assessment
- Outcomes/planning
- Implementation
- Evaluation

In addition to the nursing process steps, overarching *operational process points* help the trauma team enact a systematic and standardized approach to the care of the trauma patient:

- Preparation and triage
- Primary survey (ABCDE), with corresponding interventions as required (FG)
- Reevaluation (consideration of transfer)
- Secondary survey (HI), with corresponding interventions as required
- Reevaluation and post-resuscitation care
- Definitive care or transfer

General Principles

During the TNP skill stations, the learners in each group are presented with specific case scenarios:

- Each scenario includes discussion points. These points are unique to each scenario and are intended for small-group discussion and additional learning. It is expected that all learners will contribute to the discussion.
- Each scenario includes hands-on skills. It is expected that all learners will demonstrate the hands-on skills.
- The instructor will guide the learners through the scenario, answer questions, help the learners perfect their skills, and provide additional information as requested by the learners.
- During the primary and secondary survey, each learner is expected to evaluate the effectiveness of interventions that are likely to have an immediate effect on the patient (e.g., auscultation of breath sounds after intubation).

TNP Testing Principles

For the TNP testing station, evaluation will follow these principles:

- Each learner will be evaluated individually at one TNP testing station. The learner is cautioned about attempting to memorize any specific teaching scenario, as a new scenario is used each time.
- The double starred criteria (**) must be completed in order BEFORE moving to the next step.
  - These criteria usually represent a critical assessment step or an intervention as a response to a life threat identified within the primary assessment.
  - At the end of the primary survey, if any double-starred criteria (**) have been missed, the instructor may end the evaluation, review the process, and refer the learner to the course director for further instruction and retesting, if applicable.
- The single-starred criteria (*) are essential skill steps and are expected to be performed during the skill station demonstration, but their sequence is not critical.
- For successful completion, all double-starred criteria (**) must be demonstrated in order, all single-starred criteria (*) must be completed, and a score of 70% or greater is required.
- During evaluation, the instructor will answer specific questions and provide assessment data but is not allowed to provide prompts.
- The learner is expected to state and/or demonstrate both criteria if two criteria are listed with an **AND** (e.g., inspects **AND** palpates the head; states the need for administration of warmed, isotonic crystalloid with blood tubing **AND** identifies the appropriate rate).
- The learner is expected to demonstrate appropriate assessment techniques (e.g., auscultation and palpation).
  - It is not acceptable for the learner to state, "I would palpate the abdomen," without actually touching the model.
  - The correct method to auscultate breath sounds depends on whether the patient is intubated.
    - If the patient is not intubated, lung fields are immediately auscultated.
    - If the patient is intubated, watch for rise and fall of the chest while listening over the epigastrium and auscultate the lung fields.
- Some steps require a specific number of required assessments. As the learner requests the assessment information, the instructor will respond. After the learner has asked for the required number of assessments, the instructor may provide all of the remaining assessment information.

Trauma Nursing Process Skill Station

The application of the trauma nursing process through the teaching station includes the prehospital report and across-the-room-observation.

Prehospital Report

The teaching station begins with the scenario or prehospital report.

Across-the-Room Observation

The across-the-room observation is the first look as the patient arrives in the trauma room. Uncontrolled hemorrhage is a major preventable cause of death in the trauma patient, and this is the first of several identified steps to evaluate for that hemorrhage. This step enables immediate assessment for uncontrolled external bleeding and the opportunity to decide whether this patient requires reprioritizing to <C>ABC.

Primary Survey

The goal of the primary survey is to identify life-threatening situations and rapidly intervene. The elements assessed during the primary survey include the following:

- Alertness and airway with simultaneous cervical spinal stabilization
- Breathing and ventilation
- Circulation and control of hemorrhage
- Disability (neurologic status)
- Exposure and environmental control

These elements are critical in nature, and any deviations from baseline require immediate intervention. The severity of the patient's condition may require simultaneous assessment and intervention. The process is prioritized and systematic; therefore, any life-threatening situations need to be completed in the current element before moving on to the next (i.e., B is not assessed until A is addressed, and so on).

Corresponding Interventions as Required (FG)

These interventions include assessments and diagnostics to assure that all life threats are identified and a baseline is established for trending and ongoing reassessment.

- Full set of vital signs and family presence.
- Get monitoring devices and give comfort.
  - Laboratory studies to include, but not limited to, blood gases and a specimen for blood type and cross-match
  - Monitor for continuous cardiac rate and rhythm assessment
  - Nasogastric or orogastric tube consideration
  - Oxygenation and ventilation assessment, including capnography if indicated (i.e., intubated or sedated patient); consider weaning oxygen based on oximetry to avoid hyperoxia
  - Pain assessment and management, including the use of an appropriate, validated pain scale with nonpharmacologic and pharmacologic interventions combined for optimal management of traumatic pain. For patients who have been intubated using drug-assisted intubation, pain response will be indeterminate. Pain is assumed to be present based on mechanism of injury and is treated accordingly.

NOTE

With the risk of catheter-associated urinary tract infections, the insertion of a urinary catheter has been deprioritized and, if indicated, is addressed in the perineum section of the head-to-toe assessment.

Reevaluation

This step of reevaluation is included to determine whether any findings from the primary survey raise suspicion for uncontrolled internal hemorrhage, the need for emergency surgical intervention, or the need for transport to a trauma center. If so, the arrangements can begin. Additionally, with the suspicion of uncontrolled internal hemorrhage, a portable radiograph of the pelvis or a focused assessment with sonography for trauma may be performed at this time to expedite additional interventions aimed at the control of internal hemorrhage.

Secondary Survey (HI)

The goal of the secondary survey is to identify all injuries so as to determine priorities for the planning/outcomes and implementation phases of the nursing process.

- History: This can be additional information from prehospital providers, information generated by the patient or family regarding the traumatic event, and/or information from the electronic health record.
- Head-to-toe assessment: The head-to-toe assessment is an organized, detailed review of systems, using the assessment concepts of inspection, auscultation, and palpation. The purpose of a thorough head-to-toe assessment is to identify all injuries. Priority is given to any injuries found in the secondary survey that have the potential to compromise the airway, breathing, or circulation, or affect disability (neurologic status) or exposure/environmental control.
- Inspect the posterior: If pelvic or spinal trauma is suspected, imaging is recommended prior to turning the patient due to the potential for

harm from the log roll maneuver. Long thought to be an adequate precaution for spinal motion restriction, log rolling is now recognized as having the potential to cause secondary injuries. See Chapter 3, "Initial Assessment"; Chapter 8, "Abdominal and Pelvic Trauma"; and Chapter 9, "Spinal Trauma," for more information. If it is safe to turn the patient (no evidence of unstable injury identified on imaging or clinically cleared by the physician), the posterior surfaces are inspected and palpated. If the patient arrived on any transport device and it has not already been removed, it is removed now. If an unstable spine or pelvis injury has not been ruled out, alternative techniques that do not involve log rolling the patient are recommended to remove the patient from the transport device.

Diagnostic studies and interventions may be indicated that supplement the clinical assessment in the secondary survey, confirm findings, or rule out other possible injuries in preparation for the reevaluation phase. Additionally, important nursing interventions for stabilization and planning for post-resuscitation care are included at this point.

Just Keep Reevaluating: Reevaluation and Post-Resuscitation Care

At this point, the patient is evaluated for response to and the effectiveness of interventions. Identification of outcomes, planning, and implementation continue, and reevaluation of the primary survey, vital signs, pain, and all injuries is ongoing. Post-resuscitation care is continued until disposition of the patient to definitive care.

Definitive Care or Transfer

Consideration is given to all assessment criteria, identified injuries, response to interventions, and standardized transfer criteria as the decision is made for definitive care or transfer.

A TNP skill station evaluation form with required skill steps and potential interventions is included for reference during completion of the online modules and in class. Selected instructor responses or prompts are included in italics.

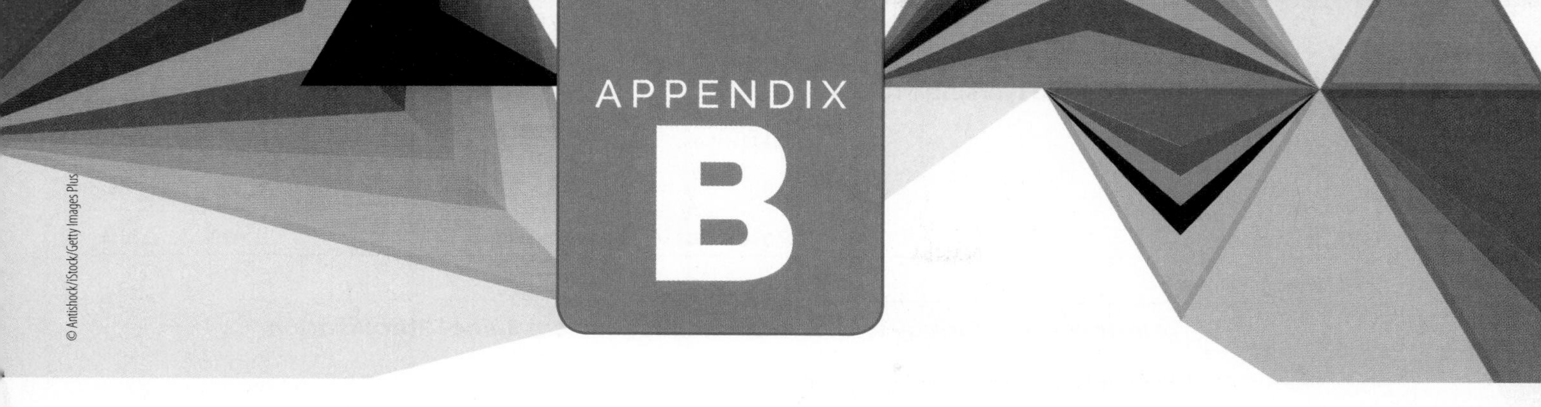

Trauma Nursing Process

Skill Steps	Potential Interventions	Demonstrated?	
		Yes	No
Preparation and Triage			
1. States the need to activate the trauma team			
"Is there any specific equipment that you would prepare?"			
2. States the need to prepare the trauma room	Equipment may include, but is not limited to, the following: › Fluid warmer › Pediatric equipment › Bariatric equipment › Difficult airway or IV equipment		
3. States the need to don personal protective equipment (PPE)	Consider potential need for decontamination or other safety threats to trauma team		
"The patient has just arrived."			
4. Assesses for obvious uncontrolled external hemorrhage	If uncontrolled hemorrhage is identified, start with "C" of the primary survey. This includes controlling uncontrolled bleeding and assessing circulation. If circulation is compromised, initiate IV fluid and blood replacement as indicated before returning to "A." With multiple team members available, airway and breathing may be assessed at this time but do *not* take priority over circulation interventions.		

(*continues*)

<table>
<tr><th rowspan="2">Skill Steps</th><th rowspan="2">Potential Interventions</th><th colspan="2">Demonstrated?</th></tr>
<tr><th>Yes</th><th>No</th></tr>
<tr><td colspan="4">Primary Survey</td></tr>
<tr><td colspan="4">Alertness and Airway with Simultaneous Cervical Spinal Stabilization</td></tr>
<tr><td>5. Assesses the patient's level of consciousness using AVPU</td><td></td><td>**</td><td></td></tr>
<tr><td>6. IF cervical spine injury is suspected, states the need for a second person to provide manual cervical spinal stabilization AND demonstrates manual opening of the airway using the jaw-thrust maneuver. If the patient is alert, it is acceptable to ask the patient to speak or open the mouth to assess the airway.</td><td>I'll maintain cervical spinal stabilization while you open the airway.</td><td></td><td></td></tr>
<tr><td>7. Demonstrates and describes techniques to determine the patency and protection of the airway, using inspection, auscultation, and palpation (identifies at least FOUR):
› Is the tongue obstructing?
› Are there any loose or missing teeth?
› Are there any foreign objects?
› Is there any blood, vomitus, or secretions?
› Is there any edema?
› Is there any snoring, gurgling, or stridor?
› Is there any bony deformity?</td><td>These may include, but are not limited to, the following:
› Suction the airway.
› Remove any loose teeth or foreign objects.
› Insert an oral or nasopharyngeal airway.
› Indicate the need for intubation.
NOTE: Patient response to any intervention is reassessed. Clear speech in an alert patient may indicate an open and maintainable airway. For learning purposes, all the assessment criteria are listed throughout the course.</td><td>**</td><td></td></tr>
<tr><td colspan="4">Breathing and Ventilation</td></tr>
<tr><td>8. Demonstrates and describes techniques for determining breathing effectiveness, using components of inspection, auscultation, and palpation (identifies at least FOUR):
› Is there spontaneous breathing?
› Is there symmetrical chest rise and fall?
› What are the depth, pattern, and general rate of respirations?
› Is there increased work of breathing?
› What is the skin color?
› Are there open wounds or deformities?</td><td>These may include, but are not limited to, the following:
› Apply oxygen.
› Provide ventilations with a bag-mask device.
› Indicate the need for intubation.
› Indicate the need for a needle decompression.
› Indicate the need for a chest tube.
NOTE: Patient response to any intervention is reassessed. Examples include, but are not limited to, the following:
› Is work of breathing improved after the intervention?
› Is there chest rise and fall with bag-mask ventilation?</td><td>**</td><td></td></tr>
</table>

Skill Steps	Potential Interventions	Demonstrated? Yes	Demonstrated? No
› Are breath sounds present and equal? › Is there subcutaneous emphysema? › Is there any tracheal deviation or jugular venous distention?	› Assessment of endotracheal tube placement (see number 9 for required steps to confirm tube placement).		
9. **IF** patient is intubated, assesses endotracheal tube placement (must identify **ALL THREE**): › Attaches a CO_2 detector device; after 5 to 6 breaths, assesses for evidence of exhaled CO_2 › Observes for rise and fall of the chest with assisted ventilations › Auscultates over the epigastrium for gurgling **AND** lungs for bilateral breath sounds	**NOTE:** If the learner chooses a capnography sensor instead of the one-time-use detection device, credit is also given in "Get Monitoring Devices." **NOTE:** If the learner chooses to insert a gastric tube, it can be done here without penalty for order. Credit is also given in "Get Monitoring Devices."	**	
10. **IF** patient is intubated, states the need to assess endotracheal tube (ETT) position by noting the number at the teeth or gums **AND** secures the ETT	*The ETT is secured and the number at the level of the teeth is documented.*		
11. **IF** patient is intubated, states the need to begin mechanical ventilation or continue assisted ventilation	*Ventilations continue.*		
Circulation and Control of Hemorrhage			
12. Demonstrates and describes techniques for determining the adequacy of circulation, using components of inspection, auscultation, and palpation (must identify **ALL THREE**): › Inspects for any uncontrolled external hemorrhage › Inspects **AND** palpates the skin for color, temperature, and moisture › Palpates a central pulse **NOTE:** Assess for capillary refill in the pediatric patient	These may include, but are not limited to, the following: › Control uncontrolled hemorrhage. › Initiate chest compressions and advanced life support (when indicated). › Anticipate emergency resuscitative thoracotomy (if appropriate). › Assess patency of prehospital IV line. › Obtain IV or IO access (two access sites). › Labs may be drawn at this time. › Administer a bolus of warmed isotonic crystalloid. › Consider the need for blood products and balanced resuscitation. › Apply a pelvic binder/sheet. › Anticipate FAST exam if the source of shock is not obvious **NOTE:** Patient response to any intervention is reassessed.	**	

(*continues*)

Skill Steps	Potential Interventions	Demonstrated? Yes	No
Primary Survey (*continued*)			
13. States the need for administration of warmed, isotonic crystalloid with blood tubing **AND** at a [controlled or bolus] rate	If circulation is adequate, learner states that fluids are indicated at a controlled rate. If circulation is **NOT** adequate, learner states that fluids or blood is indicated at a bolus rate.	**	
Disability (Neurologic Status)			
14. Describes the assessment of neurologic status using the Glasgow Coma Scale (GCS): › What is the best eye opening? › What is the best verbal response? › What is the best motor response?	These may include, but are not limited to, the following: › Indicate the need for intubation. › Indicate the need for a head computed tomography (CT) scan. › Assess bedside blood glucose.	**	
15. Assesses pupils			
Exposure and Environmental Control			
16. States the need to remove all clothing **AND** inspect for uncontrolled hemorrhage or obvious injuries	Interventions for uncontrolled bleeding and life-threatening injuries are implemented as indicated.	**	
17. States need to provide warmth (identifies at least **ONE**): › Blankets › Warming lights › Increase room temperature › Warmed fluids › Warmed oxygen			
IMPORTANT: Double-starred (**) criteria are completed in order before moving to the next step. The single-starred criteria (*) are essential skill steps and are expected to be performed during the skill station demonstration, but their sequence is not critical. **NOTE:** If the learner did not intervene to correct life-threatening findings in the primary survey and/or did not complete all double-starred criteria, the instructor may stop the station, review the purpose of the primary survey, and notify the course director.			
Full Set of Vital Signs			
18. Obtains a full set of vital signs	› BP: › HR: › RR: › T: › SpO_2:		
Facilitate Family Presence			
19. States the need to facilitate family presence			

Skill Steps	Potential Interventions	Demonstrated? Yes	No
Get Monitoring Devices and Give Comfort (LMNOP)			
20. States the need for **laboratory analysis** (blood typing, blood gases, and lactate)			
21. Attaches the patient to a cardiac **monitor**			
22. States the need to consider insertion of a **nasogastric or orogastric tube**			
23. Weans the patient from **oxygen** based on pulse **oximetry** and assessment			
24. Attaches the patient to capnography as indicated (e.g., intubated, sedated)			
25. States the need to assess **pain** using an appropriate pain scale		*	
26. Gives appropriate nonpharmacologic comfort measures (identifies at least **ONE**): › Applies ice to swollen areas › Repositioning › Places padding over bony prominences › Offers verbal reassurance			
27. States the need to consider obtaining an order for analgesic medication			

Reevaluation for Transfer to Trauma Center or Definitive Treatment

"At this time, is there a need to consider transfer to a trauma center or preparation for definitive treatment?"

Secondary Survey

Skill Steps	Potential Interventions	Yes	No
History			
28. Obtains pertinent history (identifies at least **ONE**): › Prehospital report › Past medical history (patient- or family-generated; from electronic health record)			
Head-to-Toe			
NOTE: The learner describes and demonstrates the head-to-toe assessment by describing appropriate inspection techniques and demonstrating appropriate auscultation and palpation techniques.			
29. Inspects **AND** palpates head for injuries			
30. Inspects **AND** palpates face for injuries			
31. Inspects **AND** palpates neck for injuries			

(continues)

Skill Steps	Potential Interventions	Demonstrated? Yes	No
Secondary Survey (*continued*)			
32. Inspects **AND** palpates chest for injuries			
33. Auscultates breath sounds			
34. Auscultates heart sounds			
35. Inspects the abdomen for injuries			
36. Auscultates bowel sounds			
37. Palpates all four quadrants of the abdomen for injuries			
38. Inspects **AND** palpates the flanks for injuries			
39. Inspects the pelvis for injuries			
40. Applies gentle pressure over iliac crests downward and medially			
41. Inspects the perineum for injuries			
42. States the need to assess for indications and contraindications for placement of a urinary catheter			
43. Inspects **AND** palpates all four extremities for neurovascular status and injuries			
Inspects Posterior Surfaces			
NOTE: If the patient has a suspected spinal or pelvic injury, imaging is obtained *prior* to turning the patient. The log roll maneuver may cause secondary injuries, including spinal injury or hemorrhage. In these patients, the preferred method for removing a patient from the spine board is the lift and slide technique.			
44. Inspects **AND** palpates posterior surfaces (not required if suspected spinal or pelvic injury)		*	
45. States the need to consider removal of transport device			
46. Identifies all simulated injuries	Instructor summarizes identified injuries and provides an opportunity for review if needed.	*	
"What interventions or diagnostics can you anticipate for this patient?"			

Skill Steps	Potential Interventions	Demonstrated? Yes	No
47. Identifies at least **THREE** interventions or diagnostics	These may include, but are not limited to, the following: › Imaging (radiographs, CT, ultrasound [US], interventional radiology) › Consults › Psychosocial support › Antibiotics › Pain medication and sedation › Social services › Law enforcement › Laboratory studies › Wound care › Splinting › Tetanus immunization		
Just Keep Reevaluating			
"What findings will you continue to reevaluate while the patient is in your care?"			
48. States the need to reevaluate primary assessment			
49. States the need to reevaluate vital signs			
50. States the need to reevaluate pain			
51. States the need to reevaluate all identified injuries and effectiveness of interventions			
Definitive Care or Transport			
"What is the definitive care for this patient?"			
52. States consideration of transfer to a trauma center or admission to hospital			
"Is there anything you would like to add at this time?"			

Double-starred (**) criteria to be done in order—assessments and interventions must be completed prior to moving to the next step:

**Airway and alertness

**Breathing and ventilation

**Circulation

**Disability

**Exposure

Single-starred (*) criteria to be done—sequence is not critical:

*Reassessment of primary survey interventions

*Pain assessment using an appropriate scale

*Inspects posterior surfaces (unless contraindicated by suspected spine or pelvis injury)

Skills Performance Results

Evaluation Form

Evaluator ______________________________

Learner ______________________________

Demonstrated points		Number	Percentage
Total possible	=	________	/ 100%
Learner demonstrated	=	________	________

Demonstrated all ** steps in order ❑ Yes ❑ No

Demonstrated all * items ❑ Yes ❑ No

❑ Station successfully completed

- At least X of X points (points vary per scenario—passing score is 70%)
- All ** critical steps demonstrated in order
- All * steps demonstrated

❑ Incomplete; needs minimal instruction before reevaluation

❑ Incomplete; needs considerable instruction before reevaluation

Potential instructor (must achieve 90%) ❑ Yes ❑ No

Note: Double-starred (**) criteria are completed in order before moving to the next step. The single-starred criteria (*) are essential skill steps and are expected to be performed during the skill station demonstration, but their sequence is not critical.

Index

Note: Page numbers followed by *f* and *t* denotes figures and tables, respectively.

B

J

K

L

T